ESSENTIALS OF
BASIC SCIENCE IN SURGERY

ESSENTIALS OF
BASIC SCIENCE IN SURGERY

EDITED BY

EDWARD B. SAVAGE, M.D.

STEVEN J. FISHMAN, M.D.

LEONARD D. MILLER, M.D.

DEPARTMENT OF SURGERY
UNIVERSITY OF PENNSYLVANIA MEDICAL CENTER
PHILADELPHIA, PENNSYLVANIA

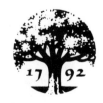

J.B. Lippincott Company
PHILADELPHIA

Acquisitions Editor: Lisa McAllister
Assistant Editor: Emilie Moyer
Cover Designer: Fuiano Art & Design
Production Manager: Janet Greenwood
Production Service: NB Enterprises
Production Coordinator: Lori Bainbridge
Compositor: Carole Desnoes
Printer/Binder: R.R. Donnelley & Sons Company
Cover Printer: John P. Pow Company

6   5   4   3   2   1

ISBN 0-397-51168-X

Library of Congress Cataloging-in-Publication Data
Essentials of basic science in surgery / [edited by] Edward B. Savage,
  Steven J. Fishman, Leonard A. Miller; with 31 additional
  contributors.
         p.   cm.
  Includes bibliographical references and index.
  ISBN 0-397-51168-X
  1. Human physiology. 2. Physiology, Pathological. 3. Surgery-
  -Physiological aspects.
  [DNLM: 1. Physiology. 2. Surgery. QT. 104 E765]
RB 113. E85 1993
616.—dc20
DNLM/DLC
for Library of Congress   92-17502
                                           CIP

The author and publisher have exerted every effort to ensure that drug selection and dosage set forth in this text are in accord with current recommendations and practice at the time of publication. However, in view of ongoing research, changes in government regulations, and the constant flow of information relating to drug therapy and reactions, the reader is urged to check the package insert for each drug for any change in indications and dosage and for added warnings and precautions. This is particularly important when the recommended agent is a new or infrequently employed drug.

CONTRIBUTORS

David L. Bartlett, M.D.
Resident in Surgery
University of Pennsylvania Medical Center
Philadelphia, Pennsylvania

Michael F. Beers, M.D.
Research Associate, Institute for
*   Environmental Medicine*
Attending Physician, Medical Intensive
*   Care Unit*
University of Pennsylvania Medical Center
Philadelphia, Pennsylvania

Patrick J. Brennan, M.D.
Assistant Professor of Medicine
Hospital Epidemiologist
Director of Infection Control
Hospital of the University of Pennsylvania
University of Pennsylvania Medical Center
Philadelphia, Pennsylvania

Charles R. Bridges, M.D., Sc.D.
Fellow in Cardiothoracic Surgery
University of Pennsylvania Medical Center
Philadelphia, Pennsylvania

Steven R. Buchman, M.D.
Fellow in Plastic Surgery
Clinical Instructor of Plastic Surgery
University of Pennsylvania Medical Center
Philadelphia, Pennsylvania

David J. Callans, M.D.
Fellow in Cardiology
University of Pennsylvania Medical Center
Philadelphia, Pennsylvania

Linda S. Callans, M.D.
Postdoctoral Research Fellow
Harrison Department of Surgical Research
Instructor in Surgery
University of Pennsylvania Medical Center
Philadelphia, Pennsylvania

Jeffrey P. Carpenter, M.D.
Assistant Professor of Surgery
University of Pennsylvania Medical Center
Philadelphia, Pennsylvania

Alex C. Cech, M.D.
Resident in Surgery
University of Pennsylvania Medical Center
Philadelphia, Pennsylvania

Michael A. Choti, M.D.
Assistant Professor of Surgery
Johns-Hopkins Hospital
Baltimore, Maryland

David H. Deaton, M.D.
Chief Resident in Surgery
Instructor of Surgery
University of Pennsylvania Medical Center
Philadelphia, Pennsylvania

M. Pia DeGirolamo, M.D.
Fellow in Infectious Disease
University of Pennsylvania Medical Center
Philadelphia, Pennsylvania

Stephen W. Downing, M.D.
Resident in Surgery
University of Pennsylvania Medical Center
Philadelphia, Pennsylvania

Steven J. Fishman, M.D.
Chief Resident in Surgery
Instructor of Surgery
University of Pennsylvania Medical Center
Philadelphia, Pennsylvania

Jonathon Freeman, M.D.
Postdoctoral Research Fellow
Department of Pathology
Brigham and Women's Hospital
Boston, Massachusetts

Irene D. Feurer, M.S. Ed.
Research Coordinator
American Psychiatric Association
Washington, DC

Robert C. Gorman, M.D.
Resident in Surgery
University of Pennsylvania Medical Center
Philadelphia, Pennsylvania

C. William Hanson III, M.D.
Assistant Professor of Anesthesia
University of Pennsylvania Medical Center
Philadelphia, Pennsylvania

Steven C. Hendrickson, M.D.
Resident in Surgery
University of Pennsylvania Medical Center
Philadelphia, Pennsylvania

Michael D. Lieberman, M.D.
Chief Resident in Surgery
Instructor of Surgery
University of Pennsylvania Medical Center
Philadelphia, Pennsylvania

James D. Luketich, M.D.
Resident in Surgery
University of Pennsylvania Medical Center
Philadelphia, Pennsylvania

James F. Markmann, M.D., Ph.D.
Resident in Surgery
University of Pennsylvania Medical Center
Philadelphia, Pennsylvania

Donald J. Moyer, M.D.
Resident in Neurosurgery
Assistant Instructor in Neurosurgery
University of Pennsylvania Medical Center
Philadelphia, Pennsylvania

Michael L. Nance, M.D.
Postdoctoral Research Fellow
Harrison Department of Surgical Research
University of Pennsylvania Medical Center
Philadelphia, Pennsylvania

Jon Odorico, M.D.
Resident in Surgery
University of Pennsylvania Medical Center
Philadelphia, Pennsylvania

Eline Luning Prak, A.B.
Ph.D. Candidate
Department of Allergy and Immunology
University of Pennsylvania School of
*   Medicine*
Philadelphia, Pennsylvania

Kathleen J. Reilly, M.D.
Resident in Surgery
University of Pennsylvania Medical Center
Philadelphia, Pennsylvania

David Rigberg, B.A.
Research Assistant
Harrison Department of Surgical Research
University of Pennsylvania Medical Center
Philadelphia, Pennsylvania

Michael F. Rotondo, M.D.
Assistant Professor of Surgery
University of Pennsylvania Medical Center
Philadelphia, Pennsylvania

Russell F. Sassani, R.P.H., M.D.
Postdoctoral Research Fellow
Harrison Department of Surgical Research
University of Pennsylvania Medical Center
Philadelphia, Pennsylvania

Edward B. Savage, M.D.
Chief Resident in Surgery
Instructor of Surgery
University of Pennsylvania Medical Center
Philadelphia, Pennsylvania

Joseph B. Shrager, M.D.
Postdoctoral Research Fellow
Harrison Department of Surgical Research
University of Pennsylvania Medical Center
Philadelphia, Pennsylvania

W. Roy Smythe, M.D.
Resident in Surgery
University of Pennsylvania Medical Center
Philadelphia, Pennsylvania

Paul J. Turek, M.D.
Resident in Urology
Instructor of Urology
University of Pennsylvania Medical Center
Philadelphia, Pennsylvania

FOREWORD

I was delighted when I learned that selected contributions by the University of Pennsylvania surgical residents, originally prepared for oral delivery at a weekly teaching conference, were to be collected and edited for publication by J.B. Lippincott. The subject matter of a volume based on this conference held at 7:00 A.M. every Saturday morning since its inception 15 years ago might have taken several forms. A debate format over controversial issues was used with great success by Dr. Alden Harken, the original faculty moderator of the conference. Subsequently, Drs. John Rombeau, Moritz Ziegler, V. Paul Addonizio, Michael Torosian, Donald Dafoe, and Jon Morris succeeded to the role of faculty advisor as the format changed from debate to didactic lectures on clinical topics, to a textbook review, and finally to the present one, in which basic science topics predominate.

We believe the weekly teaching conference is one of the most important educational exercises in our program. A constant over the fifteen years of the conference has been that the presentations are assigned, prepared, and delivered by residents. This takes advantage of two well-known principles: (1) that the most effective teachers of a subject are frequently those only a year or two ahead of their students on the educational ladder; and (2) that it is the teachers who learn most from lectures rather than the students. Over the course of seven years in the program, each resident learns in considerable depth the topics assigned for presentation to his or her peers.

The interest of the residents in educating themselves in the basic sciences derived in part from the emphasis of this subject matter in the annual in-service exam for surgical residents, which has proven to be quite predictive of success on Part One of the American Board of Surgery examination. Nine years ago, when I became

director of the residency program, it was clear that some of our residents were not scoring well on this in-service exam, despite the fact that many of the program's graduates were obtaining faculty positions and achieving prominence in academic medicine. Mainly because of my own anxiety over their performance (since few of our residents ever actually failed the ABS exam), I defined minimum acceptable scores on the in-service exam below which remedial measures were to be taken. This maneuver had an immediate beneficial effect on the scores, but institution of a prize for the top score was probably even more effective. Eight years ago a score in the 96th percentile was sufficient to win this prize, but in each of the last three years, a score above the 99th percentile has been required. In 1991, 39% of our general surgery residents scored over the 90th percentile, and 3 over the 99th percentile.

Drs. Savage and Fishman are to be congratulated for thinking of this publication, for selling the idea to Lippincott with the help of Dr. Leonard Miller, and for the tremendous effort that has gone into editing it. They selected the authors not only on the basis of the best conference presentations of important topics, but, in many cases, because the resident authors had studied these topics during the two-year laboratory rotation customary for our residents, or because they were already recognized experts. For example, James Markmann, a PGY III resident and the author of the immunology section, did his Ph.D. work in this field. Dr. Bridges' doctorate is from MIT where he studied biomedical transport phenomena. Dr. David Callans, one of the few authors who is not a surgical resident, is a fellow in cardiac electrophysiology. Drs. Savage and Fishman both spent their research rotations in distinguished laboratories of cardiovascular physiology.

It is our hope that this collection will be especially

helpful to medical students and residents in studying for exams, and as a survey of basic science topics to guide these and other groups to more complete study. Many faculty members and practicing surgeons are in more need of such a review than residents, since they are further removed from their medical school education. For all of us, learning and reviewing the status of modern biological science is crucial to the twin goals which we should all share: (1) the attainment of new knowledge; and (2) providing optimal care to our patients.

Clyde F. Barker, M.D.
Professor and Chairman
Department of Surgery
Hospital of the University
of Pennsylvania

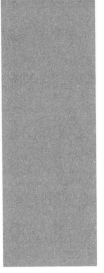

PREFACE

In recent years, the role of the surgeon in patient care has often been perceived by our nonsurgical colleagues, as well as the general public, to be limited to the technical performance of surgical procedures. To the contrary, most of us, as surgeons, pride ourselves on being complete physicians. The importance of basic science to the practice of surgery has long been promoted by the American College of Surgeons. The College has recently reaffirmed its emphasis on basic science by a mandate that all residency programs incorporate a formal basic science curriculum into their training programs. The concept for this book was derived in part from the weekly basic science course of the Department of Surgery at the University of Pennsylvania.

It is difficult to define exactly what constitutes "basic science" to surgeons. In the preparation of this text, we sought to present a concise review of those topics which we feel serve as a foundation for understanding the pathophysiology of the bulk of disease entities we encounter, as well as provide the rationale underlying the therapeutic interventions we prescribe and perform. The text is intended to provide a review of fundamental knowledge for both practicing surgeons and surgeons in training. Contributing authors were specifically requested to avoid presentation of newly developing theories or current research. In-depth, comprehensive presentations are available in other sources. Suggested references providing more detailed presentations are provided at the end of each chapter.

The majority of the contents concentrate on normal physiology and the perturbations that lead to disease. No attempt is made to describe or catalog clinical conditions, except when used to illustrate normal or abnormal physiology. Similarly, diagnostic tests are described where they assist in demonstrating physiologic principles.

The chapters are organized by physiologic function, rather than by organ system. For example, the gastrointestinal section encompasses chapters on motility, exocrine function, endocrine function, and absorption, in contrast to the more traditional presentation of separate chapters on each gastrointestinal organ. In addition to the sections dealing with physiology, we have included discussions of several ancillary topics which we believe assist in our ability to fully understand and treat our patients. These topics include principles of anesthesia, radiation therapy, chemotherapy, infectious disease, pharmacology, and statistics.

We would like to express our deepest gratitude to Dr. Leonard Miller for his wholehearted support of this project from its conception. His continued guidance, input, and encouragement have mirrored his career-long support of resident education. He has provided the stimulus for many surgeons to appreciate the art and science of surgery.

We would also like to thank the contributing authors, many of whom are residents, for their enthusiastic response in support of this book. The assistance of Mary McGlinchey, Julie Carter, Fran Ramirez, Chris DiPietro, Mary Toelke, and Carla Tolino-Panaccio in preparing the manuscript is most appreciated. Without the effort and assistance of Lisa McAllister at J.B. Lippincott Company, this text would not have been possible.

Most importantly, we would like to thank Susan and Jennifer Savage and Laurie Newman for their love, support, understanding, and patience during the completion of this project.

Finally, we would like to unofficially dedicate this work to Dr. James Mullen, whose insistence that it could *not* be accomplished was in fact a strong motivation for its actual completion.

Edward B. Savage
Steven J. Fishman
Philadelphia, Pennsylvania

CONTENTS

Michael A. Choti

1 MOLECULAR AND CELLULAR BIOLOGY

The cell is the unit of living structure. The tissues that form the body consist entirely of cells and extracellular material elaborated by cells. In order to understand the function of organs and other structures of the body, it is essential that we first understand the basic organization of the cell and the function of its parts.

Cell Structure

Advances in the understanding of the cell structure and function have been made through the use of the techniques of modern cellular and molecular biology. Although no cell is typical, a number of structures are common to most cells (Figure 1-1).

CELL MEMBRANE

The outer boundary of the cell, the cell membrane, is a continuous bilayer structure made up of a sheet of phospholipid molecules (7–10 nm) with embedded proteins. The phospholipids are oriented in such a way that the hydrophilic phosphate portion is exposed to the aqueous surfaces and the insoluble hydrophobic portions are in the interior of the membrane. A special feature of the lipid bilayer is its fluid character, allowing for movement and diffusion of bound proteins. Unlike prokaryotes, the animal eukaryotic cell membranes also contain cholesterol, the amount of which affects membrane fluidity. Additionally, the cell membrane has variable permeability, and thus the capacity to control the entrance and exit of molecules into the cell. Membrane proteins are globular units that can be attached to the inner or outer surface of the membrane, or protrude through as a transmembrane protein. These proteins are mostly glycoproteins and their membrane location and orientation depend on their hydrophilic and hydrophobic properties. There are many different types of membrane proteins including **carrier proteins,** pumps that actively transport ions across the membranes; passive ion channels, or pores; **receptors;** and **enzymes,** which catalyze reactions at the surface of the cell.

INTRACELLULAR CONNECTIONS

Two types of junctions form between the cells that make up tissue: junctions that fasten cells together, and junctions that allow the passage of molecules from one cell to another. The junctions that hold cells together include **desmosomes,** focal connections that provide general intercellular adherence; and **tight junctions,** which characteristically are located around apical margins of epithelial cells and maintain epithelial integrity. **Gap junctions** are focal connections between cells that allow passage of molecules from cell to cell without entering the extracellular space. They function to per-

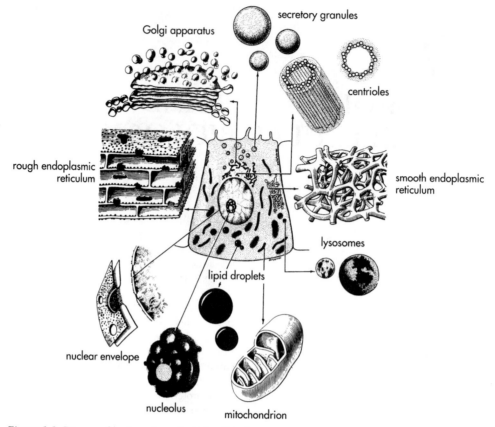

Figure 1-1 Diagram showing a hypothetical cell in the center as seen with the light microscope. It is surrounded by various organelles. (After Bloom and Fawcett. Reproduced from Junqueira LC, Cameiro J, Long JA. *Basic histology.* 5th ed. Norwalk, CT: Appleton & Lange, 1986.)

mit exchange of cellular chemical messengers as well as the propagation of electrical activity from cell to cell.

NUCLEUS

A nucleus is present in all eukaryotic cells that divide. The nucleus contains chromosomal **deoxyribonucleic acid (DNA),** packaged into chromatin in association with histone proteins. The nucleus is surrounded by a **nuclear membrane** or envelope. This membrane is a double layer with large permeable "nuclear pores." The nucleus also contains a **nucleolus,** a collection of granules rich in **ribonucleic acid (RNA),** where ribosomes are assembled (see below). Nucleoli are prominent in growing cells and nuclei can often contain more than one.

ENDOPLASMIC RETICULUM

The endoplasmic reticulum (ER) is a complex series of flattened sheets of membrane, extending throughout the cytoplasm and in structural continuity with the nuclear membrane. It specializes in synthesis and transport of lipids and membrane proteins. The **rough ER** is the portion studded with ribosomes on the cytoplasmic side and engaged in protein synthesis, whereas the **smooth ER** is free of ribosomes and functions in lipid metabolism, steroid synthesis, and detoxification.

GOLGI APPARATUS

The Golgi apparatus is a specialized portion of the ER composed of a system of stacked membrane-bound sacs (cisterns). The Golgi apparatus is involved in modifying and packaging macromolecules for delivery to other organelles and for external secretion. As expected, this apparatus is prominent in secretory cells and is located in the area of the cell from which the secretory substances are extruded.

MITOCHONDRIA

Mitochondria are the power-generating organelles of the cell. They are sausage-shaped structures and can be quite variable in size and shape. The mitochondrion is made up of two lipid bilayers: an outer membrane and an inner membrane that is folded into "shelves" called **cristae.** The outer membrane contains enzymes involved with biologic oxidation. In the interior, the matrix space contains water-soluble enzymes that convert acetyl coenzyme A (CoA) to CO_2 and water via the citric acid cycle. Attached to the cristae are oxidative enzymes and protruding globules of adenosine triphosphate (ATP) synthetase. These enzymes are responsible for transfer of electrons along the respiratory enzyme chain and oxidative phosphorylation, converting ADP to ATP. They are arranged in such a way that products of one reaction are immediately available to the next enzyme. High-energy ATP is transported out of the mitochondrion to meet cellular energy requirements. Mitochondria are self-replicating cytoplasmic organelles that contain their own mitochondrial DNA and share many similarities with free-living prokaryotic organisms.

LYSOSOMES

Lysosomes are membrane-bound cytoplasmic structures that contain hydrolytic enzymes. They function as a form of digestive system for the cell. These organelles can merge with phagocytic vacuoles to degrade exogenous material, form autophagic granules, or aid in autolysis when the cell dies. When one or more enzymes are congenitally absent, lysosomes become engorged with material that is normally degraded, resulting in characteristic lysosomal storage diseases.

CYTOSKELETON

Most eukaryotic cells contain an array of protein filaments in the cytosol, making up the cytoskeleton. These structures include **microtubules, actin fila-**ments, and **intermediate filaments.** The microtubules and microfilaments provide cell shape and motility. They also play key roles in nerve growth and in the structure and function of cilia, and make up the centriole and mitotic spindle involved in cell division.

Genetic Control of Cell Function

A gene can simply be defined as the amount of information on DNA necessary to specify a single protein molecule. The human genome contains 50,000–100,000 genes encoded in its DNA sequence. It is the differential expression of these genes that determines characteristics as varied as animal speciation and cellular and tissue function. A myriad of complex protein-nucleotide interactions occur in the process of gene expression that ultimately results in specific protein synthesis. Initially, DNA is copied to RNA in a process called **transcription,** and the RNA is then used as a template for protein synthesis in a process called **translation** (Figure 1-2).

STRUCTURE OF DNA

In the cell, DNA is condensed into chromatin and packaged into chromosomes, with each cell having two copies of the genome (diploid). Information is encoded in DNA by the precise ordering of four nucleotide bases of two types: purines, **adenine (A)** and **guanine (G)**; and pyrimidines, **thymine (T)** and **cytosine (C).** These bases are linked together by a backbone made up of phosphoric acid and deoxyribose. The DNA molecule consists of two complementary strands of opposite polarity as determined by the orientation of backbone, 5′ and 3′. The strands are held together by weak hydrogen bonds with A always paired with T, and G with C. The resulting structure is that of a long double helix.

TRANSCRIPTION

The enzyme **RNA polymerase** copies gene sequences into single-stranded messenger **RNA (mRNA)** using four monomeric nucleotides similar to those used in DNA. In RNA, **uracil (U)** replaces thymine as one of the bases. Ribonucleic acid also differs from DNA by a single substitution of a hydroxyl group for hydrogen at the 2′ position of the ribose molecule. In the typical

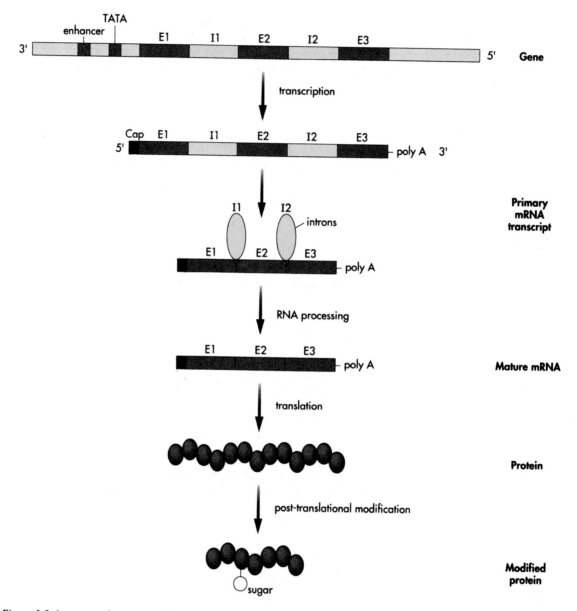

Figure 1-2 Important elements in eukaryotic gene expression. El, E2, E3 are exons. Il, I2 are introns. TATA promoter. (Modified from Baxter JD. Principles of endocrinology. In: *Cecil textbook of medicine.* 16th ed. WB Saunders, Philadelphia, 1982.)

eukaryotic gene, the transcription unit of the gene is flanked by segments on either end. Segments "upstream" often contain a "TATA" nucleotide sequence **(promoter)** as well as additional enhancers and GC-rich regions further upstream (Figure 1-2). Ribonucleic acid polymerase binds to the promoter site and catalyzes transcription proceeding from 3' to 5' on the DNA. Segments of the gene dictating formation of protein are usually separated into segments called **exons,** with intervening segments that are not translated **(introns).** These introns are clipped out during post-transcriptional modification of the mRNA in the nucleus of the cell.

TRANSLATION

The mature processed mRNA is transferred to the cytoplasm as the substrate for protein synthesis. Translation occurs on large protein-RNA structures called **ribosomes,** consisting of two unequal subunits in the eukaryote. They bind mRNA in the presence of **transfer RNA (tRNA)** and direct amino acid polymerization into protein molecules. In the genetic code, a series of triplet nucleotides or **codons** serve as recognition sites for specific amino acid charged tRNA, with each amino acid represented by at least one triplet. The first amino acid codon of every mRNA is for methionine (AUG), and all cells require this "initiation codon" to begin translation. The ribosome translocates from 5' to 3' in an energy-dependent reaction and at each codon the respective charged tRNA contributes its amino acid covalently to the growing polypeptide chain. Many ribosomes can attach to the same mRNA simultaneously, resulting in a "polyribosome." Termination codons UAA, UAG, and UGA are signals for the cessation of protein synthesis.

Posttranslational modification of the protein molecule often is required for biologic activity. Examples of posttranslational modification include glycosylation, phosphorylation, and proteolytic cleavage.

REGULATION OF GENE EXPRESSION

With the same genetic material determining a wide variety of phenotypes and functions, the cell must regulate gene expression at many different levels. Regulation at the transcription level occurs as genes are "switched" on or off. Certain DNA sequences called enhancers can be found preceding transcription units. These are thought to be the targets for regulatory DNA binding proteins that act to enhance or suppress transcription. Addition of methyl groups to DNA (DNA methylation) can regulate gene expression, as well as the degree to which the gene is condensed into chromatin. Regulation also occurs at the level of mRNA processing, translation, and posttranslational modification.

CELL DIVISION

A necessary property of all growing cells is the ability to duplicate and pass along identical copies of genetic information. Growing somatic cells undergo a cell cycle. The cycle includes the period of cell division, or **mitosis,** and the period between cell divisions or **interphase** (Figure 1-3). The replication of DNA occurs only during the **synthetic (S) phase** of interphase. During this phase, the two DNA strands separate and each serves as a template for the synthesis of a new complementary strand, catalyzed by **DNA polymerase.** The S phase is preceded and followed by two gap periods of interphase—G_1 and G_2 respectively—in which no net synthesis of DNA occurs. During G_2 the cell contains two times the amount of DNA present in the original diploid

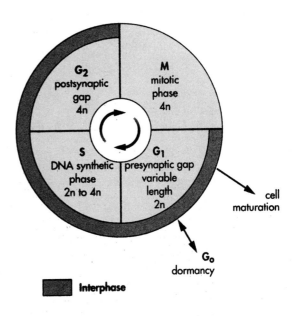

Figure 1-3 Cell cycle.

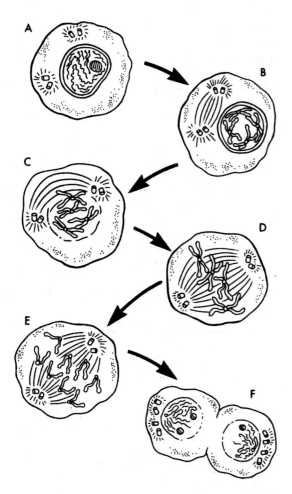

Figure 1-4 Phases of mitosis. **A,B,** Prophase. **C,** Prometaphase. **D,** Metaphase. **E,** Anaphase. **F,** Telophase. (See text for details.)

cell. Throughout interphase, continued cell growth and synthesis of RNA occurs. Cells that are not growing and dividing are halted in the diploid part of interphase (G_1), termed G_o.

The series of events that make up mitosis begins at the end of the G_2 period and terminates at the beginning of the new G_1 period. The major phases of mitosis are **prophase, prometaphase, metaphase, anaphase,** and **telophase** (Figure 1-4). During prophase, the chromatin condenses to form distinctive chromosomes and the **centrioles** migrate to opposite poles of the cell as the **mitotic spindle** forms. Prometaphase begins with the dissolution of the nuclear membrane, as each chromosome becomes attached to the mitotic spindle at its centromere region. In metaphase, the chromosomes align on the equatorial plane and are held in place by the spindle. As the cell progresses into anaphase, the two daughter chromatids separate. Telophase begins at the end of the polar migration of the chromosomes. The chromosomes then uncoil, the nuclear membranes form, and **cytokinesis,** the process of cleavage and separation of the cytoplasm, occurs. In the case of germ cells, reduction division **(meiosis)** takes place. Each mature germ cell contains only one half the amount of chromosomal material found in somatic cells.

Bibliography

Alberts B, Bray D, Lewis J, Raff M, Roberts K, Watson JD. *Molecular biology of the cell.* 2nd ed. New York: Garland, 1989.

Baserga R. *The biology of cell reproduction.* Cambridge, MA: Harvard University Press, 1985.

Beach D, Basilico C, Newport J, eds. *Cell cycle control in eukaryotes.* Cold Spring Harbor, NY: Cold Spring Harbor Laboratory, 1988.

Lewin B. *Genes.* 3rd ed. New York: Wiley, 1987.

Watson JD, Hopkins NH, Roberts JW, Steitz JA, Weiner AM. *Molecular biology of the gene.* 4th ed. Menlo Park, CA: Benjamin-Cummings, 1987.

James D. Luketich and Eline Luning Prak

2 BIOCHEMISTRY OF METABOLISM

Metabolism refers to the physical processes and biochemical pathways that enable cells to maintain homeostasis. This chapter is intended as a brief review of metabolism, including a discussion of the synthesis and degradation of proteins, carbohydrates, fats, and other important macromolecules.

Proteins and Amino Acids

Proteins are involved in all aspects of cellular function including enzymatic catalysis, intercellular communication, cell locomotion, cellular transport and storage, mechanical support, and immune system function. Proteins are generally synthesized from combinations of twenty amino acids (Table 2-1). Structurally, the amino acids possess a central carbon atom, an α-carboxyl group, an β-amino group, and a side chain designated R (Figure 2-1).

Essential amino acids are those that cannot be synthesized in sufficient quantities to meet the body's needs; therefore, a dietary source of these amino acids is required. **Nonessential amino acids** may be synthe-

TABLE 2-1. Commonly Occurring Amino Acids

Nonessential	Essential
Glycine (Gly)	Valine (Val)
Alanine (Ala)	Leucine (Leu)
Proline (Pro)	Isoleucine (Ile)
Aspartate (Asp)	Arginine (Arg)
Glutamate (Glu)	Lysine (Lys)
Asparagine (Asn)	Phenylalanine (Phe)
Glutamine (Gln)	Tryptophan (Trp)
Cysteine (Cys)	Histidine (His)
Tyrosine (Tyr)	Methionine (Met)
Serine (Ser)	Threonine (Thr)

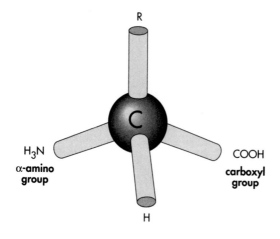

Figure 2-1 Anatomy of an amino acid.

TABLE 2-2. Biologic Roles of Selected Amino Acids

Amino Acid	Possible Roles
Cysteine	Oxidation to taurine; component of some bile acids Converted to pyruvic acid
Glutamate	Precursor of γ-aminobutyric acid Transamination to oxaloacetic acid
Glycine	Contributes to the bile salt glycocholate Part of hippurate and glutamate Contributes to purine and pyrimidine synthesis Formed from or converted to serine
Histidine	Precursor of ergothioneine, carnosine, and anserine Precursor of histamine
Methionine	Initiation codon in protein synthesis Precursor of cysteine Component of S-adenosyl methionine
Tryptophan	NAD synthesis Precursor of 5-HT (serotonin)
Tyrosine	Precursor of dopamine, norepinephrine, and epinephrine Polymer forms melanin Precursor of thyroxin

sized from precursors and thus are not required in the diet. Amino acids may also be classified according to various properties of their R groups. For example, aspartate and glutamate have acidic side chains, whereas lysine, arginine, and histidine have basic side chains. Other amino acids have characteristic chemical constituents, for example, the sulfur atom in cysteine and methionine. Phenylalanine and tyrosine have an aromatic side chain. Valine, leucine, and isoleucine have branched hydrocarbon side chains. While the functional correlates of each R group are not fully understood, some confer important biologic properties to the amino acid (Table 2-2).

The **branched chain amino acids (BCAAs)** deserve special mention in this regard. Under conditions of stress (sepsis, trauma), BCAAs are preferentially mobilized from skeletal muscle, and they act to stimulate protein synthesis and exert a nitrogen-sparing effect. Currently, the clinical importance of BCAAs remains uncertain.

SYNTHESIS AND STRUCTURE

Protein synthesis involves transcription, translation, and several modifying steps described in Chapter 1. Protein structure can be described at various levels. **Primary structure** refers to the linear arrangement, or sequence, of amino acids along the peptide backbone. Amino acids are linked by peptide bonds joining the carboxy end of one amino acid to the amino end of the adjacent amino acid. The amino acid sequence of a protein is numbered from the N-terminus (amino group end) on the left to the C-terminus (carboxy end) on the right. The molecular weights of proteins range from a few thousand to several million daltons. Smaller proteins constructed of only a few amino acids are referred to as peptides. Examples of peptides include oxytocin, vasopressin, and somatostatin.

The three-dimensional arrangement of a protein is essential to its biologic activity. This structure is specified by the primary amino acid sequence of the protein. For example, when a complex protein such as ribonuclease is treated with urea and B-mercaptoethanol, it unfolds and loses its three-dimensional conformation and biological activity, but its primary sequence remains intact. When reoxidized, the protein spontaneously refolds, regaining its conformation and biological activity. Refolding occurs through a series of interactions specified by the primary sequence, which results in the formation of secondary and tertiary structural relationships.

Secondary structure refers to the steric relations that develop between amino acids in close proximity to one another along the peptide backbone. These interactions set up important intermediates in the folding process leading to the final structure. **Tertiary structure** is similar to secondary structure but occurs as a consequence of steric forces (sulfhydryl bonding and hydrogen bonding) between amino acids that are further apart on the peptide backbone. The above interactions can give rise to regularly repeating conformations of polypeptide chains such as the α-helix or β-pleated sheet. **Quaternary structure** is defined by the relationship between different polypeptide chains (subunits) within a single complex protein.

PROTEIN DEGRADATION

Proteins are broken down into amino acids and released from tissues into the circulation. Amino acids can be taken up by other tissues and utilized in the synthesis of new proteins. In contrast to fats and carbohydrates, excess amino acids not used in synthetic reactions cannot be stored. They must be degraded into metabolic fuels. Degradation occurs primarily in the liver by **transamination** reactions that remove the α-amino group from the amino acid. The resulting carbon skeleton has many fates. In addition to some of the specialized functions listed in Table 2-2, the carbon skeleton may be converted to acetyl coenzyme A (CoA), acetoacetyl CoA, pyruvate, oxaloacetate, α-ketoglutarate, succinate, and fumarate.

The transamination reaction commonly involves **glutamate transaminase.** This enzyme catalyzes the transfer of the amino group from the amino acid to α-ketoglutarate, forming an α-keto acid and glutamate. Glutamate is oxidatively deaminated to form an ammonium ion with the regeneration of α-ketoglutarate. The ammonium ion has two possible fates: A small amount will be used in the biosynthesis of nitrogen compounds, whereas the majority will be converted to urea via the urea cycle and excreted by the kidneys. Like the transamination described above, the urea cycle takes place mainly in the liver. Secondary sites of urea formation include the kidneys and the brain. The urea cycle is a series of chemical reactions that incorporates nitrogen in an energy-dependent manner into urea (H_2N–CO–NH_2).

ENZYMES

Enzymes are polypeptides or proteins that catalyze various biological reactions by lowering their **activation energy.** Coenzymes are nonprotein molecules that contribute to the activity of some enzymes, for example, a heme or heavy metal. The nomenclature of enzymes consists of two parts: The first refers to the substrate or product of the reaction and the second describes the reaction. For example, the enzyme pyruvate carboxylase catalyzes the addition of a carboxyl group to the substrate pyruvate to form oxaloacetate.

The rate of enzyme-catalyzed reactions depends not only on the concentration of enzyme and substrate but on the presence of various regulatory substances that act as inhibitors and activators. For example, phosphofructokinase (PFK) catalyzes the rate-limiting step of glycolysis and is modulated by several intermediates. When the energy charge of the cell is low, adenosine monophosphate (AMP) is present in high concentrations and is an activator of PFK. Conversely, if the energy charge is high, increased levels of adenosine triphosphate (ATP) and citrate act as inhibitors.

Carbohydrates

Carbohydrates are polyhydroxylated molecules with a carbon skeleton having at least three carbon atoms. Monosaccharides, the simplest carbohydrates, have an empirical formula of $(CH_2O)n$. Disaccharides are formed from two monosaccharides joined by a glycosidic bond. Sucrose is a dimer of glucose and fructose; maltose consists of two glucose molecules; and lactose is galactose plus glucose. Oligosaccharides contain 2 to 10 monosaccharides. Carbohydrate polymers consisting of greater than 10 monosaccharide units are referred to as polysaccharides. **Glycogen** is a polysaccharide comprised of glucose. It is the major storage form of glucose in humans.

Entry of glucose and other simple sugars into various metabolic pathways depends largely upon the energy charge of the cell. A low level of available energy in the cell shunts glucose into **degradative pathways.** Under **aerobic conditions** glucose is broken down

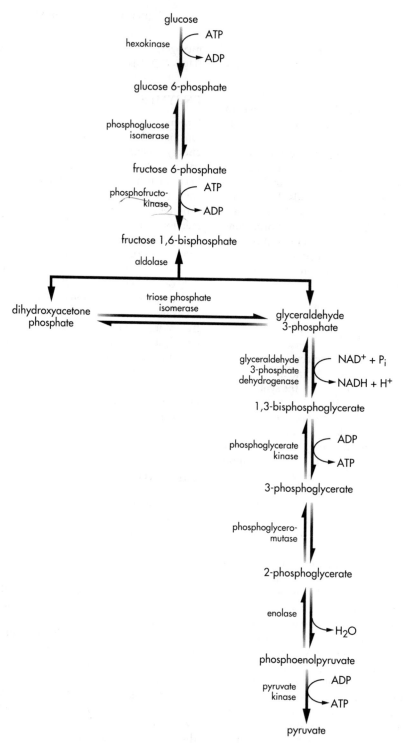

Figure 2-2 Glycolysis.

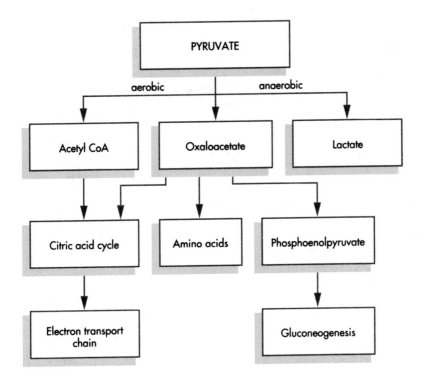

Figure 2-3 Possible fates of pyruvate.

into pyruvate by glycolysis (Figure 2-2), pyruvate is oxidized to acetyl CoA (Figure 2-3), and acetyl CoA enters the citric acid cycle (Figure 2-4). This results in the production of ATP and the generation of reducing equivalents (NADH, FADH$_2$), which donate electrons to oxygen and produce ATP via a complex series of reactions in the mitochondria referred to as oxidative phosphorylation. Under **anaerobic conditions**, the glycolytic pathway continues to oxidize glucose into pyruvate but oxidative phosphorylation at the mitochondrial level stops. If oxygen debt continues, glycolysis must become the major source of ATP. This requires a continued source of NAD$^+$ which, in the absence of oxidative phosphorylation, is supplied by the reduction of pyruvate to lactate. The goal of these degradative pathways is energy production in the form of high-energy phosphate bonds (i.e., the conversion of AMP and ADP to ATP). This can be accomplished directly by substrate-level phosphorylation, producing ATP during glycolysis or guanosine triphosphate (GTP) in the citric acid cycle; or indirectly by converting energy stored in reducing equivalents (NADH, FADH$_2$) to yield ATP.

A high level of energy in the cell inhibits the degradative glucose pathways. Under these conditions glucose enters into synthetic pathways for glycogen or into the pentose phosphate pathway (see below) to provide cells with important molecules for biosynthesis.

GLYCOLYSIS

Glycolysis consists of 10 cytosolic reactions that convert glucose into pyruvate with the concomitant production of ATP (see Figure 2-2). In this pathway, two molecules of ATP are consumed and four are produced, with a net production of two ATP for each glucose molecule. Although there are several minor steps that can influence the rate of glycolysis, PFK is the key regulatory enzyme. Phosphofructokinase is inhibited by a high-

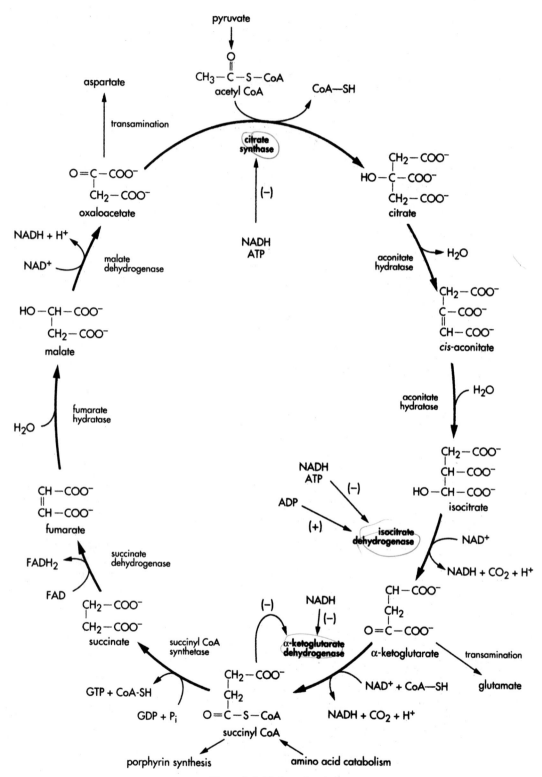

Figure 2-4 Citric acid cycle.

energy charge in the cell (i.e., an increased ATP:AMP ratio), as well as by citrate, an early intermediate in the citric acid cycle. Likewise, PFK is activated by a low-energy charge in the cell (i.e., a decreased ATP:AMP ratio).

PYRUVATE

Pyruvate formed during glycolysis has several possible fates. The pathway followed is largely dependent upon the energy charge and biosynthetic needs of the cell (see Figure 2-4). If the energy charge of the cell is low with decreased levels of NADH, ATP, and acetyl-CoA, and AMP is increased, pyruvate dehydrogenase is activated. Pyruvate dehydrogenase requires five coenzymes: thiamine pyrophosphate, lipoic acid, CoASH, FAD^+, and NAD^+. Pyruvate is decarboxylated by this enzyme complex to form acetyl-CoA. Acetyl-CoA enters the citric acid cycle, producing ATP and reducing equivalents for the electron transport chain. Conversely, if the energy charge of the cell is high, the pyruvate dehydrogenase complex is inhibited and pyruvate is carboxylated to form oxaloacetate. In the setting of high-energy charge, oxaloacetate acts as a source of atoms for synthesis of amino acids and does not enter the citric acid cycle. Oxaloacetate can also be decarboxylated and oxidized to form phosphoenolpyruvate and enter the gluconeogenic pathway.

In actively contracting muscle, the rate of oxidation of glucose may exceed the rate of pyruvate conversion to acetyl-CoA and its entry into the citric acid cycle. During these periods of relative oxygen deprivation, excess pyruvate is converted to lactate with the net anaerobic production of two ATP molecules. Lactate is essentially an end product in metabolism; it must enter the bloodstream and be oxidized to pyruvate in the liver before it can enter the gluconeogenic pathway or the citric acid cycle.

CITRIC ACID CYCLE

The citric acid, or Krebs, cycle completely oxidizes acetyl-CoA to carbon dioxide with the **generation of high-energy phosphate bonds and reducing equivalents** (see Figure 2-4). This cycle is the final common pathway for energy-yielding oxidation of carbohydrates, proteins, and fats. Each acetyl-CoA molecule that enters the citric acid cycle produces three NADH molecules, one $FADH_2$ molecule, and one GTP molecule; these

various forms of stored energy are the equivalent of 12 ATP molecules. **Intermediates for biosynthetic pathways,** such as α-ketoglutarate for amino acid synthesis and succinyl-CoA for porphyrin synthesis, are also provided by the citric cycle.

Regulation of the citric acid cycle is important. Citrate synthetase catalyzes the first committed step of the cycle and is an important control point; ATP and NADH inhibit this enzyme. Isocitrate dehydrogenase is another rate-controlling enzyme; it is stimulated by ADP and inhibited by ATP and NADH. A third control point is α-ketoglutarate dehydrogenase, which is inhibited by succinyl-CoA and NADH.

GLUCONEOGENESIS

Gluconeogenesis is the synthesis of glucose from non-carbohydrate sources including lactate, amino acids, and glycerol. It plays an important role in the formation of glucose during starvation and prolonged exercise. During starvation, glucose stores (principally glycogen) are only able to supply glucose for about 24 hours. After this, glucose-dependent tissues, such as skeletal muscle, brain, and red blood cells, depend on gluconeogenesis for energy. Primary sites of gluconeogenesis include the liver, kidneys, and intestines.

Although glycolysis converts glucose into pyruvate and gluconeogenesis converts pyruvate into glucose, gluconeogenesis cannot be considered a simple reversal of glycolysis. **Three of the ten enzymatic steps of glycolysis are not reversible:** these are catalyzed by hexokinase, PFK, and pyruvate kinase. Two enzymes, pyruvate carboxylase and phosphoenolpyruvate carboxykinase, are required to bypass the pyruvate kinase step of glycolysis. Fructose-1,6-diphosphatase and glucose-6-phosphatase bypass the glycolytic reactions catalyzed by PFK and hexokinase.

GLYCOGEN METABOLISM

Glycogen is a **storage form of glucose** found primarily in the liver and skeletal muscle. Structurally, glycogen is an α-1,4-glucose polymer with α-1,6 branches occurring every 8–12 glucose residues. This storage form of glucose is synthesized from uridine diphosphate (UDP)-glucose. Uridine diphosphate-glucose is an activated form of glucose synthesized from glucose-1-phosphate and UTP in a pyrophosphate-liberating reaction. Uridine diphosphate-glucose is then added to a growing glycogen chain by glycogen synthetase.

Glycogen is degraded to glucose-1-phosphate by glycogen phosphorylase, which removes glycosyl residues from the polymer. Other important enzymes needed for complete degradation of glycogen include a transferase and α-1,6-glucosidase (debranching enzyme).

Phosphoglucomutase converts the liberated glucose-1-phosphate into glucose-6-phosphate. Glucose-6-phosphate is then converted to glucose by glucose-6-phosphatase. Unphosphorylated glucose is free to diffuse out of the cell. Glucose-6-phosphatase is absent in glucose-dependent tissues such as the brain and skeletal muscle.

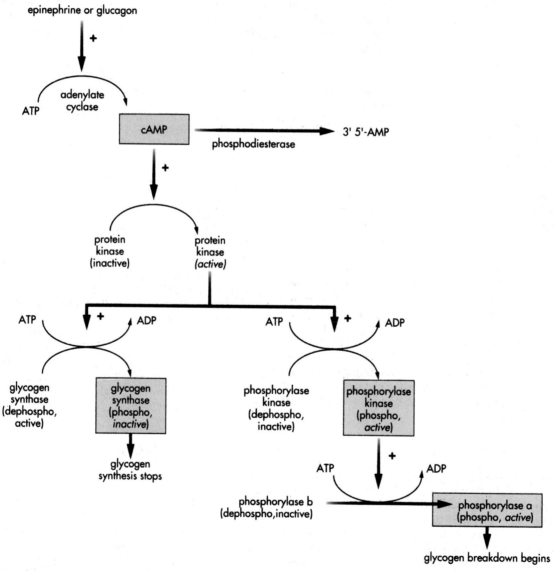

Figure 2-5 Reaction cascades and the control of glycogen metabolism. Epinephrine and glucagon promote glucose liberation from glycogen by suppressing glycogen synthase and activating glycogen phosphorylase.

Glycogen synthesis and degradation employ distinct enzymatic pathways that facilitate precise modulation. During periods of hypoglycemia or stress, glycogenolysis is stimulated and glucose is released. This response is stimulated by glucagon and epinephrine, which also inhibit glycogen synthesis.

This complex regulation of glycogen metabolism occurs through a cyclic AMP (cAMP)-mediated cascade (Figure 2-5). In this cascade, cAMP is referred to as a **second messenger;** the first messenger is the hormone. This regulatory cascade prevents glycogen synthesis and glycogen degradation from operating simultaneously.

Insulin is another important hormone that regulates glycogen metabolism. A high glucose concentration in the bloodstream stimulates the release of insulin from the β-cells of the pancreas. Insulin stimulates glycogen synthetase promoting glycogenesis. It also dephosphorylates and inactivates the glycogenolytic enzymes activated by epinephrine and glucagon, preventing concurrent glycogenolysis. In addition to its effects on glycogen metabolism, insulin suppresses gluconeogenesis and increases flow through the glycolytic pathway. However, under these "fed state" conditions, the acetyl-CoA generated during glycolysis enters into the synthesis of fatty acids and energy storage rather than into the citric acid cycle for the generation of high-energy compounds. Insulin also stimulates the synthesis and storage of triacylglycerols in adipose tissue and promotes protein synthesis.

PENTOSE PHOSPHATE SHUNT

The pentose phosphate shunt produces a supply of reducing equivalents in the form of **NADPH for biosynthetic reactions,** provides **pentoses for nucleotide synthesis,** and facilitates interconversion of hexoses and pentoses.

Lipids

Lipids are hydrophobic molecules. There are several common but structurally distinct lipids including fatty acids, phospholipids, and steroids. Lipids play a major role in the structure and function of biologic membranes, hormone synthesis, and energy storage.

FATTY ACIDS

A fatty acid is a long hydrocarbon chain with a terminal carboxylic acid moiety (Figure 2-6). Most fatty acids contain an even number of carbon atoms, commonly between 14 and 24. Carbon atoms are numbered beginning at the carboxyl terminus; carbon atoms 2 and 3 are referred to as α and β; the methyl carbon at the distal end is the ω carbon. Fatty acids can be **saturated,** with no double bonds in the hydrocarbon chain, or **unsaturated,** containing a variable number of double bonds. The length and degree of saturation are important in determining the physical characteristics of fatty acid containing compounds. Shorter hydrocarbon chain length and greater degrees of unsaturation confer greater fluidity.

FATTY ACID SYNTHESIS

Fatty acid synthesis occurs in the cell cytoplasm. Acetyl-CoA, primarily supplied by the cleavage of citrate, combines with bicarbonate in an ATP-consuming reaction to produce malonyl-CoA. This reaction is catalyzed by **acetyl-CoA carboxylase and is the rate-controlling step in fatty acid biosynthesis** (Figure 2-7). In the fed state, there is an abundance of citrate and isocitrate; both allosterically upregulate acetyl-CoA carboxylase. The process of fatty acid synthesis is orches-

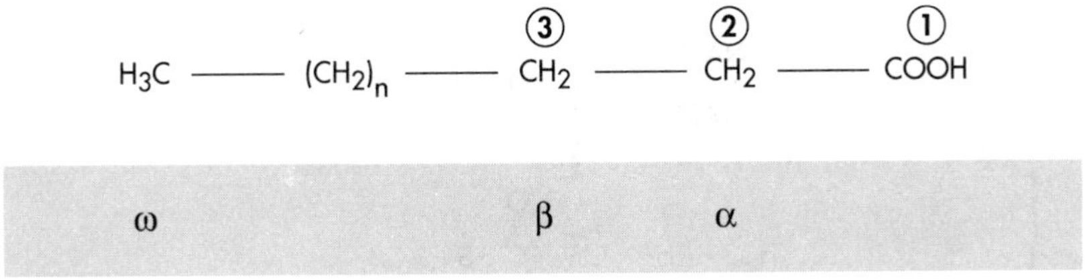

$$H_3C \longrightarrow (CH_2)_n \longrightarrow \overset{\text{\textcircled{3}}}{CH_2} \longrightarrow \overset{\text{\textcircled{2}}}{CH_2} \longrightarrow \overset{\text{\textcircled{1}}}{COOH}$$

$$\omega \qquad\qquad \beta \qquad \alpha$$

Figure 2-6 Anatomy of a fatty acid.

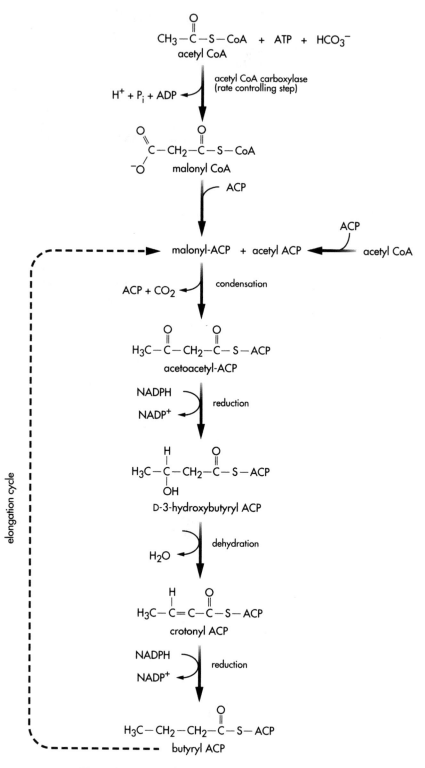

Figure 2-7 Fatty acid synthesis. ACP, acyl carrier protein.

trated by fatty acid synthetase, a cytoplasmic multienzyme complex.

Each round of elongation increases the fatty acid chain length by two carbon units and consumes two NADPH and one ATP. This synthetic cycle can continue until the nascent fatty acid chain reaches the length of palmitate (sixteen carbon atoms). Other enzyme systems control fatty acid elongation beyond this point. There are also specialized enzymes for introducing double bonds into fatty acid chains.

β-OXIDATION OF FATTY ACIDS

Fatty acid degradation occurs primarily through **β-oxidation in the mitochondria.** A carnitine transport system facilitates fatty acid entry into the mitochondria from the cytosol. Once inside the mitochondria, fatty acyl-carnitine is converted to fatty acyl-CoA and carnitine returns to the cytoplasm. Fatty acyl-CoA undergoes **β-oxidation via sequential oxidation, hydration, oxidation, and thiolysis** (Figure 2-8). Each round of degradation produces one acetyl-CoA, one $FADH_2$, and one NADH molecule. Fatty acids with an odd number of carbon atoms are degraded to propionyl-CoA, which can be converted to methylmalonyl-CoA via a carboxylation reaction. Methylmalonyl-CoA can be converted to succinyl-CoA, which, in turn, is converted into oxaloacetate. Oxaloacetate can then enter the citric acid cycle, amino acid synthesis, or the gluconeogenic pathway.

TRIGLYCERIDES AND PHOSPHOLIPIDS

Fatty acids can be incorporated into or liberated from **triglycerides,** their **primary storage form.** During incorporation into triglycerides, fatty acids are activated to fatty acyl-CoA in a reaction requiring two ATP molecules. In the liver and adipose tissue, two fatty acyl-CoA molecules combine with glycerol-3-phosphate to form a phosphatidic acid. The phosphate is cleaved from the phosphatidic acid and another fatty acyl-CoA is added to the diglyceride to complete the triglyceride.

Phospholipids are similar to triglycerides except that a phosphate atom replaces one of the fatty acid chains on the glycerol.

Fatty acid liberation from triglycerides is catalyzed by plasma lipoprotein lipase and adipocyte hormonesensitive lipase. Lipolytic enzymes are stimulated by glucagon, norepinephrine, epinephrine, and adrenocor

ticotropic hormone. Insulin inhibits lipolysis. During lipolysis of a triglyceride, three fatty acids and a glycerol molecule are mobilized. Glycerol can be phosphorylated to glycerol-3-phosphate and used in glycolysis or triglyceride formation.

KETONE BODY METABOLISM

The **ketone bodies include acetoacetate, acetone, and β-hydroxybutyrate.** Acetyl-CoA generated from fatty acid oxidation normally enters the citric acid cycle to yield metabolic energy. However, during prolonged fasting intermediates for the citric acid cycle, for example oxaloacetate, become deficient. Acetyl-CoA can no longer enter these pathways and instead enters into the synthesis of ketone bodies (Figure 2-9). The ketone body, acetoacetate, is also an important source of fuel under normal conditions in heart muscle and the renal cortex. Acetoacetate can be converted to two acetyl-CoA units in a reaction that requires succinyl-CoA.

During starvation, cellular metabolism shifts from the use of glucose to ketone bodies as a primary energy source. If this shift to a fat-burning state did not occur, muscle protein breakdown would continue at a high rate to supply amino acids for gluconeogenesis. Thus, ketone bodies facilitate the preservation of muscle protein during starvation. However, some cells cannot use ketone bodies and require a consistent source of glucose.

Diabetics become ketotic because transport of glucose into cells is deficient. Intracellular glucose stores are depleted and catabolism shifts to proteins and fats. Oxaloacetate becomes depleted and acetyl-CoA cannot enter the citric acid cycle; instead ketone bodies are formed.

CHOLESTEROL

Cholesterol, as a representative steroid, is pictured in Figure 2-10. Cholesterol is synthesized in several steps. First, two acetyl-CoA molecules combine to form acetoacetyl-CoA, which is converted to 3-hydroxyl-3-methyl-glutaryl-CoA (HMG-S-CoA) (see Figure 2-9). The HMG-S-CoA is reduced to mevalonic acid in the **rate-limiting step of cholesterol biosynthesis, catalyzed by HMG-CoA reductase.** Cholesterol is then synthesized by a series of reactions combining six subunits derived from mevalonic acid. HMG-CoA reductase is a site for the action of antihyperlipidemic drugs.

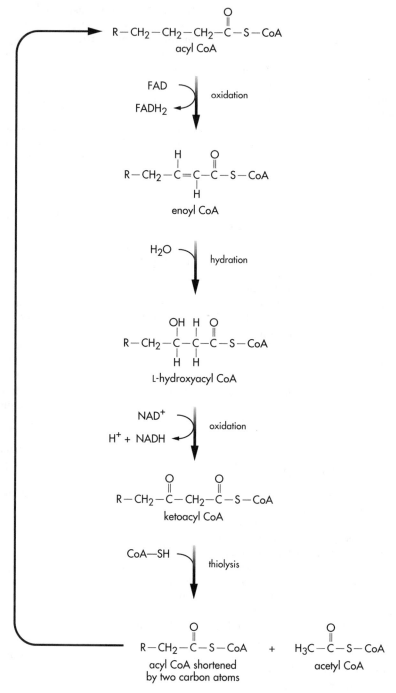

Figure 2-8 β-Oxidation of fatty acids.

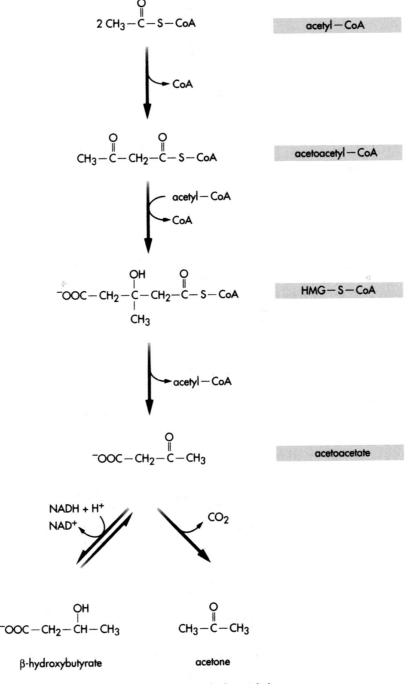

Figure 2-9 Ketone body metabolism.

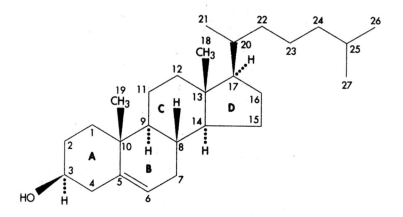

Figure 2-10 Cholesterol.

Dietary cholesterol suppresses the synthesis of HMG-CoA reductase.

Cholesterol is the parent compound for glucocorticoids, mineralocorticoids, sex steroids, bile acids, and vitamin D (see Figure 27-6). Cholesterol, a C_{27} sterol, gives rise to pregnenolone (C_{21}) and the progestagens. In the adrenal zona glomerulosa, progestagens (C_{21}) can be converted to mineralocorticoids (C_{21}) such as aldosterone. In the adrenal cortex, progestagens can be converted to glucocorticoids (C_{21}) such as cortisol and 11-deoxycorticosterone (DOC). Androgens (C_{19}) and estrogens (C_{18}) can also be formed from the progestagens. Glycocholate, the major human bile salt, is synthesized from cholesterol. Another cholesterol derivative, 7-dehydrocholesterol, is converted to vitamin D_3 by ultraviolet light. Vitamin D_3 is activated by successive hydroxylations occurring in the liver and the kidneys to the hormone 1,25-dihydroxyvitamin D.

Most cholesterol is delivered to the periphery by low density lipoprotein (LDL) particles. Low density lipoprotein cholesterol is largely esterified to linoleic acid, a polyunsaturated fatty acid. High density lipoprotein (HDL) particles return cholesterol from the periphery to the liver for degradation, storage, and other synthetic uses. Low levels of HDL particles and high levels of LDL have both been implicated in the pathophysiology of atherosclerosis.

MEMBRANES

Phospholipids, glycolipids, and cholesterol play an important role in the structure and function of biological membranes. Membrane lipids tend to be amphipathic, containing both a hydrophilic region and hydrophobic region. Depending on their concentration in aqueous solution, these amphipathic molecules can form micelles or bilayered sheets. The hydrophilic portions align toward the aqueous solution and the hydrophobic moieties remain isolated from the solution in a protected core. This orientation results in sheetlike structures composed of a lipid bilayer. The lipid bilayer and its asymmetric constellation of proteins are described by the **Fluid Mosaic Model.**

Functionally, membranes serve as semipermeable barriers and solvents for membrane proteins. Lipid bilayers have a low permeability to ions and most polar molecules; water and small nonpolar molecules readily traverse the membrane. Membrane fluidity depends on several factors including cholesterol content, degree of fatty acid saturation, and conformations about the fatty acyl bonds. Membrane proteins serve specialized functions as ion channels and pumps, receptors, transporters, and enzymes.

ESSENTIAL FATTY ACIDS

Most of the fatty acids needed for biological function and structure can be synthesized by the human body. However, mammals lack the enzymatic machinery to introduce double bonds beyond C-9 in the hydrocarbon chain and therefore cannot synthesize **linoleic** and **linolenic acids.** These two fatty acids must be supplied by the diet and are considered **essential fatty acids** (EFAs). Their presence is required for the synthesis of prostaglandins. Lack of these two fatty acids in the diet leads to a deficiency state characterized by dermatitis, decreased resistance to physical stress, and impaired lipid transport resulting in a fatty liver.

Purine and Pyrimidine Metabolism

Purines and pyrimidines are nitrogeneous heterocyclic bases found in genetic material. Important purine bases are adenine, guanine, xanthine, hypoxanthine, and uric acid. The pyrimidines include uracil, found only in RNA; thymine, found only in DNA; and cytosine. Purines or pyrimidines linked to the pentose sugar ribose are called nucleosides, which are phosphorylated to form nucleotides. The nucleotides ATP and GTP are high-energy intermediates with approximately 7.3 kcal/mol available in each phosphate bond. Cyclic AMP and GTP are involved in signal transduction as second messengers and G-protein ligands.

Purines and pyrimidines can be synthesized de novo, or enter the nucleotide pool via salvage pathways.

De novo synthesis of the purine ring begins with the activation of ribose-5-phosphate by ATP to 5-phosphoribosyl-1-pyrophosphate (PRPP) (Figure 2-11), which then combines with glutamine. This is the committed step in purine biosynthesis and is driven forward by the hydrolysis of pyrophosphate from PRPP. Next, a series of reactions forms the purine ring from several precursors including glycine, aspartate, glutamine, carbon dioxide, and activated carbon derivatives from tetrahydrofolate (Figure 2-12A). The pyrimidine ring is synthesized from carbamoyl phosphate and aspartate (Figure 2-12B) by a multifunctional enzyme complex. PRPP is also utilized in the synthesis of NAD, NADP, FMN, FAP, and the amino acids tryptophan and histidine.

External salvage brings nucleotides into the pool from dietary sources. Internal salvage uses nucleotides from endogenous degradation. Nucleotide catabolism converts nucleotides to nucleosides or bases and sugars. Bases can be recycled via internal salvage or excreted by the kidneys as uric acid.

Energetics

The extraction of energy and other building blocks from food has been described in three stages (Figure 2-13). First, large molecules in food are broken down into smaller units. Proteins are hydrolyzed into amino acids and taken up by the liver and peripheral tissues for protein synthesis. Polysaccharides and oligosaccharides are broken down into simple sugars such as glucose. Fats, such as triacylglycerols, are hydrolyzed into fatty acids

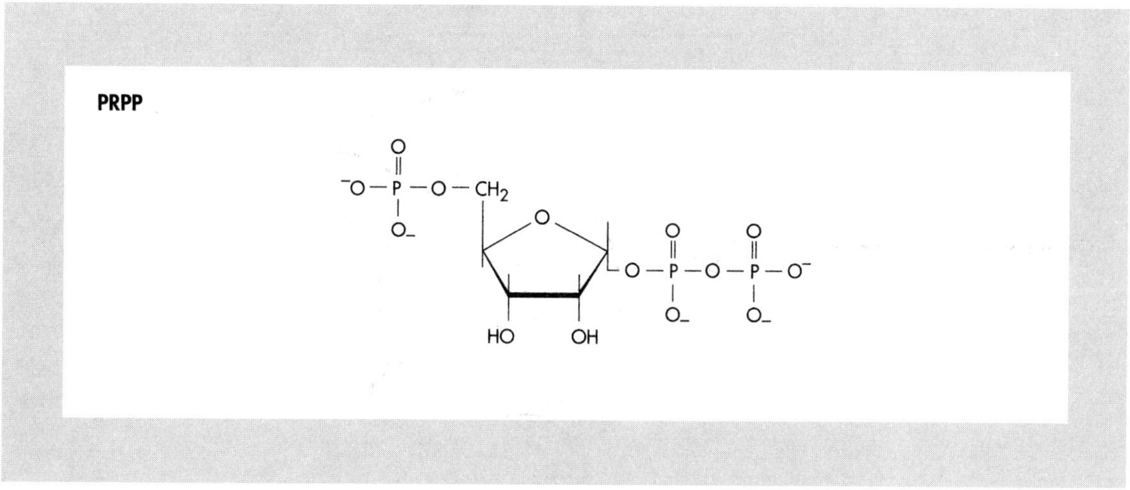

Figure 2-11 5-Phosphoribosyl-1-pyrophosphate (PRPP).

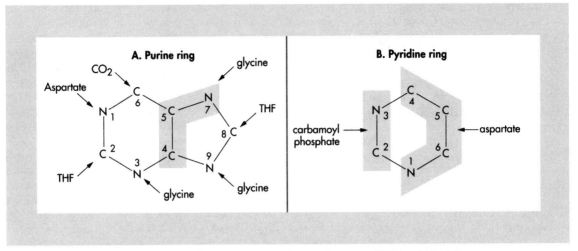

Figure 2-12 Origin of atoms in purine and pyrimidine rings. THF, tetrahydrofolate.

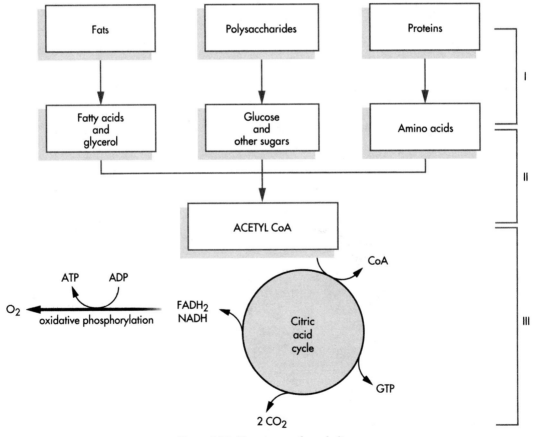

Figure 2-13 Three stages of metabolism.

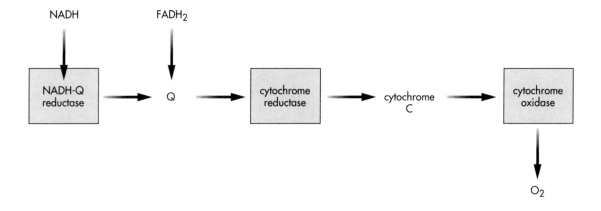

Figure 2-14 Electron transport chain. Boxed enzymes indicate sites of proton pumping (see text).

and glycerol. Essentially no usable energy is produced in this initial stage. In the next stage, many of these small molecules are converted into the acetyl unit of acetyl-CoA. Although some energy is produced in this stage, only a fraction of the potentially available energy is released.

The third stage includes the citric acid cycle and mitochondrial oxidative phosphorylation. Energy is extracted as acetyl units are oxidized to CO_2 in the citric acid cycle. Reducing equivalents are generated and carried by NADH and $FADH_2$. The majority of ATP is produced by the mitochondrial electron transport chain as electrons flow from these carriers to oxygen.

MITOCHONDRIAL ELECTRON TRANSPORT CHAIN

Mitochondria are membranous oval-shaped organelles found within the cytoplasm of cells. Important structural components include an outer membrane and an inner membrane consisting of numerous internal folds called cristae. There are two compartments created by this two-membrane system: an intermembrane space between the inner and outer membranes, and the matrix that is bounded by the inner membrane. Oxidative phosphorylation takes place within the inner membrane; the reactions of the citric acid cycle and the β-oxidation of fatty acids occur within the matrix.

Within the inner mitochondrial membrane, a series of cytochromes facilitate the transfer of electrons from NADH and $FADH_2$ to oxygen (Figure 2-14). The transfer of electrons from NADH to oxygen is a highly exothermic reaction, yielding a free-energy change of -52.6 kcal/mol. This free-energy change is utilized by the cytochromes to pump protons across the inner mitochondrial membrane. **The resultant proton gradient drives the synthesis of ATP by an ATPase complex.** Oxidation of NADH to NAD+ yields three ATP, whereas $FADH_2$ oxidation yields only two ATP.

Uncoupling of the oxidation-generated proton gradient and ATP generation may occur with the subsequent loss of potential energy as heat. This process of uncoupling occurs under certain physiologic and pathologic conditions. In newborn humans and other mammals requiring large amounts of heat to maintain body temperature, brown fat is present. These small pads of brown fat produce heat at the expense of energy (thermogenesis) by uncoupling the mitochondrial proton gradient from ATP production. Other uncouplers include dinitrophenol, excess thyroid hormone, and large doses of aspirin. Agents such as cyanide and antimycin A inhibit electron transport by blocking the mitochondrial electron carriers rather than uncoupling the proton gradient from ATP production.

Bibliography

Creighton TE. *Proteins: structures and molecular properties.* New York: WH Freeman, 1984.

Friedman PJ. *Biochemistry.* Boston: Little, Brown, 1987.

Ganong WF. *Review of medical physiology.* Norwalk: Appleton & Lange, 1987.

Loudon M. *Organic chemistry.* Reading, MA: Addison Wesley, 1984.

Ottaway JH, Apps DK. *Biochemistry.* London: Bailliere Tindall, 1984.

Rombeau JL and Caldwell MD. *Enteral and tube feeding.* Philadelphia: WB Saunders, 1984.

Segel IH. *Biochemical calculations.* New York: John Wiley, 1976.

Stryer L. *Biochemistry.* New York: WH Freeman, 1988.

Edward B. Savage

3 FLUID BALANCE AND ELECTROLYTES

Fluid and electrolyte management is one of the cornerstones of surgical care. Normally, fluid balance, electrolyte concentrations, and pH are tightly controlled by the endocrine, pulmonary, and renal systems. Imbalance in this regulation is induced by many of the diseases and injuries treated by a surgeon as well as by the surgical interventions necessary to remedy these problems.

Physiology of Body Fluid Compartments

ANATOMY OF THE BODY FLUID COMPARTMENTS

Though it varies with age, activity level, and body composition, 50–70% of total body weight is water. In order to understand the distribution of water it is useful to divide the body into compartments (Figure 3-1). **Total body water (TBW)** is distributed between **intracellular water (ICW)** and **extracellular water (ECW).** Extracellular water is comprised of **interstitial fluid (ISF)** and **plasma.** Interstitial fluid has two distinct components: (1) a rapidly equilibrating pericellular space (90%), and (2) **transcellular fluids** (10%) (water contained in connective tissue, secretions, joint space fluids and cerebrospinal fluid).

The percentage of total body mass comprised of water is primarily dependent on body composition. While skeletal muscle has a relatively high water content, the water content of adipose tissue is low. As the proportion of muscle mass relative to adipose tissue decreases, so does the percentage of body weight comprised of water. Therefore, a newborn's total body weight is 80% water, a normal adult's body weight is 50–60% water, and an elderly adult's body weight is 40–50% water. Similarly, a normal male's body weight is 60% water, and a normal female's body weight is 50% water.

The Third Space

The third space refers to a pathologic fluid compartment. Specifically, it refers to fluid that is sequestered in

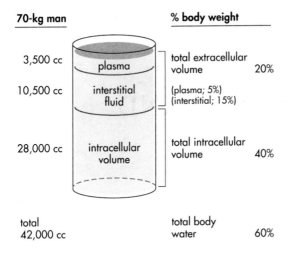

70-kg man | **% body weight**

3,500 cc — plasma — total extracellular volume 20% (plasma; 5%) (interstitial; 15%)

10,500 cc — interstitial fluid

28,000 cc — intracellular volume — total intracellular volume 40%

total 42,000 cc | total body water 60%

Figure 3-1 Functional compartments of body fluids. (Reproduced from Shires TG, Canizaro, PC. Fluid and electrolyte management of the surgical patient. In Sabiston DC Jr, ed. *Textbook of surgery: the biological basis of modern surgical practice.* 13th ed. Philadelphia: WB Saunders, 1986:64.)

certain tissues or cavities in response to inflammation or injury. This fluid is of similar composition to that of the extracellular fluid, from which it is derived. The third space is important because the losses of extracellular fluid must be adequately replaced to maintain extracellular volume.

DISTRIBUTION OF ELECTROLYTES WITHIN THE FLUID COMPARTMENTS

The term "**electrolyte**" refers to the negatively charged (anions) and positively charged (cations) particles distributed in the various fluid compartments. As outlined in Figure 3-2, the various fluid compartments have markedly different ionic compositions. These differences are maintained by the selective permeability of the cell membrane and by the active transport of ions across the cell membrane. Sodium is the major extracellular cation and potassium is the major intracellular cation. Chloride and bicarbonate are the major extracellular anions, while phosphates and proteins are the major intracellular anions.

Since ions can freely diffuse within a compartment, the sum of the cations equals the sum of the anions, and

electrical neutrality is maintained within that compartment. The plasma and interstitium have similar total ionic concentrations and cation compositions; however, their anionic makeups differ. This difference is a result of the **selective permeability** of the capillary membrane, which is permeable to water and inorganic ions but impermeable to protein. Selective permeability creates a concentration gradient of inorganic anions across the capillary membrane, promoting the flow of diffusible anions from the interstitial fluid to the plasma. To maintain electrical neutrality within each compartment, cations must diffuse with the anions. This anion gradient will eventually be balanced by developing cation and particle gradients. A steady state is reached called the **Gibbs-Donnan equilibrium** (Figure 3-3). Equilibrium is reached when the product of the concentrations of any two ion pairs is equivalent across a membrane: $[Na^+]_1 [Cl^-]_1 = [Na^+]_2 [Cl^-]_2$.

Though the relationship between the plasma and interstitial fluid is relatively simple, that between the interstitial fluid and the intracellular fluid is much more complex. As demonstrated in Figure 3-2, the ionic composition of these compartments is markedly different. The composition of the intracellular space is maintained by selective permeability of the cell membrane and **active transport** of ions. A membrane-bound **Na+, K+-ATPase** plays a dominant role in the maintenance of these gradients by exchanging three intracellular sodium ions for two extracellular potassium ions. The concentration gradients maintained by these mechanisms create transmembrane potential differences; -90 mV in skeletal muscle and -79 mV in neurons. These transmembrane potentials are important for nerve, muscle, and cardiac function as detailed in Chapters 8 and 26.

TERMS TO DESCRIBE SOLUTE CONCENTRATIONS WITHIN COMPARTMENTS

Many terms are used to describe the concentration of a solute within a compartment. A **mole** represents a constant number of molecules of a substance. One mole is the mass in grams numerically equivalent to the molecular weight of a substance. For example, one mole of NaCl is 58 grams. **Molarity** is the number of moles present per unit volume (moles/liter). **Molality** is the number of moles per 1000 grams of solvent. **Equivalents** or

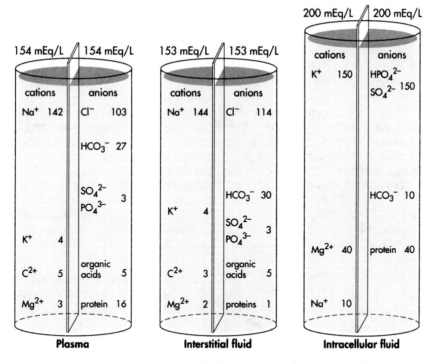

Figure 3-2 Chemical composition of body fluid compartments. (Reproduced from Shires TG, Canizaro, PC. Fluid and electrolyte management of the surgical patient. In: Sabiston DC Jr, ed. *Textbook of surgery: the biological basis of modern surgical practice.* 13th ed. Philadelphia: WB Saunders, 1986:64.)

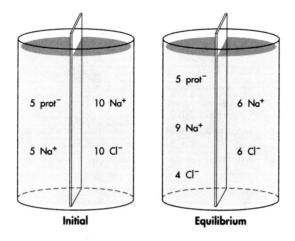

Figure 3-3 Gibbs-Donnan equilibrium. (Reproduced from Gann DS, Amaral, JF. Fluid and electrolyte management. In: Sabiston DC Jr., ed. *Sabiston's essentials of surgery.* Philadelphia: WB Saunders, 1987:33.)

milliequivalents (mEq) per liter represents the number of electrical charges per unit volume. Since sodium and potassium are univalent, 1 millimole of each is also 1 milliequivalent. However, magnesium and calcium are divalent and 1 millimole of each is 2 milliequivalents. In solution, the milliequivalents of cations and anions are equal.

Osmoles or milliosmoles (mosm) refers to the number of osmotically active particles. Osmolarity and osmolality are the concentrations of osmotically active particles per liter and per 1000 grams of water, respectively. One mole of a nonionizable substance contributes 1 osmole to solution. However, if a substance ionizes into 2 ions (as sodium chloride ionizes to a sodium and a chloride ion), 1 mole of the substance contributes 2 osmoles to solution.

The osmolality of plasma, though directly measurable, can be estimated from the concentration of the principle solutes: salts, glucose, and urea. The total plasma osmolality (P_{osm}) is approximated by the following formula:

$$P_{osm} = 2[Na^+] + [glucose]/18 + BUN/2.8.$$

In a healthy person, the contribution of glucose and urea to plasma osmolality is small because both substances are present at relatively low concentrations and urea diffuses across cell membranes. However, if either is elevated, as in diabetes or renal failure, the contribution of these solutes to plasma osmolality becomes significant.

MOVEMENT OF WATER BETWEEN COMPARTMENTS

Osmosis is the movement of water across a membrane in response to osmotic forces. Simply stated, water moves from an area of low solute concentration to an area of high solute concentration. Concentration gradients in the body are created and maintained by semipermeable membranes, as discussed above. Pressure applied across the membrane will oppose osmosis; the amount of pressure required to oppose osmosis is called the osmotic pressure.

The direction of osmosis is related to the relative tonicity of fluid compartments. Tonicity of a fluid can be defined in terms of the response of a normal body cell placed in that fluid. Cells placed in an isotonic fluid will neither shrink nor swell. Cells placed in a hypotonic environment will swell with water; cells placed in a hypertonic environment will lose water and shrink. Consider the hypothetical situation of two fluid compartments separated by (1) a completely permeable membrane or (2) a membrane permeable to water but not to solutes. A hypertonic solution is added to one compartment. In the first case, both solute and water will pass through the membrane into the second compartment and both compartments will expand in volume equally; this is an isotonic fluid shift. However, if the membrane is permeable only to water as in the second case, the hypertonicity of the compartment will result in water being *drawn* from the second compartment, thus expanding the volume of the first compartment and shrinking that of the other; this is a nonisotonic fluid shift.

DETERMINANTS OF FLUID DISTRIBUTION BETWEEN THE PLASMA AND INTERSTITIAL FLUID: THE STARLING HYPOTHESIS

The capillary membrane is permeable to water and inorganic salts but impermeable to protein. Thus, protein content is the principal determinant of osmotic pressure across the capillary membrane. The pressure exerted by protein is called the colloid osmotic or oncotic pressure.

The main determinants of fluid flux across the capillary membrane are colloid osmotic and hydrostatic pressure. Their relationship to fluid flux is described by Starling's Law:

$$Q_f = K_f [(P_c - P_i) - \sigma(\pi_c - \pi_i)]$$

in which Q_f is total flow, K_f is a fluid filtration coefficient, P_c is capillary hydrostatic pressure, P_i is interstitial hydrostatic pressure, σ is a reflection coefficient (the capacity of the capillary membrane to act as a barrier to protein movement), π_c is capillary or plasma oncotic pressure and π_i is interstitial osmotic pressure. This relationship is demonstrated in Figure 3-4. There is a net positive pressure at the arterial end of the capillary, Q_f is positive and net flux is into the interstitium. There is a net negative pressure at the venous end of the capillary, Q_f is negative and net flux is into the capillary. For the entire capillary, the mean hydrostatic pressure is 17 mm Hg; therefore, there is a net pressure of 0.3

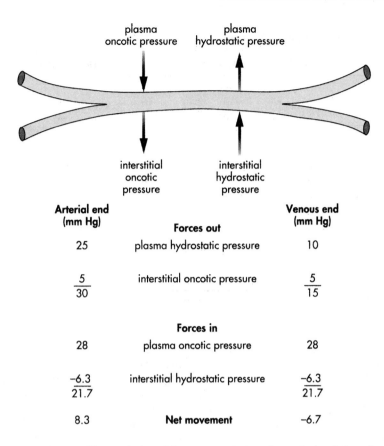

Arterial end (mm Hg)		Venous end (mm Hg)
	Forces out	
25	plasma hydrostatic pressure	10
$\dfrac{5}{30}$	interstitial oncotic pressure	$\dfrac{5}{15}$
	Forces in	
28	plasma oncotic pressure	28
$\dfrac{-6.3}{21.7}$	interstitial hydrostatic pressure	$\dfrac{-6.3}{21.7}$
8.3	**Net movement**	−6.7

Figure 3-4 Starling equilibrium. (Adapted from Gann DS, Amaral, JF. Fluid and electrolyte management. In: Sabiston DC Jr., ed. *Sabiston's essentials of surgery.* Philadelphia: WB Saunders, 1987:34. Data derived from Guyton AC. *Textbook of medical physiology.* 7th ed. Philadelphia: WB Saunders, 1986.)

mm Hg {[17 − (-6.3)] − [28 − 5]} favoring flow of fluid into the interstitium.

Fluid and Electrolyte Balance

INTAKE EQUALS OUTPUT

To maintain homeostasis, gains and losses of water and electrolytes must by closely balanced. Sources of water include oral intake of fluids and solids and the water produced by oxidative metabolism. Water losses include **sensible** losses in stool (250 mL/day), urine (variable), and sweat (100 mL/day) and the **insensible** loss of water vapor through the lungs and skin (750 mL/day). Mandatory daily water losses include insensible losses and a minimum urine output of 500–800 mL/day to excrete products of metabolism (600 mosm). Diet is the source of electrolytes, and electrolytes are lost via the skin, intestine, and kidneys. The third space, discussed above, is another source of water and electrolyte loss in surgical patients.

Obligate sodium loss is about 30 mEq/day and obligate potassium loss is about 40–60 mEq/day. The kidney, in response to aldosterone (see Chapter 25) can

TABLE 3-1. Electrolyte Composition of the Transcellular Fluids

Fluid	Na⁺ (MEq/L)	K⁺ (MEq/L)	CL⁻ (MEq/L)	HCO₃⁻ (MEq/L)	Volume (L/day)
Saliva	30	20	35	15	1.0–1.5
Gastric juice, ph < 4.0	60	10	90	—	2.5
Gastric juice, ph > 4.0	100	10	100	—	2.0
Bile	145	5	110	40	1.5
Duodenum	140	5	80	50	—
Pancreas	140	5	75	90	0.7–1.0
Ileum	130	10	110	30	3.5
Cecum	80	20	50	20	—
Colon	60	30	40	20	—
Sweat	50	5	55	—	0–3.0
New ileostomy	130	20	110	30	0.5–2.0
Adapted ileostomy	50	5	30	25	0.4
Colostomy	50	10	40	20	0.3

Reproduced from Gann DS, Amaral JF. Fluid and electrolyte management. In: Sabiston DC Jr., ed. *Sabiston's essentials of surgery.* Philadelphia: WB Saunders, 1987:42.

reduce urinary sodium excretion to less than 5 mEq/day. However, this increases potassium wasting. Daily administration of 1 mEq of sodium per kilogram body weight per day will replace sodium losses and suppress aldosterone secretion. Similarly, 0.5–1 mEq of potassium per kilogram body weight per day will replace potassium losses.

In addition to obligate losses, many surgical patients lose fluid and electrolytes from other sources. These losses can be replaced based on their composition (Table 3-1).

MAINTENANCE OF HOMEOSTASIS

Fluid and electrolyte homeostasis is maintained principally by the kidney. The function of the kidney and the influence of many neural and endocrine response mediators on the kidney is discussed in Chapter 25. Extracellular fluid volume is not regulated directly but rather indirectly via its relationship to circulating plasma volume, total body sodium, and plasma osmolality. Arterial and renal **baroreceptors** and **atrial stretch receptors** sense changes in effective circulating volume. Sodium concentration is monitored by the **macula densa** in the kidney. Plasma osmolality is monitored by **osmoreceptors** in the central nervous system and the

liver. These various sensors control the effectors of homeostasis including atrial naturetic factor, adrenocorticotropic hormone, growth hormone, β-endorphin, vasopressin, renin, epinephrine, glucagon, and the autonomic nervous system. The characteristics and functions of many of these effectors are detailed in other portions of this book.

Abnormalities of Serum Electrolytes

SODIUM

The normal range for serum sodium is 136–145 mEq/L. Sodium is the predominant extracellular cation. Abnormalities in serum sodium are manifested primarily by central nervous system signs and symptoms. Symptoms are related to the degree of the abnormality and the rate at which it develops, and are caused by swelling or shrinkage of cerebral cells.

Hyponatremia

Hyponatremia is defined as serum sodium greater than 130 mEq/L. Though hyponatremia is often associated with volume overload, it can also be associated with euvolemia or hypovolemia and can be caused by an excess of other solutes such as glucose or mannitol. Symptoms of mild to moderate hyponatremia (120–130 mEq/L) include apathy, confusion, lethargy, anorexia, nausea, muscle twitching, and hyperactive tendon reflexes. However, many patients will not manifest symptoms if the hyponatremic state developed slowly. Severe hyponatremia (<120 mEq/L) is generally symptomatic—with symptoms including convulsions, loss of reflexes, and coma—and can lead to death.

Hypernatremia

Hypernatremia is associated with a serum sodium greater than 155 mEq/L. Symptoms include dry, sticky mucous membranes and neurological symptoms that range from lethargy, restlessness, twitching, and tremulousness to ataxia, seizures, dementia, delirium, and strokes (subarachnoid and suborbital hemorrhages secondary to shear forces on vessels due to dehydration and shrinkage). Though usually associated with hypovolemia, hypernatremia can develop in the euvolemic and hypervolemic patient.

POTASSIUM

The normal range for serum potassium is 3.5–5 mEq/L. Potassium is predominantly intracellular; thus serum levels may be less reflective of total body stores. Potassium plays a major role in the function of neural and muscle tissue. As a result, the principal manifestations of abnormalities in serum potassium levels are related to the gastrointestinal, cardiovascular, and musculoskeletal systems.

Hypokalemia

Hypokalemia (<3.0 mEq/L) can result from excessive loss from the kidney or gastrointestinal tract, transfer into cells, and inadequate intake. Hypokalemia can produce alkalosis because hydrogen ion excretion is increased in the absence of potassium. Likewise, **alkalosis** promotes hypokalemia because greater amounts of potassium are exchanged for sodium reabsorption in the absence of hydrogen ions. Signs and symptoms of hypokalemia include ileus, vomiting, and constipation; low ECG voltage, flattened T waves, depressed

ST segments, and widening of the QRS; and lethargy, hyporeflexia, cramps, weakness, confusion, and paralysis.

Hyperkalemia

Hyperkalemia (>5.5 mEq/L) can result from reduced excretion (e.g., renal failure), excessive tissue release, and exogenous administration. Hyperkalemia is exacerbated by **acidosis** and **hypocalcemia.** Symptoms do not usually appear until the level is greater than 6.0 mEq/L. However symptoms will appear at lower concentrations when the level rises quickly. Symptoms include nausea, vomiting, colic, and diarrhea; peaked T waves, widened QRS complex, and depressed ST segments; and at higher serum levels, loss of T waves, heart block, and diastolic cardiac arrest.

CALCIUM

The normal range for serum calcium is 9–11 mg/dL. Most calcium is stored in bone. Calcium is excreted predominantly via the gastrointestinal tract, less so via the kidney. Of the calcium in the serum, 40% is bound to protein, 10–15% is bound to ions, and 50% is free or ionized. The **free** or **ionized calcium** maintains muscular stability. Measurement of this fraction (1.12–1.13 mmol/L, normal range) is becoming more common in clinical practice.

Pseudohypocalcemia

Hypocalcemia secondary to **hypoalbuminemia** is termed pseudohypocalcemia. Though measured total calcium is low, the ionized calcium is normal. In general, total measured serum calcium will decrease 0.8 mg/dL for every 1 g/dL decrease in albumin.

Hypocalcemia

The causes of hypocalcemia (serum Ca^{2+} < 8.0 mg/dL; ionized Ca^{2+} < 1.0 mmol/L) include pancreatitis, fistulas, massive soft tissue infections, hypomagnesemia, hypoparathyroidism, hypophosphatemia, vitamin D deficiency, drugs, and toxins. Symptoms include numbness and tingling in the circumoral region and at the tips of the digits; mental status changes, seizures,

TABLE 3-2. Acidosis-Alkalosis

	Defect	*Common Causes*	$\dfrac{BHCO_3}{H_2CO_3} = \dfrac{20}{1}$	*Compensation*
Respiratory Acidosis	Retention of CO_2 (decreased alveolar ventilation)	Depression of respiratory center by morphine CNS injury Pulmonary disease— emphysema, pneumonia	↑ Denominator Ratio < 20:1	Renal Retention of bicarbonate, excretion of acid salts, increased ammonia formation Chloride shift into red cells
Respiratory Alkalosis	Excessive loss of CO_2 (increased alveolar ventilation)	Hyperventilation: emotional disturbances, severe pain, assisted ventilation, encephalitis	↓ Denominator Ratio > 20:1	Renal Excretion of bicarbonate, retention of acid salts, decreased ammonia formation
Metabolic Acidosis	Retention of fixed acids or loss of base bicarbonate	Diabetes, azotemia, lactic acid accumulation, starvation Diarrhea, small bowel fistulas	↓ Numerator Ratio < 20:1	Pulmonary (rapid): increased rate and depth of breathing Renal (slow): as in respiratory acidosis
Metabolic Alkalosis	Loss of fixed acids Gain of base bicarbonate Potassium depletion	Vomiting or gastric suction with pyloric obstruction Excessive intake of bicarbonate Diuretic	↑ Numerator Ratio > 20:1	Pulmonary (rapid): decreased rate and depth of breathing Renal (slow): as in respiratory alkalosis

Reproduced from Shires TG, Canizero PC. Fluid and electrolyte management of the surgical patient. In: Sabiston DC Jr, ed. *Textbook of surgery*. Philadelphia: WB Saunders, 1986:69.

extrapyramidal movement disorders, tetany, paresthesias; myopathies; hypotension, lengthened Q-T interval, and occasionally ventricular dysrhythmias.

Hypercalcemia

Most cases of hypercalcemia (serum Ca^{2+} > 10.5 mg/dL; ionized Ca^{2+} > 1.25 mmol/L) are caused by malignancy or hyperparathyroidism. Thyrotoxicosis, tuberculosis, sarcoidosis, Pagets' disease, Addison's disease, thiazide diuretics, hypophosphatemia, milk-alkali syndrome, vitamin A intoxication, and vitamin D intoxication are less common causes. Manifestations include weakness, fatigue, lethargy, confusion, polydipsia, headache, impaired concentration and memory, and can progress to somnolence, stupor, and coma; polyuria, nephrocalcinosis, nephrolithiasis, and acute and chronic renal failure; anorexia, nausea, vomiting, and constipation; and bradycardia and heart block.

PHOSPHATE

The normal range for serum phosphate is 3–4.5 mg/dL. Most phosphate is found in bones and teeth. Of that found in plasma, 15% is protein bound. The rest is in solution as PO_4^{3-}, HPO_4^{2-}, and $H_2PO_4^{-}$.

Hypophosphatemia

Hypophosphatemia (<2.5 mg/dL) can result from inadequate intake or external loss of phosphate, or from redistribution of phosphate from extracellular to intracellular pools. Inadequate intake can result from poor diet, malabsorption, and the use of aluminum-containing antacids. Diuretics, alcoholism, burns, and primary hyperparathyroidism cause excessive phosphate loss. Glucose infusion, insulin and catecholamine administration, and respiratory alkalosis promote redistribution of phosphates into cells. Severe hypophosphatemia (<1 mg/dL) may lead to rhabdomyolysis. Other signs and symptoms include weakness, fatigue, obtundation, seizure, coma, and respiratory arrest.

Hyperphosphatemia

Hyperphosphatemia (>5 mg/dL) is uncommon with normal renal function. However, hyperphosphatemia can result from exogenous administration (enemas, laxatives, parenteral administration), endogenous sources (e.g., rhabdomyolosis), acute and chronic renal failure, hypoparathyroidism, thyrotoxicosis, hypovolemia, and an excess of growth hormone. Hyperphosphatemia rarely causes symptoms, although acute hyperphosphatemia may cause hypocalcemia which can result in tetany and even death.

MAGNESIUM

The normal range for serum magnesium is 1.8–3.0 mg/dL. Approximately one half of total body magnesium is stored in bone, the rest is predominantly intracellular. Magnesium is excreted predominantly in the feces, the kidney serving as alternate route. Magnesium is an important component of Na^+, K^+ ATPase and is necessary for parathyroid hormone secretion.

Hypomagnesemia

Isolated hypomagnesemia (<1.8 mg/dL) is unusual; more commonly it occurs with a deficiency of other vitamins, minerals, and nutrients. It is generally associated with inadequate intake, excessive loss of gastrointestinal fluids, pancreatitis, alcoholism, ketoacidosis, and aldosteronism. Signs and symptoms are primarily of neuromuscular, cardiovascular, and gastrointestinal origin. They include weakness, vertigo, ataxia, seizures, coma, mood changes, psychosis, arrhythmias, anorexia, vomiting, dysphagia, and anemia.

Hypermagnesemia

Hypermagnesemia (>2.9 mg/dL) is unusual in the presence of normal renal function. However, hypermagnesemia can occur when renal function is impaired and is worsened by acidosis. Antacids, laxatives, burns, tissue injury, and severe extracellular volume deficit can also cause hypermagnesemia. In general, symptoms do not usually occur until the blood level is greater than 4 mg/dL. Excess magnesium exerts a depressant effect on the function of the central nervous system and neuromuscular function. Neurologic symptoms include lethargy, weakness, and loss of deep tendon reflexes progressing to somnolence, coma, paralysis, and death. The cardiovascular effects include peripheral vasodilatation and ECG changes, and cardiac function alterations similar to those seen in hyperkalemia. Other symptoms include nausea, vomiting, and cutaneous flushing.

Acid-Base Balance

Metabolism produces large amounts of organic and inorganic acids each day. Despite this, the body fluid pH is maintained relatively constant. The acid produced is neutralized by multiple buffering systems and eventually excreted via the lungs and kidneys. A buffer is a weak acid or base and its related salt. By binding hydrogen ions released by strong acids and donating hydrogen ions to strong bases, a buffer reduces the change in pH. The important buffers are **proteins** and **phosphates,** which are the principal intracellular buffers; **hemoglobin,** which is the primary intracellular buffer for erythrocytes; and the **bicarbonate-carbonic acid system,** which is the principal extracellular buffer.

The bicarbonate-carbonic acid buffer system is principally responsible for the maintenance of extracellular pH and the excretion of acid via the lungs and kidneys. It performs these functions through a series of chemical reactions:

$$H_2O + CO_2 <\text{--}> H_2CO_3 <\text{--}> H^+ + HCO_3^-.$$

Carbon dioxide combines with water to form carbonic acid which can ionize to a hydrogen ion and bicarbonate. The blood level of CO_2 can be controlled by ventilation. Bicarbonate can be reabsorbed, manufactured, or excreted by the kidney.

The relationship of a buffering acid and its salt relative to pH is summarized by the **Henderson-Hasselbalch equation:**

$$pH = pK + \log\frac{[HCO_3^-]}{[H_2CO_3]}$$

where pK is the dissociation constant of the acid. The pK for carbonic acid is 6.1. Thus, to maintain a body pH of

TABLE 3-3. Respiratory and Metabolic Components of Acid-Base Disorders

	Acute (Uncompensated)			Chronic (Partially Compensated)		
	pH	PCO_2 (respiratory component)	Plasma HCO_3^{-a} (metabolic component)	pH	PCO_2 (respiratory component)	Plasma HCO_3^{-a} (metabolic component)
Respiratory Acidosis	↓↓	↑↑	N	↓	↑↑	↑
Respiratory Alkalosis	↑↑	↓↓	N	↑	↓↓	↓
Metabolic Acidosis	↓↓	N	↓↓	↓	↓	↓
Metabolic Alkalosis	↑↑	N	↑↑	↑	↑?	↑

[a]Measured as standard bicarbonate, whole-blood buffer base, CO_2 content or CO_2-combining power. The *base excess value* is positive when the standard bicarbonate is above normal, and negative when the standard bicarbonate is below normal.

Reproduced from Shires TG, Canizaro, PC. Fluid and electrolyte management of the surgical patient. In: Sabiston DC Jr., ed. *Textbook of surgery. The biological basis of modern surgical practice.* 13th ed. Philadelphia: WB Saunders, 1986:70.

7.4, the ratio of [HCO_3^-] to [H_2CO_3] is maintained at 20:1. Acid entering the extracellular fluid compartment binds with bicarbonate to form carbonic acid, and is then converted to water and carbon dioxide and eliminated by increasing ventilation. When acid production is chronically increased in this manner, the lost bicarbonate must be replaced. The kidney creates bicarbonate by creating carbonic acid, reclaiming bicarbonate ions and excreting hydrogen ions (see Chapter 25).

The four main types of acid-base disturbances are detailed in Tables 3-2 and 3-3. To determine the type of acid-base disturbance, the pH, bicarbonate concentration, and PCO_2 must be directly measured. Though the above mechanisms will act to correct primary acid-base disturbances, it is important to remember that physiologic mechanisms cannot overcompensate for an acid-base disturbance, and that excessive compensation implies a mixed disturbance.

Respiratory Acidosis: Reduced ventilation with an attendant increase in PCO_2 are the principal characteristics of respiratory acidosis. Acutely, pH falls and can be restored to normal by improved ventilation. With chronic respiratory acidosis, renal production of bicarbonate increases to correct the pH.

Respiratory Alkalosis: Hyperventilation, regardless of the inciting cause, leads to a reduction in the PCO_2 and increased pH. Chronically, bicarbonate concentration falls to correct pH.

Metabolic Acidosis: Metabolic acidosis results from the addition of acid to, or the loss of base from, the system. Causes of increased acid production or retention include diabetic ketoacidosis, lactic acidosis, and azotemia. Causes of increased base loss include diarrhea and fistulas. Acutely, hyperventilation partially compensates for acidosis by removing carbon dioxide produced by the bicarbonate-carbonic acid buffering system. More chronically, acid is excreted by the kidney, if it is functional.

Metabolic Alkalosis: Metabolic alkalosis results from the addition of base to, or loss of acid from, the system. Causes include persistent vomiting or gastric suction, hypokalemia, and volume depletion. These entities can be separate but often are interrelated. For example, in the presence of pyloric obstruction, gastric suction depletes sodium, potassium, and water, and, to a greater extent, hydrogen ions and chloride. Loss of hydrogen ions creates a primary alkalosis. Alkalosis and chloride depletion cause a loss of sodium and bicarbonate in the urine. As the volume deficit increases, hydrogen and potassium ions are secreted and bicarbonate is reabsorbed by the kidney, in an effort to conserve sodium. This causes a **hypochloremic, hypokalemic metabolic alkalosis** with associated "paradoxic aciduria." This can usually be corrected with isotonic volume and potassium repletion, but if refractory, may require correction of the chloride deficit with an infusion of hydrochloric acid.

Bibliography

Andreoli, TE. Disorders of fluid volume, electrolyte, and acid-base balance. In Wyngaarden JB, Smith LH Jr., eds. *Cecil textbook of medicine.* 17th ed. Philadelphia: WB Saunders, 1985.

Beck LH. Body fluid and electrolyte disorders. *Med Clin North Am* 1981; 65:24.

Falk JL, Rackow EC, Weil MH. Colloid and crystalloid fluid resuscitation. In: Shoemaker WC, Ayres S, Grenvik A, Holbrook PR, Thompson WL, eds. *Textbook of critical care.* 2nd ed. Philadelphia: WB Saunders, 1989.

Gann DS, Amaral JF. Fluid and electrolyte management. In: Sabiston DC Jr., ed. *Sabiston's essentials of surgery.* Philadelphia: WB Saunders, 1987.

Guyton AC. *Textbook of medical physiology.* 7th ed. Philadelphia: WB Saunders, 1986.

Mengoli LR. Excerpts from the history of postoperative fluid therapy. *Am J Surg* 1971;121:311.

Shires TG, Canizario PC. Fluid and electrolyte management of the surgical patient. In: Sabiston DC Jr., ed. *Textbook of surgery. The biological basis of modern surgical practice.* 13th ed. Philadelphia: WB Saunders, 1986.

Jon Odorico and Steven J. Fishman

4 ERYTHROCYTE PHYSIOLOGY

Red blood cells (RBCs) are the most numerous of all cells of the body, numbering approximately 5,000,000 cells/mm³. Although erythrocytes lack nuclei and cell surface major histocompatibility antigens, they do not lack in complexity. The principal function of erythrocytes is to transport hemoglobin, facilitating oxygen delivery to tissues. The goals of this chapter are (1) to describe the factors regulating the production and destruction of erythrocytes, (2) to describe the formation of the heme and hemoglobin molecules as well as the pathophysiologic consequences of carboxyhemoglobin generation, and (3) to review the functions of hemoglobin and oxygen-hemoglobin interactions.

Red Blood Cell Production

Early in embryonic life, primitive nucleated RBCs are produced in the yolk sac. Later, during the middle trimester of gestation, the liver is the main organ of erythropoieisis; the spleen and lymph nodes contribute at this time as well. During the latter part of gestation and after birth, the bone marrow becomes the exclusive site of production. As an individual ages, the marrow of most long bones becomes fatty and erythropoiesis continues solely in membranous bone.

Erythropoiesis begins in the bone marrow with the differentiation of pluripotent hematopoietic stem cells into **proerythroblasts,** each of which eventually divides several times to form 8 to 16 mature RBCs. The first generation of these new cells, **basophilic erythroblasts** or **normoblasts,** contain large amounts of DNA and nuclear material and therefore stain with basic dyes. Gradually, the cells accumulate more hemoglobin and their nuclei condense. At this stage they are termed **orthochromatic erythroblasts.** As the condensed nucleus is extruded, **reticulocytes** are formed, which then pass into capillaries by diapedesis. The basophilic material in reticulocytes (residual cytoplasmic apparatus) disappears within 2 days, resulting in mature erythrocytes. As a consequence of the short life span of circulating reticulocytes, their concentration in the blood reaches only 1–2%. The normal life span of an RBC is approximately 120 days; however, the life span of senescent, diseased, and stored red cells may be considerably shorter as a result of increased fragility.

Mature circulating RBCs are biconcave discs approximately 8 μ in diameter. Since the cells have excess membrane phospholipid, deformation does not cause rupture upon passage through narrow capillaries. This unique deformability accounts for the decreased viscosity relative to many other cells (e.g., white cells are 2000 times more viscous than red cells), and confers a rheologic advantage to red cells. In the capillaries, deformability of the red cell is the primary rheologic determinant of blood viscosity and flow. Abnormal disease states in which poor red cell deformability results in increased blood viscosity include sickle cell disease and hereditary spherocytosis.

The total circulating red cell mass is regulated within very narrow limits. **Erythropoietin (EPO)** is the primary regulator of erythrocyte production in the bone marrow. Within minutes to hours after a hypoxic stimulus, EPO synthesis increases and reaches maximal levels within 24 hours. New RBCs, however, only begin to appear in the circulation 5 days later. From experimental studies, it has been determined that EPO stimulates the production of proerythroblasts from stem cells in the bone marrow and causes these cells to mature more rapidly. In the absence of EPO, few RBCs are formed by the bone marrow. Between 90% and 95% of all EPO is formed in the kidneys. Patients who are anephric or have end-stage renal disease generally suffer from severe anemia because the 5–10% of EPO formed in other tissues (primarily the liver) stimulates only 30–50% of the usual red cell production needed by the body. The primary determinant of EPO production is tissue hypoxia. Factors that decrease tissue oxygenation tend to increase EPO levels. These include acquired and congenital heart disease, pulmonary disease states associated with alveolar hypoventilation, abnormal hemoglobin states, anemia, hypovolemia, decreased renal blood flow, and chemicals that interfere with oxidative metabolism.

Cobalamin (Vitamin B_{12}) and **folic acid** are essential nutrients for all cells of the body. Their depletion profoundly affects RBC production, resulting in a megaloblastic anemia. Clinically, cobalamin deficiency usually results from derangements in gastrointestinal absorption. Decreased absorption can result from (1) lack of intrinsic factor secretion by gastric parietal cells, as seen in pernicious anemia and after total gastrectomy; (2) disease or absence of the terminal ileum, as in short bowel syndrome, Crohn's disease, and tropical sprue; and (3) alterations in small intestinal flora. Cobalamin deficiency also leads to tissue folate depletion. This occurs because retention of folic acid in a cell's cytoplasm requires a cobalamin-dependent methyltransferase. Folic acid is required for the synthesis of three of the four nucleotide bases found in DNA. Folate itself is inert but is converted to tetrahydrofolate, which facilitates transfer of single carbon fragments to various intermediates in the deoxyribonucleotide synthetic pathways. Thus, megaloblastic anemia secondary to cobalamin or folate deficiency responds to the administration of folic acid alone.

Several red cell indices that may reflect alterations in RBC production are useful in classifying anemias. They include the **mean corpuscular volume (MCV)** and the **reticulocyte index.** The MCV is used to classify anemias as microcytic (e.g., iron deficiency anemia) or macrocytic (e.g., megaloblastic anemia, hemolytic anemia, and anemia of liver disease). The MCV may also increase slightly with age and smoking. The reticulocyte index provides an estimate of the rate of erythrocyte production. An elevated reticulocyte index may reflect an attempt to correct anemia, and suggests the etiology of the anemia is not due to a quantitative deficiency in RBC production.

Formation of Heme and Production of Hemoglobin

The synthesis of heme and the production of hemoglobin begins in erythroblasts and continues to the reticulocyte stage. Because they have no nucleus, mature RBCs cannot increase the amount of hemoglobin per cell. Heme production can be divided into three stages: (1) synthesis of the five-carbon ring or pyrrole, (2) formation of a tetrapyrrole, and (3) combination with iron to produce heme.

Synthesis occurs in mitochondria and begins with the production of δ-aminolevulinic acid (ALA) from glycine and succinyl-CoA by ALA synthetase (Figure 4-1A). Two molecules of ALA condense to form a monopyrrole. Four pyrrole rings then combine to form a tetrapyrrole, which is oxidized to form protoporphyrin IX. Reduced iron, Fe^{2+}, combines with protoporphyrin IX to form heme (Figure 4-1B). Four heme molecules and a 150–amino-acid protein called the globin chain condense to form a hemoglobin chain (either α or β in adults, γ in fetus). Four hemoglobin monomers, each with a molecular weight of approximately 16,000 d, associate noncovalently to form a hemoglobin tetramer. The most common form of hemoglobin in adults is a combination of two α-chains and two β-chains ($\alpha_2\beta_2$).

The nature of the globin chains is one of the determinants of oxygen binding affinity. An example is fetal hemoglobin: The γ-chain confers greater oxygen affinity to fetal hemoglobin than the adult counterpart, permitting the developing fetus to extract oxygen from the maternal circulation. The globin chain can also affect the response of hemoglobin to changes in oxygen tension. For example, in sickle cell disease, the amino acid glutamate is replaced by valine at one point in each of the two β-chains, which causes hemoglobin to crystalize at low oxygen tensions resulting in sickling of the cells.

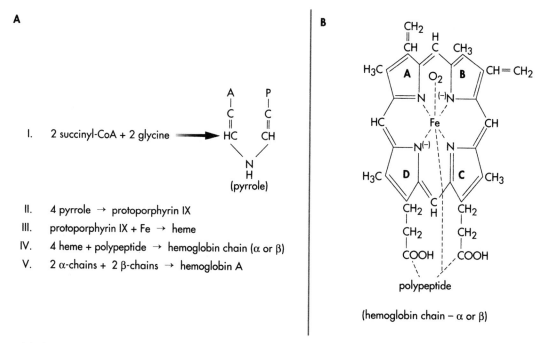

Figure 4-1 A, Formation of hemoglobin. **B,** Basic structure of the hemoglobin molecule, showing one of the four heme complexes bound with the central globin core of the hemoglobin molecule. (Reproduced from Guyton AC. *Textbook of medical physiology.* Philadelphia: WB Saunders, 1986:46.)

Red Blood Cell Destruction

The destruction of erythrocytes generally results from the entrapment of red cells by organ filtration and depends on specific features of the senescent red blood cell. As an erythrocyte ages, it loses many of its metabolic functions. This loss correlates well with the loss of structural integrity of the cell, especially its membrane. Though RBCs do not have mitochondria or endoplasmic reticulum, they retain cytoplasmic enzymes of glycolysis and the hexose monophosphate shunt, which permit glucose metabolism and adenosine triphosphate (ATP) production. ATP is required to (1) maintain pliability of the cell membrane and shape of the RBC; (2) maintain transmembrane ionic gradients by providing energy for the active transport of sodium, potassium, and calcium; (3) maintain iron in the divalent ferrous form rather than the ferric form (which causes the formation of **methemoglobin,** decreasing oxygen carrying capacity); and (4) prevent oxidation of the sulfhydryl groups of hemoglobin and other cellular proteins. As

the red cell ages, it loses the ability to generate ATP. Thus the cell cannot maintain its integrity and becomes progressively more fragile. As these fragile cells pass through the narrow (3 μ) sinuses of the red pulp of the spleen, they are fragmented and then opsonized by the reticuloendothelial system (RES) in a process called **extravascular hemolysis.** The hemoglobin released is then phagocytosed and degraded in the liver, spleen, and bone marrow.

Globin protein is degraded into its constituent amino acids, and heme is converted to **biliverdin** by the oxidative cleavage of the porphyrin ring by the microsomal enzyme, heme oxygenase (Figure 4-2). The iron released is incorporated into ferritin. Biliverdin is subsequently reduced to **bilirubin,** which enters the bloodstream, binds to albumin, and is carried to the liver. Elimination of bilirubin by the liver is discussed in Chapter 17.

Accelerated RBC destruction by extravascular hemolysis is seen in conditions where there is an abnormality of cell shape or viscosity, as in **hereditary spherocytosis** and **sickle cell anemia. Autoimmune hemo-**

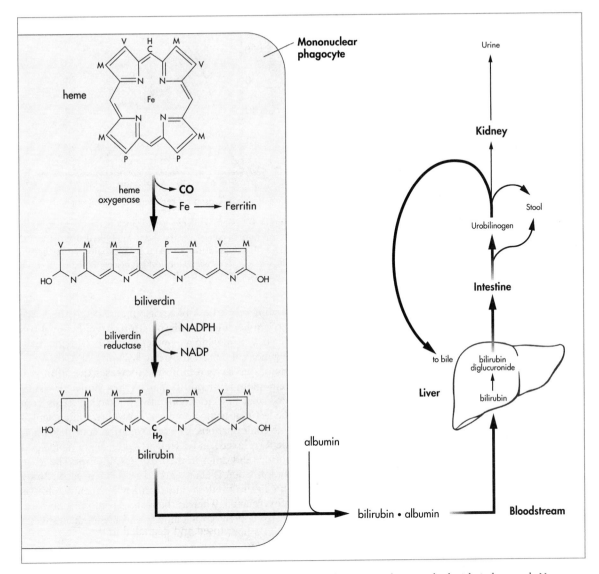

Figure 4-2 Degradation of heme. (Reproduced from Babior BM, Stossel TP. *Hematology: a pathophysiological approach.* New York: Churchill Livingstone, 1984: 100.)

lytic anemia, the most common cause of extravascular hemolysis, results from immunoglobulins coating the RBC membrane, leading to premature phagocytosis by the RES. **"Spur" cells (acanthocytes),** irregularly spiculated RBCs associated with cirrhosis, also result in accelerated extravascular hemolysis. Splenectomy has been used to ameliorate severe hemolysis in this setting. In the absence of the spleen, screening for defective erythrocytes is impaired, and RBCs with characteristic morphological abnormalities appear in the circulation. For example, cells containing **Howell-Jolly bodies** (nuclear remnants) and **Heinz bodies** (precipitates of denatured hemoglobin), as well as acanthocytes are not cleared, and constitute a poorly functional or nonfunctional, circulating pool.

Intravascular hemolysis leads to hemoglobin clearance by other mechanisms. Clinical situations producing significant intravascular hemolysis include **dis-**

seminated intravascular coagulation, **thrombotic thrombocytopenic purpura,** prosthetic heart valves, thermal injury, and the use of extracorporeal circulation devices. There are haptoglobin-dependent and haptoglobin-independent clearance pathways. **Haptoglobin** can only clear limited amounts of hemoglobin from the circulation, and is almost always overwhelmed in clinically significant intravascular hemolysis. Haptoglobin binds free hemoglobin, after which it is removed from the bloodstream by the liver. After uptake by the liver, haptoglobin levels fall. Haptoglobin, however, is an acute phase reactant and the low levels seen in hemolysis may be offset by increased production. In the absence of haptoglobin, hemoglobin is either cleared by the kidney or degraded in the plasma. In the kidney, dissociated hemoglobin dimers pass freely into the glomerular filtrate and are resorbed by the proximal tubule. Here, iron is deposited as **hemosiderin,** protein is degraded, and heme is converted to bilirubin. The proximal tubule has a limited capacity to take up dimers and if exceeded, hemoglobinuria ensues. Additional plasma hemoglobin is degraded through oxidation to **methemoglobin,** which is denatured to **ferriheme** and carried by heme binding proteins to the liver.

Oxygen Transport

The most important feature of the hemoglobin molecule is its unique ability to reversibly bind oxygen. Oxygen delivery to tissues depends on **cardiac output (CO), hemoglobin concentration (Hgb), arterial oxygen tension (P_{O_2}),** and the **saturation of arterial hemoglobin (Sa_{O_2}).** Alteration in blood **viscosity** can also affect oxygen delivery (see below, polycythemia).

Oxygen is delivered in two compartments, that dissolved in plasma and that bound to hemoglobin. The amount of oxygen carried in solution in plasma increases linearly with increasing arterial partial pressure (P_{O_2}). At physiologic temperature, plasma solubilizes 0.003 mL of oxygen in 100 mL of blood for each millimeter of mercury of oxygen tension:

Dissolved O_2 = 0.003 x P_{O_2} (mL O_2/dL blood)

Thus, at a P_{O_2} of 100 mm Hg, blood contains only 0.3 mL of oxygen dissolved per 100 mL of plasma.

The amount of oxygen bound to hemoglobin is also determined by oxygen tension; however, in this case the relationship is sigmoidal rather than linear. The oxygen

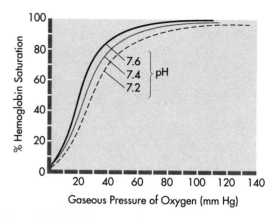

Figure 4-3 Shift of the oxygen-hemoglobin dissociation curve to the right is caused by increases in (1) hydrogen ions, (2) CO_2, (3) temperature, or (4) 2,3-DPG. (Reproduced from Guyton AC. *Textbook of medical physiology.* Philadelphia: WB Saunders, 1986:498.)

binding properties of hemoglobin are described by the **oxygen-hemoglobin dissociation curve** (Figure 4-3) . The $\alpha_2\beta_2$ hemoglobin tetramer combines with four oxygen molecules in an **allosteric** fashion; that is, the binding of one oxygen molecule increases the affinity of hemoglobin for additional oxygen molecules. The molecular basis for cooperative interaction stems from the fact that hemoglobin can exist in two interchangeable conformations. The two conformations, known as the **R (relaxed)** and **T (tense)** states, are in rapid equilibrium and differ in their oxygen affinities. The tense conformation is characterized by a low oxygen affinity and is the predominant form when hemoglobin is deoxygenated, whereas the relaxed conformation has a relatively high oxygen affinity and predominates when hemoglobin is well saturated.

At oxygen tensions below ~60 mm Hg, the oxygen-hemoglobin dissociation curve is steep, such that increasing P_{O_2} greatly increases hemoglobin saturation with oxygen. Above the inflection point of the curve, where hemoglobin is nearly fully saturated, even large increases in P_{O_2} only slightly increase the amount of oxygen bound to hemoglobin.

When fully saturated, 1 g of hemoglobin binds 1.39 mL of oxygen. The amount of oxygen carried by hemoglobin is determined by the percentage of potential sites bound:

Hemoglobin-bound O_2 = 1.39 x Hgb x Sa_{O_2}
(mL O_2/dL blood)

where Hgb represents hemoglobin concentration in grams per deciliter. Thus, with an Hgb of 15 g/dL and an SaO_2 of 97%, blood contains 19.5 mL of oxygen bound to hemoglobin per deciliter of blood.

Oxygen content (CaO_2) consists of the oxygen both dissolved in blood and bound to hemoglobin:

$$O_2 \text{ content} = (0.003 \times PO_2) + (1.39 \times Hgb \times SaO_2)$$
$$(\text{mL } O_2/\text{dL blood}).$$

Total **oxygen delivery** by the circulation is the oxygen carried per unit volume of blood multiplied by the total volume of blood circulating per minute:

$$O_2 \text{ delivery} = CO \times 10(\text{dL/L}) \times CaO_2 \text{ (mL } O_2/\text{min)}$$

where CO is cardiac output in liters per minute.

Since, under all physiologic conditions, the amount of dissolved oxygen is small relative to hemoglobin-bound oxygen, oxygen delivery is frequently expressed more simply:

$$O_2 \text{ delivery} = CO \times 10 \times (1.39 \times Hgb \times SaO_2)$$
$$(\text{mL } O_2/\text{min}).$$

It is thus clear that arterial oxygen tension (PO_2) is important in determining oxygen content and oxygen delivery only in that it determines hemoglobin saturation with oxygen. Once the PO_2 is sufficiently high to nearly completely saturate hemoglobin, further increases in PO_2 add little to carried or delivered oxygen.

Once delivered to the tissues, the amount of oxygen extracted from hemoglobin is again determined by the oxygen-hemoglobin dissociation curve. Since the oxygen tension in the peripheral tissues is lower than that in the lung, the hemoglobin tetramer changes conformation, causing oxygen to dissociate, thus liberating it for diffusion into tissues.

The **arteriovenous oxygen content difference ($C_{a-v}O_2$)** is the amount of oxygen per unit volume extracted crossing the capillary beds:

$$(C_{a-v}O_2) = 1.39 \times Hgb \times (SaO_2 - SvO_2)$$
$$(\text{mL } O_2/\text{dL blood})$$

where SvO_2 represents the oxygen saturation of mixed venous blood. In normal arterial blood, hemoglobin is 97% saturated and carries 19.5 mL of oxygen per 100 mL of blood ($1.39 \times 15 \times 0.97$). Normal SvO_2 is approximately 75%. On passing through tissue capillaries, the oxygen content is reduced to approximately 15.1 mL ($1.39 \times 15 \times 0.75$). Thus, under normal conditions about 4.4 mL of oxygen is extracted from each 100 mL of blood. Total **oxygen consumption** is defined as the amount of oxygen extracted by the body per minute:

$$O_2 \text{ consumption} = CO \times 10 \times 1.39 \times Hgb$$
$$\times (SaO_2 - SvO_2) \text{ (mL } O_2/\text{min)}.$$

The characteristics of the oxygen-hemoglobin saturation curve are frequently summarized by two numerical parameters. The first is the oxygen tension at 50% saturation, known as the **P_{50}.** This is a measure of the oxygen affinity. The higher the P_{50}, the lower the oxygen affinity. The second parameter is the **Hill coefficient,** a number derived from the binding curve. The coefficient measures the "S-ness" of the sigmoid-shaped curve. The greater the Hill coefficient, the greater the allosteric interation of the monomers; the Hill coefficient of normal hemoglobin is 3, whereas that of myoglobin is 1.

The affinity of hemoglobin for oxygen depends not only on the type of globin chain used but also on the metabolic state of the RBCs and peripheral tissues. Affinity is affected by **pH, temperature, CO_2** levels, and concentration of **2,3-diphosphoglycerate (2,3-DPG)** (Figure 4-3). The effects of pH and 2,3-DPG are responsible for most of the observed physiologic variation in oxygen affinity. A fall in pH decreases oxygen affinity by causing hemoglobin to take up protons, thereby strengthening the interaction between globin chains and stabilizing the low affinity or T state. This phenomenon, known as the **Bohr effect,** facilitates the unloading of oxygen at low pH, such as in actively metabolizing tissues. Of related importance, the ability of hemoglobin to bind hydrogen ions makes it an important constituent of the blood buffer system.

2,3-DPG is produced from 1,3-diphosphoglyceric acid, an intermediate of the glycolytic pathway, by DPG synthetase. The binding of 2,3-DPG in a cleft between the globin chains stabilizes the T conformation, and reduces the affinity of hemoglobin for oxygen. Under conditions of stress, levels of 2,3-DPG increase to promote greater release of oxygen in tissues. The increased oxygen affinity of fetal hemoglobin is partly a result of the fact that 2,3-DPG has less effect on this molecule than on adult hemoglobin. Conditions causing changes in 2,3-DPG are listed in Table 4-1.

TABLE 4-1. Conditions Causing Abnormalities in Red Cell 2,3-DPG Levels

Increase	Decrease
Alkalosis	Acidosis
Hypoxia	Shock
Anemia	Hypophosphatemia
Hepatic cirrhosis	Bank blood
Uremia	

Reproduced from Babior BM, Stossel TP. *Hematology: a pathophysiological approach.* 2nd ed. New York: Churchill Livingstone, 1984:32.

Carbon Dioxide Transport

Carbon dioxide can be transported in far greater quantities than can oxygen but, under normal resting conditions, an average of only 4 mL of CO_2 is transported to the lungs in each 100 mL of blood. The majority of CO_2 produced by cells in the peripheral tissues diffuses across the capillary membrane into erythrocytes. There, CO_2 and H_2O are converted to HCO_3^- and H^+ by **carbonic anhydrase** (Figure 4-4). The hydrogen ions produced are buffered by hemoglobin and the bicarbonate ions readily diffuse out of the cell into the plasma, while chloride ions diffuse into the red cell to maintain electroneutrality. Bicarbonate dissociates in lung capillaries and is excreted as CO_2 into alveoli. Seventy percent of the CO_2 is transported in this fashion. The remainder is primarily carried as **carbaminohemoglobin,** bound directly to hemoglobin. Only a small portion is dissolved in plasma.

Abnormal Hemoglobins

When oxyhemoglobin dissociates, the oxygen normally leaves as molecular oxygen with Fe^{2+}-hemoglobin remaining. Occasionally, oxygen dissociates abberrantly as a superoxide (O_2^-) and the iron is oxidized to Fe^{3+}. Fe^{3+}-hemoglobin or **methemoglobin** is unable to bind oxygen, leading to a decrease in the concentration of saturated hemoglobin in the serum. Circulating desaturated hemoglobin produces the striking cyanosis of acquired, acute methemoglobinemia. The process is reversible; an NADH-associated reduction of methemoglobin to Fe^{2+}-hemoglobin occurs in the RBC. Acquired methemoglobinemia is usually due to the ingestion of oxidizing

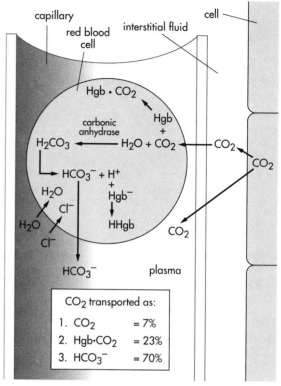

Figure 4-4 Transport of carbon dioxide in the blood. (Reproduced from Guyton AC. *Textbook of medical physiology.* Philadelphia: WB Saunders, 1986:500.)

agents, such as inorganic nitrite (NO_2^-, from contaminated well water), organic nitrites (used to produce methemoglobinemia in the treatment of cyanide poisoning), and chlorate (ClO_3^-, a constituent of safety match heads). Methylene blue, a reducing agent, can be given parenterally to treat acquired methemoglobinemia. It enters red cells and passes electrons from an NADPH-dependent reductase to methemoglobin.

Hemoglobin A1c is the result of nonenzymatic glycosylation of hemoglobin. It may account for up to 4% of total hemoglobin in poorly controlled diabetics. The percentage of hemoglobin A1c depends on the concentration of glucose in erythrocytes weeks to months prior to measurement. Hemoglobin A1c is less responsive to 2,3-DPG than is normal hemoglobin and has a lower oxygen affinity. However, whole blood oxygen-hemoglobin dissociation curves from diabetic subjects only show trivial differences compared to normals.

Carboxyhemoglobin results from the binding of **carbon monoxide** to the same heme iron binding site as oxygen, though carbon monoxide binds about 230 times more strongly than oxygen. A carbon monoxide pressure in alveoli of only 0.4 mm Hg (1/230 that of alveolar oxygen) allows carbon monoxide to compete equally with oxygen for hemoglobin. A carbon monoxide pressure of 0.7 mm Hg or 0.1% in the air can be lethal. The symptoms of carbon monoxide poisoning result from tissue oxygen deprivation. The in vivo half-life of carboxyhemoglobin can be reduced by administration of high concentrations of hyperbaric oxygen, allowing oxygen to compete with carbon monoxide for binding sites. The "cherry red" appearance of a patient suffering from carbon monoxide poisoning is due to the different peak absorbance wavelength of carboxyhemoglobin compared with oxyhemoglobin.

Physiology of Anemia and Polycythemia

Anemia is defined as a hemoglobin concentration below normal, while **polycythemia** is characterized by an hematocrit above normal. The use of these two different parameters to define the abnormal states is based on the physiologic sequelae of these conditions. Anemia may induce tissue hypoxia as a result of the low oxygen-carrying capacity of the blood. Symptoms of polycythemia are produced by the increased blood volume and viscosity.

ANEMIA

The relative tissue hypoxia caused by symptomatic or asymptomatic anemia initiates mechanisms to prevent irreversible cellular anoxia. Tissue utilization of the required oxygen leads to greater extraction of hemoglobin-bound oxygen, resulting in a lower Svo_2.

Several compensatory mechanisms are evoked in an attempt to maximize oxygen availability to tissues. The earliest and least costly adjustment is a decrease in the oxygen affinity of hemoglobin owing to increased amounts of erythrocyte 2,3-DPG.

An increase in cardiac output is another useful compensatory mechanism. It decreases the fraction of oxygen that must be extracted from circulating hemoglobin. However, metabolic demands are increased by the additional cardiac work required to augment cardiac output. A measurable increase in cardiac output

usually does not occur until the hemoglobin concentration falls below 7 g/dL.

An increase in EPO activity is the most appropriate homeostatic response to anemia. The production of EPO by the kidneys is inversely proportional to the red cell mass. The production of EPO is probably stimulated by relative renal tissue hypoxia.

POLYCYTHEMIA

Polycythemia may be relative as in the setting of dehydration, or absolute, such as when red cell mass is actually increased. Absolute polycythemia may be further divided into primary and secondary causes (Table 4-2). The EPO levels are low in primary polycythemias and elevated in secondary polycythemias.

Polycythemia vera, the most common primary polycythemia, is a chronic idiopathic myeloproliferative disorder that results in the increased production of erythrocytes, leukocytes, and platelets. Erythrocytosis, the dominant feature, results from the autonomous proliferation of a pluripotent stem cell. Erythrocytosis results in an increased blood volume and viscosity, and is responsible for many of the signs and symptoms of polycythemia. "Ruddy cyanosis" is caused by excessive deoxygenated blood flowing sluggishly through dilated

---

TABLE 4-2. Classification of Polycythemia (Erythrocytosis)

Relative
- Dehydration
- Spurious (stress or smokers) erythrocytosis

Absolute
- Primary
    Polycythemia vera
    Erythremia
- Secondary
    - Appropriate
        Altitude
        Cardiopulmonary disorder
        Increased affinity of hemoglobin for oxygen
    - Inappropriate
        Renal tumor and cyst
        Hepatoma
        Cerebellar hemangioblastoma
        Essential

Reproduced from Williams WJ et al. *Hematology.* 4th ed. New York: McGraw-Hill, 1990:428.

cutaneous capillaries. Symptoms of deficiency of cerebral blood flow or cerebral thrombosis are often observed and may be due to increased blood viscosity.

Oxygen delivery is intimately related to blood **viscosity** and at hematocrits greater than 50%, the resulting sharp increases in viscosity severely reduce oxygen transport. Over the flatter portion of the viscosity curve, oxygen delivery increases gradually as the hematocrit rises; however, in the steep portion of the viscosity curve, oxygen delivery falls because the oxygen-carrying capacity of blood is more than offset by the impedance to capillary blood flow caused by the increased viscosity.

Appropriate secondary polycythemia is a physiologic response to altitude and cardiopulmonary disorders.

In contrast, inappropriate secondary polycythemia has been associated with a number of disorders, including renal cell carcinoma, polycystic kidneys, renal cysts, hepatoma, and cerebellar hemangioblastoma.

Bibliography

Babior BM, Stossel TP. *Hematology: a pathophysiological approach.* New York: Churchill Livingstone, 1984.

Guyton AC. *Textbook of medical physiology.* 7th ed. Philadelphia: WB Saunders, 1986.

Williams WJ, Beutler E, Erslev AJ, Lichtman MA. *Hematology.* 4th ed. New York: McGraw-Hill, 1990.

W. Roy Smythe and Steven J. Fishman

5 HEMOSTASIS AND THROMBOSIS

Complex interactions between formed blood elements, plasma constituents, and the vessel wall serve to prevent undue hemorrhage, preserve vascular integrity, and maintain blood in the fluid state. A delicate balance between thrombotic and fibrinolytic processes is required to allow clotting and vascular repair at a site of injury without impairing normal blood flow to adjacent and distant sites. Although it is useful to consider separately the behavior of platelets, endothelial cells, procoagulant proteins, and fibrinolytic enzymes, it is necessary to understand that none of these factors func-

tions independently. Rather, their interaction maintains hemostatic homeostasis.

Endothelium

Until recently, the endothelium was believed to be nothing more than a passive, nonthrombogenic lining of the vascular system. It is now evident that endothelial cells are metabolically active participants not only in thrombosis and thrombolytic pathways but in many other unrelated functions, such as antigen expression and processing. The location of the endothelium at the interface between the circulating blood and the tissues imparts it with many regulatory functions. Variability of endothelial structure and function in different vascular beds and organs allows the endothelium to impart behavioral specificity to the various organs.

Endothelial properties determinine which blood components enter and leave the various tissue compartments. Molecular and cellular passage to the tissues across the endothelial monolayer may occur through intercellular clefts, transcellular channels, or by active transport mediated by intracellular vesicles.

Endothelial cells synthesize and metabolize a host of factors that regulate vascular tone, local thrombosis, and vascular repair. Arachidonic acid metabolites produced by the endothelium are major determinants of local vascular tone and thrombotic potential (Figure 5-1). Phospholipase cleaves arachidonate from endothelial membrane phospholipids. Cyclic endoperoxides and prostaglandins (PG) G_2 and H_2 are formed by the action of cyclo-oxygenase on arachidonic acid. These prostaglandins may be further metabolized to **prostacyclin (PGI$_2$)** or **thromboxane (TX) A$_2$**. These latter

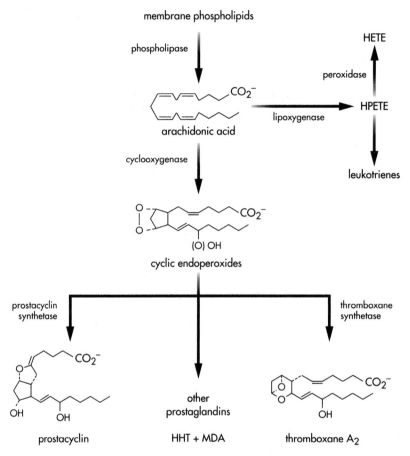

Figure 5-1 Endothelial vasoactive arachidonic acid metabolites. (Reproduced from Thompson AR, Harker LA, eds. *Manual of hemostasis and thrombosis.* 3rd ed. Philadelphia: FA Davis, 1983:6.)

two compounds have potent opposing activities. Prostacyclin is a potent vasodilator and inhibitor of platelet aggregation. Thromboxane A_2 is a potent vasoconstrictor and platelet agonist. Thus, the balance between endothelial production of PGI_2 and TXA_2 is crucial to local circulatory homeostasis. Arachidonic acid may also be processed by the lipoxygenase pathway into **leukotrienes,** which may have vasoactive effects as well, but are more characterized by their chemotactic activity in regulating inflammatory responses.

Though structurally unrelated, **endothelial-derived relaxing factor (EDRF)** and **endothelin-1** are endothelial products that have opposing activities, similar to the relationship between PGI_2 and TXA_2. Structurally similar to nitric oxide, EDRF is a potent vasodilator and

platelet inhibitor, while endothelin-1 is a protein that is the most potent known vasoconstrictor.

The endothelium synthesizes most of its surrounding milieu. On its luminal surface, it possesses proteoglycans such as heparan sulfate, which provide basal passive thromboresistance. It may also secrete plasminogen activators and thrombolytics, in addition to PGI_2 and EDRF, which more actively inhibit thrombosis. Endothelial cells can also degrade local procoagulant compounds. They actively take up and metabolize vasoactive amines and degrade the proaggregant adenosine diphosphate (ADP; see below) with a membrane-bound ADPase.

Endothelial cells also produce many of the components of the subendothelium. Collagen, fibronectin, elastin, and microfibrils contribute to the subendothelial connective tissue matrix that may stimulate thrombosis. Thus, injury to or denudation of endothelium may lead to local thrombosis as a result of both loss of the luminal thromboresistant surface and exposure of the prothrombotic subendothelium.

The Platelet

PLATELET ANATOMY

The platelet, in its most mature resting form, is an anuclear biconvex disc averaging 3–4 μ in diameter. The discoid shape is maintained by a circumferential system of microtubules. An internal cytoskeleton of microfilaments provides further structural support and suspends organelles such as mitochondria and secretory granules. A number of contractile proteins are active within the platelet. These include actin, myosin, actinin, actin binding protein, filamin, tropomyosin, and troponin.

The structure of the platelet surface is uniquely adapted for a multitude of coagulation related functions. External to the plasma membrane is a proteoglycan layer containing acid mucopolysaccharides, which promotes the adherence of platelets to other platelets and to collagen. The plasma membrane contains a number of platelet-specific membrane glycoproteins including GPIb, GPIIb, GPIIIa, and GPV. Certain phospholipids important in the generation of procoagulants and arachidonic acid metabolites are also present in the plasma membrane. An internal canalicular system, continuous with the plasma membrane, enhances the effective platelet surface area (Figure 5-2). The canalicular system interdigitates with a dense tubular system within the platelet. This system is important in the regulation of platelet function by calcium. The structure and regulatory function of the canalicular and dense tubular systems resemble those of the T-tubule and sarcoplasmic reticulum of the striated myocyte.

The response of a platelet to a stimulus is largely dependent upon the release of substances found within storage granules. Four types of storage granules are present:

1. **Glycogen granules,** which provide fuel for anaerobic glycolysis
2. **α-Granules,** which contain the platelet-specific proteins platelet factor 4 (PF4), β-thromboglobulin, platelet-derived growth factor, thrombospondin; and the plasma proteins fibronectin, albumin, fibrinogen; as well as coagulation factors V and VIII/vWF

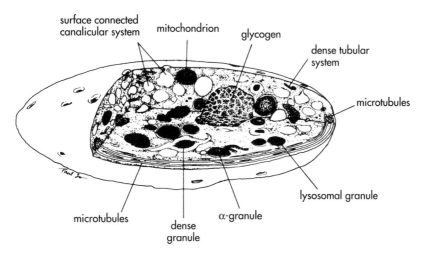

Figure 5-2 Platelet morphology. Although anucleate, the platelet possesses a complex structure that is extremely dynamic. The surface plasma membrane is continuous with a canalicular system that provides a large area for surface reactions. There are several excretory granules with varied contents, a complicated contractile protein system, cytoskeleton, and efficient energy source. (Reproduced from Thompson AR, Harker LA, eds. *Manual of hemostasis and thrombosis.* 3rd ed. Philadelphia: FA Davis, 1983:10.)

3. **Dense granules,** which contain serotonin, calcium, ADP, and other phosphates
4. **Lysosomal granules,** which primarily contain acid hydrolases.

PLATELET LIFE CYCLE AND KINETICS

As with other formed blood elements, platelet precursors are initially produced in the blood islands of the human fetal yolk sac at about 3 weeks gestation. After 3 months gestation, these platelet precursors are found almost exclusively in the bone marrow.

The stem cell precursor of the platelet is known as **CFU-Mega** (CFU, colony forming unit). The CFU-Mega precursor behaves similarly to other diploid stem precursors, exhibiting mitosis and cell division when activated. However, at some point the CFU-Mega begins to endoreplicate without cell division—a process termed polyploidization. Endoreplication begins the **promegakaryoblast** phase. Maturation of the single polyploid nucleus (predominantly 16N in humans) occurs during the **megakaryoblast** stage, as does development of the open canalicular system and the α-granule. The next stage, the **promegakaryocyte,** is one of intense cell growth and cytoplasmic development. The amount of cytoplasm and attendant complement of organelles produced is proportional to a given cell's ploidy. The **megakaryocyte** is the final platelet precursor. Synthesis of cytoplasm, organelles, and the open canalicular system continues in the early megakaryocyte stage. The development and distribution of organelles is not uniform throughout the megakaryocyte. This explains the random variation noted in size, concentration of organelles, and therefore, function of platelet progeny. Each megakaryocyte fragments into approximately 1000–1500 platelets.

Several humoral substances stimulate platelet production including thrombopoietin, erythropoietin, interleukin-3, interleukin-4, interleukin-6, granulocyte-macrophage colony-stimulating factor, thrombopoiesis- and megakaryocyte-stimulating factors, and many others. Thrombopoietin increases the rate of early precursor maturation, endoreplication, the amount of cytoplasm per megakaryocyte, and the rates of cytoplasmic maturation and platelet release. Humoral factors that inhibit platelet production include transforming growth factor β, β-, and γ-interferon, a splenic inhibitor, and acetylcholinesterase. Most of these substances act via inhibition of CFU-Mega development.

The average platelet count is 250,000 ± 60,000 platelets/µL. Two thirds of the body's platelets circulate freely, while one third are stored in a splenic pool. The platelet has a lifespan of 9–12 days and normal platelet turnover is about 35,000/µL day.

PLATELET FUNCTION

The platelet is a very dynamic blood component. Minimal mechanical stimulation of the platelet causes retractable pseudopods to develop. Further stimulation causes the platelet surface to become reversibly adhesive without further change in shape. Additional stimuli cause the platelet to contract, cluster its organelles centrally, and assume a "spiny" configuration. This sequence of events is required for expulsion of the contents of platelet granules. Energy necessary for these processes is derived from anaerobic and aerobic metabolism of glycogen from storage granules.

Injury to the vessel wall exposes subendothelial collagen types IV and V and individual microfibrils, to which platelets adhere (Figure 5-3). Required for adhesion are a platelet surface glycoprotein, **GPIb,** and **factor VIII/von Willebrand's factor (vWF).** The vWF is synthesized by endothelial cells and megakaryocytes and circulates in plasma.

Once vascular disruption occurs, a number of reactions recruit additional platelets to the area. Most notably, aggregation is facilitated by (1) **ADP** release from the dense granules of adherent platelets, (2) generation of **TXA_2** from platelet membranes, and (3) **thrombin** formation. Platelet aggregation cannot occur in the absence of **fibrinogen** or **calcium.**

ADP and TXA_2 promote the cross-linking of platelets via bound **fibrinogen.** ADP interacts with a specific platelet membrane receptor and decreases adenosine 3′–5′ cyclic monophosphate (cAMP) activity. In turn, the conformation of the membrane **glycoprotein IIb-IIIa** complex is altered to expose the fibrinogen binding site.

Thrombin generated at the site of injury may induce platelet production of ADP and TXA_2. The production of TXA_2 is via the cyclo-oxygenase pathway from platelet membrane arachidonate in a similar fashion to the endothelial cell. Though platelets contain thromboxane synthetase to produce TXA_2, they do not possess prostacyclin synthetase, and cannot produce PGI_2.

At the beginning of the aggregation phase, the marginal band of microtubules depolymerizes into component microfilaments in preparation for conformational changes during the release reaction.

In response to exposure to subendothelial connec-

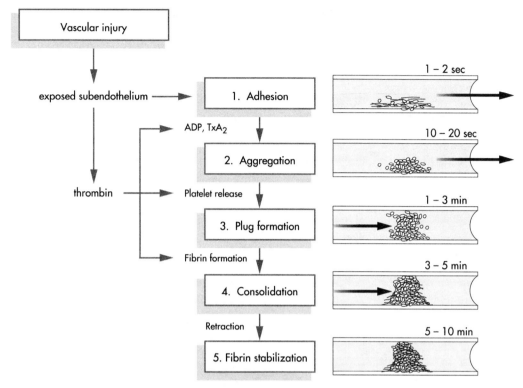

Figure 5-3 Hemostatic plug formation. The formation of a platelet plug proceeds through the following sequence: **1**, platelet adhesion to exposed subendothelial connective tissue structures; **2**, platelet aggregation by ADP and thromboxane A$_2$, and thrombin recruitment through transformation of discoid platelets into reactive spiny spheres that interact with one another through calcium-dependent fibrinogen bridges; **3**, contribution of platelet coagulant activity to the coagulation process that stabilizes the plug with a fibrin mesh; and **4**, retraction of the platelet mass to provide a dense thrombus. (Reproduced from Thompson AR, Harker LA, eds. *Manual of hemostasis and thrombosis.* 3rd ed. Philadelphia: FA Davis, 1983:11.)

tive tissue, ADP, epinephrine, and thrombin, the platelet mobilizes calcium. The calcium-calmodulin (a cytoplasmic calcium binding protein) complex then activates intracellular protein kinases which phosphorylate myosin and allow platelet contraction and release of granule contents. The α-granule requires minimal stimulation for release; the dense granule requires a somewhat stronger stimulus. In this manner, the platelet releases a wide array of granule contents. These contents include compounds that affect the coagulation process, as well as chemoattractants for phagocytic leukocytes, which eliminate platelet debris after the hemostatic plug has served its purpose.

Platelet factor 3 is a phospholipoprotein produced on the surface of aggregated platelets. Platelet factor 3 aids in activation of factor X and the conversion of prothrombin to thrombin. The surface of the aggregated platelets serves as a template for the local production of large amounts of thrombin. Platelets also participate in the direct activation of factors XII and XI.

Platelet-derived growth factor is produced by both platelets and endothelium. This protein is both mitogenic and chemotactic for fibroblasts and smooth muscle cells and is important for maintenance of vessel wall integrity.

Coagulation Factors and the Coagulation Cascade

The major plasma participants in coagulation are glycoproteins. These glycoproteins are composed of a central protein core, carbohydrate side chains, and terminal sialic acid residues. At least 12 glycoproteins, in addition to numerous cofactors and other secondary participants, are recognized. These factors interact in a complex series of reactions, referred to as the **coagulation cascade** to form an insoluble fibrin gel.

All the plasma glycoproteins are produced primarily by the hepatocyte, excepting factor VIII/vWF. Secondary extrahepatic sites of production also exist for some factors. The endothelium produces the bulk of vWF, and a lesser proportion of factor V. **Tissue factor,** a lipoprotein coagulation factor, is produced by many tissues including brain, placenta, and endothelium. Megakaryocytes produce fibrinogen, factor V, and factor XIII; and the macrophage produces prothrombin, tissue factor, and factors V, VII, IX, and X. Factor VIII is thought to be produced in multiple sites including the liver, spleen, lung, and lymph nodes.

Synthesis and structure of the **vitamin-K-dependent coagulation factors** deserves special mention. These factors, including **II, VII, IX, and X,** possess γ-carboxyglutamate residues on their amino termini. Carboxylation of the amino-terminal glutamate residues occurs during the posttranslational phase in the hepatocyte. These residues have a double negative charge and allow binding to negatively charged phospholipid membranes via calcium ions (Figure 5-4).

All clotting factors involved in the coagulation cascade are either precursors of serine proteases or cofactors. The precursors are activated by proteolytic cleavage of peptide bonds. Important **cofactors** include **calcium ions, high molecular weight kininogen (HMWK), prekallikrein, tissue factor,** and **factors V** and **VIII.** Calcium is necessary for most coagulation reactions, with the exception of several contact-mediated reactions. The calcium chelators, EDTA and citrate, used for blood collection and processing, prevent clotting by rendering calcium unavailable to participate in coagulation reactions.

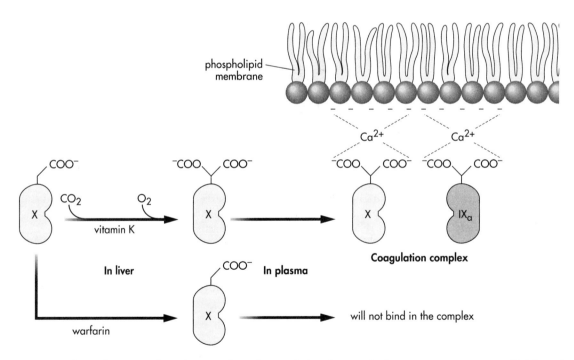

Figure 5-4 Synthesis of vitamin-K-dependent coagulation factors. Carboxylation in the hepatocyte requires vitamin K, CO_2, and O_2, and results in the formation of γ-carboxyglutamic acid residues, which have a double-negative charge at physiologic pH. These unique amino acid residues permit the coagulation factors to bind to phospholipid membranes via Ca^{2+} ions. Warfarin blocks this carboxylation step and results in the formation of abnormal clotting factors that do not function in the coagulation cascade. (Reproduced from Williams WJ, Beutler E, Erslev AJ, Lichtman MA, eds. *Hematology.* 4th ed. New York: McGraw-Hill, 1990:1286.)

Specific characteristics of the major factors and cofactors are presented in Table 5-1.

Factor VIII/vWF exists as a multimeric protein with 6–10 disulfide bond linked subsets. It is the largest factor with a molecular weight of 1–2 million. The vWF constitutes the largest portion of the conglomerate and is a carrier for the active coagulation factor VIII. A marginated pool of VIII/vWF exists, primarily in the endothelium. This noncirculating pool can be liberated by physiologic stress, such as that induced by strenuous exercise or increased epinephrine, or by drugs such as desmopressin acetate (DDAVP), and may double the plasma level and coagulant activity of VIII/vWF.

Factor VII has the shortest half-life and lowest plasma concentration, explaining why an elevated prothrombin time (PT; see below) is usually dependent on factor VII depletion when hepatic failure or warfarin derivatives are implicated.

Three systems are recognized in the coagulation cascade: the **intrinsic, extrinsic** and **common pathways** (Figure 5-5). It is important, however, to note that the following discussion of these pathways represents what

TABLE 5-1. Properties of Human Clotting Factors

Clotting Factor (Synonym)	Molecular Wt. (No. of Chains)	Normal Plasma Conc. (µg/mL)	$T_{1/2}$ Elimination (Hrs)	Active Form
Intrinsic System				
Factor XII (Hageman factor)	80,000 (1)	29	60	Serine protease
Prekallikrein (Fletcher factor)	80,000 (1)	50	?	Serine protease
High mol. wt. kininogen (Fitzgerald factor)	120,000 (1)	70	?	Cofactor
Factor XI (Plasma thromboplastin antecedent)	160,000 (2, dimer)	4	65	Serine protease
Factor IX (Christmas Factor)	57,000 (1)	4	20	Serine protease
Factor VIII/VWF (Antihemophilic factor/ von Willebrand factor)	1–2,000,000*a* (series of 6–10 subunits)	7 (vWF)	10 (VIII:C)	Cofactor
Extrinsic System				
Factor VII (Proconvertin)	55,000 (1)	1	5	Serine protease
Tissue factor (Tissue thromboplastin)	45,000 (1)	0		Cofactor
Common Pathway				
Factor X (Stuart-Prower factor)	59,000 (2)	5	65	Serine protease
Factor V (Proaccelerin)	330,000 (1)	5–12	25	Cofactor
Prothrombin (Factor II)	70,000 (1)	100	100	Serine protease
Fibrinogen (Factor I)	340,000 (6: Aα_2, Bβ_2, γ_2)	2500 (250 mg/dL)	120	Clot structure
Factor XIII (Fibrin stabilizing factor)	300,000 (4: a$_2$ b$_2$)	10	150	Transglutaminase

*a*Subunit molecular weight of factor VIII/vWF is around 200,000 with a series of multimers found in circulation.
Reproduced from Thompson AR, Harker LA, eds. *Manual of hemostasis and thrombosis.* 3rd ed. Philadelphia: FA Davis, 1983:22.

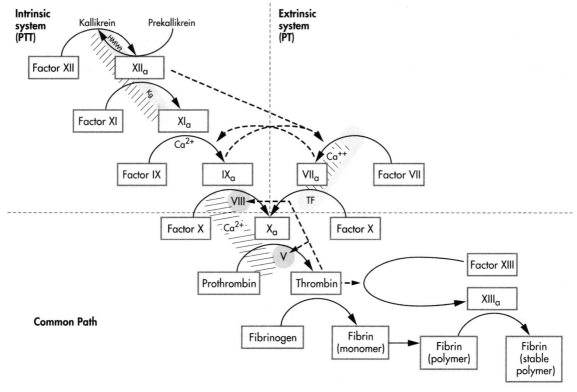

Figure 5-5 The in vitro coagulation cascade. The intrinsic and extrinsic pathways culminate in a common path and finally clot stabilization. A number of cofactors are necessary and are indicated by *shaded areas* (protein) and *hatched areas* (phospholipid). The *dotted lines* indicate interactions that may exist between the three pathways. HMWt, high molecular weight kininogen; TF, tissue factor. (Reproduced from Thompson AR, Harker LA, eds. *Manual of hemostasis and thrombosis.* 3rd ed. Philadelphia: FA Davis, 1983:25.)

is known about in vitro interactions between coagulation factors. In truth, the sequence of coagulation reactions in vivo is probably much more complex and yet to be determined.

The initiation of the sequence of reactions in the intrinsic pathway is known as **contact activation.** **Factor XII** is activated by adherence to a negatively charged surface. Activated factor XII converts **prekallikrein** to **kallikrein** and activates **factor XI.** Reciprocal activation of factor XII by kallikrein also occurs. The HMWK cofactor binds prekallikrein and factor XI, holding them at the negatively charged surface. **Factor IXa** and **factor VIII/vWF** from the intrinsic pathway initiate the common pathway via **factor X** activation. Factor VIII requires prior modification by a serine protease (i.e., **thrombin**) to perform this function.

The extrinsic pathway is initiated by the activation of **factor VII** by **tissue factor.** Tissue factor, largely com-

prised of lipid, provides a negatively charged template for factor VII binding. Calcium is also required for factor VII activation. Factor VIIa then activates the common pathway via the activation of factor X.

The common pathway begins with **factor X** activation. Modified **factor V** and factor Xa then combine to generate **thrombin** from **prothrombin.** Thrombin is perhaps the most active participant in the coagulation process. It interacts with **fibrinogen** and **factor XIII** to complete the cascade. In addition, it modifies factors VIII and V, activates protein C, and stimulates platelets, among other functions. Thrombin liberates two fibrin monomers from the fibrinogen precursor, **fibrinopeptides A** and **B.** These monomers may polymerize spontaneously; however, the complex thus formed is unstable and may be denatured easily unless polymerized by factor XIIIa. Factor XIIIa, following thrombin modification, is a transaminase that forms lysine-glutamine bonds between fibrin monomers, thus "cross-linking" the fibrin clot and rendering it insoluble.

A number of "checks and balances" serve to control the process of coagulation, preventing massive thrombosis. The mechanical process of blood flow removes coagulation factors from the site of formation and dilutes them in the vascular pool. Blood flow also serves to deliver factors to the liver and other sites where reticuloendothelial cells actively phagocytose them. In addition, a number of circulating protease inhibitors exist that inactivate hemostatic proteases. Lastly, some proteolytic enzymes, including plasmin and proteins C and S, have antithrombotic properties. These will be discussed in more depth in the following section.

Fibrinolysis and Inhibition of Coagulation

Hemostasis is controlled by a delicate balance between coagulation and the inhibition of its reactions and breakdown of its products. Controlled fibrinolysis is necessary for restoration of local and systemic tissue structure and functional capacity once platelet aggregation and thrombus formation is no longer necessary.

FIBRINOLYTIC ENZYMES AND PROTEASE INHIBITORS

In concert with the activation processes of coagulation, a number of proteolytic enzymes are produced that promote coagulation factor inactivation and degradation. These include **plasmin, protein C,** and **protein S.**

The Plasminogen/Plasmin System

Plasminogen is a plasma glycoprotein synthesized by the liver that shares structural homology with the contact activation procoagulant factors. Its activated form is plasmin. Plasminogen may be activated by three different types of mechanisms—**physiologic, intrinsic,** and **exogenous.** The two primary physiologic activators of plasminogen are the serine proteases **tissue-type plasminogen activator (tPA)** and **urokinase-type plasminogen activator (uPA).** Endothelium is the major site of tPA production. It has also been isolated from a number of malignant cell lines. A number of stimuli cause in vivo release of tPA from endothelial cells including venous stasis, exercise, thrombin, and administration of DDAVP. Both tPA and uPA cleave plasminogen, resulting in activated plasmin. The tPA must bind with fibrin in order to cleave plasminogen; whereas uPA can activate plasminogen in the fluid phase, without prior binding to fibrin. The uPA is found in human urine, plasma, and many normal tissue cell lines. Although uPA does not bind avidly to fibrin, it still has fibrin-specific thrombolytic activity, and its presence in urine is important for clot dissolution in the extrarenal collecting system.

A number of factors may participate in the activation of plasminogen in conjunction with activation of the intrinsic coagulation system. Participants include factor XIIa, kallikrein, and HMWK. Kallikrein activates uPA from a single chain to a more active double chain form, and factor XIIa is necessary for conversion of pre-kallikrein to kallikrein with the help of HMWK.

Exogenous activation of plasminogen to the active plasmin form involves administration of urokinase, streptokinase or tPA, which are now produced via bioengineering/recombinant DNA techniques.

Plasminogen may be converted to plasmin by virtue of specific disulfide bond cleavage. Lysine-lysine and arginine-valine bonds are commonly broken with subsequent production of plasmin molecules of varying length. All of these plasmin molecules are double-chain endopeptidases, which hydrolyze arginine and lysine bonds in protein at neutral pH. In addition to fibrin and fibrinogen, plasmin may hydrolyze factors V and VIII, complement components, ACTH, growth hormone, and glucagon.

Plasmin actively degrades both fibrinogen and fibrin at sites of fibrin deposition. Cleavage of fibrin complexes may occur at any point during polymerization, but is slowed once fibrin cross-linking by factor XIII has occurred. Insoluble fibrin complexes may eventually be rendered soluble by selective bond breakage, and a number of fibrin degradation products (FDPs) result. The smallest FDP that is liberated from cross-linked fibrin is known as the D-D dimer. Substantial elevation in D-D dimer often indicates ongoing pathologic disseminated intravascular coagulation. Larger X and Y fibrin degradation fragments exert some anticoagulant effects. Smaller fragments are rapidly cleared from the circulation and have little activity.

Plasmin may be rapidly inactivated by the potent protease inhibitor α_2-antiplasmin. α_2-Macroglobulin may also inactivate plasmin, but less readily.

The plasminogen/plasmin fibrinolytic system is finely regulated, especially at the level of the microcircula-

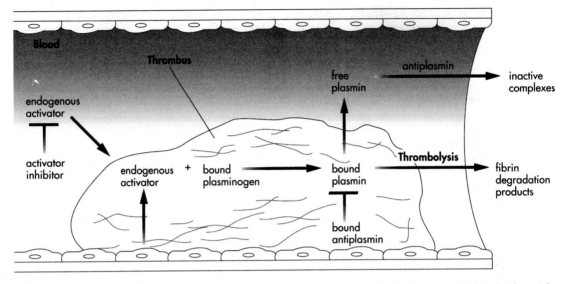

Figure 5-6 Physiologic thrombolysis at the microcirculatory level. Large local amounts of endogenous activator (tPA), antiplasmin, and fibrin allow for fine local control without development of a systemic proteolytic state. (Reproduced from Williams WJ, Beutler E, Erslev AJ, Lichtman MA, eds. *Hematology.* 4th ed. New York: McGraw-Hill, 1990:1317.)

tion where the ratio of endothelial cells (and thus plasminogen activator and plasmin inhibitors) is high relative to the exposed surface of the fibrin thrombus (Figure 5-6).

Nonplasmin Fibrinolytic Mechanisms

Proteins C and **S** are produced in the liver as are the vitamin-K-dependent procoagulants II, VII, IX, and X, with which they share structural homology. Protein C is a zymogen that requires activation by thrombin. Thrombin bound to thrombomodulin at the forming clot cleaves and activates protein C. Activated protein C may then cleave and inactivate factors V and VIII. It may also serve as a positive effector of the plasmin fibrinolytic system. Protein S is not a zymogen, but acts as a cofactor for activated protein C by aiding in localization of protein C at the phospholipid surface (Figure 5-7). The actions of protein C are limited by a number of factors including protein C inhibitor and factors Xa, V, IXa, and VIII. These complex agonist and antagonist feedback interactions between procoagulant factors and inactivating proteins demonstrate the intricate balance that allows finely tuned localized thrombosis where necessary, without inappropriate regional or distant clot formation or propagation.

A number of naturally occurring circulating protease inhibitors exist that inactivate a variety of proteases. **Antithrombin III** forms stable high molecular weight complexes with all serine proteases involved in the coagulation cascade. This effect of antithrombin III is amplified by binding exogenously administered heparin. **C_1 esterase inhibitor** is an avid inactivator of plasma kallikrein as well as factors XIa and XIIa. **α_2-Antiplasmin**, which can inactivate all unbound contact proteases in hemostasis, is also the most potent inactivator of plasmin. **α_2-Macroglobulin** and **α_1-antitrypsin** can also inhibit most of the serine proteases of the coagulation cascade.

Hemoactive Drugs and Mechanisms of Action

ANTITHROMBOTIC AGENTS

Coumarin and Indandione

Derivatives of these two families of anticoagulants act on the vitamin-K-dependent coagulation factors II, VII, IX, and X. Coumarin derivatives include dicumarol, phenprocoumarin, warfarin potassium, and warfarin sodium. Anisindione is an indandione derivative.

These drugs block vitamin-K-dependent carboxylation of amino-terminal glutamyl residues. These factors are then produced lacking a double negative charge necessary to complex with calcium ions and phospholipid membranes (Figure 5-4). Coumarin effects may be antagonized by exogenous vitamin-K administration.

Heparin

Heparin exists in the human body as an anionic sulfated glycosaminoglycan in mast cell granules. Commercially produced derivatives include heparin sodium and heparin calcium.

Heparin acts as a catalyst to inhibit the effects of a number of serine proteases, especially thrombin, VIIa, IXa, Xa, and XIa. It catalyzes the inhibitory effects of antithrombin III on these factors. Bound heparin enhances the reactivity of a specific arginine (+) residue on antithrombin III. This residue binds with aspartate (-) sites on the serine protease coagulation factors forming covalent complexes.

Streptokinase

Streptokinase is a highly antigenic nonenzymatic single-chain polypeptide produced naturally by group C β-hemolytic streptococci. Recombinant DNA techniques allow mass production of this protein. Although it lacks enzymatic activity, streptokinase promotes thrombolysis by forming equimolar complexes with plasminogen, which then enzymatically convert other plasminogen molecules to plasmin.

Urokinase

Urokinase is an enzyme isolated from human urine and embryonic renal cell culture. Urokinase directly converts plasminogen to plasmin, thus effecting fibrinolysis. Urokinase lacks the antigenicity of streptokinase, preventing the adverse consequences of sensitization, anaphylaxis, allergic reaction, and inhibition of effect by blocking antibody that may complicate streptokinase therapy.

Tissue Plasminogen Activator

Tissue plasminogen activator is produced by cell culture and recombinant DNA techniques. Tissue plas-

minogen activator promotes fibrinolysis by direct conversion of plasminogen to plasmin, and tPA has high fibrin affinity and greatly increased activity in the presence of fibrin. Most tPA circulates in a complex with an inhibitor.

Acylated Plasminogen: Streptokinase Activator Complex

The acylated plasminogen streptokinase activator complex (APSAC) is a second-generation fibrinolytic that consists of a biochemically altered streptokinase-plasminogen complex. The complex activates free plasminogen molecules to plasmin. APSAC has a half-life greatly exceeding that of streptokinase and urokinase and may be given by bolus rather than constant infusion.

Aspirin and Other Nonsteroidal Anti-Inflammatory Agents

Aspirin acts to inhibit hemostasis by virtue of its effect on platelet function. Aspirin irreversibly acetylates and inhibits the enzyme cyclo-oxygenase. As described above, this enzyme converts arachidonic acid to the endoperoxide PGG_2 (see Figure 5-1). The PGG_2 is converted to prothrombotic thromboxane A_2 in platelets and primarily to antithrombotic prostacyclin in endothelial cells. Lacking nuclei, platelets are unable to synthesize new cyclo-oxygenase. Endothelium, however, can regenerate cyclo-oxygenase to replace what was permanently acetylated by aspirin. High-dose continuous aspirin administration can significantly impair endothelial prostacyclin production. Consequently, small doses of aspirin are usually recommended to obtain an antithrombotic effect. Other nonsteroidal anti-inflammatory agents, such as indomethacin and sulfinpyrazone, reversibly inhibit cyclo-oxygenase.

Dipyridamole

Dipyridamole inhibits platelet phosphodiesterase, thus decreasing degradation of cAMP to AMP. The resultant elevated cAMP levels potentiate prostacyclin's ability to inhibit formation of the platelet plug.

This drug has been used alone and in combination with aspirin and coumarin derivatives to prevent thromboembolic phenomena. The clinical efficacy of dipyridamole alone has not been well established.

Ticlopidine

This drug is a thienopyridine that prolongs bleeding time and markedly inhibits in vitro aggregation of platelets. It is thought to inhibit the interaction of fibrinogen and vWF with platelet membrane glycoproteins.

Prostacyclin

Prostacyclin (PGI_2) is an endogenous prostaglandin that markedly inhibits platelet aggregation and adhesion and also acts as a local vasodilator. Prostacyclin analogues have been recently synthesized and are now in experimental clinical usage.

Dextran

Dextran is a hydrolyzed glucose polymer originally used as a plasma expander that increases bleeding time by inhibiting platelet function. The mechanism of action is not well characterized, but may be due to an alteration of platelet membrane properties.

PROCOAGULANTS

Vitamin K

Vitamin K is a fat-soluble vitamin required for hepatic synthesis of several coagulation factors (II, VII, IX, X). Deficiency of vitamin K may lead to profound coagulopathy. This may result from inadequate exogenous intake, which occurs with malnutrition and malabsorption, or inadequate endogenous production by gastrointestinal flora, as may occur with prolonged use of antibiotics.

Protamine Sulfate

Protamine is a basic nuclear histone that binds to heparin and renders heparin ineffective immediately. However, its short half-life may necessitate repeated administration to prevent "rebound" heparin effect.

Desmopressin Acetate

Desmopressin acetate (DDAVP) is a synthetic polypeptide related structurally to arginine vasopressin or antidiuretic hormone. It has comparable antidiuretic effects but diminished vasopressive action.

Desmopressin acetate stimulates release of vWF from natural tissue stores—primarily endothelium. Following administration, an increase in factor VIII/vWF multimers may result. This drug has clinical utility in treatment of hemophilia A, von Willebrand's disease, and uremic coagulopathy.

ε-AMINOCAPROIC ACID

ε-Aminocaproic acid (EACA) is a synthetic monoaminocarboxylic acid that behaves as a procoagulant via inhibition of fibrinolysis. It inhibits plasminogen and plasmin-induced degradation of fibrin and fibrinogen. The inhibition of plasminogen activation to plasmin may result from competition for plasminogen lysine binding sites. Also, EACA may alter the fibrin substrate, rendering it less susceptible to plasmin degradation.

Diagnostic Evaluation of Hemostatic Mechanisms

The complex interactions between formed blood elements, endothelium and plasma constituents that control hemostasis cannot be assessed with a single test. However, understanding the limitations of and the information available from the various diagnostic tests affords greater comprehension of the system as whole.

WHOLE BLOOD COAGULATION/ CLOT OBSERVATION

Although whole blood coagulation evaluation is rarely used at present, some useful information may be obtained by inspection of active clot formation.

Venous blood is collected and agitated at 37°C. When gross clots form, the test is complete. The clots may then be reinspected 1 hour and 12–24 hours later.

The normal value observed for initial clot formation is 4–8 minutes. Clot retraction should occur by 1 hour with reduction by 50% of original volume considered normal. Thrombocytopenia, thrombasthenia, and erythrocytosis may impede retraction. Ragged clot formation or clot dissolution at 1–24 hours may indicate pathologic fibrinolytic states.

BLEEDING TIME

Prolonged bleeding time after a controlled superficial injury may indicate platelet dysfunction. A small incision is made with a lancet or controlled depth template device. Excess oozing blood is removed at regular intervals with filter paper until it ceases—making sure the platelet plug beneath is undisturbed. The Ivy method uses 40 mm Hg tourniquet pressure proximal to the test site on the volar forearm. The test is operator dependent, but 3–6 minutes is generally considered a normal bleeding time. The test time will be elevated with both platelet dysfunction and thrombocytopenia. One can calculate the expected bleeding time using the following equation:

$$\text{Bleeding time} = \frac{30.5 - \text{platelet count}}{3850}$$

A bleeding time in excess of that predicted by the platelet count may indicate platelet dysfunction.

PROTHROMBIN TIME

This test measures the function of the extrinsic and common pathways of the coagulation cascade (fibrinogen, prothrombin, factors V, VII, X).

The test is performed by adding citrated plasma to ionized calcium and tissue thromboplastin (brain extract). The tissue thromboplastin reacts with factor VII and initiates the extrinsic cascade, activating factor X and culminating in fibrin formation (Figure 5-5).

Test values vary, but 11–15 seconds is considered normal in most laboratories. A more accurate method of reporting the result may be yielded by comparing the obtained value directly with a control and expressing a percentage comparison. Human brain extract is commonly used in European countries, and thus the results differ from those obtained in the United States, where where rabbit brain thromboplastin is commonly used.

The PT measures the function and concentration of the foregoing coagulation factors, but is most sensitive to low levels of factor VII. It is thus most often used to follow coumarin derivative therapy. An elevated PT is also often an indication of diminished hepatic synthetic function as a result of severe liver disease.

PARTIAL THROMBOPLASTIN TIME

This test evaluates the intrinsic and common pathways of the coagulation cascade. It may detect deficiencies of all coagulation factors except VII and XIII, and is considered more sensitive than the PT to detection of minor deficiencies.

The partial thromboplastin time (PTT) test is performed by addition of calcium and phospholipid (without tissue factor—thus the name "partial thromboplastin") to plasma. Without phospholipid the test is known as the recalcification time. The addition of phospholipid corrects for the variability of platelet surface activation, which may vary with the platelet count. Activation is dependent upon contact between the blood and the glass surface of the test container. The ratio of the blood volume to container surface area can affect this test. To prevent this variability, a negatively charged particulate substance (kaolin or celite) that rapidly activates contact-sensitive substrate can be added. The addition of this substance deems the test an activated partial thromboplastin time (APTT).

The PTT (or APTT) may be prolonged by deficiency of any coagulation factor, excepting VII and XIII. It can also be prolonged by the presence of inhibitors of these factors, such as heparin or the lupus anticoagulant. The PTT is used to monitor heparin therapy. The case of a lupus anticoagulant is an example where the in vitro assessment of coagulation does not necessarily represent physiologic function. Though the lupus anticoagulant prolongs the PTT, it may cause pathologic **hyper**coagulability.

When an elevated PTT is detected, a mixing test may be performed to differentiate the deficiency of a coagulation factor from the presence of an inhibitor. The patient's plasma is mixed in a 50:50 fashion with normal plasma. When the defect is attributable to a factor deficiency, the APTT will shorten significantly—this is termed "correction." If the abnormality is due to a strong inhibitor such as a lupus anticoagulant, the test value of the mixture will remain prolonged. The mixing test is less helpful if the APTT is only minimally elevated or if a weak inhibitor is present.

THROMBIN TIME

Thrombin directly converts fibrinogen to fibrin. After addition of thrombin to plasma, the time elapsed prior to clot formation is termed the thrombin time. The result is prolonged with quantitative and qualitative deficits in fibrinogen, and in the presence of inhibitors such as heparin or fibrinogen degradation products. Since fibrinogen may now be measured directly, the thrombin time (TT) test is infrequently necessary.

ACTIVATED CLOTTING TIME

The activated clotting time (ACT) is simply the whole blood clotting time with the addition of celite, a fine clay. Celite provides a dispersed surface area for the coagulation factors, shortens the clotting time, and reduces test variability. Normal blood clots within 100 seconds following the addition of celite.

This is an excellent test for monitoring the effectiveness of anticoagulation during extracorporeal circulation such as that used during cardiac surgery. Repeated bedside measurements allow for immediate adjustments in anticoagulation. The test is not suitable for intermittent laboratory monitoring, as it must be performed immediately after phlebotomy.

EUGLOBULIN LYSIS TIME

This test is an indirect measure of systemic fibrinolytic activity. Dilute plasma is acidified with acetic acid, promoting the precipitation of "euglobulin" (fibrinogen, plasminogen, plasminogen activator—without antiplasmin activity). Thrombin is added to the precipitant and the time taken to lyse a clot is termed the euglobulin lysis time (ELT). Thrombin converts fibrinogen to fibrin, thus activating plasminogen.

Normal results vary from 1.5 to 6 hours. Fibrinolytic states will shorten lysis time. However, reduced fibrinogen will also lower the value, making the test difficult to interpret.

TESTS FOR THE PRESENCE OF FIBRIN DEGRADATION PRODUCTS

These tests measure the presence of fibrin degradation products (FDPs) and may be useful for diagnosis and monitoring of disseminated intravascular coagulation. These tests employ monoclonal antibodies and latex agglutination techniques. Currently two tests exist, one for all FDPs, and a more specific test for the D-dimer. The D-dimer test is more sensitive in the diagnosis of disseminated intravascular coagulation. With fibrinolytic therapy, FDPs may be present, while the D-dimer test is negative unless pathologic thrombolysis is occurring.

MISCELLANEOUS FACTOR DEFICIENCY TESTS

Specific quantification tests, most utilizing monoclonal technology, exist for proteins C and S, antithrombin III, factor VIII, vWF, and antiplatelet antibodies. Mixing tests may be performed to diagnose rarer coagulation factor deficiencies. Plasma from the patient is mixed with known-factor-deficient samples and normal specimens. Continued prolongation of coagulation time with known-factor-depleted specimens and normalization with control samples provides evidence for that particular factor's absence in the patient's blood.

Thrombosis and Thromboembolism

Thrombus formation is a natural and beneficial response to threats to the integrity of the vascular system; however, a number of situations exist where the thrombotic process may become detrimental.

In 1899, Welch defined a thrombus as a solid mass or plug formed in the living heart or vessels from blood components. A clot, however, is defined as extravascular or postmortem endovascular coagulation.

The thrombus is a mixture of platelets, fibrin, leukocytes, and erythrocytes. White or **conglutination thrombi** consist primarily of platelets and fibrin with few leukocytes. Red or **coagulation thrombi** consist mainly of erythrocytes enmeshed in a fibrin network. These are dark, red, and elastic and resemble the in vitro clot. Intermediate forms are termed **mixed.** The platelet content is directly related to flow in the vessel where the thrombus occurs. In the arterial system, thrombi tend to have a larger platelet component. Also, platelets tend to deposit on the upstream side of the thrombus creating a conglutination type thrombus with coagulation-type thrombus downstream. This produces a white "head" and a red "tail."

The postmortem clot consists of fibrin gels in which the formed elements of blood become trapped. These clots are dark red, moist, and elastic, and may conform to the lumen of the vessel.

Virchow's triad describes the basic requirements for the thrombotic process—alterations of vessel wall integrity, blood coagulability, and blood flow. Thrombogenic factors and protective mechanisms now recognized are summarized in Table 5-2.

Damage to the vessel wall exposes the subendothelium, to which platelets are readily adherent. Platelet aggregation leads to formation of a platelet plug. These processes may contribute to the activation of coagulation by either the intrinsic, extrinsic, or common path-

TABLE 5-2. Thrombogenic Factors and Protective Mechanisms

Thrombogenic Factors
 Vessel wall damage
 Stimulation of platelet aggregation
 Stasis
 Activation of coagulation

Protective Mechanisms
 Intact endothelium
 Protease inhibitors
 Dilution by blood flow
 Hepatic coagulation factor degradation
 Fibrinolysis

way. Factor XII may become activated by exposure to damaged endothelium or prosthetic material, and tissue thromboplastin released from damaged areas activates factor VII. Platelet procoagulant activity may directly activate factor X.

Damage to the vessel wall may also change the dynamics of regional blood flow. Stasis prevents dilution of coagulation factors and delivery of factors to sites of degradation such as the liver.

Both local and systemic mechanisms exist to protect against thrombosis. Local dilution of factors by blood flow is extremely important in smaller vessels. Numerous antithrombotic substances are produced locally by the endothelial cell including PGI$_2$, thrombomodulin, and heparin. Systemic protective mechanisms include circulating protease inhibitors and the plasminogen/plasmin fibrinolytic system. Hepatic degradation of coagulation factors occurs by hepatic protease inhibitors and active phagocytosis by Kupffer cells.

Although thrombi may occur in the microcirculation, it is rare, due to ongoing fibrinolysis. Thrombi that do occur in the venules, capillaries, and arterioles are simple in nature. Direct injury usually produces pure platelet thrombi; hypercoagulable states produce simple fibrin thrombi; and low flow states lead to red cell aggregates (sludge).

Regardless of the nature of the inciting event—stasis, vascular wall injury, hypercoagulability, or excessive stimulation of the coagulation cascade—a thrombus may be dissolved, continue to **propagate, organize** and/ or possibly **embolize**.

Although even the simplest capillary platelet plug can be onerous, depending on its location, vascular occlusion and distal embolic sequelae usually result

from a thrombus that continues to propagate. Thrombi usually extend downstream, but can extend in an upstream (retrograde) fashion. Propagation of the thrombus becomes self-driven at some point as platelets adhere to the exposed thrombus, the thrombus grows to partially occlude the vessel, and creates stasis—promoting more thrombosis in the area of stagnant flow.

Freshly formed and forming fibrin are most sensitive to dissolution via the plasmin system. Once factor XIII begins to cross-link the fibrin strands, fibrinolysis is greatly slowed, allowing propagation and organization. Fibrinolytic activity may be much higher in the venous then the arterial system.

Whether or not a propagated thrombus will organize is determined within 48 hours. During this period the thrombus loosens and fibrin interdigitates into interstices between adherent platelets. Neutrophils and mononuclear cells appear and secrete proteolytic enzymes. Within a week, the total fibrin content of the thrombus is greatly diminished, neutrophils disappear, and monocytes increase in number—phagocytosing debris and even whole platelets. During the same time period, elongated cells similar to smooth muscle cells penetrate and cover the thrombus under the influence of platelet mitogens such as platelet-derived growth factor. The adjacent endothelial cells then begin to grow over the mass from its margins.

By 2 weeks, the organizing thrombus consists of a partial covering of endothelial and smooth muscle cells, an underlying layer of granulation tissue with a mixture of collagen and, below this, a layer of residual debris. During the following weeks, complete endothelialization occurs, thrombogenesis ceases at the site, and the underlying tissue becomes a mixture of smooth muscle and collagen with some elastic fibrils. The organized thrombus may persist as a mural plaque or be completely incorporated and nondiscernible from the vessel wall.

The rate of organization may be greatly influenced by the dynamics of the vessel wall. Active inflammation at a viable vessel wall may speed up the process of organization, whereas a severely damaged, low-viability vascular wall (thick atherosclerotic plaque, ventricular aneurysm, fibrotic aneurysmal wall of vessel) may preclude total organization and lead to the development of masses of inspissated fibrin, which are prone to embolization.

New channel formation in the organizing occlusive thrombus is termed **recanalization**. These channels usually result from a combination of thrombus retrac-

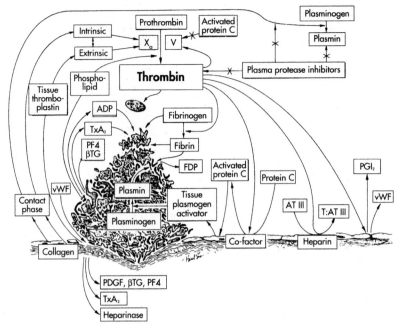

Figure 5-7 Interactions among hemostatic components. (Reproduced from Thompson AR, Harker LA, eds. *Manual of hemostasis and thrombosis.* 3rd ed. Philadelphia: FA Davis, 1983:42.)

tion and fibrinolysis, and mural components may reform if flow is vigorous.

A thromboembolus is a thrombus or portion of a thrombus dislodged by flow or mechanical force. Most emboli show few or no signs of organization, since an organized thrombus is less likely to break apart or dislodge. Unorganized thromboemboli may therefore be removed quickly by the fibrinolytic system if the insult caused by embolism and occlusion does not threaten survival.

Conclusion

It is important to understand that the various components of the hemostatic system—platelets, endothelium, coagulation factors, and fibrinolytics—do not function alone. These constituents maintain hemostatic homeostasis by virtue of a complicated, interrelated system of concurrent interdependent events (Figure 5-7).

It is also important to remember that the majority of the foregoing descriptions of component function have

been elucidated by in vitro techniques. There is strong evidence to suggest that in vivo hemostatic function may differ greatly, and that many interactions between and within components have yet to be discovered.

Bibliography

Colman RW, Hirsch J, Marder VJ, Salzman EW, eds. *Hemostasis and thrombosis: basic principles and clinical practice.* 2nd ed. Philadelphia: JB Lippincott, 1987.

Goth A, ed. *Medical pharmacology: principles and concepts.* 11th ed. St. Louis: CV Mosby, 1984.

McEvoy GK, ed. *AHFS drug information 90.* Bethesda: American Society of Hospital Pharmacists, 1990.

Rick ME. Protein C and protein S: vitamin K-dependent inhibitors of blood coagulation. *JAMA* 1990;263(5):701–703.

Thompson AR, Harker LA, eds. *Manual of hemostasis and thrombosis.* 3rd ed. Philadelphia: FA Davis, 1983.

Widmann FK. *Clinical interpretation of laboratory tests.* 9th ed. Philadelphia: FA Davis, 1984.

Williams WJ, Beutler E, Erslev AJ, Lichtman MA, eds. *Hematology.* 4th ed. New York: McGraw-Hill, 1990.

Michael F. Rotondo

6 PHYSIOLOGY OF TRANSFUSION THERAPY

The first successful transfusion was performed over 300 years ago by Richard Lower in 1669. Since then, the practice of transfusion has developed on a foundation of tradition rather than on physiologic rationale. The purpose of this chapter is to discuss the indications for transfusion based on the physiology of blood cells and clotting factors. Furthermore, the complications of this therapy with regard to immunity, infection, and metabolism are discussed.

Indications for Transfusion

The indications for transfusion can be divided into two broad categories. The most common indication is to enhance the oxygen-carrying capacity of blood by expanding the red cell mass. The second broad indication is to replace clotting factors, either lost, consumed, or not produced.

ENHANCEMENT OF OXYGEN-CARRYING CAPACITY

The majority of arterial blood oxygen binds with hemoglobin reversibly. This allows the hemoglobin molecule to serve as a carrier for oxygen, which can be released to the tissues on demand. If cardiac output is adequate, increasing the red cell mass will increase the oxygen-carrying capacity of blood. However, it's not quite this simple. Release of oxygen to the tissues is dependent on many factors. The oxygen saturation of hemoglobin is probably the most important. The saturation of hemoglobin molecules with oxygen determines the binding affinity. As the degree of saturation increases, the binding affinity decreases and the release of oxygen to the tissues is enhanced. The partial pressure of oxygen required to saturate 50% of the hemoglobin molecules is called the P_{50} value (see Figure 4-3). The P_{50} value is increased with fever, acidosis, and increased 2,3-diphosphoglycerate (2,3-DPG); thus oxygen is released to the tissues with greater ease under these conditions. However, with hypothermia, alkalosis, and decreased 2,3-DPG, oxygen-binding affinity is increased and release to the tissues is decreased.

Adequate tissue oxygenation is not only dependent upon adequate oxygen delivery, but also on tissue oxygen demands. Under normal circumstances, a large physiologic reservoir exists between oxygen delivery (1000 cc/min) and oxygen consumption (250 cc/min). Despite this large reserve, clinical circumstances, such as massive multisystem injury and sepsis, occur in which oxygen consumption outstrips oxygen delivery.

What then, is the best level of red cell mass such that oxygen delivery meets tissue oxygen demands? Hemoglobin normally ranges from 12 to 18 g/dL depending on the age, sex, and pre-existing medical condition.

Traditionally, a hemoglobin concentration of 10 g/dL has been considered to be the minimal acceptable level of hemoglobin prior to elective operative procedures. However, the limits of acceptability for hemoglobin concentration are currently being challenged. It is well known that a hemoglobin concentration of 6–7 g/dL is well tolerated in patients with chronic renal failure. Furthermore, it has been demonstrated that oxygen supply to the tissues during limited normovolemic hemodilution is well tolerated. A hemoglobin concentration of 7–8 g/dL has been demonstrated to be adequate except in patients with coronary artery disease or chronic obstructive pulmonary disease. Though the issue of best hemoglobin concentration is far from settled, it is clear that the rate and magnitude of blood loss, the state of tissue perfusion, and pre-existing cardiopulmonary disease all affect the ability of a patient to tolerate lower concentrations of hemoglobin.

One other important factor bears mentioning when considering transfusion of stored blood to enhance oxygen-carrying capacity. As previously noted, decreased levels of 2,3-DPG increase oxygen-hemoglobin binding affinity. In fact, 2,3-DPG levels may decrease by 30% in blood stored for greater than 2 weeks, and by 60–70% in 3 weeks. When transfused, this "old" blood has a significantly diminished ability to release oxygen to the tissues. Furthermore, in vivo restoration of 2,3-DPG can take as long as 24 to 48 hours in patients with metabolic abnormalities. Therefore, length of storage is a consideration when utilizing transfusions to enhance oxygen-carrying capacity. Fresh whole blood, citrate-phosphate-dextrose-adenine blood less than 14 days old, and cryopreserved red cells have enough 2,3-DPG for nearly normal oxygen release.

ENHANCEMENT OF HEMOSTASIS

The second most common indication for transfusion of blood products is for the repletion of hemostatic agents. An understanding of the pathophysiology of hemostasis (detailed in Chapter 5) is required prior to the use of replacement products. It is not safe practice to simply correct abnormal laboratory values or to blindly abide by traditional surgical dictums of transfusion. Replacement products should be used only in preparation for elective surgery or with clinically significant abnormalities in hemostasis. These abnormalities include disorders of consumption or production of fibrinogen, extrinsic or intrinsic coagulation factor defects, and platelet dysfunction.

Replacement Products

Appropriate use of replacement products is dependent upon knowledge of their physiologic effects and an understanding of their preparation for use. For example, consider the use of fresh whole blood as a replacement product. Fresh, warm, whole blood effectively restores red cell mass and plasma volume while providing hemostatic agents, including hormones, coagulation factors, and antibodies. It seems ideal. However, it is simply not feasible to have donors of each type available at a blood bank at a moment's notice. Furthermore, screening of blood for hepatitis B and acquired immunity deficiency syndrome (AIDS) necessitates a certain period of storage and time for testing. Therefore, though fresh whole blood appears to be the ideal product based on its physiologic properties, practical considerations concerning preparation preclude its use.

PRODUCTS THAT ENHANCE OXYGEN-CARRYING CAPACITY

Packed Red Blood Cells

Packed red blood cells are prepared by removing 200 cc of plasma from fresh whole blood to achieve a final hematocrit of 70–80%. Packed cells are anticoagulated with citrate-phosphate-dextrose (CPD) or Adsol (adenine, glucose, mannitol, and sodium chloride) and stored in liquid state at 4°C or frozen at -80°C.

Several factors affect the therapeutic efficacy of packed cell transfusions. The length of storage time determines the in vivo post-transfusion red cell survival. The longer the storage, the lower the rate of survival. Immediately transfused packed red blood cells yield a 90% 24-hour in vivo red cell survival rate. However, after 6 weeks of storage, survival is decreased to 65%. Furthermore, there is considerable variability in the volume and the hemoglobin concentration in a "standardized blood product unit." Prior to plasma extraction, volume can vary from 400 to 500 cc and concentration can range from 12 to 17 g/dL. It is easy to see then that the variability in volume, concentration, and cell survival affects the therapeutic efficacy of transfusion.

Cryopreserved Red Blood Cells

Cryopreservation may represent the best technique for storage of red blood cells. This technique utilizes rapid cooling of the packed cell to -80°C in a 40% glycerol solution. The 24-hour post-transfusion red cell survival of cryopreserved red cells is 80–90%, while 2,3-DPG levels are near normal and antigenic immune reactions are minimized. Furthermore, large quantities of red cells can be stockpiled for many years. However, this technique is not yet readily employed by most hospital blood banks.

Autotransfusion

Autotransfusion involves the collection and immediate reinfusion of the patient's own blood for volume repletion and increase in red cell mass. Patients with massive exsanguination from either blunt or penetrating trauma, without gross contamination with enteric contents, are usually the most appropriate candidates for autotransfusion. This method has obvious advantages regarding the elimination of risk of histocompatibility reactions and transmission of infectious disease.

The autotransfusion process is performed when massive amounts of shed blood are collected in a container, filtered, anticoagulated, and immediately returned to the patient at infusion rates as high as 700–800 cc/min. A processor can be added to this circuit that washes the cells to remove debris. In the process, plasma cofactors and oncotic proteins of blood are removed and saline is added. This portion of the cycle adds approximately 15 minutes in turnaround time to transfusion.

As with all therapeutic maneuvers, autotransfusion is not without risk. The most common complication is thrombocytopenia. When patients receive greater than 4 L of autologous processed blood, the platelet count may drop below 50,000. In addition, plasma-free hemoglobin is elevated and the risk of acute tubular necrosis is increased. This is of particular importance when accompanied by shock or acidosis. Other complications include air embolism, particulate microemboli, and disseminated intravascular coagulation.

Pre-Donation

Pre-donation of blood products prior to elective surgery has recently increased with the rise in public awareness of transmission of infection with blood transfusion. This concept has significant advantages to the patient regarding alloimmunization and transfusion reactions. Blood storage in pre-donation is similar to storage of packed red blood cells (42 day maximum in Adsol). Con-

traindications for pre-donation include significant coronary artery disease, chronic obstructive pulmonary disease, and the existence of a primary hematologic disorder.

Red Cell Substitutes

Currently, two acellular oxygen carriers are being evaluated as red cell substitutes. They are polymerized or pyridoxylated hemoglobin solution, and fluorocarbon emulsion (Fluosol-DA-20%). Experimental models have demonstrated that both products can maintain normal levels of oxygen consumption, carbon dioxide production, and circulatory dynamics in the virtual absence of red blood cells. Although both of these solutions satisfy the most important criteria for a red cell substitute, their safety and efficacy has not yet been established. Therefore, neither product can be used for standard care in patients with hemorrhagic shock or chronic anemia, or in those who refuse blood transfusion.

PRODUCTS THAT ENHANCE HEMOSTASIS

Fresh Frozen Plasma

Fresh frozen plasma is the plasma component of whole blood. It is separated within 6 hours of collection and frozen at 8°C. This temperature has been chosen to protect Factors V and VIII in particular. Fresh frozen plasma contains components of the **coagulation, fibrolytic** and **complement** systems. It is useful in the treatment of deficiencies in Factors II, V, VII, VIII, IX, X, and XI. Furthermore, it is useful in warfarin-induced anticoagulation, antithrombin III deficiency, and to treat humoral immunologic deficiencies. Fresh frozen plasma is a single donor product with the same risk of hepatitis and AIDS as packed red blood cells. Since it contains the major anti-A, B, and Rh antibodies, type- and Rh-specific plasma should be used. Certain allergic reactions may occur, ranging from urticaria to fatal noncardiac pulmonary edema, with the administration of fresh frozen plasma.

Cryoprecipitate

Cryoprecipitate is the second most commonly used coagulation enhancer available in the blood bank. It is formed as a plasma concentrate that consists primarily of **factor VIII** (100 clotting units) and **fibrinogen** (250 mg). In addition, it contains factor XIII, von Willebrand's factor, and fibronectin. Cryoprecipitate is stored at 37°C. Temperatures in excess of this destroy factor VIII. Cryoprecipitate is used to replenish factor VIII or fibrinogen. Its main disadvantage lies in the greater risk of disease transmission due to multiple donors and a slightly increased risk for hemolytic reactions due to the small amounts of anti-A, anti-B, and Rh antibodies leftover in product preparation.

Platelets

Platelets are collected by repeated centrifugation of fresh whole blood and subsequent suspension in 30–50 cc of plasma at 22°C. They are preserved in liquid form, remain viable for up to 5 days, and are most efficacious if used within 24–48 hours of pooling. After that time, they lose their ability to produce **thromboxane A_2**, a potent vasoconstrictor and platelet aggregator.

As with packed red blood cells, the number of platelets present in a "unit" is variable, thereby yielding variable therapeutic effectiveness with transfusion. The number of platelets can vary from 6×10^{10} to 22×10^{10} platelets per unit. The risk of infectious complications is directly proportional to the number of donors. In all instances, donor plasma is present and platelets must be ABO and Rh compatible with the recipient's blood.

Coagulation Factor Concentrates

Coagulation factor concentrates exist in commercially prepared forms for patients in need of factor VIII (hemophiliacs) and for patients with prothrombin complex factor deficiencies (II, VII, IX, X). With the excep-

TABLE 6-1. Coagulation Factor Concentrates

Factor	Required Replacement Level (%)	Product Form
II	15–20	PRBC/Concentrate
VII	5–30	PRBC/Concentrate
VIII	30	FFP/Concentrate/ Cryoprecipitate
IX	20–30	PRBL/FFP/Concentrate
X	15–20	PRBL/Concentrate

Adapted from Schwartz SI et al. *Principles of surgery.* 4th ed. New York: McGraw-Hill, 1984:107.

tion of factor VIII, most coagulation factor concentrates are rarely used in elective surgical patients (Table 6-1).

Complications of Transfusion

Complications associated with transfusion of blood and its companion products can be serious and sometimes fatal. These complications can be divided into immunologic reactions, metabolic disturbances, and infectious complications (Figure 6-1).

IMMUNOLOGIC REACTIONS

Red Cell Type

Immediate hemolytic reactions occur when red blood cells of Group A or B are infused into a recipient normally lacking that blood group antigen. These are most often caused by errors in sample labeling or patient misidentification. Only a small percentage result from laboratory failure of the type and cross-match. The clinical signs and symptoms of an immediate hemolytic reaction begin soon after the transfusion has been started. These manifestations include change in mental status, shortness of breath, hypotension, back pain, or substernal chest pain. Moreover, facial flushing, distention of neck veins, cyanosis, tachycardia, and profound shock can follow shortly thereafter. This process may end in disseminated intravascular coagulation, acute renal failure, and death.

It was initially believed that acute renal failure in this setting was due to precipitation of hemoglobin within the renal tubules. Under normal circumstances, circulating haptoglobin is capable of binding free hemoglobin in the plasma. This complex is cleared by the reticuloendothelial system. If the haptoglobin binding capacity is exceeded, free hemoglobin circulates and combines with albumin to form methemalbumin. When this mechanism for hemoglobin clearance is overcome, hemoglobinuria occurs, and a small amount of hemoglobin is precipitated within the renal tubules. More importantly, hypotension and vasoconstriction cause a reduction in renal blood flow and subsequent fibrin thrombi deposition in the renal tubules. Stroma-antibody complexes released into circulation exacerbate this process and renal failure ensues. The range of renal failure can vary from mild to severe, ending in complete renal failure with bilateral renal cortical necrosis.

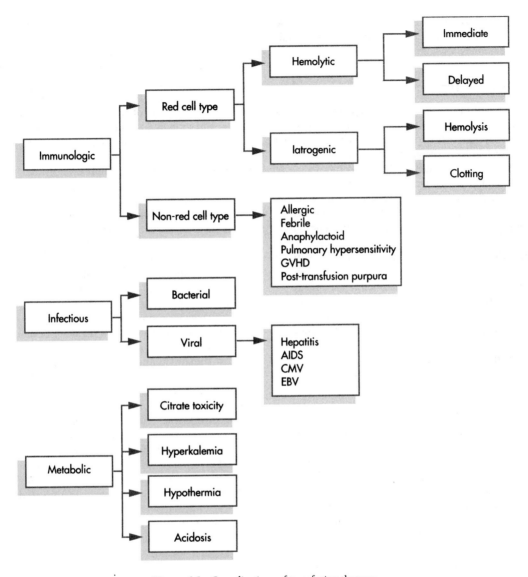

Figure 6-1 Complications of transfusion therapy.

A **delayed form** of hemolytic transfusion reaction infrequently seen is related to red cell antigens other than A and B. It can occur 3–21 days after blood is infused and symptoms include malaise and fever. Laboratory studies demonstrate a low hemoglobin and elevation of the indirect bilirubin fraction. The Coomb's test will be positive though no serologic incompatibility is present. The etiology of this reaction is likely to be an anamestic response related to prior transfusion or pregnancy, and not a primary immunologic response.

Two other forms of red cell reactions are worth mentioning. **Iatrogenic hemolysis** is induced if blood is administered with 5% dextrose and water, rather than with saline. These patients will present with signs and symptoms of immediate massive hemolysis. **Iatrogenic clotting** will occur if blood is administered with a calcium containing solution such as lactated ringers. If these clots are pushed into the circulation, massive pulmonary emboli will result.

Non–Red-Cell Type

Allergic reactions are caused by the passive transfer of sensitizing antibodies or the transfusion of antigens to which the recipient is hypersensitive. These reactions may occur following the administration of packed red blood cells, plasma, or factor VIII concentrates and are usually manifested by urticaria chills, itching, and fever. This simple allergic reaction occurs relatively frequently, accounting for reactions in 2% of transfusions. In rare instances, the reaction may be severe enough to cause anaphylactic shock.

Febrile reactions represent the vast majority of untoward transfusion reactions and are seen in approximately 7% of all blood product recipients. This reaction is due to antileukocyte antibodies that develop as a result of prior transfusions. The frequency of this reaction increases with repeated transfusions. The presenting manifestations include fever, chills, flushing, and tachycardia. This may progress to hypertension, cyanosis, and a syndrome of self-limited fibrinolysis. On rare occasions, this reaction can progress to complete cardiovascular collapse. The total number of leukocytes contained in the blood product, the rate of transfusion, and the level of recipient antibody titers all determine the severity of the nonhemolytic febrile reaction. Though this is the most common form of transfusion reaction, one must rule out red cell incompatibility and bacterial contamination when it occurs.

Anaphylactoid reactions can occur when the recipient is sensitized to IgA, a common immunoglobin. These patients present with a spectrum of clinical manifestations including fever, chills, bronchospasm, diarrhea, abdominal pain and total vascular collapse.

Pulmonary hypersensitivity reactions can also occur. The exact etiology of this phenomenon is unclear. Leukocyte antigen, as well as microaggregates accumulated in stored blood, have been implicated. The patients present with normovolemic pulmonary edema. Animal models have demonstrated an increase in shunt fraction and a diminished pulmonary diffusing capacity after transfusion. It is unclear if these same alterations in normal physiology occur during a pulmonary hypersensitivity reaction in man. In this regard, the exact role of blood transfusions and the development of pulmonary dysfunction in man remains unclear.

Graft-vs-Host Disease (GVHD) occurs following the infusion of donor lymphocytes in an immunocompromised recipient. Consequently, the infused donor lymphocytes initiate rejection of the host's normal tissue. Conversely, the recipient is incapable of rejecting the foreign cells. Patients with cell-mediated immune deficiency, recipients of allogeneic bone marrow transplants, and individuals with primary immunodeficiencies who receive viable immunocompetent lymphocytes are at particular risks for acute GVHD. Blood products containing these insighting lymphocytes include: packed red blood cells, buffy coats, granulocytes, fresh plasma, and platelets. Clinical manifestations involve many organ systems including skin, liver, gastrointestinal tract, and bone marrow. These reactions begin as generalized erythroderma beginning first on the face, and spreading to the trunk and extremities. This can be followed by bullous formation and skin slough. Biopsy will demonstrate extensive lymphocyte infiltration. Shortly thereafter, anorexia, nausea, vomiting, diarrhea, hepatocellular degeneration, and pancytopenia can occur. Ultimately, death occurs as a result of bone marrow aplasia, hypoplasia, and failure of regeneration.

Post-transfusion purpura occurs in patients lacking PL^{A1} antigen, which is present in 99% of the normal population. It can occur up to one week after blood transfusion and results from an acute hemorrhagic thrombocytopenia. The classic presentation is that of an older female (age 30–70) with a previous history of pregnancy without history of prior transfusions. The clinical manifestations include skin and mucous membrane bleeding with a platelet count less than 10,000. This thrombocytopenic state may last from 10 days to 2 months and seems to be somewhat mitigated by exchange transfusion and plasmapheresis. Platelet replacement is contraindicated, and indeed exacerbates the situation by inducing an autoimmune thrombocytopenia and severe febrile reactions.

INFECTIOUS COMPLICATIONS

Bacterial Contamination

Nineteen percent of all fatal transfusion reactions involve blood products with significant contamination. Its been reported that 1–2% of all blood product units may be contaminated with bacteria. The most common cold-growing, endotoxin-producing, gram-negative organisms are **klebsiellae** and **pseudomonads,** identified in 68% of the reported reactions. Gram-positive organisms responsible for bacterial infections are most commonly staphylococci. Contamination arises from bacteremia in the donor, organisms on the skin of the donor, or from airborne organisms. Patients will present with symptoms including hypotension, fever, abdominal or extremity pain, and at times, with a complete picture of sepsis. The onset of symptoms occurs shortly after transfusion begins, and if the patient survives the acute episode, temperature spikes and pain recur at 12-hour intervals. Though this may be difficult to differentiate from a red cell hemolytic reaction by symptomatology, hemolysis does not usually occur with a bacterial infection reaction. Therefore, the absence of the hemoglobin in the urine and the presence of bacteria in the donor blood product confirms the diagnosis. Despite aggressive supportive measures and cessation of the transfusion, mortality ranges from 50 to 80%.

Viral Contamination

Hepatitis is the most commonly transmitted disease related to the use of blood products. The transmission rate is affected by the geographical area in which the donor products are obtained, and ranges from approximately 2.5–8% risk per unit transfused. This risk increases as the number of transfusions increases. The ability to prevent transmission of hepatitis is limited by the inability to detect all sero-types of hepatitis in the donor blood product. So far, four types of hepatitis have been identified: infectious (type A), serum (type B), delta (type D), and type non-A, non-B. Sensitive assays for antibodies associated with types A and B are easily identified and the viruses are well characterized. For this reason, types A and B hepatitis associated with transfusion are rare. An assay is currently available for the delta agent responsible for hepatitis D. Therefore, hepatitis D represents a small risk to the recipient. The most common form of hepatitis transmitted is the non-A, non-B type, responsible for 85–98% of post-transfusion hepatitis cases. Its insidious course includes an incubation period up to eight weeks and generally presents as mild elevations of liver enzymes in anicteric, asymptomatic patients. However, the clinical presentation varies along a spectrum from mild symptoms to a fulminant hepatitis. Non-A, non-B hepatitis may persist in its chronic from in 50% of patients. In 1989, the blood-borne agent responsible for non-A, non-B hepatitis, identified as hepatitis C virus (HCV) was isolated. Furthermore, the immunoassay to detect specific anti-HCV antibodies has been developed. Early studies indicate that routine screening of blood donors for anti-HCV antibody should prevent approximately half the cases of transfusions associated hepatitis.

Though the transmission of **(AIDS)** may occur with blood transfusion, the risk is rather low. The estimated per unit risk for developing AIDS is approximately 0.02–0.03 %. In fact, only 1-2% of all AIDS cases result from transfusion of blood products. It is believed that with improved screening of donors with known risk factors and testing of donated blood products for the human immunodeficiency virus (HIV), the rate of transmission will decrease even further. The main difficulty in screening donors, as well as blood products, is the existence of viremia for up to 6 weeks without clinically detectable antibody production.

Other viral infections such as **cytomegalovirus** and **Epstein-Barr virus** are associated with transfusion infections. They occur most commonly in immunocompromised patients including premature infants and transplant recipients. Presentation of the virus can vary from a self-limited mild febrile illness in the healthy individual to extensive disseminated disease in the immunocompromised patient.

METABOLIC DISTURBANCES

Metabolic complications of transfusions occur most frequently in the setting of rapid exsanguination necessitating infusion of large amounts of blood products. This is a common scenario in the patient suffering from penetrating trauma to a vital vascular region or complex, blunt, multisystem injury. **Massive transfusion** is defined as replacement equal to the recipient's blood volume over a short period of time. In fact, it is not uncommon for patients to receive replacement of multiple blood volumes within hours after admission. Soon after, patients may develop obvious signs of coagulopathy. This is predominantly a dilutional effect resulting from the transfusion of packed red blood cells devoid of platelets, factor V, and factor VIII. It can be countered by the concurrent administration of fresh frozen plasma and platelets. Moreover, under these extreme conditions, the metabolic effects of multiple transfusions become apparent.

Citrate Intoxication

Citrate toxicity occurs as a result of the anticoagulation agents used in the preservation of banked blood. Normally, plasma citric acid concentration is approximately 1 mg/dL. The addition of CPD or Adsol increases the concentration of citrate significantly. Under normal circumstances, during the transfusion of small amounts of blood in healthy, warm, and well-perfused patients, the citrate load is easily metabolized. However, in the setting of massive transfusion, when the exsanguinating patient is hypothermic and in shock, citrate toxicity becomes a significant clinical entity.

Citrate binds calcium on a molar basis, which can result in near complete binding of ionized calcium and severe hypocalcemia. This may be manifested as cardiac electrical instability. Electrocardiographic changes, including prolongation of the QT interval, pulses alternans, and depression of P and T waves, may precede irreversible ventricular fibrillation. Moreover, citrate has a direct myocardial depressant effect, independent of its calcium-binding capabilities.

These toxic effects can be minimized by the administration of replacement calcium during massive transfusion. The precise amount and rate of replacement has been a source of controversy in the past. With the refined techniques of serum ionized calcium quantification, calcium supplementation can be determined based on measured levels. However, in the setting of rapid exsanguination and massive transfusion, measurement of ionized serum calcium may not be practical. In this case, empiric supplementation at a rate of 1 gram of calcium chloride for every 4-6 units of packed red blood cells transfused should take place.

Potassium Abnormalities

Post-transfusion hyperkalemia exists as a theoretical possibility. As a consequence of adenosine-triphosphate–pump inactivation, which occurs during prolonged periods of blood storage, potassium levels of stored blood can reach up to 70 mEq/L. This is due to shift of potassium out of red cells. The degree of potassium migration is dependent upon the type of anticoagulation used and the length of storage. Upon the transfusion of the blood product, the transfused red cells take up the previously released potassium so that the true transfused potassium load is relatively small. Moreover, if the potassium concentration is 70 mEq/L and each unit of blood contains approximately 100 cc of plasma, then 10 units of blood must be transfused to achieve infusion levels of 70 mEq/L of potassium. When hyperkalemia does result after mass transfusion, it is most likely secondary to other factors such as hypothermia, uncontrolled acidosis, and shock.

Hypothermia

One telling side effect of mass transfusion is hypothermia that can occur with infusion of blood normally stored at 4°C. Infusion of cold solutions can lower core temperatures significantly and predispose the patient to ventricular arrhythmias. Furthermore, hypothermia causes a leftward shift in the hemoglobin-oxygen dissociation curve thereby decreasing oxygen release to the tissues. Moreover, citrate metabolism is impaired and the binding of ionized calcium is intensified. This can be avoided by warming all fluids given prior to infusion, particularly blood. A simple well-known technique involving a mixture of normal saline heated to 38°C with cold blood, results in a blood infusion temperature of 21°C without detrimental effects in the red blood cells. Rapid infusion of warmed blood will help alleviate the deleterious effects of massive transfusion hypothermia.

Acid-Base Abnormalities

Theoretically, transfusion of large quantities of blood, in and of itself, can result in acidosis because of the nature of some anticoagulation agents used for storage. This concern has diminished with the use of packed red blood cells anticoagulated with CPD. Most often, persistent metabolic acidosis after massive transfusion indicates a prolonged period of hypoperfusion rather than iatrogenic acidosis secondary to administration of blood products.

Bibliography

Choo QL, Kuo G, Weiner AJ, Overby LR, Bradley DW, Houghton M. Isolation of a DNA clone derived from a blood-borne non-A, non-B viral hepatitis genome. *Science* 1989;244:359–62.

Civetta JM, Taylor RW, Kirby RR. *Critical care.* Philadelphia: JB Lippincott, 1988.

Esteban JI, Gonzalez A, Hernandez JM, Viladomiu L, Sanchez C, Lopez-Talavera JC, Lucea D, Martin-Vega C, Vidal X, Esteban R, et al. Evaluation of antibodies to hepatitis C virus in a study of transfusion-associated hepatitis. *N Engl J Med* 1990;18:323(16):1107–12.

Food & Drug Administration, Records on Transfusion Fatalities, 1979–1985.

Gould SA, Moss GS. Red cell substitutes: an update. *Ann Emerg Med* 1985;798:803.

Gould SA, Rice, CL, Moss GS. The physiologic basis of the use of the blood and blood products. *Surg Annu* 1984;16:13.

Jarrell BE, Carabasi III RA, eds. *Surgery*. Pennsylvania: Harwal Publishing, 1986.

Lyons AS, Petrucelli II JR. *Medicine: an illustrated history*. New York: Harry N. Abrams, 1978.

Mattox KL., Moore EE, Feliciano DV, eds. *Trauma*. Connecticut: Appleton & Lange, 1988.

Messmer K, Sunder-Plassman C, Jesch F, et al. Oxygen supply to the tissues during limited normovolemic hemodilution. *Res Exp Med* 1973;159:152.

Sabiston Jr DC. *Textbook of surgery: the biological basis of modern surgical practice*. Philadelphia: WB Saunders, 1986.

Schwartz SI, Shires GT, Spencer FC, Storer E, eds. *Principles of surgery*. 4th ed. New York: McGraw-Hill, 1984.

Woodson, RD. Importance of 2,3-DPG in banked blood: new data in animal models. In Collins JA, Murowski K, Shafer AW. *Massive transfusion in surgery and trauma*. New York: Alan R. Liss, 1982:69–78.

Joseph B. Shrager

7 HOMEOSTATIC MECHANISMS IN SHOCK, TRAUMA, AND SEPSIS

The human body contains a wide array of complex systems that function to maintain a stable internal milieu, allowing optimal function of each of the various organ systems and contributing to the survival of the organism. These homeostatic systems act continuously under normal conditions, when the body is not stressed by external forces to any great degree. The mechanisms underlying these normal physiologic responses are detailed throughout this book. This chapter traces the responses of these systems as the body is subjected to the most severe challenges to the maintenance of homeostasis—trauma, shock, and sepsis.

The array of metabolic and physiologic responses that initiate and aid recovery from a major stress, although quite complex, follow a general pattern. This pattern includes a general acceleration of body metabolism with degradation of muscle protein (negative nitrogen balance) and the generation of extra energy substrates from endogenous sources, the restitution of decreased circulating blood volume via temporary derangements in normal electrolyte and water balance, and the production of new cells and molecular products that contribute to host defense and healing. The current understanding of both the mechanisms of successful restoration of normal physiology and the deleterious side effects of these mechanisms will be reviewed.

Responses to Trauma and Sepsis: An Organ System Approach

PULMONARY AND CARDIOVASCULAR RESPONSES

Shock is the end result of overwhelming trauma or sepsis. It can be defined as inadequate tissue perfusion or inadequate oxygen delivery. Even in preshock traumatic or septic states, oxygen is in great demand. It is essential to the efficient metabolism of the energy that is required to support reparative processes. Without sufficient oxygen delivery, glycolysis with lactic acid generation takes place, often accompanied by clinical deterioration. Thus, **a cardiopulmonary response must occur which increases oxygen delivery dramatically.** This is accomplished by (1) increased blood flow in essential tissues largely as a result of local stimuli to arteriolar vasodilatation; (2) shifts in the HbO_2 dissociation curve that promote oxygen release, secondary to changes in tissue temperature and pH; (3) increased cardiac output secondary to increases in heart rate, preload, and contractility; and (4) increased oxygenation of blood passing through the lungs.

The most commonly employed therapeutic intervention to increase cardiac output is raising the preload with volume infusions. In a patient with a normal heart whose preload is decreased by hemorrhage, third space fluid accumulations, or decreased peripheral vascular tone, higher preload will result in increased cardiac output until the transition point on the Frank-Starling curve is reached. It is difficult to reach this point in otherwise healthy patients who are in hypovolemic shock after trauma. In contrast, in septic patients, who may have diminished myocardial contractility secondary to circulating toxic agents, volume alone may not have a significant effect. It is in these patients that inotropic agents generally become necessary.

In the lung, it is the pathologic rather than physiologic responses to injury which are most prominent. Adult respiratory distress syndrome or noncardiogenic pulmonary edema may follow a number of initiating events, including sepsis, aspiration, chest trauma, and even ischemic bowel disease. This diversity of initiating events suggests several pathways to a common injury. It is currently believed that agents or events that trigger inflammatory reactions with the release of vasoactive agents and the stimulation of abnormally armed leukocytes play a central role in the pathogenesis of this disorder. The end result of this blood-borne injury is disruption of the capillary endothelium and alveolar epithelium, resulting in alveolar flooding, hypoxemia, and diminished functional residual capacity and compliance.

RENAL RESPONSE—FLUIDS AND ELECTROLYTES

A reduction in effective circulating volume occurs in virtually all injuries and sepsis, either from hemorrhage, pump failure, diminished vascular tone, or third space losses. **The neuroendocrine response to injury (described below) induces alterations in renal and circulatory functions that tend to return the patient toward salt and water balance.** First, catecholamines cause prompt vasoconstriction, reducing capillary hydrostatic pressure. This alters the Starling forces such that interstitial salt and water return to the intravascular space. In the kidney, there are a number of changes that result in net reabsorption of salt and water, including (1) autoregulation to maintain the glomerular filtration rate (GFR) despite reduced renal perfusion pressure, (2) increased tubular salt and water reabsorption, and (3) redistribution of blood flow from cortical nephrons to "salt saving" juxtamedullary nephrons.

A severe hemorrhagic or septic insult sometimes overwhelms renal autoregulatory mechanisms, causing marked reductions in both the renal blood flow and GFR, resulting in oliguria and decreased clearance of waste. This may culminate in acute renal failure. A less severe low-flow insult to the kidneys may result in nonoliguric renal insufficiency.

Mild to moderately injured patients generally display a metabolic alkalosis as a result of hydrogen wasting in the distal tubules. It is only with severe hypoperfusion and resultant anaerobic metabolism that metabolic acidosis from lactate production supervenes.

Although the kidneys and cardiovascular system do their utmost to restore effective circulating volume, these responses are often inadequate in severe injuries. For this reason exogenous fluids are administered. An ongoing debate has raged regarding the relative benefits of **crystalloid versus colloid** solutions. It has been argued that albumin, blood, and other colloids are optimal resuscitation fluids, since they restore intravascular oncotic pressure and thereby reduce or reverse transcapillary fluid efflux, secondarily reducing lung water and improving oxygenation. Such a suggestion is based on the assumption that albumin will remain in the vascular space, but this assumption may be invalid, particularly in patients with sepsis or in shock who manifest increased vascular permeability. It is clear that approximately twice as much crystalloid as colloid is required to maintain normal filling pressures in shock patients. Available studies show, however, no increase in lung water in animals or humans when crystalloid is used. In fact, there is some evidence from clinical trials of albumin supplementation that albumin may accumulate in the lung interstitium and that it may cause a deleterious fall in GFR due to increased osmotic pressure within the glomeruli. Hetastarch is a plasma volume expander which appears to stay in the vascular space for several days. However, it causes prolongation of the partial thromboplastin time and for this reason has been used with caution. Finally, fluorocarbons have been proposed as a blood substitute that expands plasma volume and carries and releases oxygen to the tissues, but clinical applicability of this solution is pending.

In summary, it would seem that there is no clear advantage to using colloid over crystalloid. Further rationale for the use of crystalloid does exist. First, in shock states there is loss not only of shed blood or intravascular volume, but also of functional extracellular volume as interstitial fluid moves into muscle cells. To restore both of these spaces, a salt solution would be most appropriate. Secondly, crystalloids such as Ringer's lactate may partially correct any metabolic acidosis that may be present in severe shock. Finally, they decrease blood viscosity and may enhance perfusion of the microvasculature.

METABOLIC RESPONSE

More than 50 years ago Cuthbertson divided the metabolic response to injury into a short lived "ebb" phase during which there are no marked alterations in energy handling, and a longer "flow" phase characterized by **catabolism** and a **negative nitrogen balance.** Metabolic changes associated with shock and illness are detailed in Figure 7-1. Septic patients exhibit a state similar to the "flow" phase of trauma. The maximal increase in resting energy expenditure in injured patients occurs approximately 1 week post-injury and coincides with the maximal rate of protein catabolism. Postulated mechanisms for this increased heat production include resetting hypothalamic regulatory mechanisms and inefficient recycling of glucose and triglycerides, causing adenosine triphosphate hydrolysis; a process known to occur at an increased rate in trauma patients. The mechanisms of metabolism of each of the individual substrates—glucose, fat, ketone and protein—are altered in the integrated metabolic response to trauma and sepsis.

Sepsis and the immediate posttraumatic ebb phase are characterized by **hyperglycemia.** This is initially the result of increased glycogenolysis, but later it stems from increased glucose production in the liver coupled with reduced peripheral utilization. During the flow phase, glucose levels fall to normal or slightly elevated levels. This **conversion of fuel reserves into glucose** would seem to have adaptive value in trauma and sepsis, as a number of vital organs—including the brain, peripheral nerves, renal medulla, red and white cells, and inflammatory tissue—all utilize glucose as a primary fuel.

Lipolysis is enhanced immediately after injury despite hyperglycemia and elevated insulin levels. Worsening sepsis is frequently accompanied by a progressive fall in the respiratory quotient, suggesting increased lipid oxidation.

In severe sepsis and trauma, the normal production of ketone bodies in response to starvation is blunted. Thus, there are minimal ketones circulating to serve as an alternative energy substrate to glucose, and for this reason gluconeogenesis must proceed vigorously from protein. In severe trauma, both synthesis and catabolism of protein are increased, with the latter outstripping the former. This is the exact opposite of the situation in starvation where both synthesis and catabolism are reduced. Considerable increases in the rate of skeletal muscle breakdown have been demonstrated in traumatized and septic patients, while at the same time there is a net increase in the production of hepatic structural and secretory proteins. Teleologically speaking, the body appears to degrade muscle tissue in order to provide amino acids to the liver for the purposes of gluconeogenesis and the synthesis of acute phase proteins essential to host defense and healing.

The optimal nutritional support of septic and traumatized patients is a subject of ongoing investigation. Despite recent advances, a positive nitrogen balance cannot be achieved in septic or severely injured patients by current hyperalimentation protocols, although reductions in the net rate of protein loss have been achieved.

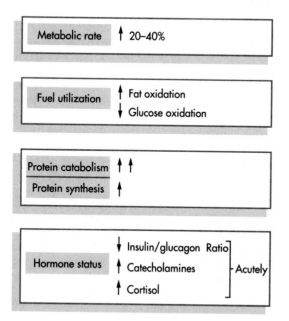

Figure 7-1 Summary of the metabolic changes associated with critical surgical illness. (Reproduced from Douglas RG, Shaw JHF. Metabolic response to sepsis and trauma. *Br J Surg* 1989;76:115–122, by permission of the publishers, Butterworth-Heinemann, Ltd.)

The Afferents: Stimuli and Receptors

The general changes and priority shifts of each organ system in response to injury and sepsis are, in part, initiated by various stimuli and mediators. Any injury can be understood as a collection of adverse stimuli to which the patient's systems must react in order to maintain homeostasis. These stimuli must be sensed by receptors and transmitted by afferent nerves to central processing centers where they can be integrated prior to the evocation of efferent responses directed to counteract the stimulus (Figure 7-2). Stimuli that have been demonstrated to play a role in this process include pain, volume status, oxygenation, osmolality, temperature, and substrate changes.

Pain

Peripheral nociceptive fibers sense pain and employ Substance P as their primary neurotransmitter. Stimulation of these fibers results in signal transmission to the thalamus and hypothalamus, which increases sympathetic outflow and produces increased secretion of antidiuretic hormone (ADH), adrenocorticotropic hormone (ACTH), opiates, catecholamines, cortisol, and aldosterone. Emotion has similar effects, mediated via the limbic system. Spinal cord section inhibits the normal catecholamine, steroid, and autonomic nervous

system response to a traumatic injury below the level of section, demonstrating the enormous role that neural afferents play in modulation of neuro-pituitary-adrenal responses.

Volume Status

The direct loss of blood, sequestration of fluid formerly in the vascular space into "third spaces," and dehydration all can decrease the effective circulating volume. This decrease is sensed by high pressure baroreceptors in the aorta, carotid arteries, and renal arteries, and by low pressure or volume receptors in the atria. When activated, these receptors exert a tonic inhibition on many hormone systems. A decrease in the effective circulating volume reduces this inhibition and increases the secretion of ACTH, ADH, renin, growth hormone, endogenous opiates, and catecholamines, as well as increased sympathetic nervous outflow and decreased parasympathetic outflow; all of which tend to restore

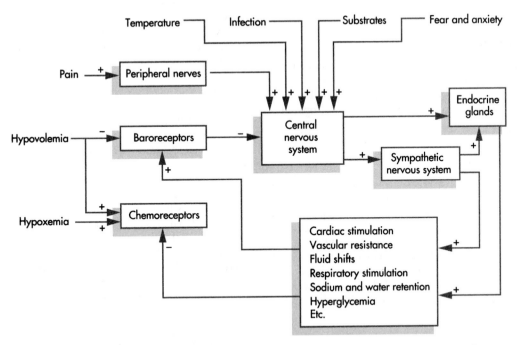

Figure 7-2 Overview of the neuroendocrine reflexes induced by shock and injury. There are at least seven stimuli consequent to injury that elicit neuroendocrine reflexes. These include hypovolemia; pain; changes in pO$_2$, pCO$_2$, pH; infection, emotional arousal; changes in substrate availability; and changes in temperature. The most common of these are hypovolemia and pain. (Reproduced from Gann DS, Amaral JF. Endocrine and metabolic responses to injury. In: Schwartz SI, Shires GT, Spencer FC, eds. *Principles of surgery*. 5th ed. New York: McGraw-Hill, 1989:4.)

the effective circulating volume. The net effect of these responses is termed the baroreceptor reflex.

Oxygen, Carbon Dioxide, and pH

Chemoreceptors located in the carotid and aortic bodies sense changes in oxygen, hydrogen ion, and carbon dioxide concentrations in the blood. These receptors do not exert a tonic influence analogous to the baroreceptors. Rather, they are activated by reductions in oxygen concentration or by increases in hydrogen ion or carbon dioxide concentration, and such activation results in stimulation of the respiratory center in the central nervous system, among other less important effects.

Osmolality

Alterations in plasma osmolality are sensed by osmoreceptors located in the hypothalamus. An increase in osmolality is the primary stimulus for ADH secretion from the neurohypophysis, which results in increased water reabsorption in the kidney.

Temperature

Sensed in the preoptic area of the hypothalamus, changes in temperature lead to alterations in the secretion of many hormones, including ACTH, ADH, cortisol, epinephrine, growth hormone, aldosterone, and thyroxine.

Substrate Changes

Plasma glucose concentration is sensed by receptors in the ventromedial nucleus of the hypothalamus and in the pancreas. Decreased concentrations stimulate the release of catecholamines, growth hormone, cortisol, ACTH, endorphins, and ADH via central pathways. The release of glucagon and inhibition of insulin is mediated by peripheral pathways. There are also complex, and as yet incompletely understood, relationships between the concentrations of various amino acids and hormone secretion.

Infection

The mechanism by which infection induces a response has been elusive. However, monokines are now known to play a central role and are discussed in detail below.

Integration

Major injury or sepsis subjects the individual to multiple stresses and stimuli simultaneously. The homeostatic response to the injury is the summation of the responses to each of these stresses and stimuli. The complex integration of the response to injury ensures that the overall response is appropriate and well regulated. Neural pathways within and around the hypothalamus, which control ACTH and ADH secretion, have been delineated in some detail, and it appears likely that the control of other hormones is analogous.

Afferents from baroreceptors and pain stimuli converge in the A1 region of the medulla as well as in the dorsal pons. This is thought to be the first site of interaction of pain and volume signals to form an integrated neuroendocrine response. Fibers in the A1 region then project to the periaqueductal gray area of the dorsal pons. Inhibitory and stimulatory fibers from this region project to various hypothalamic nucleii, exerting a controlling effect over the secretion of releasing factors, which, in turn, govern the secretion of anterior pituitary hormones.

An instructive example of the complex processing involved in a response to injury is that of the catecholamine response to hemorrhage. Stimulation of low- or high-pressure baroreceptors individually results in potent sympathetic nervous activity but little adrenal catecholamine secretion, whereas if both are stimulated simultaneously, adrenomedullary secretion increases markedly. This effect is thought to result from interaction between afferent fibers of the two receptor systems in their shared pathways through the nucleus tractus solitarius. Some control is also exerted at the receptor level. Catecholeamines, for example, increase the responsiveness of baroreceptors.

The neuroendocrine response to a given stimulus has been shown to depend upon the duration, intensity, and timing of the stimulus. For example, in experimental models, significant hemorrhage evokes a large increase in plasma epinephrine concentration, and when the blood loss occurs rapidly, the rise is greater than if it had occurred more slowly.

The Efferents: Effectors of the Response

Effectors integral to the physiologic response to injury are **hormones, cytokines, and the autonomic nervous**

system. The mechanism by which a particular effector exerts its effect is determined by its chemical nature. Among the hormones, steroid hormones diffuse through the target cell's membrane and bind to cytosolic receptors. The receptor-hormone complex translocates to the nucleus, where it binds nonhistone proteins, thereby modulating the transcription of certain genes. Since the effects of steroids are transcription-dependent, there is a several hour delay in onset of most of the primary actions of steroid hormones. Nonsteroid hormones generally act by binding cell surface receptors, which then act through a "second messenger" system such as the cyclic adenosine monophosphate cascade or alterations in calcium metabolism. Since these hormones act via activation of already existing enzymes rather than through synthesis of new proteins, their actions are of faster onset and shorter duration than steroid hormones.

β_1- And β_2-receptors, which are stimulated by the adrenergic nervous system and circulating catecholamines, function via activation of a membrane-bound adenylate cyclase, causing increased cyclic adenosine monophosphate levels, which, in turn, activate a protein kinase that then activates a phosphorylase kinase via phosphorylation. This phosphorylase kinase phosphorylates, and thus activates, a regulatory enzyme, thus resulting in the particular effect.

α_2-Receptor activation, in contrast, proceeds via inhibition of a membrane-bound adenylate cyclase. It results in an increase in phosphatidylinositol turnover which causes increased intracellular calcium concentrations, thereby activating the calcium-binding protein calmodulin, which, in turn, activates an inactive protein or phosphorylase kinase.

HORMONES

Catecholamines

The two catecholamines norepinephrine and epinephrine are synthesized at sympathetic nerve endings by the conversion of tyrosine to dopamine, norepinephrine, and finally epinephrine. Epinephrine is made and secreted by the adrenal medulla and functions primarily as a hormone, whereas norepinephrine is primarily a neurotransmitter. Normal plasma levels of these catecholamines are less than 50 pg/ml, but in patients with sepsis or in shock, values in excess of 200 pg/mL are usually found. These increases begin immediately after injury and achieve peak at 24–48 hours

after injury, from which point they gradually fall to baseline. In nonsurvivors, high levels of catecholamines may be sustained until just before death.

Actions of catecholamines can be categorized as hemodynamic, metabolic, and modulatory. The hemodynamic effects are well known and include α_1-receptor–mediated arteriolar vasoconstriction; β_2-receptor–mediated arterial vasodilation in muscle; and β_1-receptor–mediated cardiac effects which increase cardiac output. These all tend to increase blood pressure and effective circulating volume. The metabolic effects include stimulation of glycogenolysis, gluconeogenesis, lipolysis, ketogenesis, and inhibition of the action of insulin on peripheral tissues, all of which contribute to hyperglycemia. Modulation of other hormones by catecholamines include stimulation of renin, parathyroid hormone, and glucagon secretion.

ACTH and Adrenocortical Steroids

In trauma or sepsis, ACTH values rise to 40-90 pg/mL from normal values of 4–20 pg/mL. In burn patients, values as high as 185 pg/mL have been recorded. Similarly, cortisol concentrations in unstressed humans range from 6–15 mg/dl but in traumatized patients rise to 40–80 mg/dl, and the levels may remain elevated from a few days to as long as a month, depending on the severity of the insult.

Unexplained hemodynamic instability in patients stressed by trauma or infection with fever, hypoglycemia, hyponatremia and hyperkalemia can occasionally be ascribed to acute Addisonian crisis (hypoadrenalism), with measured blood cortisol concentrations of less than 10 mg/L. The most common cause of this syndrome is suppression of the hypothalamo-pituitary-adrenal axis by chronic steroid use, though a few patients have been found to have adrenal hemorrhage as the etiology.

The actions of adrenocortical steroids, which render them so indispensable in the severely stressed state, are several. At the slightly supraphysiologic levels seen in stressed states, cortisol induces gluconeogenesis and lipolysis in the liver and inhibits insulin mediated glucose uptake while increasing amino acid release in skeletal muscle, thus contributing to substrate availability in the face of crisis. Cortisol also promotes urinary sodium retention, helping to restore circulating volume, although aldosterone, discussed below, is clearly the more important steroid hormone in this regard.

At pharmacologic doses, corticosteroids stabilize cell

membranes, and for this reason have been therapeutically in shock. These studies have not demonstrated any change in mortality or morbidity, perhaps due to impairment of immune function that also occurs with large doses.

Endogenous opiates

β-Endorphins and enkephalin (the endogenous opiates) are fragments of the precursor which they share in common with ACTH, pre–pro-opiomelanocortin. They too increase in stressed states. Aside from altering the psychological state, these substances contribute to stress-induced hyperglycemia, potentiate catecholamine release, and have direct cardiovascular effects including a hypotensive effect of β-endorphin and a hypertensive effect of the enkephalins. The opiate antagonist naloxone has been shown to cause a dose-dependent increase in cardiac parameters in experimental shock, though clinical trials are inconclusive.

Renin, the Angiotensins, Antidiuretic Hormone, and Aldosterone

These hormones are related via a complex system initiated by hypotension, hypovolemia, and/or inadequate perfusion (Chapter 25, Figure 25-4). Any insult that causes hypotension causes renin to be secreted by the juxtaglomerular apparatus of the kidneys. This occurs directly in response to reduced renal blood flow; and indirectly via sensation of decreased chloride concentration in the distal nephron, and by the increased adrenergic activity that occurs with shock through the baroreceptor reflex. Circulating renin enzymatically cleaves angiotensinogen, produced by the liver, to angiotensin I. Angiotensin I is then altered by angiotensin converting enzyme in the lung to angiotensin II. Angiotensin I has some activity that contributes to homeostasis in the face of shock, including potentiation of catecholamine release and redistribution of renal blood flow to "salt-saving" cortical nephrons. However, angiotensin II is the more powerful effector of the two. Angiotensin II is a vasoconstrictor and cardiac stimulant. It affects fluid and electrolyte balance, promoting volume expansion by stimulating aldosterone and ADH (vasopressin) secretion and by increasing thirst. In addition, it has metabolic effects which promote glucose mobilization.

Although one stimulus to the release of ADH from the neurohypophysis is angiotensin II, its primary stimulus is increased serum osmolality, and its secretion is increased to some extent by nearly all of the stimuli discussed above. Surgery causes plasma ADH levels to rise from a baseline of less than 5 pg/mL to peaks of near 100 pg/mL. Antidiuretic hormone exerts its osmoregulatory effect by promoting reabsorption of free water in the distal tubules and collecting ducts of the kidney. Less prominant effects include peripheral vasoconstriction and promotion of glucose mobilization. Both the syndrome of inappropriate secretion of ADH, beyond that needed for homeostasis, and insufficient secretion (diabetes insipidus) may occur following head injury.

Aldosterone, synthesized in the adrenal zona glomerulosa, undergoes plasma level increases of up to 600% with insults as relatively minor as cholecystectomy. This increase is mediated by increases in angiotensin II, ACTH, and potassium which accompany injury. Aldosterone's primary action is to increase reabsorption of sodium and chloride and secretion of potassium in the distal convoluted tubule, thus helping restore circulating volume.

Insulin and Glucagon

Whereas plasma insulin levels vary between approximately 10 and 30 microunits (μU)/mL in the normal fasting and fed states, posttraumatic or septic patients have levels that may be high or low, depending on whether the patient is hyperdynamic and compensated, or in shock. Patients with elevated cardiac indices can be hyperglycemic despite insulin levels of 40–102 μU/mL, presumably due to insulin resistance. In true shock states, elevations of serum glucose are still found, with insulin levels averaging only 6.1 μU/mL. This hypoinsulinemia in shock is thought to be due to intense sympathetic activity, as catecholamines suppress insulin secretion. The major actions of insulin on carbohydrate, protein, and lipid metabolism are discussed in Chapter 18.

Glucagon, normally in the range of 200 ± 95 pg/mL in blood, rises to concentrations in excess of 400 pg/mL in severely injured patients. The timing of the rise varies with the type of stress. Similar to the fall in insulin levels in injured patients, rises in glucagon levels are thought to be secondary to sympathetic activity and elevated levels of circulating catecholamines. In contrast to βα-cells (insulin), α-cells (glucagon) have a greater density of stimulatory α-adrenergic receptors than inhibitory β-adrenergic receptors. The main physiologic actions of glucagon are the stimulation of glycogenolysis and gluconeogenesis, thus contributing to hyperglycemia. However, peak glucagon levels do not correlate with peak glucose levels, suggesting an incomplete role in the genesis of the hyperglycemia associated with the stressed state.

Growth Hormone

The concentration of this hormone is increased following injury as a result of decreased effective circulating volume. Levels remain elevated for approximately 24 hours following the insult. Growth hormone is yet another factor contributing to postinjury hyperglycemia via its catabolic effect on carbohydrate and lipid metabolism, perhaps via second messengers called somatomedins.

Thyroxine

Perhaps unexpectedly, given the increased basal metabolic rate in the posttraumatic state, after most injuries concentrations of thyroid hormones are normal or depressed. It appears that, though the presence of thyroid hormone is necessary for normal function of organs in response to stress, elevated levels are not necessary. Specifically, the peripheral conversion of T4 to T3 is impaired following injury, and there is also increased conversion of T4 to the inactive molecule, reverse T3. Finally, recent evidence has shown that thyrotropin releasing hormone may be important in the response to shock, as recent studies have shown improved blood pressure, respiratory rate, pulse rate, and survival in experimental animals given thyrotropin releasing hormone during hemorrhagic shock.

CYTOKINES AND OTHER HUMORAL FACTORS

Cytokines are protein or glycoprotein hormones derived from a wide variety of cells which, unlike the hormones described above, tend to act locally, in a paracrine manner. Lymphokines are cytokines derived from lymphocytes, while monokines are those derived from monocytes. Among the more important cytokines in severely stressed states are tumor necrosis factor and the interleukins. The complex interrelationship of these cytokines with the classical endocrine hormone system and a wide variety of other mediators stimulates inflammatory responses which, when well-regulated, help restore homeostasis. In some circumstances, however, the deleterious effects of these factors clearly predominate, resulting in spiralling illness and ultimately multiorgan system failure.

Tumor Necrosis Factor/Cacechtin

This macrophage product has been identified as a central mediator in a diverse range of protective, as well as toxic, events in sepsis and inflammation. Tumor necrosis factor (TNF) is produced within 2 minutes of infusion of bacterial endotoxin and its levels fall to normal within minutes thereafter, suggesting that it serves a protective role in endotoxemia. Tumor necrosis factor has been shown to increase leukocyte adherence to tissues, stimulate the production of oxygen free radicals by neutrophils, and enhance phagocytosis, all of which contribute to the local reaction against pathogens. If these processes are uncontrolled, however, it is apparent how they might contribute to tissue injury. Further, TNF induces fever (both directly and through stimulation of interleukin-1 [IL-1]) which is thought to play an immunoenhancing role in host defense. From a metabolic standpoint, TNF has been shown to cause increased peripheral muscle and fat breakdown while stimulating hepatic protein synthesis, contributing to the hyperglycemia of stress and allowing for the synthesis of the acute phase proteins essential to the host response. Experimentally, mice given sublethal doses of TNF can survive what would otherwise be lethal doses of certain microorganisms.

Despite the above protective effects, it is clear that in cases of uncontrolled sepsis, whether it be a primary infectious process or one superimposed upon a trauma or postoperative situation, TNF's systemic, harmful effects become manifest. Sufficient doses of bacteria, endotoxin, or TNF injected into experimental animals result in hypotension, anuria, respiratory arrest, acidosis, disseminated intravascular coagulation, acute renal failure, pulmonary edema, myocardial dysfunction, and intestinal ischemia. These reproducible effects can be blocked by pretreating the animals with monoclonal antibody to TNF. Broken down into components, this clinically familiar septic syndrome can be explained in part by the following effects of TNF:

1. It is a direct mediator of the decreased skeletal muscle membrane potential seen in sepsis, presumably indicative of a generalized cell membrane defect.
2. It induces capillary leak. These effects are major con-

tributors to the accumulation third space fluid and resultant hypotension.

3. It contributes to the development of disseminated intravascular coagulation by stimulating expression of an endothelial cell surface factor that has procoagulant activity while suppressing synthesis of tissue plasminogen activator.

4. Its effects on leukocyte adherence and potency described above may cause tissue injury via direct toxic effects to organs.

Finally, it must be noted that TNF is entwined with the classical hormone system in a number of ways: TNF has a major upregulating effect on the secretion of ACTH and cortisol, epinephrine and norepinephrine, and glucagon, thus contributing to the rise of these hormones in the severely stressed state.

Interleukin-1

Interleukin-1 is produced primarily by macrophages, but also by some other cells, in response to endotoxin or TNF. Similar to TNF, IL-1 also has both protective and deleterious effects. Its protective effects include immunoenhancement, inducing differentiation and activation of T lymphocytes, and production of interferon, colony stimulating factor, B-cell growth factor, and IL-2. Interleukin-1 promotes the growth of several cell types, including fibroblasts and vascular smooth muscle cells. Further, IL-1 is an endogenous pyrogen and stimulates hepatic synthesis of acute phase proteins. Like TNF, IL-1 stimulates procoagulant activity of endothelial cells and induces neutrophil adherence and activation. Although IL-1 and TNF act synergistically in most regards, the adverse effects of IL-1 are not as dramatic as those of TNF.

Eicosanoids

These products of arachidonic acid metabolism have also been implicated in the pathogenesis of septic shock. Arachidonic acid liberated from cell membrane phospholipids by phospholipase A_2 is metabolized via one of two pathways: the cyclo-oxygenase pathway results in the production of the prostaglandins and thromboxanes, while the lipoxygenase pathway yields the leukotrienes (Figure 7-3). These factors exhibit a number of biological effects which implicate them in the genesis of septic shock. Among these are vasodilatation or constriction, increased vasopermeability, platelet aggregation, myo-

cardial depression, chemotaxis, and leukocyte adhesion. Platelet aggregation and vasoconstriction, caused by thromboxane A_2, are characterstic of adult respiratory distress syndrome, and some believe this to represent a pathogenetic link. Interestingly, TNF and IL-1 stimulate the biosynthesis of a number of eicosanoids, suggesting that the latter may in part serve as mediators of cytokine activity. In fact, cyclo-oxygenase inhibitors mitigate some of the in vivo toxicity of TNF in experimental systems. The fact that cortisol largely blocks eicosanoid production is a major impetus for the therapeutic trials of steroids in shock.

Complement Components

The complement system (see Chapter 20) is another source of restorative, but potentially toxic humoral factors. Once initiated by either the classic (by immune complexes) or alternative (by bacteria or trauma) pathways, the cascade products include the anaphylatoxins (C3a and C5a) and the terminal membrane attack complex. The former, in particular, have been shown to cause many of the effects described above for TNF, IL-1, and eicosanoids. Animals passively immunized against C5a do much better following gram-negative bacterial infusion than controls, perhaps most notably with regard to their lungs, which develop neither pulmonary edema nor adult respiratory distress syndrome. The membrane attack complex, on the other hand, has been implicated in direct tissue toxicity resulting in organ system failure. Again, to highlight the complex interrelationship between these systems, it should be noted that C5a stimulates leukocyte synthesis of TNF and IL-1.

The Hemostatic Cascade

This also is a system that produces responses that contribute to homeostasis in most circumstances, but in situations of severe trauma or sepsis it may become pathologic. In trauma situations that threaten hemorrhagic shock, the body's normal hemostatic mechanism is among the most important responses in the maintenance of homeostasis. Details of this cascade are described in Chapter 5. Some tissue injuries and infections, however, initiate pathologic responses in the hemostatic system, resulting in the potentially devastating microcirculatory thrombotic process, **disseminated intravascular coagulation**. This syndrome is characterized pathologically by the presence of platelet/fibrin thrombi in arterioles, capillaries, and venules. It is

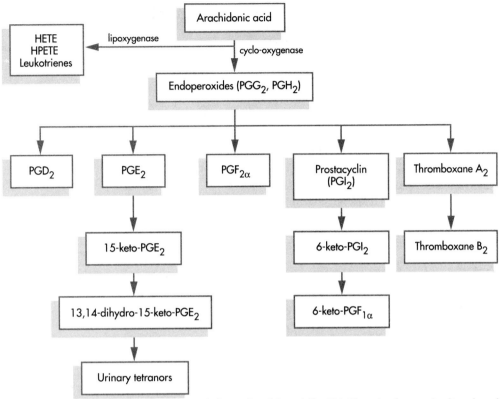

Figure 7-3 Prostaglandin products of arachidonic acid. (Reproduced from Jaffee BM. The role of prostaglandins, thromboxane, and leukotrienes in surgery. In: Sabiston DC, ed. *Textbook of surgery*. 15th ed. Philadelphia: WB Saunders, 1991:466.)

thought to result from "free" thrombin in the circulation which causes deposition of fibrin, trapping of platelets, consumption of clotting factors, and activation of fibrinolysis with the appearance of elevated levels of the degradation products of fibrinogen and fibrin in the plasma. These changes result paradoxically in both diminished blood flow to vital organs, which may contribute to the development of multiorgan system failure, and a bleeding diathesis. Disseminated intravascular coagulation is evoked through complex mechanisms. In trauma, thromboplastin is released from areas of extensive tissue damage, serving as a continuing stimulus to thrombin generation via the alternate pathway, thus initiating the vicious cycle of thrombosis, lysis, and bleeding. In infection, a number of organisms—but primarily endotoxin-producing gram-negative bacteria—trigger the syndrome by unknown mechanisms. Treatment includes eliminating the cause (i.e., specific antimicrobial therapy or local wound care), restoring hemostatic

balance (by replacement therapy with fresh frozen plasma and platelets), and, potentially, inhibiting circulating thrombin by heparin administration (though this has met with only limited clinical success).

Kinins

Levels of these plasma factors also increase in shock and may serve diverse roles in such states. Circulating kininogens are converted to kinins by kallikrein, which may be activated by tissue injury, factor XII, or complement. Bradykinin infusion causes hypotension and increased cardiac output experimentally, and also has the effect of increasing bronchial resistance.

Serotonin and Histamine

Released by platelets and gut enterochromaffin cells after tissue injury, serotonin is a potent veno- and bronchoconstrictor (possibly significant in the pathogenesis of adult respiratory distress syndrome), and platelet aggregator. Histamine, which rises abruptly in the serum following administration of endotoxin to animals, has been implicated in actions as diverse as vasodilatation and increased vascular permeability, bronchoconstriction, and increased myocardial contractility, in addition to its well-known effect on gastric acid production.

THE AUTONOMIC NERVOUS SYSTEM

The autonomic nervous system is closely intertwined with the hormonal response to injury. Sympathetic neural outflow is a major stimulus to the secretion of many of the hormones discussed above, most notably catecholamines and glucagon. It is probably most appropriate to consider the autonomic nervous system and hormone systems together, as a single neuroendocrine system which mounts a large portion of the overall response to injury.

Bibliography

Brown JM, Grosso MA, Harken AH. Cytokines. Sepsis and the surgeon. *Surgery Gynecol Obstet* 1989;169:568–575.

Clowes GHA Jr, ed. *Trauma, sepsis, and shock: The physiological basis of therapy.* New York: Marcel Dekker, 1988.

Douglas RG, Shaw JHF. Metabolic response to sepsis and trauma. *Br J Surg* 1989;76:115–122.

Gann DS, Amaral JF. Endocrine and metabolic responses to injury. In: Schwartz SI, Shires GT, Spencer FC, eds. *Principles of surgery,* 5th ed. New York: McGraw-Hill, 1989.

Richardson JD, Polk HC Jr, Flint LM, eds. *Trauma: clinical care and pathophysiology.* Chicago: Year Book Medical Publishers, 1987.

Shires GT III, Canizaro PC, Carrico CJ, Shires GT. Shock. In: Schwartz SI, Shires GT, Spencer FC, eds. *Principles of surgery.* 5th ed. New York: McGraw-Hill, 1989.

Siegel JH, ed. *Trauma: emergency surgery and critical care.* New York: Churchill Livingstone, 1987.

Tracey KJ, Lowry SF. The role of cytokine mediators in septic shock. *Adv Surg* 1990; 23:21–56.

David J. Callans

8 ELECTROPHYSIOLOGY OF CARDIAC FUNCTION

The electrophysiologic properties of the heart have been studied at all levels of organization—from the measurement of individual ion fluxes through single channels in isolated myocytes, to high resolution recording of potentials from the body surface. The breadth of these studies now provides us with the unique opportunity of integrating the findings from several investigative avenues to explain cardiac arrhythmias encountered in clinical practice. This chapter will focus on the following topics: (1) the structure and function of the various components of the cardiac conduction system; (2) the physiology of impulse generation and propagation; and (3) our present understanding of the cellular mechanisms of arrhythmogenesis, and how antiarrhythmic agents can effect this process.

Anatomy of the Specialized Conduction System

Although all myocytes have electrical properties, a distinction is made between cells that are designed primarily for contraction and those that are designed for conduction. The latter group of cells are organized into a **specialized conduction system,** which provides the temporal coordination necessary for the heart to function as an effective pump (Figure 8-1). In addition, it is primarily through contact with the conduction system that the autonomic nervous system influences cardiac function.

SINUS NODE

In man, the sinus node is 10–20 mm long by 2–3 mm wide and is composed of a thick collection of cells that are closely packed within a matrix of connective tissue. It is located just beneath the epicardial surface of the lateral, superior aspect of the right atrium, near the junction of the base of the atrial appendage and the root of the superior vena cava. Clusters of nodal cells, a subtype of small, ovoid, poorly staining cells within the center of the structure, are thought to be the origin of the normal cardiac impulse. These cells are richly interconnected by intercellular gap junctions, which allow electrical continuity: thus, no single cell, but rather an entire region of cells acts as the "pacemaker." Other cell

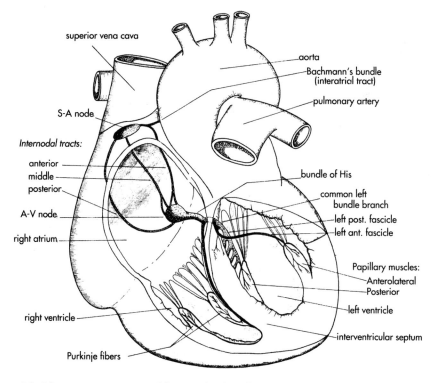

Figure 8-1 Schematic representation of the specialized conduction system of the heart. The normal cardiac impulse originates in the sinus node and is conducted throughout the atria. The impulse is delayed slightly at the atrioventricular (AV) node, then continues to the His bundle, the bundle branches, and through the Purkinje network to the ventricular myocardium. (Reproduced from Dunn MI, Lippman BS. *Lippman-Masse clinical electrophysiology.* 8th ed. Chicago: Year Book Medical Publishers, 1989:9.)

types within the node, transitional cells and atrial muscle cells (indistinguishable from those located elsewhere within the atrium), transmit the sinus impulse to the remainder of the atrial myocardium.

The blood supply to the node is the centrally located sinus node artery, which is a proximal branch of the right coronary artery in 55–60% of cases, and of the left circumflex in 40–45% of cases. An extensive network of postganglionic adrenergic and cholinergic nerve terminals enter the nodal region. Parasympathetic stimulation via the vagus nerve slows the sinus discharge rate and prolongs conduction within the node, potentially even to the point of block. Sympathetic stimulation increases heart rate and improves intranodal conduction. Thus, the chronotropic state of the heart is determined by the interaction of these two inputs on the sinus node. For example, tonic vagal stimulation causes a greater decrease in sinus rate in the presence of background sympathetic stimulation (accentuated antagonism).

INTERNODAL TRACTS

The presence of preferential pathways for conduction of impulses from the sinus node to the atrioventricular (AV) node has been suggested, mostly on the basis of anatomic studies. Anterior, middle, and posterior internodal tracts, named according to their course relative to the superior vena cava and the intra-atrial septum, all originate in the sinus node and give off branches to the AV node and the left atrium. The cells of these "tracts" have never been demonstrated to possess unique histologic or physiologic properties. In contrast, Bachmann's bundle, a collection of muscle fibers that course posteriorly around the aorta to connect the atria, probably does provide a specialized pathway for conduction.

ATRIOVENTRICULAR NODE

The AV node is located just beneath the right atrial endocardium at the apex of a triangle (Koch's triangle) formed by the tricuspid valve annulus, the sinus septum, and the membranous septum (Figure 8-2). Several cell types coexist in a complex three-dimensional architecture within this region. Although they are easily distinguished histologically, their functional properties depend on their position within the node and their orientation relative to the activation wavefront, as well as on their morphology. Atrioventricular nodal cells are relatively isolated electrically, by the absence of gap junctions and the presence of connective tissue between adjacent cells. This isolation and the type of action potentials generated in this region are responsible for the slow conduction of the AV node. Atrioventricular node conduction delay coordinates atrial and ventricular systole and slows the ventricular response to supraventricular tachycardia.

In 80–90% of cases, the AV nodal artery arises from the right coronary artery after a peculiar "U-turn" at the posterior intersection of the atrioventricular and inter-ventricular grooves; it originates from the left circumflex in the remaining cases. The AV node receives a rich supply of sympathetic and parasympathetic innervation. Vagal inputs lead to an increase in the time required for AV nodal conduction, and can frequently cause conduction block in the node. Adrenergic stimulation improves conduction. In addition to autonomic input, AV nodal conduction also varies with the intrinsic heart rate; at faster rates, conduction time through the AV node gradually prolongs to the point of block.

HIS BUNDLE

The His bundle is formed by the continuation of the AV node fibers as they pass through the central fibrous body and the membranous portion of the interventricular septum. Distally, the His bundle gives rise to the left and right bundle branches. Proximal His cells resemble cells of the compact portion of the AV node; the distal His bundle is composed of cells that are histologically identical to Purkinje fibers. Arterial blood is supplied by an arcade of septal perforators from the left anterior descending and the posterior descending

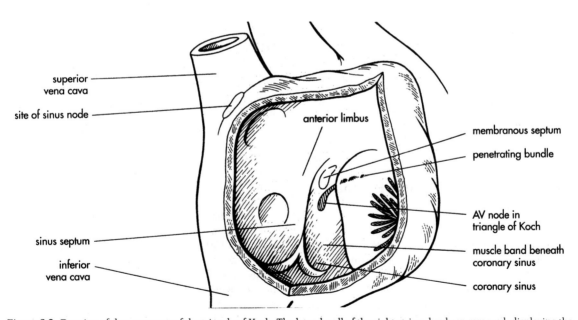

Figure 8-2 Drawing of the structures of the triangle of Koch. The lateral wall of the right atrium has been removed, displaying the anatomic relations of the atrioventricular (AV) node and the His bundle with other right atrial structures. (Reproduced from Becker AE et al. Functional anatomy of the cardiac conduction system. In: Harrison DC, ed. *Cardiac arrhythmias: a decade of progress.* Boston: GK Hall, 1989:10.)

branch of the right coronary artery. This dual blood supply protects this critical junction of the conduction system from all but massive myocardial infarction. His bundle impulse conduction is not affected by autonomic nervous system input, and its conduction time is fairly constant (normally 35–55 milliseconds) irrespective of heart rate. Intracardiac recordings from this region during electrophysiologic study display atrial and ventricular depolarizations as well as a separate high-frequency His bundle spike. The relative timing of these three events is helpful in determining the site of AV conduction disorders and in distinguishing supraventricular from ventricular arrhythmias.

BUNDLE BRANCHES, PURKINJE SYSTEM

The distal His bundle divides at the superior margin of the muscular interventricular septum to give rise to a discrete **right bundle branch** and a fanlike network of tissue, collectively called the **left bundle branch.** The right bundle runs within the septal myocardium to the right ventricular apex. Separate components of the left bundle branch, the anterior and posterior fascicles, are useful conceptual and electrocardiographic constructs, but are not distinct anatomical structures. The left anterior descending coronary artery supplies the bundle branches along with the septal myocardium; bundle branch block is often observed with anterior infarction. Both bundle branches further subdivide to form the Purkinje network, which penetrates the inner third of the endocardium throughout both ventricles. Due to the extensive ramifications of the Purkinje system, the endocardium is activated in an orderly fashion from apex to base within 30–50 milliseconds in the normal heart.

Generation of the Action Potential

THE CELL MEMBRANE

An essential property of electrically active cells is the presence of a selectively permeable outer membrane. The cell membrane, or sarcolemma, is a phospholipid bilayer oriented such that the polar heads of the lipid molecules face outwards and the nonpolar tails face toward the center. This nonpolar, hydrophobic core provides a high resistance to the flow of ionic species across the membrane. Because ions are charged, the flow of ions across the membrane generates electric cur-

rent (see below). Ions can pass through the membrane only at certain sites, called channels, which are formed by transmembrane proteins. Channels are relatively ion-specific. They allow passage of one ionic species almost to the exclusion of all others.

The basis for this selectivity is poorly understood, but it seems to be related to factors other than just molecular size and charge; a potassium ion is 1000 times more likely to enter the cell through the potassium channel than a sodium ion, even though the ionic charge and the hydrated molecular radius of the two ions are essentially identical. Ion passage through channels can be regulated such that the ability for an ion to enter the cell through its channel, and thus the total membrane permeability for that ion, can change under various conditions. Another way of stating this is that channels are "gated." The probability of a channel being "open" (for the passage of a specific ion) is not constant. Changes in the channel gating status can occur with changes in the transmembrane voltage (voltage-dependence), or with passage of time from an event, such as the initiation of an action potential (time-dependence). The channel properties of ion selectivity and gating are thought to result from conformation changes in the three-dimensional structure of the transmembrane proteins that form the channel.

THE RESTING MEMBRANE POTENTIAL

The unique features of the sarcolemma allow for a distinct separation of intracellular and extracellular conditions. Extracellular electrolyte concentrations mirror those of the intravascular space. Thus, measurement of serum electrolytes provides an accurate assessment of the extracellular environment. Because the movement of polar and larger nonpolar molecules is restricted, concentration gradients are established across the membrane. Sodium is the major extracellular cation; its concentration is almost 10-fold greater outside the cell (145 mM) than inside (15 mM). Potassium is the primary intracellular cation, with a similar concentration differential (150 mM inside, 4 mM outside). These concentration gradients are formed and maintained by energy-dependent, active transport mechanisms within the cell membrane. The most important of these is the Na-K "pump," which transports 3 sodium ions out and 2 potassium ions into the cell at the expense of energy derived from high-energy phosphate bonds in adenosine triphosphate. The action of this pump is blocked by digitalis, leading to an intracellular excess of sodium which drives exchange for calcium mediated by a separate transport protein. The major extracellular anion is chloride, and large, negatively charged proteins, sulfates, and phosphates are the primary intracellular anions.

Because ions carry charge, the generation of a concentration gradient also produces a separation of charges or an electric field. The inside of normal myocardial cells is 50–95 mV negative relative to the outside. This voltage difference is constant in the absence of electrical impulses, and is called the resting membrane potential. Thus, how an ion is distributed (i.e., its relative intra/extracellular concentration) is determined by the force of the electric field, the concentration gradient of the particular ion, and the membrane permeability for that ion. To illustrate how membrane permeability influences the distribution of ions, it is helpful to consider the extreme conditions. If the membrane is absolutely impermeable to an ionic species (e.g., negatively charged large protein molecules), any difference in intracellular vs. extracellular concentration will be maintained, even in the absence of a specific mechanism (such as a pump). Alternatively, if the membrane offers little resistance to ion passage, its distribution will be determined by the balance of forces generated by the electric field and the concentration gradient. At steady state, the membrane is highly permeable to potassium ions, i.e., there is a high probability that an individual potassium channel will be open. A potassium ion tends to be driven outside the cell by osmostic force based on its concentration gradient, but tends to remain within the electrically negative cell because it is positively charged. Eventually, potassium ions distribute across the membrane until the forces are balanced—the system is then in electrochemical equilibrium. This is expressed in a mathematical form by the **Nernst equation** (see Chapter 26). If the membrane is permeable to a certain ion, eventually an equilibrium will be reached such that a given transmembrane voltage will result in a specific concentration gradient and vice versa. Solving the Nerst equation for the measured concentration gradient for potassium yields a value of -96 mV, which is very close to the observed membrane potential in His-Purkinje tissue and ventricular myocardium. In other words, potassium is the key ionic determinant of the resting membrane potential.

Few sodium ions can diffuse into the cell in the resting state despite the fact that both electrical and osmotic forces would favor this flux. This is because the membrane permeability to sodium is very low at resting membrane potential (sodium channels are gated closed). Solving the Nerst equation for sodium yields a value of +40 mV. In other words, the observed concentration gradient for sodium would result in equilibrium conditions if the transmembrane voltage was +40 mV (inside positive). This contrast illustrates that a particular ion contributes to the resting potential relative to its membrane permeability in the resting state. This is mathematically expressed in the Goldman constant field equation, a simultaneous solution of the Nerst equation for different ions with different permeabilities. For practical purposes, however, the membrane at rest acts as a potassium electrode, and the influence of other ionic species can be ignored.

THE ACTION POTENTIAL

The electrical activity of a single myocyte cell can be recorded by inserting a glass microelectrode. If the tip of the electrode is sufficiently thin (0.5 μm), the cell membrane will seal around it such that the cell will not be damaged. If this electrode is inserted into a resting Purkinje cell, it records the transmembrane potential, -90 mV relative to the outside. Current can be injected through the electrode into the cell to make the transmembrane potential less negative (depolarizing current, the inward movement of positive charges) or more negative (hyperpolarizing current, the outward movement of positive charges). If the current injected depolarizes the cell to a threshold value (-70–65 mV in Purkinje tissue), a sudden change in voltage occurs that is disproportionate to the strength of the stimulus. This "all or none" response is the cardiac **action potential** (Figure 8-3).

RAPID DEPOLARIZATION (PHASE 0)

The upstroke of the action potential (V_{max}) is caused by a sudden increase in sodium permeability (Figure 8-4A). When a suprathreshold stimulus is applied, sodium channels are suddenly opened and sodium ions enter the cell, driven by the force of the concentration gradient and the electrical field. The membrane potential approaches equilibrium at a value predicted by solving the Nerst equation for sodium (i.e., inside positive relative to outside). However, the membrane conductance for sodium does not remain high indefinitely: The sodium channel closes and the membrane becomes relatively impermeable to sodium after 1–2 milliseconds. Our understanding of the properties of the sodium

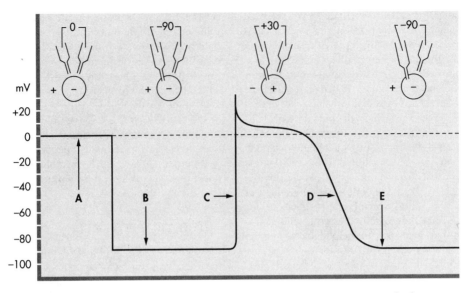

Figure 8-3 Demonstration of microelectrode recordings of the cardiac action potential. The *upper row* shows the cell (represented as a circle), the two microelectrodes, and the transmembrane voltages recorded during activation and recovery. **A,** Both electrodes are outside the cell, and no potential difference exists. **B,** One microelectrode is inserted into the cell to record transmembrane potential (-90 mV). **C,** The cell depolarizes as the action potential upstroke is recorded. **D,** After a period of depolarization, the membrane returns to its previous resting potential **(E).** (Reproduced from Cranefield, PF. *The conduction of the cardiac impulse.* Mt. Kisco NY: Futura Publishing Co., 1975:5.)

channel that determine these changes in sodium permeability is incomplete. Hodgkin and Huxley suggested a hypothetical model to explain the gating behavior of the sodium channel. It proposes that the probability of the sodium channel remaining open progressively decreases as the transmembrane voltage becomes positive and as time passes since action potential onset. When the channels close, the membrane is no longer permeable to sodium, and phase 0 is complete.

It is important to realize that the voltage change of phase 0 occurs with the passage of very few sodium ions (4×10^{-12} mol/cm^2). Because of this, even after hundreds of action potentials, the sodium concentration gradient remains intact, and does not need to be regenerated for the cell to return to resting membrane potential.

EARLY RAPID REPOLARIZATION (PHASE 1)

Following the "overshoot" when the cell's interior becomes transiently positive, the membrane quickly repolarizes to near 0 mV. This change in voltage is due

to the inactivation of the inward sodium current as well as to a repolarization current carried by outward movement of potassium ions and/or inward movement of chloride ions.

PLATEAU (PHASE 2)

The presence of a plateau phase distinguishes cardiac from neural cells; it is marked by a low membrane conductance to all ions. The transmembrane potential may remain near 0 mV for more than 100 milliseconds. Small inward fluxes of chloride are balanced by a background slow inward current carried by calcium ions. In addition, the Na-K pump makes a small contribution to repolarization; since it exchanges 3 sodium ions out for each 2 potassium ions in, the net effect is the outward flow of positive charges, which makes the interior more negative.

RAPID REPOLARIZATION (PHASE 3)

Rapid repolarization to a transmembrane voltage near the resting potential is largely due to two currents: slow

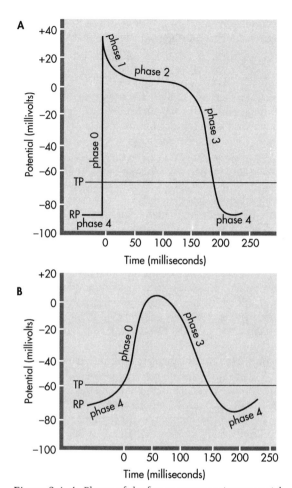

Figure 8-4 A, Phases of the fast response action potential. Once a stimulus depolarizes the membrane to threshold potential (TP), the cell responds with a sudden change in voltage mediated by fast inward sodium current (phase 0). Following a short period of rapid repolarization (phase 1) and an extended plateau period (phase 2), the cell gradually repolarizes (phase 3) to resting potential (RP; phase 4). Very slow diastolic depolarization may occur in Purkinje cells, but not in normal atrial or ventricular myocytes. **B,** Phases of the slow response action potential. Threshold is frequently attained spontaneously during phase 4 depolarization, particularly in sinus nodal cells. A slower voltage change of less magnitude results (phase 0) from slow inward current carried by calcium ions. Phase 1 and 2 are not distinct, and phase 3 is prolonged, returning the membrane to a resting potential of approximately -70 mV. The slope of phase 4 depolarization, as well as the relative voltages at resting and threshold potential, determine the period of automaticity. (Reproduced from Hurst JW. Recognition and treatment of cardiac arrhythmias and conduction disturbances. In: Hurst JW, ed. *The heart.* 4th ed. New York: McGraw-Hill, 1978:639.)

inward current (calcium ions moving into the cell) is inactivated, and an outward movement of positive charges (carried by potassium) is activated. Sodium channels are still closed during this period, and thus an action potential cannot occur, regardless of the intensity of the stimulus. The amount of time before the sodium channels have the capacity to open again is called the absolute refractory period—the minimal time period between action potentials.

DIASTOLIC DEPOLARIZATION (PHASE 4)

The membrane potential returns to -90 mV at the conclusion of phase 3. In atrial and ventricular muscle, the transmembrane voltage remains constant throughout diastole under normal conditions. Certain cells have the capacity to spontaneously depolarize and may reach threshold in the absence of an external stimulus, leading to another action potential. The ionic basis of the current(s) responsible for diastolic depolarization is complex. This phenomenon is called automaticity, and is responsible for the ability of cells in several locations (sinus node, AV node, His-Purkinje system) to act as "pacemakers" for the remainder of the heart.

SLOW RESPONSE FIBERS

The action potential is not identical in all cardiac cells (Figure 8-4B). The "fast response" action potential described above occurs in atrial and ventricular myocardium and in His-Purkinje tissue under normal conditions. Action potentials recorded from cells in the sinus or AV nodes have a different morphology, are caused by different currents, and are called "slow response" action potentials.

In nodal tissue, the concepts of resting membrane and threshold potential still apply; however, the upstroke of the action potential (phase 0) is not mediated by sodium current, but by the slow inward current carried by calcium. The channel responsible for this current opens and closes slowly, thus recovery of excitability (i.e., ability for the Ca^{2+} channel to open in response to another stimulus) is prolonged and the absolute refractory period is longer. In addition, the slow upstroke of the action potential in nodal tissue results in low conduction velocity, and explains the "physiologic delay" which is provided by the AV node and is necessary for the synchrony of atrial and ventricular pump function.

Impulse Propagation

Once an action potential is generated, it provides a stimulus to depolarize adjacent patches of cell membrane to threshold so that a wave of activation spreads sequentially to all nonrefractory tissue. The velocity of this transmission, and in fact whether or not it will occur, depends on several factors which are described by the local circuit theory.

In order for the current generated in phase 0 to affect portions of the membrane downstream, a circuit must be formed. Our present understanding of this process is called the local circuit theory. Positive charges crossing the membrane into the cell during the action potential upstroke must eventually return to the current source. Since cells are interconnected by gap junctions which allow the passage of ions, this collection of positive charges can flow throughout the intracellular space. Alternatively, some of these charges cross the cell membrane to return to the source and complete the circuit. This extracellular movement of ions is recorded at the body surface as the electrocardiogram. The conduction velocity of an impulse is a reflection of the ability of a local action potential to depolarize adjacent patches of membrane to threshold, resulting in perpetuation of the spread of action potentials downstream. It is directly related to the magnitude of the current generated in phase 0, and indirectly related to the degree of resistance offered by the intracellular space; the greater the resistance, the more current will "leak" to the extracellular space and not be available to depolarize other portions of the membrane. Electrolyte and acid/base disturbances, tissue ischemia and cellular death, as well as antiarrhythmic drugs can affect either or both of these parameters and thus alter conduction velocity and make arrhythmias either more or less likely to occur.

Mechanisms of Arrhythmogenesis

Cardiac arrhythmias are generally considered to be disorders of impulse formation or of impulse conduction, or a combination of both. Often the precise mechanism for a clinically observed arrhythmia cannot be proven; however, based on the clinical behavior of the arrhythmia and its response to interventions, it can usually be classified within one of the broad categories discussed below. Both brady- and tachyarrhythmias can cause symptoms by interfering with ventricular systolic and diastolic function, leading to inadequate cardiac output.

DISORDERS OF IMPULSE FORMATION

The usual focus of impulse formation is the sinus node. Normal sinus rhythm has a rate of 60–100 impulses per minute and is under the control of the autonomic nervous system. As such, sinus tachycardia or bradycardia is only a response to a perceived need, recognized by the autonomic nervous system, rather than a sign of sinus node dysfunction. This response can be appropriate and helpful (e.g., increases in rate associated with exercise) or seemingly inappropriate (extreme bradycardia and hypotension with vagal reactions). Other cardiac cells are capable of automaticity as well. Lower pacemakers usually do not reach threshold because of overdrive suppression by the more rapidly depolarizing sinus nodal cells. In the event of failure of sinus node automaticity, as may occur with degenerative diseases (sick sinus syndrome), cells of the AV node (40–60 beats/min), His bundle (30–50 beats/min), or Purkinje system (15–40 beats/min) may provide an escape rhythm, each with its own characteristic rate.

A distinction is made between failure of the normal automatic mechanism and abnormal automaticity, the occurrence of phase 4 depolarization in cells that are not capable of it under ordinary circumstances. Many conditions, such as acute ischemia, electrolyte imbalance (particularly hyperkalemia), and digoxin intoxication, can cause the resting membrane potential in atrial and ventricular muscle cells to reach less negative values and even achieve threshold. Although the resultant action potential will be abnormal (because the sodium channel is less responsive at less negative transmembrane voltages), it may be conducted slowly, depending on the state of the surrounding tissue. If the discharges from this abnormal tissue occur at a rate faster than that of the fastest working normal pacemaker focus, a sustained ectopic tachycardia may result. Clinical examples of this mechanism are certain atrial tachycardias, accelerated junctional tachycardia (in the setting of valve surgery, ischemia, or digitalis overdosage), and certain idioventricular rhythms.

Other mechanisms of abnormal impulse formation, such as parasystole and triggered activity due to early and delayed afterdepolarizations, may exist, but their physiology is more complex. Triggered activity has been demonstrated in experimental preparations of tissue made abnormal by ischemia, digitalis intoxication, and excess catecholamine infusion. The relationship of these observations to clinically relevant arrhythmias is unclear.

DISORDERS OF IMPULSE CONDUCTION

Slow conduction and conduction block can lead to either bradyarrhythmias or tachyarrhythmias; the former occurs when asystole or a slow escape rhythm ensues after block, the latter when abnormal conduction allows for the formation of a re-entrant circuit.

Raising the membrane potential to less negative values results in a sluggish sodium current during phase 0 because of relative voltage-dependent inactivation of the sodium channels. In addition, various conditions (ischemia, infarction, certain drugs) influence intracellular resistance to current flow, either by effects at the level of the individual cells (a decrease in cellular coupling) or by replacing communicating cells with electrically inactive collagen scar. A reduction in sodium current or the ease with which it influences adjacent cells decreases the conduction velocity through the affected tissue, and also may lead to conduction block. If this block occurs proximally within the conduction system, i.e., before at least a portion of the ventricles are depolarized, the resultant ventricular rhythm will depend on the function of escape pacemakers distal to the site of block.

RE-ENTRY

Under normal circumstances, a sinus impulse is carried along the specialized conduction system until every cell within the heart is activated. At this point, all cells will be refractory, and the impulse extinguishes. If conduction block prevents an area of tissue from being depolarized, this protected region may be able to conduct impulses when the remainder of the heart is refractory. A delayed wave of activation may pass through this region and serve to reactivate the rest of the myocardium just after it recovers from refractoriness and long before the next sinus impulse is due.

For this phenomenon to occur, three conditions must be present (Figure 8-5). First, there must be two distinct anatomic or functional pathways of conduction, joined at their proximal and distal ends. Second, the propagating impulse must block in one pathway. Third, conduction must be sufficiently slow in the other pathway to allow enough time for recovery of the tissue of the first pathway proximal to the site of block, allowing

for the formation of a re-entrant circuit. If continuous re-entry occurs, the resulting impulse generated by the circuit may be conducted to the rest of the heart. Most clinically important tachyarrhythmias are thought to be caused by re-entry. Common examples include AV nodal re-entry, AV reciprocating tachycardia in the Wolff-Parkinson-White syndrome, and ventricular tachycardia arising from the border zone of surviving tissue near an area of a prior infarction.

Antiarrhythmic Agents

As discussed above, disorders of impulse formation and impulse conduction are more likely to occur in areas of myocardium with abnormal cellular electrophysiology. Antiarrhythmic agents further alter conduction and/or the propensity for automaticity in cardiac tissue. This is why, in certain cases, antiarrhythmic drugs can have a proarrhythmic effect. That is, they can facilitate rather that prevent arrhythmias. However, because they tend to affect abnormal tissue to a greater extent than normal tissue, and because they affect impulses conducted at excessive rates more than those conducted at normal

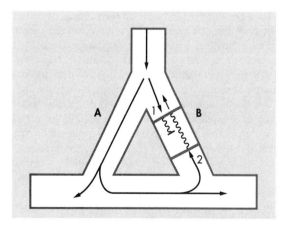

Figure 8-5 A model of re-entry. An impulse enters a bifurcation at point A. It blocks proximally in the pathway on the left (point B), but is conducted in the other branch, eventually to the distal point of insertion of the first pathway. If this impulse is conducted slowly enough for the proximal limb of the left pathway to recover, retrograde activation of the tissue proximal to the site of block can occur and a circuit may be formed. (Reproduced from Hoffman BF, Rosen MR. Cellular mechanisms for cardiac arrhythmias. *Circ Res* 49:1,1981:9.)

TABLE 8-1. Classification of Antiarrhythmic Drugs

Class I

Drugs that reduce V_{max} owing to block of inward sodium current in fast response tissue

- *Class IA* drugs reduce V_{max} at all heart rates and increase action potential duration (quinidine, procainamide, disopyramide).
- *Class IB* drugs have little effect on V_{max} in normal tissue and at slow rates but exert a greater effect on V_{max} in partially depolarized tissue or at faster rates; minimal effect on action potential duration or refractoriness (lidocaine, tocainide, mexiletine).
- *Class IC* drugs decrease V_{max} in normal tissue and at normal rates and have a minimal effect on action potential duration (flecainide, encainide).

Class II

Beta-adrenergic receptor antagonists that decrease impulse formation and conduction especially in nodal tissue (propranolol, metoprolol)

Class III

Agents that prolong action potential duration in fast response tissue (amiodarone, bretylium)

Class IV

Calcium channel antagonists that decrease action potential upstroke in slow response fibers, decreasing conduction velocity in these tissues and increasing refractoriness (verapamil, diltiazem, nifedipine)

V_{max} is the upstroke of the action potential (phase O).

rates (use dependence), they usually have a beneficial effect.

The major classes of antiarrhythmic drugs and representative examples are listed in Table 8-1. They are classified by their predominant actions: block of sodium, potassium, or calcium channels; or block of β-adrenergic receptors. Class I agents slow conduction by blocking sodium channels and decreasing the magnitude of the action potential upstroke. The agents within class I are subdivided based on their effects on action potential duration and duration of refractoriness, effects that are mediated by blocking potassium channels to a greater or lesser extent. The class II agents interfere with β-adrenergic receptors. Their effects are directed primarily at major sites of sympathetic nervous system innervation, primarily the sinus and AV nodes, where they cause a reduction in the rate of impulse formation and conduction. Class III drugs block potassium channels and thus prolong the time needed for repolarization and recovery from refractoriness. Finally, members of class IV interfere with slow inward calcium current. Digoxin is typically not included in this schema. It blocks the sodium-potassium pump, leading to less negative cellular resting potentials and thus slow conduction or conduction block. Similarly, atropine is also usually not classified with the remainder of the antiarrhythmic drugs. It blocks the action of parasympathetic innervation at the sinus and AV nodes and can lead to improved nodal conduction.

Bibliography

Atlee JL. *Perioperative cardiac dysrhythmias: mechanisms, recognition, management.* Chicago: Year Book Medical, 1985.

Berne RM, Levy MN. *Cardiovascular physiology.* 4th ed. St. Louis, CV Mosby, 1981.

Hodgkin AL. *The conduction of the nervous impulse.* Springfield, IL: Charles C Thomas, 1964.

Josephson ME, Buxton AE, Marchlinski FE. The bradyarrhythmias. In: Braunwald E, Isselbacher KJ, Petersdorf RG, et al., eds. *Harrison's principles of internal medicine.* New York: McGraw-Hill, 1987.

Josephson ME, Buxton AE, Marchlinski FE. The tachyarrhythmias. In: Braunwald E, Isselbacher KJ, Petersdorf RG, et al., eds. *Harrison's principles of internal medicine.* New York: McGraw-Hill, 1987.

Zipes DP. Genesis of cardiac arrhythmias: electrophysiologic considerations. In: Braunwald E, ed. *Heart disease.* Philadelphia: WB Saunders, 1988.

Stephen W. Downing

9 PHYSIOLOGY OF CARDIAC PUMP FUNCTION

This chapter will discuss the heart as a pump, and the major factors that modulate its performance. The discussion includes anatomy and physiology from the gross to subcellular levels, and the pathophysiology of common cardiac diseases. The principles of some major diagnostic modalities will also be described.

Anatomy

The heart is situated in the chest with the apex pointing anteriorly and to the left. It is rotated such that the right ventricle (RV) is the most anterior cardiac structure, and the left atrium is the most posterior.

At the entrance of the inferior vena cava into the right atrium, there is a variably present flap of tissue—the Eustachian valve—which minimizes venous reflux during atrial contraction. Medial to that the coronary sinus (with its own Eustachian valve) opens immediately above the posterior leaflet of the tricuspid valve.

Blood flow through the ventricles is smooth and ordered, minimizing inertial changes and turbulence which would waste significant amounts of energy. It tends to follow a "V" pattern in both ventricles. Blood enters the RV posteriorly, flowing down across the tricuspid valve, and exits up and anteriorly into the pulmonary outflow tract. The leaves of the tricuspid valve, and the muscular trabeculae, are important in maintaining this pattern. Analogously, left atrial blood enters posteriorly and exits anteriorly and superiorly. In addition to directing flow, the mitral valve/papillary muscle complex contributes to ventricular contraction by "pulling" the mitral valve in, aiding ejection. In theory, this complex also serves to idealize **stress** (force per unit area) distribution across the ventricle, thus maximizing efficiency. For these reasons many surgeons advocate preserving the mitral apparatus during valve replacement.

The RV is relatively thin-walled, and its crescentic cavity wraps around the right side of the much thicker left ventricle (LV). It is easily compressed by the surgeon's hand or pericardial collections.

The LV walls vary considerably in thickness from the base to the apex. They are most substantial where the intracavitary radius is the largest, thinning toward the narrower apex. Stress is directly proportional to the radius (law of Laplace); it is also inversely proportional to the wall thickness. Thus, this architecture provides for a relatively uniform distribution of stress throughout the ventricle. This fine balance is disturbed with infarction, which alters both wall thickness and ventricular geometry.

A well-developed network of extracellular connective tissue is present in the myocardium. There are relatively large collagen fibers that run from the fibrous base to the apex where they terminate en masse. There is another finer network of fibrillar extracellular collagen that enwraps the individual myocardial fibers. Functionally, this arrangement behaves in a manner similar to that of a cargo net. At low volumes these fibers are slack and somewhat random, offering no resistance to ventricular distention. Beyond a certain volume they become aligned in a very ordered crisscrossing pattern, resisting further distention. This point, at which resistance to enlargement increases exponentially, coincidently occurs when the sarcomeres have been stretched to their physiologic maximum length 2.2 μm.

Ventricular muscle fibers are arranged in an ordered syncytium. In general they run from base to apex, curving in a counterclockwise direction. The degree of this curving varies layer by layer, such that a section through the wall at any one point reveals fibers running in multiple directions. This arrangement makes herniation impossible. It also orients the pull of myocyte contraction along several axes simultaneously, so that the ventricle can contract in three dimensions. This also causes the heart to experience some mild torsion during systole; with a motion akin to that of a towel being wrung. The contribution of torsion to the ejection of blood is unknown.

Myocytes are long, slender, polynuclear cells with plentiful mitochondria. They are attached end-to-end by structures called intercalated discs. These are the load-bearing junctions. There are no lateral connections of any mechanical significance. The cell surface membrane, the sarcolemma, has multiple invaginations called T tubules that penetrate deep into the cell. This insures that even remote structures have rapid access to the depolarizing signal, which is carried on the sarcolemma. The T tubules terminate near the Z bands (see below). Here they lie in close proximity to the terminal cisternae of the **sarcoplasmic reticulum**, though there is no direct contact between these structures. The sarcoplasmic reticulum is a large network of internal branching tubules that runs throughout the myocyte, enveloping and enmeshing the contractile elements. The sarcoplasmic reticulum stores large amounts of calcium for use during contraction.

The contractile elements of the myocytes are made

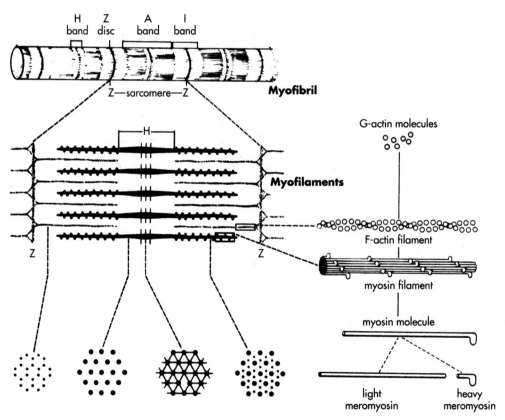

Figure 9-1 Diagram of the organization of skeletal muscle from the gross to the molecular level. (Reproduced from Fawcett DW, ed. *A textbook of histology.* 11th ed. Philadelphia: WB Saunders, 1986:282.)

of **actin, myosin, troponin,** and **tropomyosin.** The so-called "thin" fibers are composed of actin, and anchor to one another at the Z lines (Figure 9-1). They interdigitate with the "thick" fibers, which are composed of woven chains of myosin subunits. A sarcomere is considered to run from Z line to Z line. The I (isotropic) band is the area on either side of the Z line; it contains only actin. The A (anisotropic) band is the area in the middle of the sarcomere containing both actin and myosin. The H zone is the center of the A band, and is composed solely of myosin. It is visible only when the muscle is partially stretched (otherwise the actin ends overlap into this region). When a myocyte is elongated, the I band and the H zone increase; the A band does not change, for its length depends on the length of the myosin chain, which is unaltered. The area that is chemically active during contraction is the A band—excepting the H zone.

Protruding off the myosin chains are heads composed of subfragments called heavy meromyosin. These are notable because they contain the adenine triphosphatases (ATPases) which provide the energy for fiber movement, and they are the sites that bind to actin when contraction is initiated. Tropomyosin is woven in and around actin, and inhibits its interaction with myosin. Troponin is a protein that is in intimate association with tropomyosin. It serves to regulate the conformation of tropomyosin and together these two proteins form the trigger mechanism for contraction.

Excitation and Contraction

As the wave of depolarization spreads across the cell, the **slow calcium channels** are opened and a small amount of Ca^{2+} moves across the sarcolemma. This occurs during phase 2, or the plateau phase of the action potential (see Figure 8-4). This modest amount of calcium is the trigger for a **massive release of Ca^{2+}** from the sarcoplasmic reticulum into the cytosol. The cytosolic calcium then binds to the troponin. The tropinin then "disinhibits" the tropomyosin, altering its conformation such that it no longer blocks the interaction of actin and myosin. With the loss of inhibition the myosin head binds to the actin, and ATP is hydrolyzed. The myosin head has four active sites in series on its surface (Figure 9-2). The initiation of binding at one site increases the affinity for binding at the next. The increased binding affinity and energy from ATP allows

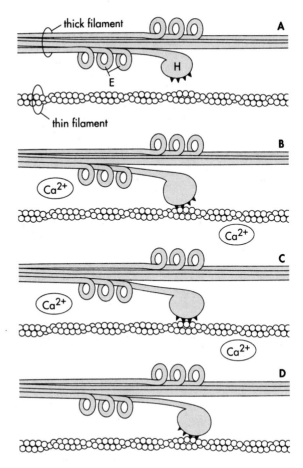

Figure 9-2 Proposed mechanism of actin and myosin interaction to allow muscle contraction. The thick filament is composed of myosin molecules; the thin filament is actin with troponin (not shown) and tropomyosin (not shown). **A,** At rest, the myosin is free with bound ATP. **B,** Ca^{2+} binds troponin, allowing filament interaction (see text). **C, D,** ATP is hydrolyzed and the myosin head rolls forward. E, Elastic element. H, Myosin head.

the myosin head to roll forward along the actin filament. These actin-myosin crosslinks are formed and reformed many times during each contraction and combine with many other actin-myosin crossbridges to contract the sarcomere, bringing the Z lines closer together.

Relaxation begins with the reuptake of Ca^{2+} into the sarcoplasmic reticulum. This is driven by an ATP-dependent Ca^{2+} pump. The rate of relaxation is dependent on the rate of Ca^{2+} reuptake, which is governed by a number of factors which are just now being elucidated. Defects of relaxation probably occur in many diseases.

The force of contraction is determined by the number of actin/myosin crossbridges that are formed during each beat. According to classic sliding filament theory, this is determined by the alignment of the fibers before contraction begins. When the Z lines are close together (1.5 μm) there is a significant fiber overlap, decreasing the number of effective sites for crossbridge formation. As the sarcomere is drawn out, there is an increase in the number of active sites, reaching a maximum at 2.2

μm. Theoretically, beyond the maximum, the number of potential crossbridge sites decreases again as the fibers are pulled farther apart. However, even with high end-diastolic pressures, cardiac sarcomeres beyond 2.2 μm are rarely noted.

The relationship between sarcomere length and developed force is directly linear (Figure 9-3A). In contrast, the relationship between resting length and the pressure or tension required to achieve that length (preload) is curvilinear (Figure 9-3B). Thus, the relation between preload and developed force is curvilinear. (Figure 9-3C). The concept that preload determines

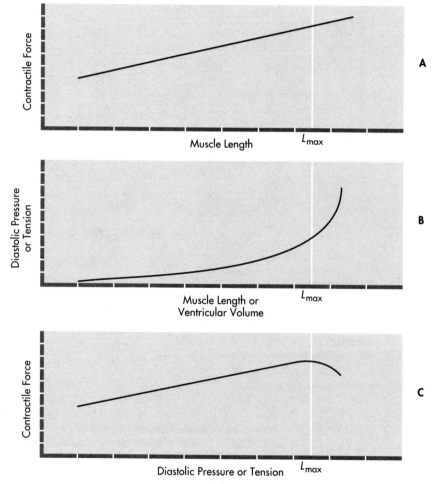

Figure 9-3 Note that while the relationship between muscle length (preload) and contractile force is linear over the physiologic range (**A**), the relationship between diastolic pressure and muscle length (or ventricular volume) is curvilinear (**B**). Thus, in vivo, the relationship between diastolic pressure and contractile force is also curvilinear (**C**).

contractile force is the basis of the **Frank-Starling law.** There is debate as to whether or not one can "go over the top" of the Frank-Starling curve. While it is true that developed force per unit preload decreases near the sarcomere's upper limits, the passive force (tension) is increasing exponentially at that time. Since the total force is the sum of the resting and developed forces, a nearly linear relationship is maintained between force and length in the physiologic range. This is summarized in Figure 9-4.

The other major determinant of contractile force is **intracellular Ca^{2+}**. The total velocity and force of contraction is directly proportional to the intracellular Ca^{2+} released during a given cardiac cycle. All the major inotropes appear to work by increasing intracellular Ca^{2+}. This includes digitalis, which acts indirectly through the Na^+/K^+ pump to raise Ca^{2+} levels. Increases in heart rate are also associated with augmented contractility, which results from the increased cumulative intracellular Ca^{2+} owing to incomplete reuptake during the shortened diastole.

The total cellular Ca^{2+} content is regulated primarily via the Na^+/Ca^{2+} exchange pump (not to be confused with the Ca^{2+} flux associated with contraction). Thus, intracellular levels of Ca^{2+} can be affected (in an inversely proportional manner) by Na^+ concentration. Na^+ con-

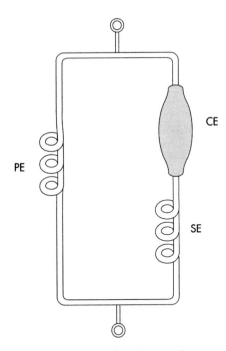

Figure 9-5 Maxwell model of cardiac muscle consisting of three elements. CE, contractile element; PE, parallel elastic; SE, series elastic. (Reproduced from Parmley WW. Mechanics of ventricular muscle. In: Levine HJ, Gaasch WH, eds. *The ventricle, basic and clinical aspects.* Boston: Martinus Nijhoff, 1985:50.)

centration, in turn, is partially related to K^+ and H^+ concentrations. This is one mechanism by which acidosis and electrolyte abnormalities affect cardiac performance.

Mechanically, the myocyte has been modeled by Maxwell as a "contractile element" attached to a "series elastic element." Working in parallel with this complex is the "parallel elastic element" (Figure 9-5). The parallel element provides resistance to extension and overextension when the muscle is in the passive state. It is what determines how much force is required to pull the sarcomere out to a given precontraction length. Structurally, this is probably the extracellular collagen and its matrix.

A useful analogy for understanding the contractile element/series elastic element relationship is one of a boy pulling a heavy rock with an elastic cord. When he stretches the cord it is put under tension, storing the energy of his arm movements. The rock, meanwhile, remains motionless until a critical level of force is reached, then it bounces forward. His arm movements can begin before the rock moves, and end before it

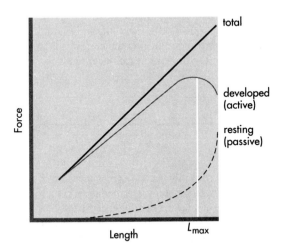

Figure 9-4 Schematic diagram of passive and active length tension curves of isolated heart muscle studied in vitro. Subtracting the resting force from the total force gives the developed force line. L_{max} is the length where developed force is maximum. (Reproduced from Parmley WW. Mechanics of ventricular muscle. In: Levine HJ, Gaasch WH, eds. *The ventricle, basic and clinical aspects.* Boston: Martinus Nijhoff, 1985:44.)

stops. The tension required to begin movement and the time required to complete this movement depend on the rock's weight.

This arrangement allows the myosin heads to roll along the actin during isovolumic contraction, creating tension, even though the muscle is not shortening. The elastic elements will release this energy when enough force has been generated to open the aortic valve and eject blood. This elastic element has not been morphologically identified, but there is general agreement on its existence.

Ventricular Function

In the following sections, function of the LV is primarily discussed; however, the same principles apply to RV function.

The cardiac cycle is traditionally divided into several phases: isovolumic or isometric contraction, isotonic contraction or ejection, isovolumic or isometric relaxation, and periods of rapid and slow ventricular filling (see Figure 10-1). The period of **isovolumic contraction** begins with the onset of systole. It is a time of rapidly increasing wall tension, but without ejection of blood. This period is not without movement. The ventricular walls rapidly thicken, and the mitral valve closes. This alters cavitary shape, without inducing a net volume change. This is known as **isovolumic rearrangement.** Because the impulse for contraction begins at the cardiac apex and spreads toward the base (over a period of milliseconds), the apical region begins contracting before the basal. This transiently increases the pressure on the noncontracting myocardium, augmenting the preload in those regions. This is called the "idioventricular kick."

Isotonic contraction begins with the opening of the aortic valve and the ejection of blood. While the heart contracts in all three dimensions, the greatest contribution comes from changes along the short axes. Wall thickening during contraction also aides ejection by further diminishing LV cavitary size. At end systole the ventricular cavity is at its absolute minimum volume.

Isovolumic relaxation begins with a drop in cavity tension and aortic valve closure. The ventricular wall, which had been compressed at end systole, rebounds to its somewhat larger resting size. This creates a negative pressure or "ventricular suction," drawing blood in through the mitral valve. This is the period of **rapid ventricular filling.** As the pressure differential between atrium and ventricle decreases, diastolic filling slows. The ventricle will begin to resist filling as it nears its volume limits. Diastole is ended by the atrial contraction, which provides the **atrial kick,** to top off the preload. The importance of this kick will vary directly with the stiffness of the LV.

Determinants of Cardiac Output

Cardiac output is determined by four factors: preload, afterload, contractility, and heart rate.

Preload is the force that determines the length of the sarcomeres prior to systole. The global correlate of sarcomere length is ventricular volume. Ventricular stroke work varies linearly with end-diastolic volume in the physiologic range: The greater the volume, the greater the stroke work. Clinically, however, volumes cannot be measured, so end-diastolic pressure is used as the gauge of preload. Like the correlation between tension and length in the myocyte, ventricular diastolic pressure and volume are not linearly related. Thus the relation between end-diastolic pressure and stroke work is curvilinear.

Afterload is the force applied to a muscle during contraction. The lower the afterload, the greater the stroke volume during that ejection, and therefore the greater the cardiac output. In the heart, this is roughly equivalent to the systemic vascular resistance (SVR). This is calculated as:

$$SVR = \frac{mean\ aortic\ pressure\ - mean\ right\ atrial\ pressure}{cardiac\ output} \times$$

conversion factor .

While this is clinically useful, a truer measure of afterload in a pulsatile system is impedance, which takes into account such factors as arterial elasticity, heart rate, and wave reflection. For example, in early systole the arterial tree is relatively empty and compliant, and can hold a bolus of blood. Near the end of systole the system is fuller, and its elastic components are stiffer. This reduction in compliance increases the resistance to ejection, raising pressure. Thus, resistance fluctuates during the cardiac cycle.

This increase in pressure during the latter part of systole could potentially increase ventricular wall stress.

However, at the same time that the systemic pressure is rising, LV cavitary radius is decreasing, which in turn decreases wall stress (law of Laplace). This cyclic balancing, called "impedance matching" or "ventricular-vascular coupling," is important for efficient cardiac function.

Contractility is the measure of how much work will be generated by a given preload. Contractility is difficult to determine clinically, and a Frank-Starling plot of ventricular stroke work versus end-diastolic pressure is one method of quantifying it (Figure 9-6). Factors that increase contractility will shift the curve up and to the left. Myocardial depressants shift it down and to the right. Common positive inotropes include the catecholamines and their analogs such as dobutamine and isoproterenol, as well as xanthines, calcium, glucagon, and thyroxin. Negative inotropes include β-blockers, calcium channel blockers, most antiarrythmics, most inhalational anesthetics, and barbiturates. Acidosis, hypothermia, and ischemia also have negative inotropic effects. As mentioned earlier, contractility is increased by increasing intracellular calcium. This may be accomplished directly by stimulation of β- or other receptors which produce cyclic AMP (cAMP), or indirectly by blocking cAMP breakdown. Cyclic adenosine monophosphate is believed to increase calcium flux through

the membranes during contraction and to increase protein affinities for calcium. This increased affinity produces a contraction that is more forceful, but also of shorter duration with more rapid relaxation. This permits the increase in heart rate that is usually concomitant with increases in contractility. Negative inotropes all tend to slow or decrease calcium flux.

Heart rate increases cardiac output through the following relation:

Cardiac Output = Heart Rate x Stroke Volume.

Heart rate makes the greatest contribution to cardiac output changes under normal circumstances. The rate is increased primarily by shortening diastole. Shortening systole requires increases in contractility. There is a point at which further increases in heart rate can be detrimental because, as diastole is shortened, ventricular filling is limited, decreasing preload. Increased heart rate also limits myocardial blood flow, which occurs primarily during diastole.

All of the determinants of cardiac output are interrelated, as shown in the following examples: Increasing the preload increases the force of contraction, increasing pressure and flow, which increases afterload. Increasing afterload decreases stroke volume, which

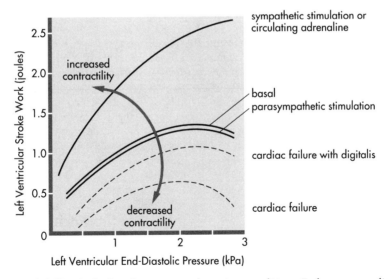

Figure 9-6 Ventricular function curves under various conditions. Each curve complies with Starling's law of the heart under the particular conditions: Within limits, the work done by the heart is proportional to the resting length of the muscle fibers. (Reproduced from Bowman WC, Rand MN. *Textbook of Pharmacology.* 2nd ed. Oxford: Blackwell Scientific, 1980: 22.40.)

increases end systolic volume, which will increase the preload of the next beat. Increasing heart rate increases flow, which increases pressure and thus resistance, but it also increases intracellular calcium, which increases contractility, and so on.

The **total work** done by the heart during the cardiac cycle is the sum of the internal and external work. The **internal work** is the amount of energy lost as heat and stored as elastic energy in the ventricular wall. It can be indirectly derived mathematically. **External work,** or stroke work can be calculated by plotting a pressure/volume loop (the closed loop graphical representation of ventricular pressure plotted against volume throughout a cardiac cycle), and integrating to derive the area of that loop. **Stroke work** varies in direct proportion to the preload or end-diastolic volume. At a constant preload, stroke work remains constant, independent of the afterload. However, the components of stroke work, **pressure work,** and **volume work** will vary with afterload. If afterload (i.e., aortic pressure) is relatively small, stroke volume will be large and a greater portion of the work done will be volume work. Conversely, if afterload is relatively large, stroke volume will be small and a greater portion of the work done will be pressure work. The importance of this difference is that for the same stroke work, pressure work uses much more energy, owing to increased internal elastic work.

Under physiologic conditions, oxygen consumption correlates nearly directly with LV wall tension. Wall tension, in turn, is dependent on LV cavity size and pressure. Ischemia alters this relation. A given wall tension will utilize more oxygen in the face of ischemia then in a nonischemic state. Thus, more oxygen is required to produce equivalent work in an ischemic heart than in a normal heart. **Power** is the work per unit time and is determined by the stroke work and the heart rate. While it is tension that determines the oxygen utilized per beat, the heart rate as well determines how much oxygen is consumed per minute.

Diastolic Function

There is currently a trend toward distinguishing systolic from diastolic heart failure. Classic congestive heart failure has a significant component of diastolic dysfunction, manifested as increased stiffness or impaired relaxation.

Diastolic function is usually graphically illustrated

by a pressure-volume (Figure 9-3B) or stress-strain curve. Stress is expressed as force per unit area, such as dynes/cm². Strain is usually expressed as Lagrangian strain, which is the percent change in dimension compared with a reference dimension.

As mentioned above, the initial determinants of diastolic filling are the rate of relaxation and the vigor of diastolic suction. The **rate of relaxation** is determined by the rate of calcium reuptake by the sarcoplasmic reticulum. This may be disturbed by temperature and metabolic abnormalities. Unusual mechanical loading conditions may also have an effect on relaxation by affecting the amount of calcium released into the cytosol. **Diastolic suction** results from elastic energy stored in the cell walls and the very ordered extracellular collagen matrix. It can be dampened by myocardial fibrosis. Minor impairments in relaxation may become highly significant at higher heart rates.

There are many other factors that will influence how the heart fills. For example, high coronary arterial pressures increase wall stiffness. This is called the "coronary erectile effect."

Diseases causing acute myocardial dysfunction, such as ischemia or sepsis, will cause an increase in the nonstressed ventricular volume (at zero pressure) causing the ventricle to appear more compliant at low pressures. However, calculation of the stress/strain relationship demonstrates that the ventricle actually is stiffer. This has clinical significance. While low pressures produce a larger ventricle, and thus a greater preload, slight volume increases beyond this are associated with very high diastolic pressures and pulmonary edema.

Aging, LV hypertrophy, and chronic coronary artery disease (with associated fibrosis) all increase myocardial stiffness. High volume venous returns during periods of demand cannot be compensated for, and pulmonary diastolic hypertension ensues. Decreased stiffness may by seen in chronic volume overload.

Effect of the Pericardium

The pericardium is generally very rigid, with strict volume limits. Over time, however, it can slowly expand in the face of chronically elevated pressures. This may be beneficial, allowing the failing ventricle to partially compensate by increasing its cavity size.

The presence or absence of the pericardium has no effect on normal filling pressures. It will protect against overdistention under extreme conditions. Significant pericardial fibrosis will obviously impair LV filling.

The pericardium also serves to magnify the effect other chambers have on LV function. With an intact pericardium, high right ventricular pressures are transmitted to the septum, shifting it over and impairing LV filling. Increases in left atrial size (as with fibrillation or mitral valve disease) will increase pericardial pressure and thus decrease LV filling.

Pump Pathophysiology

Heart failure is the inability to adequately deliver oxygenated blood to the periphery. It can divided into that caused by (1) work overload, (2) oxygen deprivation, or (3) myocardiopathy. Compensation occurs in three ways: (1) Large end-systolic volume from impaired ejection increases the preload for the subsequent beats, (2) increased adrenergic tone increases local and systemic catecholamines, and (3) the heart hypertrophies to increase muscle mass. The result is a larger and thicker heart that has a decreased ejection fraction, but is able to maintain stroke volume, and thus cardiac output.

Work overload comes in two types—pressure and volume. Pressure overload arises from hypertension or valvular stenosis. It is a systolic overload and is characterized by concentric hypertrophy. Teleologically, the heart increases wall thickness and decreases cavitary size to reduce the high wall stress that the elevated pressure has produced. Volume overload occurs with valvular incompetence and arteriovenous fistulae. It is a diastolic overload, and while some hypertrophy occurs, the primary compensation occurs through ventricular dilation. There is less depression of contractility associated with the myocardial hypertrophy of volume overload as compared with that of pressure overload. The volume overloaded heart is also more compliant during diastole, especially at lower pressures. Again teleologically, this allows the heart to handle large volumes without high filling pressures and subsequent pulmonary edema. With mitral regurgitation, ventricular wall stress does not increase greatly at the larger ventricular volume because valvular incompetence limits systolic pressure. When the incompetence is eliminated by repair, wall stress acutely increases. This is why patients with mitral regurgitation do poorly if their preoperative end-dias-

tolic volumes are greater than 160 mL/m² of body surface area.

Myocardial ischemia is characterized by focal myocyte loss and replacement fibrosis. This decreases systolic capabilities by decreasing the active myocardial mass, and alters diastolic performance by increasing resistance to filling. To compensate, the ventricle will dilate and the remaining myocytes hypertrophy as nutrient supply allows. A special case occurs when an entire region of myocardium is infarcted. This produces an alteration in ventricular geometry. For example, a large anteroapical infarction produces a segment of akinetic myocardium that with time becomes frankly dyskinetic, bulging paradoxically with each systole (an LV aneurysm). Not only does this deprive the heart of its idioventricular kick, but this bulging sac places high stresses on the normal myocardium it is attached to, producing dysfunction there as well. It is postulated that this leads to recruitment of normal tissue into the LV aneurysm. This may initiate the progressive process of ventricular dysfunction and aneurysm expansion that frequently leads to patient death.

All compensatory shifts are incomplete and will eventually fail. The hypertrophied myocardium has less force producing capability per unit volume than normal myocardium. It has known inadequacies in energy supply (separate from issues of coronary perfusion) and abnormalities of calcium metabolism. Hypertrophied muscle is also stiffer, and is often accompanied by fibrosis. This adversely affects diastolic performance. While ventricular volume elevations increase preload, they also increase afterload by increasing systolic wall stress (the cavitary radius is large throughout systole). Increased adrenergic tone depletes cardiac catecholamine stores, limiting responsiveness to stress, and raising peripheral vascular tone, increasing afterload.

Reperfusion Injury

Myocardium that has been ischemic, but which is reperfused before irreversible damage occurs, may also be dysfunctional. During the ischemic period, high-energy phosphates are lost, and membrane pumps can no longer maintain appropriate ionic and osmotic gradients. Cellular swelling results in increasing resistance to shortening when contraction resumes. There is also significant interstitial edema from capillary leakage, which, in turn, decreases ventricular compliance.

During reperfusion there is a large influx of calcium, which can cause substantial mitochondrial damage. Additionally, with the influx of oxygen, the partially uncoupled oxidative phosphorylation system produces excess oxygen free radicals. This overwhelms local free radical scavengers, allowing membrane peroxidation. The net effect is "stunned," poorly contracting myocardium. It may take greater than 48 hours to replete high-energy phosphates and restore the homeostasis required for normal contractility.

Diagnostics for Cardiac Pump Function

Noninvasive determination of cardiac function is limited by an inability to attain highly accurate, reproducible, instantaneous volume measurements. There are, however, several methods of approximation from which performance data can be derived.

The most common measurement is cardiac output. The **Fick method** actually determines RV output. Its principle is simple. If the amount of oxygen a given amount of blood extracts as it traverses the lungs (i.e., how many milliliters of O_2 are added to each milliliter of blood) and the amount of alveolar oxygen extracted by the lungs per minute are known, then the blood flow through the lungs necessary to extract that amount of oxygen can be calculated. Mathematically, this is described as

$$\text{Cardiac output (L / min)} = \frac{O_2 \text{ extraction (ml } O_2 \text{ / min)}}{\text{A-V } O_2 \text{ difference (ml / } O_2 \text{ L blood)}}.$$

Arteriovenous (A-V) O_2 difference (mL O_2 /L blood) = 13.9 x Hgb (g/dL) x (% saturation arterial – % saturation venous blood).

This calculation is limited clinically by the difficulty in determining oxygen extraction (which equals oxygen consumption in a steady state).

The Fick method has been essentially supplanted by dilutional techniques. While traditionally these methods utilized indicator dyes, the method of choice today is **thermodilution**. A bolus of cold saline is injected into the right atrium. A thermistor in the pulmonary artery records the temperature change. A plot of temperature versus time is generated. The cardiac output is calculated using a complex equation that calculates the area under the curve and a decay constant, and takes into account the temperature of the injectate, the temperature of the blood, injected volume, and specific gravity. Again, this is actually an RV output. It is not valid in conditions of tricuspid regurgitation or with intracardiac shunts. Additionally, it tends to underestimate the cardiac output in low flow states because of heating from surrounding cardiac structures. There are also errors from temperature fluctuations during respiration. In general, these techniques are accurate to within 15%.

Additional information can be obtained during **cardiac catheterization.** Using biplane ventriculography, long and short axes can be measured. Modeling the LV as a prolate ellipsoid (football) then allows LV volume calculation. Knowing end-systolic and end-diastolic volumes (ESV and EDV), **stroke volume (SV)** and **ejection fraction (EF)** can be calculated:

$$EF = \frac{EDV - ESV}{EDV} = \frac{SV}{EDV}.$$

Valve cross-sectional area can also be estimated during catheterization. The principles are based on Torricelli's law (which is derived from Bernoulli's equation). The effective valve orifice area is proportional to the flow divided by a constant times the square root of the pressure gradient. There are different constants for the aortic and mitral valves.

Radionucleotide imaging can provide two basic types of information—LV volume changes and myocardial perfusion. The first technique uses a bolus of **technitium-99.** This radioactive bolus is followed through the heart with a scintillation camera. The count rates emitted from a chamber are proportional to its volumes. The change in volume with contraction is used to calculate ejection fraction. This is called first pass radionucleotide imaging. A more precise image is obtained from tagging the patients red blood cells with the technitium-99 and allowing it to equilibrate in the circulation. The recording camera is gaited to the electrocardiogram and a picture is created at certain points in the cardiac cycle (such as end systole or end diastole) using the summation of 200–300 beats. Volume changes and regional wall motion can be monitored.

Thallium-201 is a radioactive tracer that acts as a potassium analog and is taken up by myocytes. Its distribution correlates with blood flow distribution, and can show regions of infarction, or regions with flow rates that do not increase during exercise (suggesting vascular stenosis limiting coronary blood flow reserve to those regions).

Echocardiography produces two-dimensional images based on the reflections of sound waves. Examination of the percentage wall thickening during contraction can quantify regional contractility. This is generally done to compare one region with another. Global volumes can also be approximated and ejection fraction calculated. Beat-to-beat variations cannot be exactly quantitated because of the lack of a reproducible reference point. Doppler ultrasound can calculate blood velocity by noting frequency shifts in returning signals. This is not a flow measurement per se, but coupled with knowledge of the cross-sectional area at the point of measurement, can be used to calculate flow or cardiac output. Pressure drop across a valve or stenosis can also be derived using the Holen formula:

Pressure Drop = $4(\text{maximal flow velocity})^2$.

Knowledge of the pressure in one chamber allows calculation of the pressure in a connected chamber.

Bibliography:

Huxley AF. The mechanical properties of cross-bridges and their relation to muscle contraction. In: Varga E, Köver A, Kovacs T, Kovacs L, eds. *Molecular and cellular aspects of muscle function. Advances in physiological sciences, vol 5.* Elmsford, NY: Pergamon, 1981.

Levine HJ, Gaasch WH, eds. *The ventricle.* Boston: Martinus Nijhoff, 1985.

Sabiston DC Jr, Spencer FC, eds. *Surgery of the chest.* 5th ed. Philadelphia: WB Saunders, 1990.

Schlant RC, Sonnenblick EH. Normal physiology of the cardiovascular system. In: Hurst JW, Schlant RC, eds. 7th ed. *The heart arteries and veins.* New York: McGraw-Hill, 1990.

Steven C. Hendrickson,
Charles R. Bridges, and
Edward B. Savage

10 INTEGRATED CONCEPTS OF CARDIOVASCULAR FUNCTION

Functional Anatomy
Oxygen Delivery
Myocardial Oxygen Consumption
Coronary Blood Flow
Pathophysiology
    Myocardial Ischemia
    Myocardial Infarction
    Shunts
    Hypertrophy
    High-Output Congestive Heart Failure
    Low-Output Congestive Heart Failure

This chapter will emphasize the integration of the cardiovascular system with body function to maintain homeostasis. The normal physiology of the heart and circulation will be discussed along with pathological alterations in function.

Functional Anatomy

Four rings of dense connective tissue form the fibrous skeleton of the heart. Two are the atrioventricular valve (AV) rings of the mitral and tricuspid valves. The atria are fastened to the superior surface of these rings. The mitral and tricuspid valves are similar in structure. The mitral valve is functionally bicuspid, consisting of large anteromedial and posterolateral cusps with corresponding chordae tendinae and papillary muscles. The tricuspid valve also consists primarily of two large septal and posterior cusps and a smaller anterior cusp with associated papillary muscles and chordae tendinae.

The other two rings suspend the semilunar aortic and pulmonary valves. These valves both consist of three symmetrical cusps. Behind each aortic valve cusp is a sinus of Valsalva. The right and left coronary arter-

ies originate from the right and left (anterior) sinuses. The posterior sinus lies behind the noncoronary cusp and no coronary artery originates from this sinus.

The ventricles are fastened to the entire circumference of this fibrous skeleton of the heart. Each ventricle consists of sheets of myocardial fibers wrapped around the ventricular chamber in a complex orientation. The overall pumping function of the heart is the summation of the contraction and relaxation of individual myocardial muscle fibers. The tension generated by each muscle fiber is determined by the cardiac cycle, the fiber length, the tension applied across the fiber, and the inotropic state of the muscle. For a three-dimensional vessel like the left ventricle, the determinants of fiber length and applied tension are the left ventricular volume or preload and the aortic pressure or afterload.

The period from onset of one cardiac contraction to the onset of the next cardiac contraction is known as the cardiac cycle. There is both an electrical cycle and a mechanical cycle which are coupled with a fixed temporal relationship. During a normal cardiac contraction, the electrical cycle begins with spontaneous generation of an action potential in the sinoatrial (SA) node leading to depolarization and contraction of the right and left atria. The impulse then travels through the AV node, the bundle of His, and then rapidly through the Purkinje fibers to the ventricles, resulting in the initiation of the mechanical cardiac cycle.

The mechanical cardiac cycle can be divided into a period of contraction called systole and a period of relaxation called diastole. Figure 10-1 illustrates the components of a normal cardiac cycle. Blood flows continually from the vena cava and pulmonary veins into the right and left atria, respectively. The diastolic interval ends as the wave of excitation spreads over the atria, resulting in atrial contraction. The earliest phase of sys-

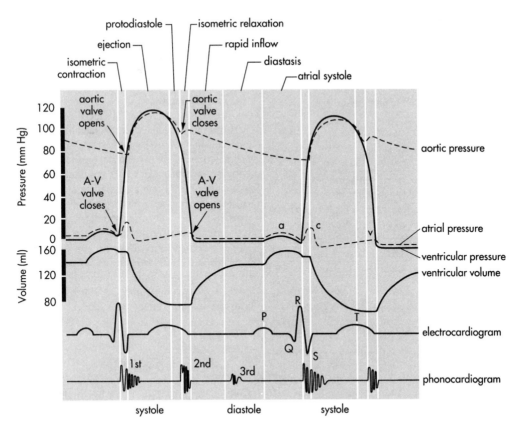

Figure 10-1 The events of the cardiac cycle, showing changes in left atrial pressure, left ventricular pressure, aortic pressure, ventricular volume, the electrocardiogram, and the phonocardiogram. (Reproduced from Guyton AC. *Textbook of medical physiology.* 6th ed. Philadelphia: WB Saunders, 1981:154.)

tole occurs as the electrical activity extends along the Purkinje system to the endocardial fibers and papillary muscles. Contraction of the papillary muscles apposes the atrioventricular valve leaflets, closing the valve. As the wave of excitation passes from the endocardium to the epicardium, the entire ventricular muscle mass becomes involved in the contraction, and cavity pressure begins to rise. The semilunar valves remain closed, since the pressure in the ventricles is less than aortic or pulmonary artery pressure. During this period, all four valves are closed, and, since blood is an incompressible fluid, contraction of the ventricular muscle elevates ventricular pressure without a change in intraventricular volume (**isometric contraction**). When the pressure in the left and right ventricles exceeds aortic and pulmonary artery pressures, respectively, the semilunar valves open, resulting in rapid ventricular emptying

(**ejection**). During the last one fourth of ventricular systole, the velocity of flow from the ventricles decreases substantially, although the muscles remain contracted (**protodiastole**).

At the end of systole, ventricular relaxation begins and the semilunar valves close; ventricular pressure falls while ventricular volume remains constant (**isovolumic relaxation**). When ventricular pressures fall below their associated atrial pressures, the atrioventricular valves open, resulting in rapid filling of the ventricles during the first third of diastole (**rapid inflow**). During the middle third of diastole, filling slows as blood flows directly from the great veins through the atria and into the ventricular chambers (**diastasis**). During the final third of diastole, the atrium contracts, emptying its contents into the ventricle (**atrial systole**).

During the cardiac cycle there are characteristic

pressure changes in the atria. The **a wave** represents atrial contraction. The **c wave** corresponds to the bulging of the AV valves into the atria at the onset of ventricular contraction. The **v wave** corresponds to the slow build up of blood in the atria while the AV valves are closed during ventricular systole.

Oxygen Delivery

Oxygen delivery is determined by the amount of blood delivered to the tissues and the amount of oxygen carried by the blood. Therefore, oxygen delivery (DO_2) equals the oxygen content of arterial blood (CaO_2) x **cardiac output (CO)**. The components of CaO_2 are the hemoglobin concentration (Hgb), the oxygen saturation of hemoglobin (SaO_2) and plasma dissolved oxygen (PaO_2).

$$CaO_2 = 1.39 \times (Hgb) \times SaO_2 + 0.003 \times PaO_2$$

where $1.39 = mL\ O_2/g\ Hgb$.

Since the amount of oxygen dissolved in plasma is relatively small, its contribution is not clinically significant. Therefore, for practical purposes the oxygen content of arterial blood can be expressed as follows:

$$CaO_2 = 1.39 \times (Hgb) \times SaO_2.$$

Therefore, for a normal individual with a Hgb = 15 g/dL and an SaO_2 = 100%,

$$CaO_2 = 1.39 \times 15 \times 100\% = 21\ mL\ O_2\ /dL\ blood.$$

Cardiac output is the other factor contributing to oxygen delivery. With a normal cardiac output, DO_2 is approximately 900–1100 mL O_2/min. DO_2 can also be expressed in terms of **cardiac index (CI)**: CO/body surface area. With a normal CI of 3.0 L/min/m², the DO_2 would be approximately 600 mL O_2/min/m². Again, these normal values are calculated assuming an Hgb = 15 g/dL and 100% SaO_2.

Myocardial Oxygen Consumption

At rest, the myocardium extracts approximately 10 mL of oxygen per 100 grams of tissue per minute. This is 70–75% of the available oxygen and results in an arteriovenous oxygen difference of 11 mL O_2/dL of blood and a coronary venous PO_2 of 20 mm Hg. Increased car-

diac metabolic activity associated with accelerated heart rate or greater myocardial contractility increases myocardial oxygen consumption.

Myocardial oxygen consumption is also related to the amount of work performed by the ventricle. When the work increases, so does oxygen consumption. The amount of the increase is related to the type of work performed. An increase in cardiac output against a constant aortic pressure (volume work) produces a relatively small increase in myocardial oxygen consumption. In contrast, pressure work (i.e., maintaining the same cardiac output against an increased systemic pressure) produces a much greater increase in oxygen consumption. This is because the primary determinant of myocardial oxygen consumption is **myocardial wall tension.** Oxygen demand increases in direct proportion to wall tension. Since wall tension (T) is directly proportional to intracavitary pressure (P) and radius (R) of the cavity (T::PR), oxygen consumption increases with increased pressure work and left ventricular dilatation.

Coronary Blood Flow

Blood is supplied to the heart by the right and left coronary arteries. The right coronary artery supplies the right ventricle and, usually, the posterior left ventricle (80–90% of hearts). The anterior and lateral portions of the left ventricle are perfused by the left coronary system. The main source of blood to the posterior wall and posterior septum is variable. The right coronary artery is dominant 67% of the time, the left 15% of the time, and in 18% the flow is about equal. The venous drainage from the left ventricle is predominately through the coronary sinus (75% of coronary flow). The right ventricle primarily drains via the anterior cardiac veins into the right atrium. A small amount of blood drains directly into the cardiac chambers through the **thebesian veins.** The average coronary blood flow at rest is 70–80 milliliters per 100 grams of cardiac muscle per minute; approximately 225 mL/min, or 4–5% of cardiac output.

Flow through the left coronary artery is phasic. During systole there is cessation and even reversal of blood flow due to compression of the intramuscular branches by the contracting myocardium. With diastolic relaxation, extravascular resistance is decreased and blood flow rapidly increases. Thus, the heart is the only organ that receives the majority of its blood flow during diastole. Flow to the right ventricle also has a phasic pattern, but the forces involved are not as great and the ratio of diastolic to systolic blood flow is much smaller.

Extravascular resistance to flow during systole is not uniform through the ventricular wall. During systole all layers of the heart squeeze toward the lumen to eject the blood. This creates a gradient of pressure within the myocardium, with the pressure being greatest in the subendocardium and least in the subepicardium. Because of this gradient, the subendocardium receives almost no flow during systole. The subendocardium compensates for this by having larger vessels which offer less resistance to flow during diastole.

Control of coronary blood flow is primarily a local phenomenon (**autoregulation**). In response to an increased myocardial oxygen demand, the coronary vessels dilate, and flow increases proportionally. The exact cause of the coronary vasodilatation is unknown, but the most likely scenario is that the relative oxygen deficit causes the release of vasodilator substances from the myocardial cell. **Adenosine** is a vasodilator released by myocytes under conditions of relative ischemia and may be the primary substrate of autoregulation. Other vasodilators include potassium and hydrogen ions, CO_2, bradykinin, and prostaglandins.

Autonomic stimulation also affects coronary blood flow. The direct effects of sympathetic stimulation are dependent on whether α- or β-receptors are stimulated. α-Receptors predominate in the epicardial coronary vessels and mediate vasoconstriction. β-Receptors are more common in the intramuscular arteries and mediate vasodilatation. The direct effects of sympathetic stimulation are minor compared with the indirect effects. Increases in heart rate and contractility cause increased myocardial oxygen consumption, which results in increased coronary flow by autoregulatory mechanisms. Therefore, the net effect of sympathetic stimulation is to increase coronary blood flow. Parasympathetic stimulation has no direct effect on the coronary arteries, but by decreasing heart rate and contractility, myocardial oxygen consumption is reduced, indirectly producing coronary vasoconstriction.

Pathophysiology

MYOCARDIAL ISCHEMIA

Myocardial ischemia occurs when myocardial oxygen demand exceeds the oxygen supply. The most common cause of myocardial ischemia and myocardial infarction is **coronary artery atherosclerosis.** Less common causes include coronary vasospasm (Prinzmetal's or variant angina), aortic stenosis, hypertrophic cardiomyopathy, embolism, aortic dissection, and inflammatory diseases of the coronary arteries (i.e., Kawasaki's disease).

Though the pathogenesis of atherosclerosis is discussed in Chapter 12, several points merit emphasis for this discussion. Most atherosclerotic lesions of the left coronary system occur within 6 cm of the origin and at branch points. The majority of these lesions are discrete, being less than or equal to 5 mm in length. These characteristics are important, since lesions that fit these criteria are usually amenable to treatment with percutaneous transluminal coronary angioplasty or coronary artery bypass grafting. Lesions of the right coronary artery are more often diffuse and involve the proximal and middle thirds of the artery. The left anterior descending artery is the most commonly affected artery, being involved by 45% of lesions, followed by the right coronary artery (27%), the left circumflex (23%), and the left main coronary artery (5%). The posterior descending coronary artery is seldom involved. Hemodynamically significant stenosis requires greater than or equal to 70% narrowing of the cross-sectional area of the lumen.

As stated previously, myocardial ischemia occurs when oxygen supply is insufficient to meet demand. Since the heart extracts approximately 70% of oxygen from arterial blood at rest, the only way to increase oxygen delivery is to increase blood flow. In the normal heart, autoregulation of coronary blood flow ensures that cardiac oxygen demand will not exceed supply even with heavy exercise.

With **aortic stenosis**, myocardial oxygen demand exceeds supply despite normal coronary arteries. Hypertrophied muscle and increased wall tension increase oxygen demand. The increased extraluminal resistance to coronary blood flow, which is due to the elevated intracavitary pressure, and decreased aortic root diastolic pressure (coronary perfusion pressure) reduce coronary blood flow beyond the limits of autoregulation. These two aspects combine to reduce the ratio of oxygen supply to oxygen demand to a critical level.

Coronary perfusion pressure is reduced distal to a stenosing or occluding lesion. Coronary vascular resistance is reduced by autoregulatory mechanisms to maintain adequate distal flow and oxygen delivery at rest. Since the vascular bed is dilated at rest, the reserve for further dilitation with increased oxygen demand is reduced. When resistance is maximally reduced (i.e., the vessels are maximally dilated), the distribution of myocardial blood flow, once dependent on active autoregulation, becomes passively dependent on coronary perfusion pressure (CPP).

The diastolic pressure-time index (DPTI) summarizes the factors that determine myocardial blood flow when autoregulatory mechanisms have been exhausted. The DPTI represents the area between the curves of CPP and left ventricular diastolic pressure (LVDP). Factors that affect DPTI are the length of diastole and the proportion of the cardiac cycle spent in diastole. Normally, LVDP is negligible compared with the CPP and has little effect on blood flow. However, with a proximal coronary stenosis, the difference between CPP and LVDP is reduced, and increases in LVDP, such as with left ventricular distention, can have a profound effect on subendocardial perfusion.

A less common cause of myocardial ischemia is **coronary vasospasm,** which produces the clinical syndrome of **Prinzmetal's (or variant) angina.** Vasospasm occurs in the epicardial coronary arteries, resulting in transmural ischemia. It is usually superimposed on a pre-existing atherosclerotic stenosis, but may also occur in an otherwise normal coronary artery. Vasospasm is produced by α-adrenergic stimulation. The underlying abnormality making the artery hypersensitive to stimulation is unknown.

Myocardial ischemia secondary to coronary atherosclerosis and vasospasm can be differentiated clinically. Angina pectoris secondary to coronary atherosclerosis is typically associated with exertion (when subendocardial flow is compromised) and is reproducible. The subendocardial ischemia is reflected by ST segment depression on the electrocardiogram (ECG). Variant angina, on the other hand, is due to transmural ischemia resulting in ST segment elevation on the ECG. It also characteristically occurs at rest, often during the early morning hours. Vasospasm can be induced during cardiac catheterization with ergonovine stimulation (an α-adrenergic agonist).

Relief of myocardial ischemia is based on decreasing oxygen demand or increasing oxygen delivery. **Nitrates** relax vascular smooth muscle, dilating epicardial coronary arteries and increasing coronary blood flow. Venous vasodilation decreases ventricular preload and wall tension. Systemic arterial vasodilation decreases cardiac afterload, further lessening myocardial oxygen demand. **β-Adrenergic blocking agents** competitively inhibit circulating and synaptic

catecholamines, decreasing heart rate and contractility. These effects combine to greatly diminish myocardial oxygen consumption. However, β-blockers may exacerbate vasospasm by allowing unopposed α-adrenergic stimulation. **Calcium channel blockers** inhibit influx of calcium ions into vascular and cardiac smooth muscle during membrane depolarization. By doing so they decrease systemic vascular resistance and produce coronary vasodilatation, alleviating vasospasm or increasing flow through a stenotic artery. Calcium channel blockers also slow conduction through the AV node, decreasing heart rate.

MYOCARDIAL INFARCTION

An **acute myocardial infarction** occurs when prolonged myocardial ischemia leads to irreversible coagulative necrosis of myocytes. The extent of a myocardial infarction depends on the severity of the ischemia, the area supplied by the obstructed artery, the oxygen demands of the myocardium at risk, and the extent of coronary collateral blood flow. A myocardial infarction may be either **transmural,** involving the full thickness of the muscle, or **subendocardial,** involving less than 50% of the wall thickness. Infarct **extension** refers to new myocardial cellular necrosis at the border of the myocardial infarction. Extension is probably due to microvascular vasoconstriction near the infarct secondary to local cathecholamine release. Infarct **expansion** refers to thinning and an increase in the surface area of an infarct without new necrosis. Expansion may be due to disruption of myocardial cells, but a more likely cause is destruction of the connective tissue framework of the heart. Left ventricular aneurysm formation and ventricular rupture can occur as a result of expansion.

The morphologic features of an acute myocardial infarction do not become apparent until approximately 6 hours after the myocardial infarction occurs. Coagulative necrosis is marked by loss of striations in the myocytes, hypereosinophilic staining, hyaline change, nuclear karyolysis, pyknosis, and karyorrhexis. At 12–24 hours, neutrophils migrate into the infarcted region. Neutrophil infiltration increases up to the fourth day. Edema and focal areas of hemorrage are present during this period. Capillaries and fibroblasts migrate into the infarct at approximately the seventh postinfarct day. After 8–10 days there is thinning of the infarct as debris is cleared by mononuclear cells. Granulation tissue begins to form at 8–10 days and is present throughout the infarcted area by 3–4 weeks. A thin scar develops, and it becomes firm by 6 weeks.

The majority of acute myocardial infarctions (greater than 90%) occur when an acute obstruction is superimposed on a pre-existing atherosclerotic lesion. Three mechanisms can potentially cause this acute occlusion: **thrombosis, plaque rupture, and vasospasm.** Fresh thrombus at the site of a critical stenosis has been found in up to 90% of patients studied by cardiac catheterization at the time of myocardial infarction. Thrombosis has been linked to increased platelet aggregability. This is the basis for thrombolytic reperfusion therapy with **streptokinase** and **tissue plasminogen activator (TPA).** These agents, if used within the first 6 hours after a mycardial infarction, may lyse the acutely occluding thrombus and restore blood flow to the region at risk.

Atherosclerotic plaque rupture is another potential source of acute occlusion. Evidence of plaque rupture has been noted in 78–93% of obstructing lesions at autopsy. Rupture of a plaque could result in total obstruction by one or all of the following mechanisms:

1. Exposure of underlying collagen to circulating platelets,
2. Release of tissue thromboplastin,
3. Mechanical obstruction of the lumen by plaque contents.

Most likely, obstruction associated with plaque rupture is due to the first two mechanisms causing thrombosis at the site of the plaque. It has been hypothesized that plaque rupture is brought about by rupture of small vessels within the plaque itself. However, it is not likely that the forces generated in this manner could overcome the intraluminal pressure in the coronary artery.

Vasospasm may result in disruption of the intimal covering of the atheroma, leading to plaque rupture. Vasospasm may also occur at a site of stenosis, leading to stasis and thrombus formation. It may also produce obstruction of a coronary artery independent of the other two mechanisms, usually at a site of partial obstruction. Vasospasm in an otherwise normal coronary artery accounts for 7% of acute myocardial infarctions. Other causes of acute occlusion of a coronary artery include embolism and aortic dissection involving the coronary ostia, but these mechanisms are rare.

Acute coronary occlusion results in transmural ischemia. There is a **gradient of ischemia** within the ventricular wall from the subendocardium to the subepicardium. Myocardial necrosis occurs in a sequential fashion from the inner to the outer layers of the heart wall. To limit the size of a myocardial infarction, flow must be restored before cell death occurs, within 6 hours of the onset of the myocardial infarction. After 6 hours all the ischemic myocardium necroses irreversibly. Flow to ischemic myocardium can be re-established through collateral circulation or by reopening the occluded segment. Coronary collaterals are seldom well enough developed in the human heart to prevent a myocardial infarction. However, collaterals may supply flow adequate enough to salvage the less severely ischemic subepicardium, converting a potential transmural infarction into a subendocardial myocardial infarction.

The diagnosis of a myocardial infarction is made on the basis of ECG changes and elevated serum levels of enzymes released from necrotic cells. Characteristic ECG changes are the result of alterations in signal conduction and depolarization patterns secondary to cell ischemia and death. Among the enzymes released are creatine kinase (CK), lactate dehydrogenase (LDH), and serum glutamic oxaloacetic transferase (SGOT). Elevation of SGOT is nonspecific and can arise from so many different abnormalities that it is seldom used for the diagnosis of myocardial infarction. Creatine kinase and LDH are also nonspecific. However, the specificity of these enzymes for myocardial infarction is greatly enhanced by isoenzyme analysis. Creatine kinase is found in cardiac and skeletal muscle, brain, and the gastrointestinal tract. The isoenzymes of CK are the BB, MM, and MB subunits. CK-BB predominates in the brain and GI tract, CK-MM is found in both cardiac and skeletal muscle, and CK-MB is present almost exclusively in myocardial cells and is the most specific indicator of myocardial infarction. Total CK begins to rise within 6 hours of a myocardial infarction. Its activity reaches a peak at 24–36 hours and returns to normal in 48–72 hours. CK-MB follows a more rapid course being elevated in approximately 2 hours post myocardial infarction, peaking at 10–12 hours, and returning to normal in 24–36 hours. An MB fraction greater than 7–8% indicates myocardial necrosis even if total CK activity is not increased.

There are five LDH isoenzymes. LDH1 is found predominately in cardiac muscle. It is also found in smaller quantities in red blood cells, kidney, brain, stomach, and pancreas. The other isoenzymes are chiefly found in liver and skeletal muscle. The LDH1/LDH2 ratio is primarily used in diagnosing myocardial infarction. Normally, LDH2 exceeds LDH1 in serum, but with a myocardial infarction, the serum level of LDH1 becomes greater than that of LDH2, resulting in an LDH1/LDH2 ratio greater than 1.0. Renal infarction is the only other disorder that regularly causes LDH1 to exceed LDH2. LDH activity rises 12–24 hours after myocardial infarction, peaks at 3–4 days, and returns to normal levels within 2 weeks.

SHUNTS

A shunt occurs when an abnormal connection exists between the right heart/pulmonary circulation and the left heart/systemic circulation. Shunt flow may be left to right, right to left, or bidirectional. The vast majority of bidirectional shunts have a left-to-right or right-to-left component that is responsible for the clinical manifestations.

Left-to-right shunts occur in the presence of an atrial septal defect, a ventricular septal defect, or a patent ductus arteriosus. Oxygenated blood flows from the systemic to the pulmonary circulation. Left-to-right shunts result in increased pulmonary blood flow (PBF). A shunt becomes physiologically significant when PBF becomes 1.5 to 2 times greater than systemic blood flow (SBF), resulting in pulmonary congestion. Large shunts may increase PBF to 3–4 times SBF. Cardiac failure is common, but cyanosis is not a feature of left-to-right shunts.

An **atrial septal defect** results in pressure equalization between the right and left atria. The degree and direction of the shunt depends on the relative compliance of the ventricles. Since the left ventricle normally is much less compliant than the right, blood is shunted from left to right, following the path of least resistance. Pulmonary artery pressures and pulmonary vascular resistance remain low, hence Eisenmenger's physiology (see below) is rare with atrial septal defects.

The hemodynamic consequences of a **ventricular septal defect** depend on the size of the defect and the pulmonary vascular resistance. Small ventricular septal defects are usually of little hemodynamic consequence. Moderate ventricular septal defects result in a left-to-right shunt with minimal elevation of pulmonary artery pressures. In the presence of a large ventricular septal defect, there is equalization of right and left ventricular pressures, and shunt flow depends on the relative resistance in the pulmonary and systemic vascular beds. Since systemic vascular resistance is greater than pulmonary vascular resistance, left-to-right flow predominates. However, chronically increased pulmonary artery pressures and PBF cause the pulmonary vascular resis-

tance to increase. As pulmonary vascular resistance rises, flow becomes bidirectional and eventually reversal of flow (i.e., right-to-left shunting) is possible. This is **Eisenmenger's syndrome.**

Right-to-left shunts result in the flow of deoxygenated blood from the pulmonary into the systemic circulation. They are produced when there is an intracardiac septal defect and obstruction to normal blood flow into the pulmonary artery. The classic example is tetrology of Fallot, where pulmonic outlet obstruction leads to right-to-left flow through the ventricular septal defect. These shunts cause arterial hypoxemia and deficient systemic oxygen delivery manifested as cyanosis, which cause deficient oxygen transport to the body. In contrast to left-to-right shunts, cardiac output is not increased and PBF is usually reduced, so that cardiac failure is rare with right-to-left shunts.

The most prominent clinical feature of a right-to-left shunt is **cyanosis.** Five grams of deoxygenated (reduced) hemoglobin are necessary for cyanosis to be manifested. This requires a reduction in arterial oxygen saturation from 95 to 75% when the hemoglobin concentration is normal. Since cyanosis depends on the absolute (not the relative) amount of reduced hemoglobin, more severe hypoxia is needed to produce cyanosis when anemia is present. Alternatively, polycythemia can result in severe cyanosis with relatively mild hypoxemia. Exercise tolerance is limited because of the inability to increase pulmonary flow and therefore oxygen delivery in response to exercise. The classic maneuver of the patient with **tetrology of Fallot** with exercise-induced cyanosis is to squat. The squatting position increases systemic vascular resistance, which increases PBF, alleviating the hypoxemia.

Shunts are diagnosed by cardiac catheterization. Left-to-right shunts result in an oxygen step-up on the right side of the circulation and increased PBF. Right-to-left shunts are manifested by an oxygen step-down on the left side of the circulation, and decreased PBF. Oximetry is limited in that left-to-right shunts of less than 25% of SBF cannot be detected. The indicator-dilution method is more sensitive for detecting shunts. Indocyanine green is the most commonly used dye. Left-to-right shunts are detected by early appearance of dye in the pulmonary artery after injection into the left heart. Early appearance of dye in a systemic artery after injection into the inferior vena cava is indicative of a right-to-left shunt. Sequential injections can then be used to localize the level of the shunt. The shunt position is confirmed by angiography.

Flow through shunts is quantified using the Fick equation to calculate pulmonary and systemic blood flow.

$$PBF \ (L/min) = \frac{\text{oxygen consumption}}{PV \ O_2 \text{ content} - PA \ O_2 \text{ content}}$$

where   PV = pulmonary venous
PA = pulmonary arterial

$$SBF \ (L/min) = \frac{\text{oxygen consumption}}{SA \ O_2 \text{ content} - MV \ O_2 \text{ content}}$$

where   SA = systemic arterial
MV = mixed venous.

$$Shunt(L/min) = PBF - SBF.$$

Left-to-right shunts have positive values and right-to-left ones have negative values using this formula. Bidirectional shunts are quantified using the effective pulmonary blood flow (EBF):

$$EBF = \frac{\text{oxygen consumption}}{PV \ O_2 \text{ content} - MV \ O_2 \text{ content}}$$

The right-to-left component then equals SBF − EBF, and the left-to-right component equals PBF − EBF.

HYPERTROPHY

Cardiac hypertrophy is a compensatory response to chronically increased wall stress. **Hypertrophy** is the increase in size of and number of sarcomeres within a myocardial cell. **Hyperplasia,** an increase in the actual number of cells, does not occur when the heart enlarges. Lesions that produce pressure overload, such as aortic stenosis or hypertension, result in **concentric hypertrophy.** Increased afterload causes an increase in systolic wall tension. This stimulates production of new sarcomeres in parallel with existing ones. The end result is an increase in ventricular wall thickness, while the ventricular chamber remains the same or, possibly, decreases in size. This results in a reduction in ventricular wall stress. Diastolic compliance is much lower in the concentrically hypertrophied ventricle, and higher pressures (a greater preload) are necessary to fill the ventricle.

Eccentric hypertrophy refers to an increase in ventricular wall thickness accompanied by an increase in the diameter of the ventricular chamber in the setting of relatively normal end-diastolic pressures. Disorders that cause ventricular volume overload (e.g., mitral or aortic insufficiency) result in eccentric hypertrophy. It also appears in normal hearts after endurance training. The etiology is increased preload, which produces increased diastolic wall tension.

HIGH-OUTPUT CONGESTIVE HEART FAILURE

High-output congestive heart failure develops when the circulatory system is unable to meet the systemic metabolic demand despite increased cardiac output. It may be due to decreased oxygen carrying capacity (e.g., severe anemia), increased metabolic demand (e.g., hyperthyroidism), and shunting of blood from arterial to venous circulation (e.g., a systemic arteriovenous fistulae or patent ductus arteriosus). A frequent cause of high-output congestive heart failure in surgical patients is early sepsis. In early septic shock, to decrease core body temperature, cutaneous vessels dilate. Systemic vascular resistance is greatly decreased. Blood pressure falls but cardiac output rises because the heart is pumping against a reduced afterload.

LOW-OUTPUT CONGESTIVE HEART FAILURE

Low-output congestive heart failure refers to the inability of the circulatory system to provide adequate tissue perfusion because of insufficient cardiac output. Low cardiac output is defined as a cardiac index of less than 2.0 L/min/m² and may be due to primary myocardial dysfunction or secondary to other factors such as hypovolemia or late septic shock. Hypovolemia and septic shock (through hypovolemia when untreated) decrease venous return (i.e., preload), causing a reduction in stroke volume and cardiac output. Primary myocardial dysfunction may be due to ischemia, infarction, an aneurysm, cardiomyopathies, shunts, sepsis, and valvular disease, among other causes.

Cardiac failure induces a number of compensatory mechanisms that acutely serve to maintain homeostasis, but over time worsen congestive heart failure. In acute left ventricular failure, the **Frank-Starling mechanism** comes immediately into effect. When the stroke volume of a beat is decreased, it results in an increased end-systolic volume, which leads to an increased end-diastolic volume or preload. This increase in left ventricular end-diastolic volume and pressure results in a larger stroke volume with the next systole. This compensation maintains cardiac output at the expense of elevated filling pressures. With chronic failure, sodium and water are retained to increase the effective blood volume and provide the additional preload needed to maintain stroke volume near normal levels. However, this also results in increased venous pressure, which can lead to pulmonary and peripheral edema.

The autonomic nervous system also plays a role in compensation for myocardial failure. Sympathetic activity increases, releasing greater amounts of norepinephrine from sympathetic nerve terminals. Stimulation of β-1 receptors increases heart rate and myocardial contractility. Elevated plasma levels of norepinephrine contribute to generalized arteriolar vasoconstriction, which helps maintains blood pressure but increases afterload. Vasoconstriction also increases venous return, augmenting preload. Sympathetic stimulation redistributes the diminished cardiac output by maintaining cerebral and coronary blood flow and decreasing flow to the cutaneous, renal, and splanchnic vascular beds. With chronic failure, the stores of norepinephrine in the sympathetic nerve terminals are depleted and the heart becomes progressively more dependent on circulating norepinephrine. Although it improves venous return, vasoconstriction worsens the low-output state because increased afterload reduces cardiac output.

Decreased renal blood flow stimulates renin release. Renin acts on angiotensinogen in plasma to produce angiotensin I, which is converted to angiotensin II by angiotensin converting enzyme. Angiotensin II is a strong peripheral vasoconstrictor acting to maintain blood pressure by increasing systemic vascular resis-

tance. This raises afterload and has a detrimental effect similar to that of norepinephrine. Angiotensin II also stimulates thirst and aldosterone release from the adrenal glands. Aldosterone promotes reabsorption of sodium and chloride in the distal renal tubules and collecting system.

The treatment of low-output congestive heart failure is aimed at reducing the liabilities while maximizing the contribution of each component of cardiac function (heart rate and rhythm, preload, afterload, and contractility) to the heart's output. A sinus heart rhythm at 90–100 beats per minute provides optimal cardiac performance, without causing excessive oxygen consumption. Intravascular volume must be maintained at a level that will provide adequate ventricular filling but not cause tissue edema. Systemic vascular resistance can be reduced to decrease the pressure workload of the heart, but systemic pressure must be maintained at a level that ensures adequate tissue perfusion. If maximization of these parameters is not adequate, then contractility can be increased with inotropic agents. These agents function by increasing the level of cytoplasmic calcium, making it available to the contractile apparatus. Most inotropic agents are sympathomimetics, manifesting cardiac and peripheral effects, with varying affinity for α- and β-receptors. The specific effect of each type of adrenergic receptor is outlined in Table 10-1 and the affinity of the different inotropes for various receptors is outlined in Table 10-2. Inotropic agents increase myocardial oxygen consumption and should be used only when other interventions fail to correct the low output state.

Norepinephrine is a potent α-1 and β-1 agonist. It increases contractility and is a strong peripheral vaso-

TABLE 10-1. Cardiovascular Effects of Adrenergic Stimulation

Receptor Site	Heart	Systematic Arteries	Pulmonary Arteries	Veins
Alpha$_1$	0	↑ Constriction (+++)	↑ Constriction (+)	↑ Constriction (++)
Beta$_1$	↑ Rate (++) ↑ Contractility (+++) ↑ Automaticity (+++)	0	Constriction^a	0
Beta$_2$	0	Dilatation (++)	Dilatation (+)	Dilatation (++)

^{a}Indirect effect; mediated by increased renin secretion in the kidneys.
Reproduced from Rice CL. Pharmacologic support of the failing heart. In: Wilmore DW, ed. *Care of the surgical patient, vol. I.* New York: Scientific American, 1989:Sect 2, Ch 3, p 5.

TABLE 10-2. Receptor Types Stimulated by Adrenergic Agonists

Agonist	α	β₁	β₂
Epinephrine	++++	+++	++
Norepinephrine	+++	+++	0
Isoproterenol	0	++++	++++
Dopamine	++	+++	+
Dobutamine	0	++++	++
Mephentermine	+++	++	0
Metaraminol	+++	0	0
Phenylephrine	+++	0	0

From Rice CL. Pharmacologic support of the failing heart. In: Wilmore DW, ed. *Care of the surgical patient, vol. I.* New York: Scientific American, 1989:Sect 2, Ch 3, p 5.

constrictor. Increased afterload and decreased renal blood flow limit norepinephrine's clinical usefulness for the failing heart. **Epinephrine** also has both α- and β-activity resulting in increase heart rate, increased contractility, and increased systemic vascular resistance. Arrhythmias are common with epinephrine.

Dopamine is a precursor of epinephrine and norepinephrine that releases norepinephrine from sympathetic nerve terminals, binds to α- and β-receptors, and exerts primary effects by binding to dopaminergic receptors. In low doses (1–5 mcg/kg/min), its affects are mediated predominately by dopaminergic receptors, increasing renal blood flow. In moderate doses (5–10 mcg/kg/min), the β-effects predominate and contractility and heart rate increase while the increase in renal blood flow is maintained. At these doses, dopamine is less likely than epinephrine or norepinephrine to cause arrhythmias or increased oxygen demand. At higher doses (greater than 10 mcg/kg/min), the α-effects predominate and produce the same deleterious effects that are found with norepinephrine and epinephrine, namely, increased afterload, tachycardia, and arrhythmias.

Dobutamine is a synthetic analogue of dopamine. It directly stimulates β-1 receptors, producing increased contractility. Its chronotropic effect is milder than dopamine. It has some peripheral vasodilatating effects, but has no direct renal vasodilating activity. At high infusion rates, dobutamine increases myocardial irritability and arrhythmias are common. Dobutamine does not rely on releasing endogenous stores of norepinephrine from sympathetic nerve terminals, and therefore may be more effective than dopamine in patients with chronic failure who have depleted stores of norepinephrine.

Isoproterenol is a β-receptor agonist that has no significant α-activity. It produces peripheral vasodilatation (β-2 stimulation) and increased contractility (β-1 stimulation). However, it also causes myocardial irritability, and tachycardia and arrhythmias limit its usefulness.

Amrinone is a phosphodiesterase inhibitor, which sets it apart from the agents mentioned above. It increases cardiac output and results in peripheral vasodilatation, thereby decreasing both preload and afterload. It has fewer chronotropic effects than dobutamine or dopamine. Hypotension, as well as gastrointestinal side-effects and thrombocytopenia, are potential complications of amrinone.

The **intra-aortic balloon pump** reduces afterload mechanically. The balloon is positioned in the proximal descending aorta. The balloon deflates during systole, reducing afterload, and inflates during diastole, increasing coronary perfusion pressure.

Bibliography

Berne RM, Levy MN. *Physiology.* St. Louis: CV Mosby, 1983.

Guyton AC. *Human physiology and mechanisms of disease.* 4th ed. Philadelphia: WB Saunders, 1987.

Hurst JW. *The heart.* 6th ed. New York: McGraw-Hill, 1986.

Sabiston, DC. *Textbook of surgery.* 13th ed. Philadelphia: WB Saunders, 1986.

Schwartz SI. *Principles of surgery.* 5th ed. New York: McGraw-Hill, 1989.

Wilmore DW. *Care of the surgical patient.* New York: Scientific American, 1989.

Jeffrey P. Carpenter

11 PERIPHERAL VASCULAR PHYSIOLOGY AND RHEOLOGY—ARTERIAL, VENOUS, AND LYMPHATIC SYSTEMS

Physiologic Determinants of Blood Flow

ENERGY

The flow of blood is determined by differences in total fluid energy. The major component of fluid energy is usually pressure, but it is not the exclusive determinant. **Total energy** (E) is composed of **potential energy** (E_p) and **kinetic energy** (E_k). Potential energy is stored as intravascular pressure (P) and as gravitation potential energy (ρgh), where ρ is the specific gravity of the fluid, g is the acceleration owing to gravity, and h is the height above a reference point. Kinetic energy is the energy of blood resulting from its motion and is proportional to blood's specific gravity and to the square of blood's velocity (V):

$$\frac{\rho V^2}{2}.$$

Thus,

$$E = E_p + E_k = P + \rho gh + \rho\frac{V^2}{2}.$$

Bernoulli's Principle

For a fluid moving steadily (not accelerating or decelerating) the energy at any point along the streamline of fluid remains equal. Bernoulli's equation expresses this conservation of energy and establishes an important relationship among gravitational potential energy, pressure, and kinetic energy:

$$P_1 + \rho gh_1 + \rho\frac{V_1^2}{2} = P_2 + \rho gh_2 + \rho\frac{V_2^2}{2}.$$

Figure 11-1 illustrates energy and pressure relationships during flow from left to right through a diverging

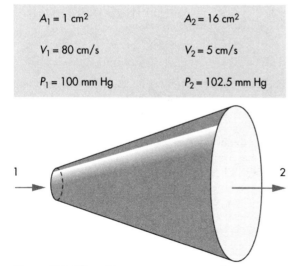

$A_1 = 1$ cm^2	$A_2 = 16$ cm^2
$V_1 = 80$ cm/s	$V_2 = 5$ cm/s
$P_1 = 100$ mm Hg	$P_2 = 102.5$ mm Hg

1   2

Figure 11-1 Effect of increasing cross-sectional area on pressure in a frictionless fluid system. While pressure increases, total fluid energy remains constant owing to a decrease in velocity. (Reproduced from Rutherford RB, ed. *Vascular surgery.* Philadelphia: WB Saunders, 1977.)

tube. Even though the pressure gradient increases during flow from left to right, the total energy remains the same. If the flow were from right to left (a converging tube) the pressure would drop, but the velocity of the fluid would increase as the potential energy of pressure was converted to the kinetic energy of motion. This equation is true for a **Newtonian liquid** in a frictionless environment. Although this is a useful concept, energy loss during flow must be taken into account.

Energy Loss

Viscous

Energy is lost mostly in the form of heat. This is generated by friction between fluid layers as a result of the attractive forces between the various fluid elements. The mathematical description of viscous energy loss is given by **Poiseuille's law:**

$$P_1 - P_2 = Q\frac{8L\eta}{\pi r^4} .$$

This describes the relationship between length (*L*) and viscosity (η) in a tube of radius *r*. The energy loss over length *L* is described by the pressure gradient from beginning to end ($P_1 - P_2$). It is expressed as the product of a flow (*Q*) and a resistance term ($8L\eta/\pi r^4$), and is analogous to the simplified expression that pressure is equal to the product of flow and resistance (see below). Energy loss increases in direct proportion to the viscosity of the fluid. The viscosity of blood increases exponentially with the hematocrit. Thus, hematocrit is the main determinant of viscous energy loss in blood.

Inertial

Poiseuille's law describes viscous energy losses during **laminar flow** through a tube. In the situation during which **pulsatile flow** occurs, the predominant source of energy loss may be inertial rather than viscous.

Inertial energy losses are due to the acceleration and deceleration of a fluid during pulsatile flow. Velocity is the sole independent determinant of this type of energy loss:

$$\Delta E = \frac{K\rho V^2}{2} .$$

These losses are most dramatic in small-diameter vessels, where velocity changes are greatest. Since velocity is a vector quantity, changes in direction of flow owing to junctions and branching of small vessels result in inertial losses as well. These losses are also significant in diseased vessels, where blood squeezes at high velocity through a small-diameter plaque to emerge at lower velocity in a less diseased vessel segment.

FLOW: LAMINAR, TURBULENT, AND PULSATILE

Under the conditions of ideal Newtonian fluid mechanics described by Poiseuille's law, flow in a tube is streamline or laminar. All motion is parallel to the walls of the tube, and the energy losses are those viscous losses incurred moving one lamina of fluid over the adjacent lamina. In the physiologic situation, pulsatile flow is the rule. The changes in velocity vectors caused by turns and branches of vessels as well as disease and pulsatile flow incur kinetic energy losses in addition to viscous losses. The occurrence of truly random velocity vectors is called **turbulent flow.** This rarely occurs in the clinical setting, as viscous forces dampen out those factors favoring turbulence. Rather, the human circulation is best described as being in a state between turbulence and laminar flow known as "**disturbed flow.**" Given this, the energy-loss equations described above for the more ideal situation serve to estimate the minimum energy lost in the actual situation of physiologic circulation.

RESISTANCE

The equation describing vascular resistance (R) is analogous to Ohm's law for electrical resistance. Resistance is the ratio of energy lost and the flow in the hemodynamic circuit.

$$R = \frac{E_1 - E_2}{Q} .$$

As discussed above, total fluid energy is determined by kinetic, gravitational, and pressure forms of fluid energy. If the system is horizontal, the gravitational term can be eliminated. In actual hemodynamic circuits, the contribution of arterial pressure to the total energy is much greater than that of kinetic energy, so that pressure (P) may be substituted for energy (E) in the above equation:

$$R = \frac{P_1 - P_2}{Q} .$$

Substituting the equation describing Poiseuille's law,

$$\frac{P_1 - P_2}{Q} = \frac{8L\eta}{\pi r^4} = R .$$

This describes resistance for an ideal fluid. When blood flows through a vessel, viscous and inertial energy losses also contribute to the resistance to flow.

Sources of resistance can be arranged in series (multiple stenoses in a single vessel) or in parallel (collateral beds). The equation for total resistance when arranged in series is

$$R_T = R_1 + R_2 + \ldots R_n$$

and in parallel is

$$\frac{1}{R_T} = \frac{1}{R_1} + \frac{1}{R_2} + \ldots \frac{1}{R_n} .$$

CONDUCTANCE

Conductance is the inverse of resistance and is a measure of blood flow through the vessel for a given pres-

sure difference. Conductance varies in direct proportion to the fourth power of the radius.

STENOSIS

Energy losses associated with stenoses are of both viscous and inertial types. Viscous losses, described by Poiseuille's law, are directly proportional to the length of the stenotic segment and inversely proportional to the fourth power of the radius of the stenosis. The inertial losses are proportional to the square of the blood velocity and occur at both the entrance (**contraction effect**) and exit (**expansion effect**) of the stenotic segment. The viscous losses are usually far less than those inertial losses incurred with contraction and reexpansion effects.

The magnitude of these losses is dependent on the geometry of the entrance and exit; if the stenosis is a smoothly tapered narrowing, the losses are much smaller than for an irregular stenosis. As stated above, inertial energy losses are described by

$$\Delta E = \frac{\rho^2 V^2}{2} .$$

Given a normal lumen of radius r, a stenotic lumen of radius r_s, a normal velocity of V, and a velocity through a stenotic segment of V_s, this becomes

$$\Delta E = \frac{\rho^2 (V_s - V)^2}{2} .$$

Assuming conservation of energy, since flows through a given cross-sectional area of the stenotic and normal segments are equal,

$$2\pi r^2 V = 2\pi r_s^2 V_s .$$

Solving for V_s and substituting V_s into the energy equation above gives the inertial energy loss across a stenosis

$$\Delta E \cong \Delta P = K \frac{\rho}{2} V^2 \left[\left(\frac{r}{r_s} \right)^2 - 1 \right]^2 .$$

The constant, K, varies with the geometry of the stenosis. A graphic representation of inertial and viscous effects along a stenotic segment of 1-in length is shown in Figure 11-2. Energy is lost as heat upon contraction

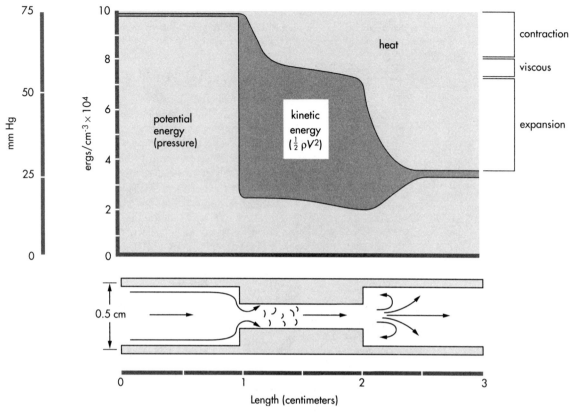

Figure 11-2 Diagram illustrating energy losses experienced by blood passing through a stenosis 1 cm long. Flow is assumed to be unidirectional and steady. Note that very little of the total energy loss is attributable to "viscous" losses. Thus, applications of Poiseuille's law greatly underestimate the pressure drop across an arterial stenosis. (Reproduced from Rutherford RB, ed. *Vascular surgery*. 3rd ed. Philadelphia: WB Saunders, 1989:24.)

at the entrance and expansion at the exit of the stenosis. Viscous losses along the stenosis itself play a smaller role in total energy lost.

WALL TENSION

Wall tension is described by **Laplace's law** for thin-walled structures,

$$T = Pr$$

where T is tangential tension in the wall, P is intraluminal pressure, and r is radius. Tangential tension increases in direct proportion to the vessel's radius. A more precise estimate of the physiologic situation is given by the tangential stress (τ), which considers pressure, radius, and wall thickness (δ);

$$\tau = Pr/\delta.$$

Tangential wall stress increases in direct proportion to pressure and radius, but is inversely proportional to wall thickness.

The application of this concept to aneurysm rupture is apparent. When the tangential wall stress exceeds the wall's tensile strength, it ruptures. The more the aneurysm expands (r increases and/or δ decreases), the more likely it is to burst. Similarly, the importance of hypertension as a risk factor is accounted for in the tangential stress equation (Figure 11-3).

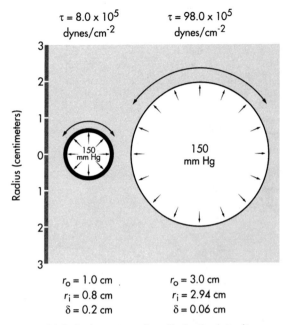

$\tau = 8.0 \times 10^5$ dynes/cm^{-2}

$\tau = 98.0 \times 10^5$ dynes/cm^{-2}

$r_o = 1.0$ cm
$r_i = 0.8$ cm
$\delta = 0.2$ cm

$r_o = 3.0$ cm
$r_i = 2.94$ cm
$\delta = 0.06$ cm

Figure 11-3 End-on view of a cylinder 2 cm in diameter before and after expansion to a diameter of 6 cm. Wall area remains the same in the two figures, but wall stress (τ) is greatly increased owing both to the decrease in wall thickness (δ) and to the increase in inside radius (r_i). (Reproduced from Rutherford RB, ed. *Vascular surgery*. 3rd ed. Philadelphia: WB Saunders, 1989:37.)

Arterial System

ARTERIAL WALL CHARACTERISTICS

Arteries are not rigid tubes. They are distensible, elastic structures, and their ability to stretch and recoil allows storage of potential energy. Their elastic properties are chiefly due to their content of elastin. Elastin content is highest in the thoracic aorta, which stores energy during systole and returns it to the system during diastole. The other main wall components are collagen and smooth muscle. Collagen is much less elastic than elastin. Peripheral arteries, like the femoral artery, have high collagen content, making them stiff blood conduits rather than reservoirs of potential energy. Arterioles have high smooth muscle content, allowing active control of diameter to regulate pressure and flow. As vessels age, their elastin content decreases, and collagen is

altered; they thicken and become atherosclerotic. All this serves to make the vessels stiffer, altering patterns of pulse wave conduction and blood flow.

THE ARTERIAL PULSE WAVE

The normal arterial pulse has a triphasic curve (Figure 11-4). Initially, as the blood is ejected from the heart there is a large positive systolic flow with a sharp upstroke. This is followed by a brief reversal of flow in early diastole, followed by a brief forward flow in late diastole, related to the elastic recoil of the aorta and closure of the aortic valve. The pulse wave is transmitted from the central circulation to the periphery, where the changes in arterial compliance modify the contour of the wave. As compliance decreases and there is a greater reflected component of the pulse wave, the systolic

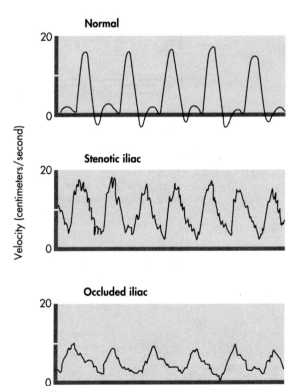

Figure 11-4 Femoral artery flow pulses from a normal subject, a patient with a stenotic external iliac artery, and a patient with an occluded common iliac artery. (Reproduced from Strandness DE Jr, Sumner DS. *Hemodynamics for surgeons*. New York: Grune & Stratton, 1975:257.)

pressure is actually amplified. Thus, the ankle systolic pressure is higher than the more central upper arm systolic pressure. In order to continue to propagate, however, the mean and diastolic pressures decrease as the wave moves to the periphery. Clinically the ratio of ankle to arm systolic pressure is called the ankle brachial index (**ABI**) and is normally 1.1. Patients with claudication have a mean ABI of 0.59; and patients with rest pain, 0.26.

The pulse wave is further modified by other effects. Heating the body causes vasodilation and a decreased resistance. This abolishes the reflected component of the pulse wave. Increased vascular resistance from cooling has the opposite effect, and the reversed-flow phase is accentuated. Stenosis causes a compensatory decrease in peripheral resistance by autoregulatory vasodilatation, which results in a wave that has no reversed-flow phase. The contour of the pulse wave demonstrates a delayed upstroke, a rounded peak, and loss of the reversed-flow phase and bowing of the downstroke away from the baseline. In the vascular laboratory the **pulse volume recordings** give waveforms for analysis as well as quantitative measurements of the pulse pressure. A more detailed analysis of the pulse wave that can examine the individual velocity components of arterial and venous flow is possible using the doppler velocity analyzer. Under laminar flow conditions all velocity components are parallel. At a stenosis the laminar flow is disturbed, causing velocity vectors to be oriented in a broad spectrum of orientations. This **"spectral broadening"** is proportional to the degree of stenosis and can be used noninvasively to define the stenosis.

CRITICAL STENOSIS

Poiseuille's law and the description of inertial energy loss above demonstrate that viscous and inertial energy losses are inversely related to the radius of a stenotic area. Thus, plots of pressure drop versus the radius of a stenosis, for a given flow, have an exponential shape. For each flow rate, there is a critical radius, such that any further decrement in radius causes a precipitous increase in the pressure gradient across the stenosis (Figure 11-5).

This is described as **critical stenosis.** In most instances this occurs when the vessel's diameter is narrowed 50%, or the cross-sectional area is narrowed 75%. As flow increases, the diminution in radius necessary to create critical stenosis becomes less. Thus high-

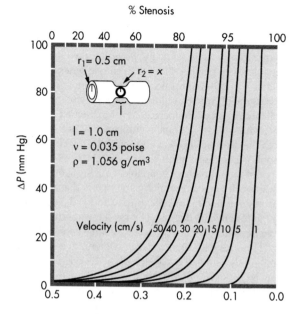

Figure 11-5 Relationship of pressure drop across a stenosis to the radius of the stenotic segment and the flow velocity. (Reproduced from Strandness DE Jr, Sumner DS. *Hemodynamics for surgeons.* New York: Grune & Stratton, 1975:109.)

flow systems (i.e., those with large runoff beds) reach the point of critical stenosis at less severe narrowing than low-flow systems. Exercise, which lowers peripheral resistance and increases flow, may cause an otherwise asymptomatic lesion to act as a critical lesion.

MULTIPLE STENOSES

Poiseuille's law indicates that viscous energy losses are proportional to the first power of the stenotic length. Thus, for two stenoses in series the viscous losses are merely doubled. However, as indicated above, the chief sources of energy loss are the entrance and exit effects of compression and expansion. For multiple stenoses in series these effects are additive as well and far exceed the viscous losses. Thus, separate stenoses of equal diameter are of far greater significance than a single stenosis of that diameter whose length is equal to the sum of the lengths of the separate stenoses. The additive effect of multiple subcritical stenoses may produce the same effect as a single critical stenosis.

COLLATERAL CIRCULATION AND RUNOFF

So far the discussion has been limited to simple hemodynamic circuits. In actuality, however, the circuits are complex with parallel rather than simple series arrangements. Blood flows through the collateral circulation to bypass the obstructed segment. The ability of the collateral circulation to compensate for the diseased segment determines the functional significance of the stenosis. Both the diseased segment and the collateral circulation supply a common runoff bed (Figure 11-6). The resistance of the runoff bed is variable, consisting of muscular arterioles and precapillary sphincters that undergo autoregulation and are responsive to local, systemic, and autonomic mediation. The resistance of the collateral circulation, consisting mainly of large and medium-sized arteries with high collagen content, is essentially fixed. Only a limited expansion of the collateral circulation is possible. An excellent example of the above model would be the lower extremity with a diseased superficial femoral artery, a profunda-geniculate collateral system, and the lower leg runoff bed. While the resistance of the superficial femoral artery is increased owing to disease, the resistance of the peripheral runoff bed decreases through **autoregulation** to maintain adequate flow through the collateral circulation. The ability of these compensatory mechanisms is limited, however, and is manifest clinically as claudication, rest pain, and ischemic lesions. As discussed above, energy loss and pressure drop across stenoses are flow dependent; higher flow (exercise) causes an exponentially higher pressure drop. In the normal limb there is almost no pressure gradient between the thigh and ankle. However, in the diseased limb, there can be a large pressure gradient, which is exacerbated with exercise. For example, in the presence of an arterial stenosis, although there is a pressure drop across the lesion at rest, flow remains normal as a result of autoregulation. Both collateral and runoff beds are dilated. During exercise there is an increase in flow to the limb but not as much as in the normal limb. The autoregulatory reserve has already been used to maintain flow at rest and is unable further to augment flow during exercise. Thus stenoses that are asymptomatic at rest become symptomatic with exercise. This is the mechanism of claudication. When the flow is reduced to the point where the severity of disease outstrips the autoregulatory reserve mechanisms, there is inadequate flow at rest and the patient develops "rest pain."

VASCULAR STEAL

In complicated hemodynamic circuits it is possible to have two runoff beds supplied by a limited common inflow source. In this case the variable resistance of each runoff bed dictates which one will best compete for the limited flow. For instance, a leg may have a lesion of both the iliac artery and the superficial femoral artery (SFA). The two runoff beds with variable resistance would be the thigh, via the profunda femoris artery, and the calf. At rest, the calf vessels are near maximally dilated as they receive flow through profunda collaterals instead of through the SFA. Thigh pressure is decreased owing to the iliac lesion and ankle pressure is further reduced from the iliac and SFA lesions. At rest, flow to the thigh is normal through the profunda but requires autoregulatory dilatation of the thigh runoff bed to maintain flow during exercise because of the proximal iliac lesion. The calf vessels, already maximally dilated, cannot increase flow; thus flow is "stolen" to the thigh through the thigh's autoregulatory process. The calf and thigh pressures drop further with exercise as a result of the energy lost with increased flow across the iliac lesion. The net effect is to decrease calf flow with exercise.

The necessary components of "steal" phenomena are a limited inflow supplying two runoff beds of variable resistance. The **subclavian steal syndrome** involves a stenotic subclavian artery proximal to the takeoff of the vertebral artery. The arm and cerebral circulations make up the two runoff beds in this scenario. Flow in the vertebral artery can actually reverse as the resistance of the arm runoff bed drops. Thus, blood is stolen from the cerebral circulation to supply the arm, and patients may have symptoms of cerebral ischemia during exercise.

TREATMENT OF ARTERIAL INSUFFICIENCY

Exercise

Exercise lowers peripheral resistance and thereby increases flow. In the ischemic situation, however, peripheral resistance is already significantly lowered to compensate for the high segmental resistance proximal to the runoff bed. Nonetheless, exercise therapy is effective in providing modest improvement in clinical symptoms for patients with mild symptoms, presumably by improving collateral flow.

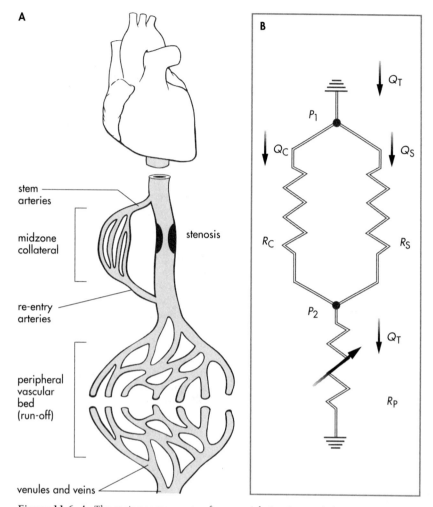

Figure 11-6 A, The major components of an arterial circuit containing a stenotic major artery. **B,** An electric analogue of this circuit. The battery at the top represents the potential energy source, i.e., the heart; ground potential, at the bottom, indicates the central veins. Q_t is total flow, Q_c is collateral flow, and Q_s is flow through the stenotic artery. Resistances are R_c, collateral; R_s, stenotic artery; and R_p peripheral "runoff" bed. R_c and R_s are relatively "fixed"; R_p is "variable." (Reproduced from Rutherford RB, ed. *Vascular surgery.* 3rd ed. Philadelphia: WB Saunders, 1989:25.)

Vasodilation

Another method of lessening peripheral resistance and increasing flow is with direct vasodilation therapy. However, as mentioned above, ischemic beds are already vasodilated through autoregulation. The net effect of vasodilators in this situation is to dilate those beds that are constricted and thereby steal blood from

ischemic beds. Currently this is not a clinically useful therapeutic modality for treatment of ischemia resulting from arterial disease.

Sympathectomy

Sympathectomy ablates sympathetic vasomotor tone, thereby decreasing peripheral resistance. It is subject to the same criticism as vasodilator therapy with respect to treatment of claudication and rest pain. However, sympathectomy is a somewhat more specific therapy in that it chiefly affects the cutaneous arterioles, shunting blood flow to the skin. Healing of cutaneous lesions is often a limiting factor in treatment of vascular disease, and for those patients whose disease process has not already rendered them maximally dilated there may be a role for sympathectomy.

Rheologics

The final component of Poiseuille's law remaining to be discussed is the viscosity of the blood. Resistance is directly proportional to viscosity, which is chiefly a function of the hematocrit. Viscosity can be lowered by decreasing the hematocrit, but this robs blood of its oxygen-carrying capacity. Low molecular weight dextran, in addition to its capacity as an antiplatelet and antiaggregation agent, decreases peripheral vascular resistance. It is also a volume expander that causes hemodilution and reduces the viscosity of blood.

Pentoxifylline is an agent whose efficacy is currently being evaluated. In addition to its antiplatelet effects it lowers viscosity by altering red blood cell membrane flexibility. It remains to be seen whether rheologic agents will be of major importance as a result of their effects on blood viscosity.

Surgery

The most apparent solution to alleviating the problems associated with arterial stenosis is removal or bypass of stenotic lesions. This can be accomplished by angioplasty, thrombectomy, embolectomy or direct arterial surgery. In multiple-level occlusive disease relief of the most proximal obstruction is usually sufficient to provide relief from symptoms, since the effects of multiple stenoses are more than merely additive. The grafts used to do arterial reconstruction are themselves subject to the same hemodynamic principles outlined above. The length of a graft is of far less consequence than its diameter, as energy losses are inversely proportional to the fourth power of the radius but only to the first power of the length. Entrance and exit effects are minimized by making graft size and native vessel size as nearly equal as possible. Discrepancies should be managed by creating smooth, tapered transitions rather than abrupt high-energy-loss anastomoses.

Venous System

Unlike the arterial system, which operates at high pressure, the venous system is a low-pressure system. The venules usually have a mean pressure of 15–20 mm Hg, which drops to 0–6 mm Hg in the right atrium. Hydrostatic pressure is one of the main components of venous pressure. With upright posture, there is a large gradient of pressure, ranging from 0 at the right atrium to 100 to 120 mm Hg at the ankle

Since veins are collapsible tubes, when tissue pressure exceeds venous pressure veins collapse. Active venous constriction does not occur in response to postural change; rather, blood that pools in the legs with upright posture is returned via the muscle pump mechanism described below. Veins do, however, constrict in response to certain stimuli, including pain, hyperventilation, exercise, hypovolemia, sympathetic stimulation, cold (allowing heat conservation), histamine, and sympathomimetic drugs. The distensibility of veins is responsible for their ability to store large amounts of blood without a noticeable rise in venous pressure. Veins are elliptically shaped in cross section at low filling volumes but distend to large-capacity circular tubes at higher filling volumes. Once they are converted to this circular conformation, further filling requires stretching of the venous wall, which results in much higher pressure. Thus the volume-pressure plot for veins has both low- and high-compliance regions (Figure 11-7). At high filling volumes venous and arterial compliances are about equal.

The distensibility of veins also means that venous resistance is dynamic. The resistance of an elliptically shaped vein (low filling volume) is much higher than the open circular tube configuration (high filling volume). Thus, as veins distend, their resistance drops, allowing increased flow. The flow of venous blood is accomplished with approximately the same pressure gradient as that of arterial blood, 15 mm Hg from the venule to the right atrium (compared with a 15 mm Hg drop from the left ventricle to the peripheral arteries). Various factors contribute to venous flow.

EFFECT OF THE HEART

During atrial systole, right atrial pressure rises, elevating central venous pressure. This causes reversal of venous blood flow. During ventricular systole the atrium relaxes, increasing forward flow by lowering central

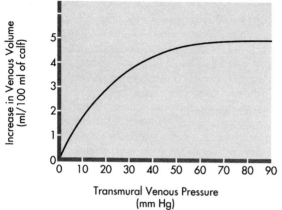

Figure 11-7 Relationship of venous volume to transmural pressure. Note that veins are very compliant at low pressure, but quite stiff at high pressure. (Reproduced from Rutherford RB, ed. *Vascular surgery. 3rd* ed. Philadelphia: WB Saunders, 1989:1484.)

venous pressure. During diastole flow initially decreases until pressure rises enough to open the tricuspid valve, allowing greatly increased flow, which again drops to zero as the cycle is completed (Figure 11-8).

EFFECT OF RESPIRATION

During inspiration intra-abdominal pressure increases owing to the descent of the diaphragm, inhibiting venous return. When the diaphragm relaxes during expiration, return flow to the heart is facilitated from the lower body. For the upper body the opposite situation is seen. During inspiration the lower intrathoracic pressure favors return flow from the head and arms. During expiration venous return falls as intrathoracic pressure rises. The pressure difference driving venous return from the head and arms is equal to the difference in peripheral venous pressure and intrathoracic pres-

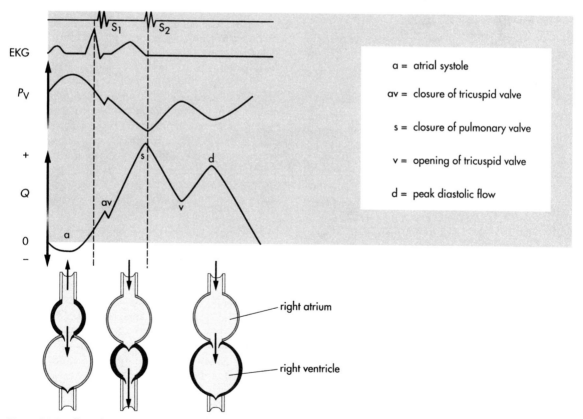

Figure 11-8 Effect of cardiac contraction on venous pressure (P_v) and venous blood flow (Q). *Vertical dashed lines* define the period of ventricular systole. First and second heart sounds are indicated by S_1 and S_2, respectively. (Reproduced from Sumner DS. In Bergen JJ, Yao JST, eds. *Surgery of the Veins.* Orlando, FL: Grune & Stratton, 1983: 3-23.)

sure. The driving pressure in the lower body is the difference of peripheral venous pressure and intra-abdominal pressure.

ANATOMY

The venous system consists of parallel superficial and deep systems connected by **perforating veins.** The superficial veins are muscular, large veins, whereas the deep veins are thin-walled vessels running parallel to (and having the same name as) the deep arteries. A particularly clinically relevant set of perforating veins are the calf perforators joining the posterior tibial deep venous system and the greater saphenous system. The role of these perforators in venous ulceration is discussed below. Veins have bicuspid valves to direct flow centrally. These valves exist in most patients to the level of the femoral vein and occasionally in the iliac veins as well.

CALF MUSCLE PUMP

Blood is also aided in its return against gravity to the central circulation by the calf muscle pump. Constriction of the muscle containing venous sinusoids raises peripheral venous pressure, favoring flow toward the heart. Competent venous valves assure unidirectional flow. When the muscle relaxes, valves above the relaxed muscle close, and the collapsed calf sinusoids fill with inflowing blood from the periphery. Even though muscle contraction in the deep compartments of the leg raises deep venous pressure higher than superficial pressure, competent valves in the perforating veins prevent reflux to the superficial system. Thus, exercising muscle has a lower venous pressure than resting muscle as the pump actively decreases venous volume. This has the end result of augmenting arterial perfusion of the muscle, since the perfusion gradient (mean arterial minus mean venous pressure) is increased. This complements the arterial vasodilation response to exercise described above. The increased return to the heart from the calf muscle pump during exercise also increases preload and thereby augments cardiac output.

THROMBOSIS AND THROMBOPHLEBITIS

The main pathologic disorders of the venous system are thrombosis and thrombophlebitis. Thrombosis is discussed in Chapter 5. The end result of thrombosis is venous obstruction. This serves to raise venous pressure and mean capillary pressure, leading to edema. Lower-extremity edema can be secondary to conditions that raise central venous pressure—for example, heart failure, pulmonary hypertension, and tricuspid valvular insufficiency. Edema from venous thrombosis is dependent on the local rise in venous pressure, and the rise in venous pressure is dependent on the adequacy of collateral pathways to the central circulation. Leg edema, dilated superficial collaterals, and painful tender veins are reliable signs and symptoms of acute venous thrombosis. In the case of near-complete acute venous thrombosis of the leg and iliac system, known as **phlegmasia cerulea dolens,** massive fluid loss from edema formation can produce shock.

Venous thrombosis and thrombophlebitis lead to destruction of venous valves, allowing blood to reflux from the deep to the superficial system. The calf muscle pump is less effective with valvular incompetence. The inability to empty the legs of blood and the concomitant increase in venous pressure leads to edema and varicosities of superficial veins.

In patients with pure venous valvular incompetence **(primary varicose veins)** the site of reflux is at the saphenofemoral junction. However, the disorder in these patients can range from congenital absence of venous valves to the more common valvular incompetence from incomplete coaptation of valve cusps. This is thought to result from chronic exposure of the valves to high venous pressure. Activities that involve straining, constant upright posture, pregnancy, etc., predispose one to varicose veins. Compression of the saphenofemoral junction prevents reflux and is the basis of surgical treatment of this disorder by ligation and stripping of the saphenous vein to the level of the saphenofemoral junction. External compression stockings are thought to facilitate valve competence by applying external pressure.

Chronic venous hypertension and the ensuing capillary hypertension cause the capillaries to become damaged. They become hyperpermeable, allowing proteinaceous fluid and red blood cells to leak into the interstitium, producing the characteristic hyperpigmented and "woody" appearance of the skin. This situation limits the oxygenation of the tissue, causing local ischemic changes and ulcerations typical of venous hypertension. Patients typically display these venous skin changes at the medial ankle, just superior and posterior to the malleolus. It is at this region that the perforating veins connect the deep leg veins to the posterior arch vein. It is hypothesized that, owing to the incompetence of the perforators, the local hypoxic effects of venous hypertension are most pronounced at this site of deep-superficial communication. Application of direct pressure to this perforator zone by compression bandages, stockings, or boots can reduce venous hypertension by decreasing perforator reflux and facilitate healing of venous ulcers. Stripping of superficial veins is only of benefit if the deep system is competent.

Lymphatic System

The lymphatic system transports fluid from the interstitial space back to the vascular system, clearing fluid and particles too large to be removed by capillaries. Lymph drains from the lower body into the cysterna chyli, then through the thoracic duct, which joins the venous system at the junction of the left internal jugular and subclavian veins. Only small amounts of lymph enter veins directly in the lower body. Lymph from the right arm, head, and neck enters the right lymph duct, which joins the venous system at the junction of the right internal jugular and subclavian veins. The lymphatic capillaries are composed of endothelial cells that have very loose cell-to-cell junctions, permitting easy passage of large proteins and particles into the lymphatic circulation. These loose junctions are arranged in such a way as to behave like one-way flap valves. The larger lymphatic channels have actual bicuspid valves serving to direct flow just as in the venous system. Lymph flow in the thoracic duct is approximately 100 cc/h. Numerous factors serve to propel lymph through to the venous circulation. The muscle pump mechanism discussed for veins above also applies to the lymphatic circulation. Arterial pulsation adjacent to lymphatics can propel lymph as well. Lymphatic smooth muscle is known to contract in response to distension. Thus, as the lymphatic distends with fluid, it contracts in response. The valves assure unidirectional flow toward the venous circulation. Factors that increase the interstitial pressure also favor flow into the lymphatics.

Edema forms when excess interstitial fluid accumulates in the tissues. This can result from a disturbance of any of the factors that determine the balance of hydrostatic and oncotic forces in the interstitial space. Lymphatic obstruction is an important cause of edema. Edema results from the impaired clearance of protein from the interstitium and elevated intralymphatic pressure. Thus, lymphatic obstruction alters both oncotic and hydrostatic forces, favoring edema formation.

Worldwide, the most common cause of lymphatic obstruction is filariasis. The extremely edematous state, produced by profound lymphatic obstruction, is called elephantiasis. Lymphatic obstruction can also be the result of surgical excisions, neoplastic invasion, radiation injury, or other inflammatory processes. Lymphedema may also be congenital or may appear during later years as a result of abnormal development of the lymphatic system (lymphedema praecox). Lymphangiography is of great benefit in determining the etiology of lymphedema and determining the type and level of lymphatic obstruction.

Bibliography

Bergan JJ, Yao JST, eds. *Surgery of the veins*. New York: Grune & Stratton, 1985.

Guyton AC. *Textbook of medical physiology*. Philadelphia: WB Saunders, 1986.

Moore W, ed. *Vascular surgery*. New York: Grune & Stratton, 1980.

Rutherford RB, ed. *Vascular surgery*. 3rd ed. Philadelphia: WB Saunders, 1989.

Strandness DE, Summer DS. *Hemodynamics for surgeons*. New York: Grune & Stratton, 1975.

Robert C. Gorman

12 ATHEROSCLEROSIS AND ATHEROGENESIS

Arteriosclerosis is a progressive disease of blood vessels that begins early in life and causes unparalleled morbidity and mortality during middle and late adulthood. Among the diseases afflicting modern, economically developed societies, arteriosclerosis is by far the most significant in terms of premature death and loss of productivity. The disorder has reached epidemic proportions, with approximately 50% of all deaths in the United States being attributed to arteriosclerosis-related disease. While any artery may be affected, there is a clear predilection for arteriosclerotic lesions to occur in the coronary circulation, the aorta and cerebrovascular systems, leaving little wonder as to why this disorder results in lethal and crippling vascular events. Although quite common, particularly among American males, arteriosclerosis occurs with varying severity among nations and individuals as well as social and ethnic groups. These variations are evidence that the disease is not an inevitable consequence of human life. Efforts to understand why arteriosclerotic disease severely affects some individuals and not others, as well as attempts to understand fully the pathogenesis of the disease, are two of the most intensely sought goals of medical research today.

The research effort focused on the natural history and pathogenesis of atherosclerosis that has developed over the past 20 to 30 years has produced an enormous quantity of both basic science and clinical information. However, the existing data on atherosclerotic vascular disease may be characterized as copious, incomplete, and at times contradictory, making a cohesive, understandable model of the disease difficult to formulate. In this chapter, an attempt has been made to formulate an organized and concise review of existing knowledge of the natural history and etiology of atherosclerotic vascular disease.

Definition

Arteriosclerosis literally means "hardening of the arteries." The term encompasses a group of disorders that have in common a thickening and loss of elasticity of the arterial wall. Three morphologic variants are included under the general category of arteriosclerosis: atherosclerosis, characterized by the formations of fibrous lipid-containing plaques (atheroma); medial calcific sclerosis, characterized by calcification of the media of muscular arteries; and arteriolosclerosis, associated with hyalinization of the walls of small arteries and arterioles, usually secondary to severe hypertension. All three of these pathologic entities are structurally and etiologically distinct. Atherosclerosis is by far the most common and clinically relevant form of arteriosclerosis; therefore, the terms are generally used interchangeably unless otherwise specified.

Atherosclerosis is a disease of muscular arteries (coronaries, carotids, femoral) and elastic arteries (aorta, iliacs). The basic lesion of the disease is the atheroma, or fibrofatty plaque. The atheroma consists of raised focal plaque within the innermost layer of the artery (intima) with a core of lipid and a fibrous cap. Plaques increase in size over time, subsequently protruding into the vessel lumen and muscular wall. These changes can compromise blood flow and cause weakening in the arterial wall, which can result in aneurysmal dilatation.

Epidemiology and Risk Factors

The epidemiologic characteristics of atherosclerosis have drawn much attention because of the varied incidence of the disease among individuals and groups. Review of these differences has provided some clues into the pathogenesis of the disease. Multiple studies have linked several patient characteristics with the development of atherosclerosis. The factors with the strongest independent association are age, male sex, family history, smoking, hypertension, hyperlipidemia, and diabetes mellitus. The presence of more than one risk factor has been found to have a synergistic effect.

Recent studies suggest that genetics plays (in a poorly characterized manner) a significant role in determining degree, time course, and severity of the atherosclerotic vascular disease.

There is a close relationship between age and the incidence and severity of atherosclerosis. This point is well illustrated by the fact that the death rate from ischemic heart disease rises continually up to age 85. The relationship between age and atherosclerosis may be related to the time required for the lesion to develop once precipitating insults have started the progression of the disease, or it may be the result of persistent exposure to other risk factors that finally causes the disease to become symptomatic.

Men develop symptomatic coronary artery disease an average of 10 years before women. When the comparison is based on proven myocardial infarction, the average age is 20 years younger. The exact reason for this association is unclear. Estrogen has been proposed to be the protective agent for premenopausal women; however, estrogen is known to exacerbate atherosclerotic disease in men taking it for the treatment of prostatic cancer. It is also well established that the rate of ischemic heart disease is increased in women on long-term oral contraceptives. While the incidence of atherosclerotic vascular disease is much lower in women, the relationship of the "modifiable" risk factors

(hyperlipidemia, hypertension, smoking, and diabetes mellitus) is as least as strong as it is in men.

Hypertension is the single most useful factor in detecting individuals at high risk for atherosclerotic disease. It is more reliable than either hyperlipidemia or smoking, especially in men over 45 years old. It now appears that both systolic and diastolic hypertension contribute to the development of the disease. There appears to be a direct linear relationship, over a wide range of blood pressures, between the risk of death owing to ischemic heart disease and blood pressure. The mechanism by which hypertension induces atherosclerotic vascular disease remains unclear. However, direct endothelial injury or dysfunction have been implicated.

While smoking is independently linked to atherosclerosis, there is a marked and unique synergy when it is combined with one or more other risk factors. The risk of developing atherosclerosis is related to the early initiation, the duration and extent of exposure, deep inhalation, and time since cessation. There is a clear dose-response relationship between peripheral vascular disease and the number of cigarettes smoked. Cessation of smoking results in a dramatic reduction in risk; incidence is reduced 50% in one year but requires a decade to approximate the level of nonsmokers.

The mechanism by which tobacco leads to atherosclerosis is uncertain; however, direct endothelial cell injury and increased fibrinogen level have been proposed as possibilities. Fibrinogen values are higher for smokers than nonsmokers, and the levels increase directly with the number of cigarettes smoked. In addition, the risk of coronary heart disease increases with fibrinogen levels in nonsmokers as well as smokers. It appears that the enhanced thrombotic tendency associated with hyperfibrinogenemia must to some extent lead to the development of atherosclerosis. The exact mechanism remains to be elucidated.

There is strong evidence that elevated serum lipids are correlated with the development of atherosclerosis, especially coronary artery disease. Populations with high serum lipid levels have a higher morbidity and mortality from atherosclerosis-related disorders. The risk of developing atherosclerosis appears to rise linearly with cholesterol level. Risk of symptomatic atherosclerotic disease is associated most strongly with cholesterol level and its carrier, low-density lipoproteins (LDL). Elevated triglycerides and the associated very-low-density lipoproteins (VLDL) are less strongly linked to atherogenesis. In contrast, high-density lipoproteins

(HDL) have been found to provide resistance to athero-sclerosis.

Hyperlipidemia may be secondary to some well-known causes such as nephrotic syndrome or hypothyroidism, or may be the direct consequence of a single gene defect, as in the familial hypercholesterolemias. Complex inheritance factors may also predispose some patients to hypercholesterolemia. Nevertheless, the level of plasma cholesterol is measurably influenced by the dietary intake of total calories of cholesterol, saturated fat, and polyunsaturated fat. Further, there is a direct relationship among diet, hyperlipidemia, and the development of coronary heart disease.

Diabetes mellitus has a well-documented association with all manifestations of atherosclerotic vascular disease. In diabetics, the incidence of myocardial infarction is twofold and the incidence of lower extremity gangrene is eightfold that of the general population. The reason for the association is obscure but seems to be independent of the high incidence of hyperlipidemia and hypertension in diabetics. There is no evidence that strict regulation of serum glucose is of benefit.

Structure of the Normal Artery

The normal large artery is a tubular structure whose primary function is to act as a nonthrombogenic conduit for blood and, at times, as a capacitor. In smaller arteries, capillaries, and venules, the vessels also serve to regulate the molecular and cellular traffic between the vascular and extravascular space.

The wall of the artery can be divided into subregions or tunics, called the intima, media, and adventitia (Figure 12-1). The intima, the innermost layer of the wall lying inside the internal elastic lamina and directly adjacent to the flowing blood, is composed of endothelium at the luminal surface and subendothelial extracellular matrix. In some vessels, one or more layers of smooth muscle cells are present; this so-called intimal cushion of smooth muscle cells might in some circumstances be the progenitor of the fibrous intimal plaque. The media, bounded by the internal and external elastic laminae, contains smooth muscle cells embedded in a matrix of collagen, elastin, and proteoglycans; in addition, elastic arteries have clearly defined lamellae of elastin interspersed with layers of smooth muscle. The adventitia lies outside the external elastic lamina and is composed of loose connective tissue, fibroblasts, capillaries, and occasional leukocytes (particularly mast cells). In very large elastic arteries with more than 28 elastic layers, a microvasculature (vasa vasorum) penetrates the media from the adventitial side and provides an alternative nutrient supply for the outer layers of the wall. In vessels containing substantial atherosclerosis, the vasa vasorum can be very well developed and extend into the intimal plaque.

Pathologic Anatomy

THE ATHEROMATOUS PLAQUE

This is the fundamental lesion of atherosclerosis. These lesions initially form in the intima; medial changes are secondary. Characteristically these plaques are whitish yellow and range in size from 0.1 to 1.5 cm in diameter; however, multiple plaques can coalesce to form larger masses.

Structurally, plaques are composed of a superficial fibrous cap and a deeper lipid-containing core. The fibrous cap is an accumulation of connective tissue made up of collagen, proteoglycans, elastic fibers, and smooth muscle cells. The central core is composed of lipid-laden foam cells, free extracellular lipids, as well as cellular debris and plasma proteins. The primary lipid in atherosclerotic plaques is cholesterol or cholesteryl esters. The so-called foam cells are lipid-filled smooth muscle and blood-derived macrophages (Figure 12-2).

While most plaques contain large amounts of lipid, there are lesions that are composed mainly of connective tissue and smooth muscle elements. These are known as fibrous plaques and have a propensity to occur in the coronary circulation.

Atheromatous plaques, whether fibrous or lipid-rich, may undergo changes that result in "complicated plaques." The nature of these lesions is outlined below:

1. *Calcification.* This complication is common in advanced disease and results in loss of the normal elastic recoil of large arteries.
2. *Ulceration.* Disruption of the endothelium over the plaque results in discharge of lipid debris into the bloodstream that act as microemboli.
3. *Thromboses.* This complication usually results over ulcerated plaque and can result in sudden vascular occlusion.

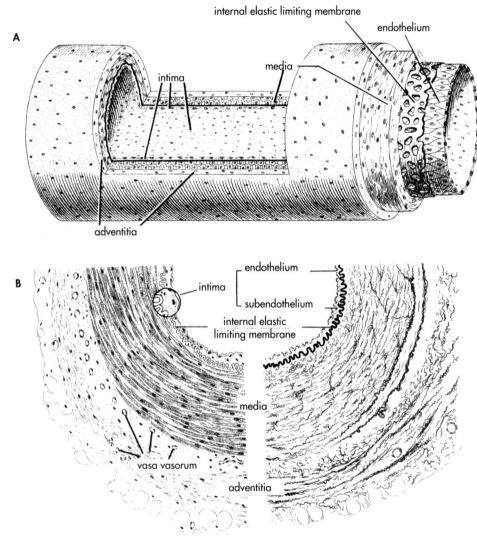

Figure 12-1 A, Drawing of a medium-sized artery (muscular artery), showing its layers. In the usual histologic preparations, the layers appear thicker than shown here. **B,** Comparative diagrams of a muscular artery prepared by hematoxylin and eosin (H & E) staining (*left*) and by Weigert's staining method for elastic structures (*right*). The medium is composed of a mixture of smooth muscle cells, collagen, and elastic fibers. The adventitia has small blood vessels (the vasa vasorum) and elastic and collagenous fibers. (Reproduced from Junqueira LC, Carneiro J. *Basic histology,* 4th ed. Los Altos, CA: Lange, 1983:250.)

4. *Hemorrhage.* Bleeding into a plaque can occur from rupture of either the overlying endothelium or small intraplaque capillaries that often exist at the margins of advanced lesions. In either case this phenomenon can lead to sudden vascular occlusion.
5. *Aneurysmal Dilatation* . While atherosclerosis is a disease of the vascular intima, the media does experience a type of "pressure atrophy" that can result in aneurysm formation.

Although any type of atherosclerotic lesion is potentially dangerous, it is the complicated plaque, particu-

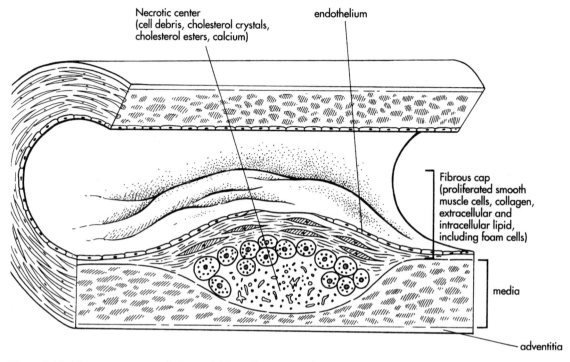

Figure 12-2 Major components of advanced (clinically important) atherosclerotic plaque. (Reproduced from Wissler RW, Vellelinovitch D. Animal models of regression. In Schettler G, et al., eds. *Atherosclerosis IV*. Berlin: Springer-Verlag, 1977:377. Courtesy of P. Constantinides.)

larly the superimposed thrombosis, that produces greatest morbidity and mortality from this disease.

In addition to the histologic structure of the atherosclerotic plaque, a knowledge of the anatomical distribution of such lesions is central to understanding both the clinical manifestations of the disease and its possible pathogenesis. The distribution of mature plaques is relatively constant and differs from that of fatty streaks (see below). The subrenal abdominal aorta and iliac arteries are most commonly involved, followed in order by the coronary arteries, the descending thoracic aorta, femoral and popliteal arteries, the internal carotids, the vertebra basilar system, and the circle of Willis. The ascending aorta and vessels of the upper extremity are usually spared, as are the mesenteric and renal arteries (except at their ostia).

THE FATTY STREAK

This lesion is important because it may be a precursor of the atherosclerotic plaque. Macroscopically, these lesions are thin (<2 mm), long (1–2 cm), flat, yellow lesions that have no hemodynamic significance. Characteristically, fatty streaks are aligned with the direction of blood flow. Fatty streaks occur in all children regardless of sex, race, or environment, and like atherosclerotic plaques, have a very predictable distribution. They first occur at approximately 1 year of age in the ascending thoracic aorta. The number of aortic lesions grows until the third decade, at which time fatty streaks may cover 30% of the aortic intimal surface. It is important to note that the distribution of fatty streaks does not correlate with the usual distribution of aortic atherosclerotic plaques. Coronary artery fatty streaks commonly are found by the age of 10 years and are located mainly in the first 2 cm of the left coronary artery. This position does correlate with atherosclerotic plaques that develop in adulthood.

The histologic appearance of fatty streaks is also characteristic. The lesion is composed of a subintimal lipid collection contained for the most part within macrophages and smooth muscle cells (foam cells). The significance of fatty streaks in the pathogenesis of atherosclerosis remains unsettled.

Pathogenesis

The exact etiologic mechanism of atherogenesis is unknown. Over the years, many models have been proposed in an attempt to synthesize a coherent mechanism that incorporates risk factors for atherosclerosis, known morphologic characteristics of atherosclerotic plaques, and an ever-enlarging body of experimental information.

The structure of the atherosclerotic plaque as described previously indicates that at least four distinct processes occur during plaque formation:

1. Intimal accumulation of macrophage and smooth muscle
2. Proliferation of smooth muscle
3. Production within the intima of extracellular matrix elements
4. Accumulation of lipids in cells and extracellular connective tissue.

THE ROLE OF LIPIDS IN ATHEROGENESIS

Plasma lipids circulate in combination with protein (lipoproteins). Lipoproteins are globular particles of varying size that are composed of a hydrophobic core (triglycerides and cholesteryl esters) and a hydrophilic shell (cholesterol, phospholipids, and apoproteins). Lipoproteins can be broken down into four types, according to their electrophoretic and sedimentation properties: (1) chylomicrons, which have the lowest density, are composed primarily of triglyceride, and are found in plasma only after a meal; (2) VLDL, which mainly transports triglycerides that have been synthesized in the liver; (3) LDL, and (4) HDL (Table 12-1).

Dietary and endogenous lipids are transported by the various lipoproteins by separate pathways (Figure 12-3). Both the endogenous and exogenous pathways contain similar types of metabolic steps:

1. Production of triglyceride-rich lipoproteins
2. Lipoprotein lipase-mediated triglyceride catabolism
3. Remnant lipoprotein catabolism.

The endogenous pathway contains two unique metabolic steps:

4. LDL metabolism
5. HDL-mediated surface catabolism.

Exogenous Pathway

After hydrolysis of dietary triglycerides in the small intestines, the resulting fatty acids and monoglycerides are combined with apoprotein B48, phospholipid, and small amounts of cholesterol to form large chylomicrons (step 1). These particles are secreted into lymphatics and reach the circulation via the thoracic duct. During flow through capillary beds, chylomicrons are

TABLE 12-1. Classification of Lipoproteins

Ultracentrifugal Designation	Electrophoretic Mobility	Major Core Lipids	Numeric Designation of Hyperlipidemia
Chylomicrons	Remain at origin	Dietary triglycerides	I (alone) V (with VLDL)
Very low-density lipoproteins	Pre-β	Hepatic triglycerides	IV (alone) V (with chylomicrons) IIb (with LDL)
Remnants (IDL)	Slow pre-β	Cholesteryl esters, triglycerides	III
Low-density lipoproteins	β	Cholesteryl esters	IIa (alone) IIb (with VLDL)
High-density lipoproteins	α	Cholesteryl esters	

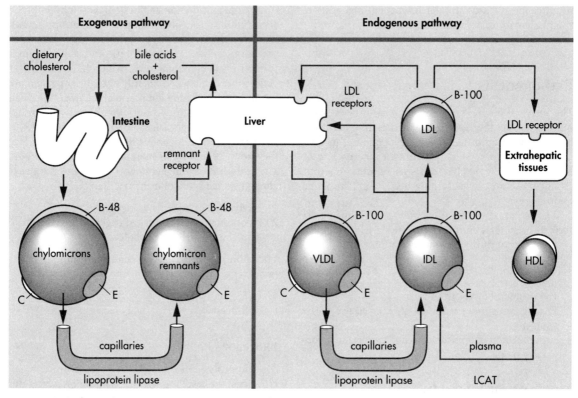

Figure 12-3 Pathways for receptor-mediated metabolism of lipoproteins carrying endogenous and exogenous cholesterol. HDL, High-density lipoprotein; LCAT, lecithin:cholesterol acyltransferase; LDL, low-density lipoprotein; IDL, intermediate-density lipoprotein; VLDL, very-low-density lipoprotein. The distinction between exogenous and endogenous cholesterol applies to the immediate source of the cholesterol in plasma lipoproteins. After the exogenous cholesterol has been delivered to the liver and has been secreted in VLDL, it is considered endogenous cholesteryl. Note that HDL is the lipoprotein that removes cholesterol from extrahepatic cells. E, C, B48, and B100 are apoproteins (see text). (Reproduced from Goldstein JL, et al.: Defective lipoprotein receptors and atherosclerosis. *N Engl J Med* 1983;309:288.)

exposed to an endothelial enzyme called lipoprotein lipase (LPL), which hydrolyzes the triglycerides, allowing delivery of fatty acids to adipose cells for storage (step 2). The interaction of lipoprotein lipase with triglyceride-rich lipoproteins requires the presence of apoprotein CII, which chylomicrons pick up from contact with HDL particles. Thus, the triglyceride-rich lipoproteins contain both substrate and activator for their hydrolysis by LPL. As the chylomicron passes through capillary beds, it becomes progressively depleted in triglycerides with a relative increase in cholesterol. These cholesteryl ester-rich chylomicron remnants are then taken up by the liver through a receptor-mediated mechanism dependent on the presence of apoprotein E (step 3). Most of this cholesterol is secreted through bile into the intestines.

Endogenous Pathway

Input of triglyceride-rich lipoproteins (step 1) also occurs from endogenous sources. Triglycerides synthesized in the liver, together with cholesteryl ester, are combined with phospholipid, unesterified cholesterol, and apoprotein B100 and subsequently secreted as triglyceride-rich VLDL. Like chylomicrons, VLDL particles are hydrolyzed during capillary flow by LPL in the presence of apoprotein CII (step 2). As VLDL particles pass through the capillary network, they also become depleted of triglyceride. They are then classified as intermediate-density lipoproteins (IDL) or VLDL remnants. Intermediate-density lipoproteins particles, through an ill-defined mechanism, acquire large quantities of cholesterol esters, lose apoprotein E, and become lipoproteins LDL (step 3). The cholesterol-rich LDL can be removed from plasma by extrahepatic tissues, where it functions as the chief source of cholesterol for membrane or steroid-hormone synthesis (step 4). Alternatively, LDL may be taken up by the liver and not used peripherally. Apoprotein B100 appears to be recognized by a specific binding site in tissues. Once bound, LDL is internalized and cholesteryl esters are released and hydrolyzed to free cholesterol. The cell is able to regulate its own cholesterol content though a feedback loop in which intracellular cholesterol inhibits endogenous cholesterol synthesis (by inhibition of HMG-CoA reductase; see Chapter 2). Cholesterol accumulation within the cell also decreases the number of LDL receptors expressed on the cell membrane.

The final aspect of lipoprotein metabolism that requires discussion is the role of HDL in catabolism of cell membranes and lipoprotein surfaces (step 5). As the core of triglyceride-rich lipoproteins is removed by the above-described pathways, the particles decrease in size, resulting in "excess" surface. High-density lipoprotein is secreted by the liver and other extrahepatic tissues and is composed of phospholipid and apoproteins AI and AII. High-density-lipoprotein particles pass through the circulation and act as receptors for excess phospholipids (mainly lecithin) and cholesterol from cell membranes as well as other lipoproteins. The enzyme lecithin-cholesterol acyl transferase (LCAT) then catalyzes the transfer of fatty acid from lecithin to cholesterol, forming cholesteryl esters, which can either be transported to the liver or other lipoproteins. In addition, HDL shuttles apoproteins CII and E to and from chylomicrons and VLDL as part of their metabolism.

The mechanism by which normal and abnormal lipoprotein metabolism promotes atherosclerosis is not well understood. It seems certain that the cholesterol in atheromatous plaques is derived from plasma lipoprotein, since both apoprotein B and intact LDL particles have been localized in atheromas. Lipids in atheromatous plaques accumulate both extracellularly and within foam cells. Foam cells are known to be of smooth muscle cell and macrophage origin; however, neither cell when exposed to normal LDL in vitro sequesters lipid. The question is, then, how do these cells become filled with lipid? Recent in vitro studies have shown that modification such as acetylation or changing the charge of the LDL particle may bypass the normal receptor-mediated uptake mechanism described above. In addition, the uptake of these so-called modified LDL

particles is not followed by the normal feedback inhibition loop so lipid is progressively accumulated. It has also been shown that in the presence of HDL the accumulation of cholesteryl esters from modified LDL is greatly reduced. This finding is in keeping with the known cholesterol-clearing properties of HDL.

Although the in vivo significance of normal and deranged lipid metabolism as well as the above in vitro results is uncertain, it appears likely that the interactions of lipoproteins with platelets, macrophages, smooth muscle cells, and endothelium are involved in the net accumulation of lipid in atheromatous plaques.

HEMODYNAMIC FACTORS

The fluid mechanics and flow characteristic of blood have long been proposed as an etiologic factor in atherogenesis. This hypothesis has been made because many plaques develop in areas where flow profiles deviate from unidirectional laminar flow. High shear stress was initially postulated to cause endothelial injury, thereby exposing the underlying vessel wall to lipids and platelets. However, experimental evidence indicates that high shear stress probably inhibits plaque formation. Low shear stress, on the other hand, has been clearly associated with the formation of plaques. Some authors have proposed that low shear rates may impede the transport of atherogenic substances away from the vessel wall, resulting in lipid deposition. Low shear rates may also be detrimental to arterial wall nutrition and endothelial metabolism.

THEORIES OF ATHEROGENESIS

Three of the most popular models of atherogenesis are presented below.

The *response-to-injury hypothesis* states that the lesions of atherosclerosis are initiated as a response to some form of injury to the arterial endothelium. This hypothesis proposes that there are three components to atherogenesis.

The first is the endothelial injury itself. Various types of experimental endothelial injury have been shown to cause proliferation of vascular smooth muscle. Such injuries include balloon denudation, immune complex deposition, irradiation, arteriovenous fistulae, and chronic hyperlipidemia. Hypertension and cigarette smoking are probably also injurious to vascular endothelium. It should be stressed that frank denudation of endothelium is not a necessary requirement for this theory; some type of endothelial cell dysfunction is probably all that is required to initiate the process of atherogenesis.

The second component of the hypothesis is smooth muscle proliferation. The proliferating cells originate from the media. Several smooth muscle mitogens have been implicated, with platelet-derived growth factor (PDGF) being the most widely studied. Whatever the stimulus, it is the smooth muscle cells that produce the extracellular constituents (collagen and proteoglycans) of plaques. It is these same cells that accumulate serum lipids and become foam cells.

The third aspect of the response to injury hypothesis

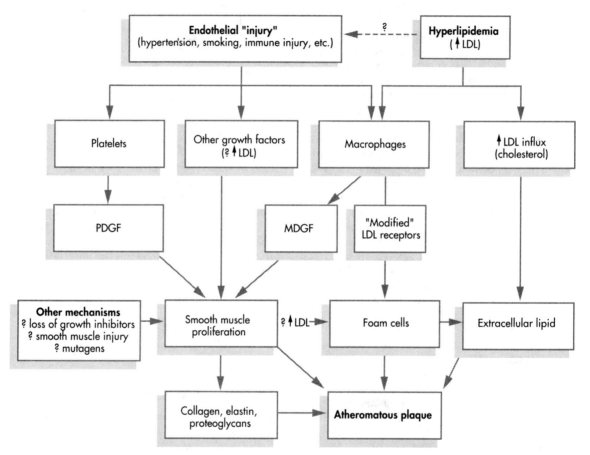

Figure 12-4 Proposed sequences involving endothelial injury, hyperlipidermia, and other mechanisms in the pathogenesis of the atheromatous plaque. Many of the mechanisms are based on in vitro studies. "?" refers to unproved or controversial sequences. Denuding or nondenuding endothelial injury causes platelet and monocyte macrophage adhesion to injured sites; factors derived from these cell types (PDGF, MDGF) or factors derived from the blood (e.g., hyperlipidemic LDL) cause smooth muscle migration and proliferation in the intima. Foam cells are derived from smooth muscle cells by as yet poorly understood mechanisms, and from macrophages in part by uptake via "modified" LDL receptors. The extracellular lipid is derived partly from direct migration from the serum and partly from breakdown of foam cells. The atheromatous plaque is composed of proliferating smooth muscle cells, their secreted extracellular matrix, foam cells, extracellular lipid, and necrotic debris. Hyperlipidemia *may* contribute to atherogenesis by (1) increasing the influx of LDL, (2) causing endothelial injury, (3) directly inducing smooth muscle proliferation, and (4) influencing the formation of foam cells. Note that smooth muscle proliferation may also be induced directly by several postulated mechanisms (left). (Reproduced from Robbins SL, Cotran RS, Cumar V. *Pathologic basis of disease*. 3rd ed. Philadelphia: WB Saunders, 1984:516.)

is its relationship to hyperlipidemia. Elevated serum lipids may interact with the vascular injury response in several ways. (1) Endothelial damage permits the entrance of plasma lipids into the vessel wall. (2) Chronic hyperlipidemia may in itself cause endothelial injury. (3) Certain components of hyperlipidemic serum may directly stimulate smooth muscle proliferation. (4) Hyperlipidemia favors platelet aggregation and release of PDGF, which in turn increases LDL receptors on smooth muscle cells and thus increases their rate of uptake of lipid. PDGF also induces migration of smooth muscle cells from the media into the intima and stimulates smooth muscle replication within the intima.

While the response-to-injury model is dependent on an endothelial event, the development of atheromatous plaques could also be explained if smooth muscle proliferation was the initial event. Two theories that implicate a primary smooth muscle dysfunction have been proposed and are briefly reviewed below.

The **monoclonal hypothesis** resulted from a study that looked at the distribution of the A or B isoenzyme of glucose 6-phosphate dehydrogenase in black women heterozygous for the enzyme. It was found that the normal aorta contained smooth muscle cells that contained both A and B isoenzymes; however, atherosclerotic areas usually contain only one of the enzymes. This monotypic nature is evidence that atherosclerotic plaques may be equivalent to benign neoplastic growth initiated by mutation. The significance of this hypothesis is unclear but has directed attention toward smooth muscle cell mutagens as possible initiators of atherogenesis.

Disturbance of growth control is the third hypothesis and implicates smooth muscle cell proliferation as the inciting event of atherogenesis. A heparinlike molecule expressed by normal aortic endothelial and smooth muscle cells has been shown to inhibit smooth muscle cell proliferation in cell culture. Presumably, focal loss of this inhibitor (possibly initiated by injury) may lead to smooth muscle proliferation. This mechanism is supported by the fact that heparin has been shown in vitro to arrest the smooth muscle cell proliferation precipitated by endothelial cell injury.

Figure 12-4 illustrates some of the proposed mechanisms of atherogenesis. Emphasis is placed on the response-to-injury model as well as the role of serum lipids.

It seems likely that atherosclerosis is not the result of any single initiating event or exclusive pathologic mechanism. Clinically significant atherosclerotic vascular disease appears to be a disease of multiple origins. Perhaps the cumulative effect of many factors is involved, as seems evident from epidemiologic studies.

Bibliography

Gotto AM, Gross HL, Fites LL. *Atherosclerosis—a scope publication.* Kalamazoo, MI: The Upjohn Company, 1977.

Kelly DE, Wood RL, Enders AC. *Bailey's textbook of microscopic anatomy.* 18th ed. Baltimore: Williams & Wilkins, 1984.

Robbins S, Cotran RS, Kumar V. *Pathologic basis of disease.* Philadelphia: WB Saunders, 1984.

White RA. *Atherosclerosis and arteriosclerosis: human pathology and experimental animal methods and models.* Boca Raton, FL: CRC Press, 1989.

Wyngaarden JB, Smith LH. *Cecil textbook of medicine.* Philadelphia: WB Saunders, 1988.

C. William Hanson III

13 PHYSIOLOGY OF RESPIRATION

Architecture
  Vascular Supply
  Thoracic Mechanics
  Lung Zones
Oxygenation
Ventilation
Mechanical Ventilators
Pulmonary Function Tests

The primary functions of the lung are respiration, oxygenation, and ventilation. It also has metabolic, endocrine, and immunologic responsibilities, which are discussed in Chapter 15. The respiratory interface comprises 2 to 600 million alveoli, with a surface area of about 100 m². In a fit young adult who is exercising strenuously, this "membrane" can effectively expose 120 liters of air to 25 liters of blood per minute.

Architecture

The design of the lung allows for the maximum interdigitation of the airways with the bloodstream. On the airway side of the circuit, there are five lobes of the lung: the right upper, middle and lower lobes, and the left upper (including the lingula), and lower lobes. They are served by up to 23 generations of branching airways. The first four generations include the main, lobar, and segmental bronchi. The 5th through the 11th generations are the small bronchi. Generations 12 through 16 are the bronchioles: the first noncartilaginous airways, with a diameter on the order of 2 mm, and a total cross-sectional airway about 30 times larger than that of the larger airways. The first airways that serve some function other than that of conduction are the respira-

tory bronchioles, the 17th through 19th generations. They begin to function in gas exchange, as do the alveolar ducts, the 20th, 21st, and 22nd generations. The alveolar sac is the 23rd and final generation (in the normal lung), and is the blind endpoint of the conducting system, although an alveolus may communicate with a neighbor through pores of Kohn, which provide collateral ventilation.

The alveolus itself is a polyhedron rather than a sphere, with flat walls forming the common wall between adjacent alveoli. There are several types of cells involved in the architecture of a given alveolus. The **capillary endothelial cells** are continuous with the major pulmonary vasculature, as metabolically active as the liver (when taken in aggregate), and form vessels wide enough, at 10 nm, to allow the passage of one red cell at a time. The **type I alveolar epithelial cells** make up the infrastructure of the alveolar wall, forming tight, albumin-impermeable junctions with neighboring cells. The **type II alveolar epithelial cells** are stem cells from which type I cells are derived, and in which **surfactant** is made. There are also several immunologically active cells that may be found in normal lungs: neutrophils, mast cells, and most importantly, alveolar macrophages. Macrophages are active in scavenging the airways of dust, bacteria, and cellular debris, and pass freely from the interstitial space through the tight junctions of the type I cells into the alveolus itself. These cells are effective in defending this vulnerable interface of the body from the environment, but have been implicated as deadly mediators in the adult respiratory distress syndrome (ARDS). Secretion of oxygen free radicals and enzymes by activated macrophages may damage the alveolar unit. Alveolar brush cells of uncertain function; Clara cells, which are metabolically active; and secretory and amine-precursor uptake decarboxylation cells

(APUD), which may have an endocrine function, complete the list of cells normally found in the lung.

Lymphatic circulation begins at the interface between the alveolar and extra-alveolar space, forms a capillary network around the airways and vessels of the lung, and drains toward the hilum and into the thoracic duct. In times of excess pulmonary lung water, the lymphatics may carry substantial amounts of edema from the interstitial space.

VASCULAR SUPPLY

The vascular supply of the lung is dual, with the pulmonary circulation subserving respiration and providing continuity between the right ventricle and left atrium, and the bronchial circulation providing nutrition to the conducting airways and accompanying blood vessels. The bronchial circulation derives from the aorta and returns, in part, to the pulmonary venous system, adding oxygen-depleted blood to arterialized blood and contributing to physiologic shunting.

The pulmonary vasculature begins with the pulmonary artery, which leaves the right ventricle and almost immediately divides to form the right and left pulmonary arteries. The vessels travel with airways after bifurcation. The pulmonary arterial system is a low-resistance, low-pressure system, with pressures one sixth to one eighth those of the systemic circulation.

The microcirculation of the lung consists of the arterioles, the capillary mesh, and the proximal venules. Arterioles have an internal diameter of 100 μm, are thin-walled and lack a medial muscular layer. They are quite similar to the pulmonary venules in structure. The capillary network is continuous and surrounds the alveoli in such a way that a red cell may traverse several alveoli in its passage from arteriole, through "one" capillary and into a venule. The venules and veins ultimately merge to form four veins that drain into the left atrium.

THORACIC MECHANICS

The infrastructure that prevents the lungs from collapsing, and permits their ready inflation, depends on the mechanics of the thoracic cavity, the elastic nature of the lung parenchyma, and on surfactant, a detergentlike molecule that is secreted by alveolar epithelial cells.

At any given point in the respiratory cycle, the lung expresses a balance between forces that tend toward collapse and those that maintain inflation. At the alveolar level, nitrogen acts from within to stent open the alveolus. It is a major constituent of air but is poorly absorbed by the blood. Note that this distending force is lost in patients breathing higher than ambient inspired concentrations of oxygen, which is well absorbed from the alveolus. Patients breathing high concentrations of oxygen may develop resorption atelectasis as a result.

Laplace's law, which states that pressure is inversely proportional to radius, indicates that smaller alveoli should have a higher internal pressure and should therefore empty into larger ones (Figure 13-1). Some cystic, emphysematous lung diseases may reflect this phenomenon. In the normal lung, however, elastic fibers that tend to collapse a single alveolus simultaneously tend to expand neighboring alveoli, opposing the effect of Laplace's law on small alveoli. More important, perhaps, is the role of **surfactant**, which consists of dipalmitoyl phosphatidyl choline, a molecule with hydrophilic and hydrophobic poles. Surface tension is defined as the force acting across a theoretical line 1 cm long on the surface of a liquid (see Figure 13-1). When suspended on saline, surfactant reduces surface tension; and for a given amount of surfactant, the reduction in surface tension is greater at smaller surface areas. As alveoli collapse, developing higher pressures by Laplace's law, surfactant will cause a greater reduction in surface tension, which opposes the tendency to collapse.

On a macroscopic scale, lung inflation is maintained by the thoracic cage. Negative intrapleural pressure maintains apposition of the parietal and visceral pleura. On normal inspiration, the diaphragm contracts, lengthening the thoracic cavity, and the external intercostal muscles contract, raising the ribs and increasing the circumference of the cavity. The accessory muscles of respiration are recruited with successively greater degrees of hyperventilation. With the addition of the scalenes, sternocleidomastoids, and vertebral column extensors, ventilation rates up to 50 L/min can be generated. The pectorals and abdominal wall muscles can be recruited for active exhalation to achieve ever higher ventilatory rates.

LUNG ZONES

An understanding of the relationship between alveolus and blood vessel is of fundamental importance to the concept of ventilation/perfusion (V/Q) match and mismatch. The V/Q ratio expresses the balance between ventilation and perfusion in a portion of the lung. Ratios approaching 1/0 represent pure dead space; and

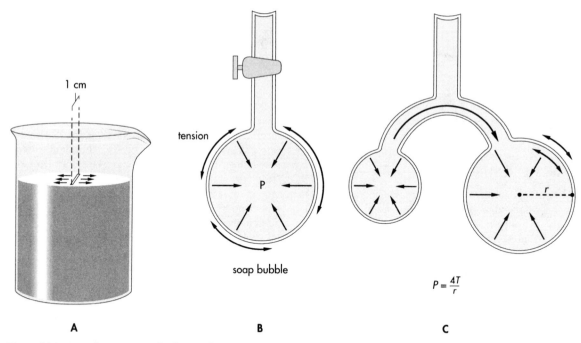

Figure 13-1 **A,** Surface tension is the force in dynes acting across an imaginary line 1 cm long in a liquid surface. **B,** Surface forces in a soap bubble tend to reduce the area of the surface and generate a pressure within the bubble. **C,** Because the smaller bubble generates a larger pressure, it blows up the large bubble. (Reproduced from West JB. *Respiratory physiology—the essentials.* 3rd ed. Baltimore: Williams & Wilkins, 1985:90.)

ratios approaching 0/1, pure shunt (Figures 13-2 and 13-3). West describes three zones of V/Q relationship (Figure 13-4). Zone 1 conditions are those at the apex of the upright lung, where the V/Q ratio is high. Zone 3 conditions prevail at the base, where the V/Q ratio is lower (zone 2 falls between zones 1 and 3). Inherent in this change of V/Q ratio is the fact that while both ventilation and perfusion increase from the top to the bottom of the lung, perfusion increases more rapidly than ventilation (Figure 13-5). Some interesting clinical correlates of ventilation and perfusion relationships are the predilection of tuberculosis for the oxygen-rich environment at the apex and the tendency of a pulmonary artery catheter to lodge in areas of the lung where zone 2 or 3 relationships exist and better blood flow is found.

Zone 1 conditions approximate those of alveolar "dead space"—areas of ventilated but unperfused lung. Normal lungs have anatomic dead space (trachea and upper airway), and alveolar dead space is small to absent. Hypovolemia and pulmonary embolism result in decreased pulmonary arterial perfusion (↓Q). Increasing intra-alveolar pressure by applying positive

pressure ventilation or positive end-expiratory pressure (PEEP) improves the V/Q ratio in some units, thereby decreasing shunt. PEEP also decreases perfusion to some areas of the lung, resulting in a higher V/Q ratio and greater dead space.

Dead space is classified into several types. **Anatomic dead space** is the volume of the conducting conduit (trachea and bronchi) and amounts to about 2 cc/kg or about 150 cc in a normal adult. **Alveolar dead space** is the gas that ventilates unperfused portions of the lungs and is negligible in the normal, well-hydrated patient. **Physiological dead space** is the combination of anatomic and alveolar dead space and can be estimated by collecting a sample of mixed expired gas and determining its partial pressure of CO_2. By Bohr's equation:

$$\frac{\text{Dead space}}{\text{Tidal volume}} = \frac{\text{alveolar } CO_2 - \text{expired } CO_2}{\text{alveolar } CO_2}$$

$$\frac{V_d}{V_T} = \frac{P_{ACO_2} - P_{ECO_2}}{P_{ACO_2}}.$$

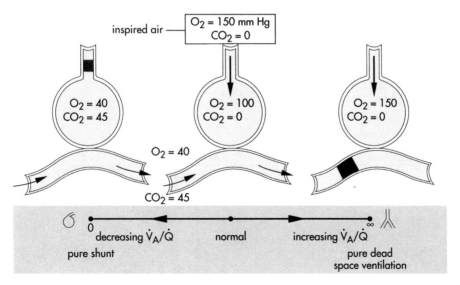

Figure 13-2 Effect of altering the ventilation-perfusion ratio on the Po_2 and Pco_2 in a lung unit. (Reproduced from West JB. *Ventilation blood flow and gas exchange.* 3rd ed. Oxford: Blackwell, 1977.)

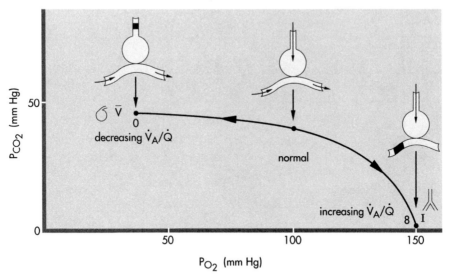

Figure 13-3 O_2-CO_2 diagram showing a ventilation-perfusion ratio line. The Po_2 and Pco_2 of a lung unit move along this line from the mixed venous point v to the inspired gas point I as its ventilation-perfusion ratio is increased. (Reproduced from West JB. *Ventilation blood flow and gas exchange.* 3rd ed. Oxford: Blackwell, 1977.)

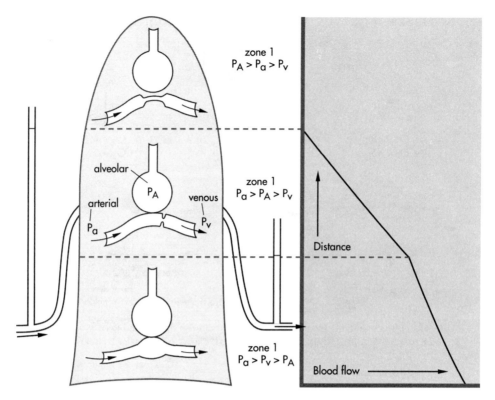

Figure 13-4 Model to explain the uneven distribution of blood flow in the lung based on the pressures affecting the capillaries. (Reproduced from West JB, et al. *J Appl Physiol* 1964;19:713.)

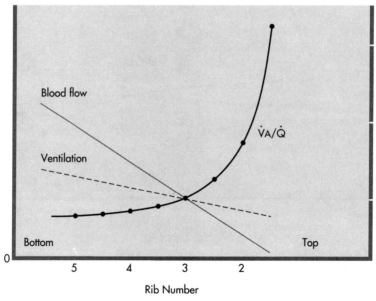

Figure 13-5 Distribution of ventilation and blood flow down the upright lung. Note that the ventilation-perfusion ratio decreases down toward the base of the lung. (Reproduced from West JB. *Ventilation blood flow and gas exchange.* 3rd ed. Oxford: Blackwell, 1977.)

The ratio of dead space to tidal volume is ordinarily on the order of 0.2–0.35. This ratio increases with advancing age, body size, and upright posture. Smokers tend to have higher ratios than nonsmokers. Pulmonary embolism and high levels of PEEP result in an increased ratio by increasing the amount of ventilated but unperfused lung.

Zone 3 conditions approach (but do not reach) those of pure shunt, with perfusion in excess of ventilation. With basilar atelectasis, for example, zone 3 will enlarge. In the absence of active redistribution of blood flow away from alveoli with low P_{O_2}, hypoxemia will result.

The term **shunt** is used to refer to the fraction of blood that enters the systemic arterial system without passing through a ventilated portion of the lung. Normal, or "physiologic," shunt sources are the bronchial circulation and blood from the Thebesian veins, which drain a small portion of the coronary circulation into the left ventricle. Abnormal causes of shunt include intracardiac shunt, arteriovenous malformations of the lung, or vasodilators like nitroprusside, which override hypoxic pulmonary vasoconstriction (see below).

Of the four causes of hypoxemia (see below), shunt is the only one that cannot be corrected by oxygen therapy. The portion of blood that is shunted never "sees" the raised F_{IO_2}, and because of the shape of the oxyhemoglobin dissociation curve, a small amount of shunted blood added to blood with a high P_{O_2} will cause significant decreases in arterial P_{O_2}.

The shunt formula is cumbersome:

$$\frac{\text{Shunt flow}}{\text{Total flow}} =$$
$$\frac{O_2 \text{ content capillary } - O_2 \text{ content arterial blood}}{O_2 \text{ content capillary } - O_2 \text{ content venous blood}}$$

i.e.,

$$\frac{Q_s}{Q_T} = \frac{Cc'_{O_2} - Ca_{O_2}}{Cc'_{O_2} - Cv_{O_2}}$$

This can, with certain assumptions, be simplified to

$$\frac{Q_s}{Q_T} = \frac{Cc'_{O_2} - Ca_{O_2}}{3.5 + \left[Cc'_{O_2} - Ca_{O_2} \right]}$$

where

$$Ca'_{O_2} = \text{Hgb x Sa}_{O_2} \text{ x } 1.39,$$

and

$$Cc'_{O_2} = \text{Hgb x Sc'}_{O_2} \text{ x } 1.39.[1]$$

A formula in use at some institutions that approximates the shunt equation is

$$\frac{Q_s}{Q_T} = \frac{\left[F_{IO_2} \text{ x } 5 \right] - Pa_{O_2}}{10}.$$

A calculated shunt of less than 10% is compatible with normal lungs, 10–20% is rarely of clinical importance, 20–30% indicates significant pulmonary disease, and greater than 30% is life-threatening and requires aggressive therapy.

Other measures of intrapulmonary shunting that are probably less reliable include the alveolar-to-arterial (A–a) P_{O_2} gradient, the a/A ratio, and the ratio between the Pa_{O_2} and the F_{IO_2}. These approximations of shunt are subject to inaccuracies owing to temperature, P_{CO_2}, and ventilation/perfusion inaccuracies.

While a shunt could theoretically raise the patient's P_{CO_2}, there is generally a full or even more than compensatory rise in minute ventilation, which normalizes the CO_2. The hyperventilation is stimulated by hypoxia that results from the shunt.

The process of active redistribution of pulmonary blood flow to maintain optimal V/Q relationships is called **hypoxic pulmonary vasoconstriction (HPV)**. Pulmonary arterial vasoconstriction occurs as the alveolar P_{O_2} of a given lung region falls below 70 torr. The exact mechanism by which local hypoxia is detected and constriction is mediated is not clear. The vasoconstriction seems to occur on the arterial side of the pulmonary capillaries. Cor pulmonale, seen in chronic obstructive pulmonary disease and sleep apnea, is probably the result of chronic pulmonary vasoconstriction resulting from chronic arterial hypoxemia. Similarly, some inhalational anesthetics and vasodilators abolish HPV, causing a shunt by increasing perfusion through poorly ventilated lung regions.

Oxygenation

The control of oxygenation is mediated by peripheral chemoreceptors—the carotid and aortic bodies. These are rapidly responding monitors of arterial blood which

---

[1]Sc'_{O_2} is assumed to be 100% and therefore equal to 1.0.

react to decreases in P_{O_2} or pH, increases in P_{CO_2}, or to absolute decreases in perfusion with an increased firing rate. They are located at the bifurcation of the carotid artery and above and below the aortic arch.

There are several cell types in the carotid body: glomus cells, afferent and efferent nerves from the glossopharyngeal nerve and the superior cervical ganglion, and sheath cells. It is not clear which cell type is responsible for the detection of hypoxemia; but it is clear that the responder cells represent the body's only source of response to hypoxemia. In the absence of these bodies (as after bilateral carotid endarterectomy), complete loss of hypoxic ventilatory drive ensues. The carotid bodies begin to fire as arterial P_{O_2} drops below 500 mm Hg, but they remain relatively quiescent until arterial P_{O_2} is reduced below 100 mm Hg, at which point firing rate increases until it maximizes at P_{O_2}'s below 50 mm Hg.

Acidemia and increases in P_{CO_2} also have stimulatory effects on the peripheral chemoreceptors, although primary control of the magnitude of response to hypercarbia is through the central, medullary control centers. In some chronically hypercapnic patients, the primary respiratory stimulus comes from the carotid bodies in response to chronic hypoxemia. These patients, known as "CO_2 retainers," seem to require the hypoxic stimulus to control respiration, and are insensitive or unresponsive to rises in CO_2. This is demonstrated clinically by increasing hypercarbia when their P_{O_2} is allowed to rise above 60 to 70 mm Hg on supplemental oxygen. Baseline arterial blood-gas analysis in these patients tends to show a well-compensated respiratory acidosis with hypoxemia. Most pulmonary physiologists feel that the central CO_2 drive becomes blunted in these patients with chronic hypercapnia. There has, however, been some recent research evidence indicating that CO_2 retention may be a result of changes in V/Q ratios rather than blunting of the central CO_2 drive.

Hypoxemia results from four different processes: **hypoventilation, diffusion gradients, shunt,** and **ventilation-perfusion mismatch.** Hypoventilation can be caused by drugs (opiates, barbiturates, etc.), mechanical impairments of the chest wall (painful incisions and binders), and paralysis of the respiratory muscles (muscular dystrophy, polio virus, and neuromuscular blockade). Since the level of alveolar P_{O_2} is a function of the balance between the source gas (alveolar ventilation) and the consumed gas (O_2 consumption), any fall in the level of ventilation will result in a fall in the alveolar (and therefore the arterial) P_{O_2}. A second consequence of a fall in alveolar ventilation will be a rise in alveolar

(and therefore arterial) P_{CO_2}. The relationship between the fall in arterial P_{O_2} and simultaneous rise in P_{CO_2} is given by the alveolar gas equation: where P_{AO_2} is alveolar partial pressure of oxygen, P_{IO_2} is the partial pressure of oxygen in inspired air and P_{ACO_2} is alveolar CO_2, which is assumed to equal arterial CO_2:

$$P_{AO_2} = P_{IO_2} - P_{ACO_2}/.8 + F$$

where F is a small correction factor that can be ignored. In a normal subject, breathing room air and sea level,

$$P_{AO_2} = 21\% \times (760 - 47) - 40/.8 = 99 \text{ mm Hg}$$

where 47 equals the vapor pressure of water in alveolar gas, P_{AO_2} represents the **ideal alveolar** P_{O_2}, and the discrepancy between that and the true arterial P_{O_2} is the A–a gradient.

An increased **diffusion gradient** causes failure of equilibration between the hemoglobin in the red cell and the gas in the alveoli it traverses. Under normal conditions the red cell has fully equilibrated with alveolar oxygen after one-third of its transit time through an alveolar capillary, allowing a significant safety margin. In interstitial lung disease, such as the collagen vascular diseases, sarcoidosis, alveolar cell carcinoma, idiopathic interstitial fibrosis, and asbestosis, diffusion impairment may become a significant cause of arterial hypoxemia.

Shunt has already been discussed as a cause of hypoxemia. It is seen commonly in young children with congenital heart disease, and then only when right-sided pressures become sufficiently high that blood "shunts" from the right heart to the left. Shunt is also seen with pulmonary arteriovenous malformations, and consolidation of the lung (e.g., pneumonia) where blood passes through unventilated lung.

Ventilation-perfusion mismatch is probably the most common cause of hypoxemia. It is seen with a variety of different pulmonary conditions and is generally a diagnosis of exclusion, i.e., when **hypoventilation, diffusion impairment,** and **shunt** have been ruled out. Ventilation and perfusion are ideally matched in zone 2 conditions; and, in normal patients, zone 2 conditions will prevail over most of the lung. Pathological conditions that affect either the ventilation or the perfusion of the alveolar unit will contribute to mismatch, either with perfusion in excess of ventilation (tending toward shunt) or ventilation in excess of perfusion (tending toward dead space).

Many patients with diseases of the lung will have

alveoli with a spectrum of ventilation-perfusion ratios, and, as a result, have both a decrease in arterial oxygen saturation and an increase in dead space. The former will be more evident clinically, because the hyperventilatory response is more efficient at eliminating CO_2 than in correcting hypoxemia (owing to the relative shapes of the CO_2 dissociation curve and the O_2 dissociation curve). The CO_2 dissociation curve is linear in the normal range, and an increase in ventilation will effectively and completely compensate for inefficiencies in CO_2 elimination. An increase in ventilation will not raise the arterial Po_2, however, because while units with an intermediate V/Q ratio will benefit from improved oxygen exchange, units with high V/Q ratios will not improve over their already adequate level, and units with very low ratios exchange gas so poorly that blood leaving these alveoli approximates mixed venous blood regardless of ventilation (Figure 13-6).

The differentiation of the four causes of hypoxia from one another can be difficult. **Shunt**, for example, is not always easy to distinguish from **ventilation-perfusion** mismatch, since they are but different points along a spectrum of ventilation perfusion ratios. Several "rules" are helpful.

Hypoventilation is always accompanied by hypercarbia and is secondary to a low minute ventilation, either on the basis of a low tidal volume or rate. The addition of supplemental oxygen to the inspired gas of a hypoventilating patient will readily overcome the hypoxia of hypoventilation.

Impaired diffusion is relatively rare and is usually seen in specific clinical settings. Differentiating diffusion gradient from V/Q mismatch is problematic—the diffusing capacity of the lung is one measure that can be used, but this is generally done only as a part of formal pulmonary function testing.

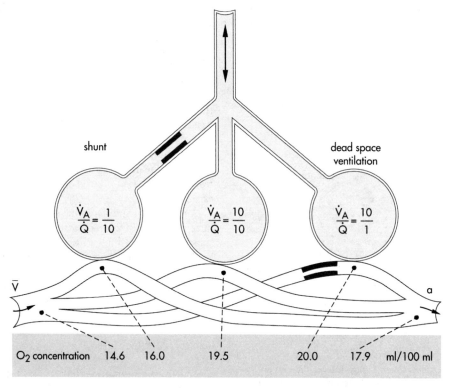

Figure 13-6 Additional reason for the depression of arterial Po_2 by mismatching of ventilation and blood flow. The lung units with a high ventilation-perfusion ratio add relatively little oxygen to the blood, compared with the decrement caused by alveoli with a low ventilation-perfusion ratio. (Reproduced from West JB. *Ventilation blood flow and gas exchange.* 3rd ed. Oxford: Blackwell, 1977.)

Shunt is the only cause of hypoxia that cannot be corrected by administration of 100% inspired oxygen—the test usually performed to diagnose its presence and magnitude. The equation to calculate the magnitude of shunt in a given patient is discussed above.

Ventilation-perfusion mismatch is diagnosed primarily by the exclusion of the other three causes of hypoxia and can be conceived of as in an analogy provided by West. He describes a mixing chamber in which dye and water are added at different rates and allowed to equilibrate, as ventilation and perfusion allow for equilibration between partial pressures of gases in air and blood (Figure 13-7). In each case, the final concentration of the effluent mix, or the saturation of arterialized blood by analogy, is a function of the ratio of the rate of addition of dye (or ventilation) to water (or perfusion). Hypoxia occurs because blood from units with adequate ventilation and poor perfusion have less absolute blood flow than well-perfused units and therefore contribute less to the final concentration of the effluent. In addition, the shape of the oxyhemoglobin dissociation curve demonstrates that units with higher ventilation and resulting higher partial pressures of oxygen will have a minimal incremental increase in the amount of oxygen carried over the flat portion of the curve (see Figure 4-3). The ultimate saturation of the effluent blood will therefore be weighted more toward the low oxygen saturation of the poorly ventilated, well-perfused units that have greater absolute blood flow.

Positive end-expiratory pressure (PEEP) is used to convert lung units with low ventilation-to-perfusion ratios to those with higher or normal ratios, thereby improving oxygenation. Several effects of PEEP are felt to contribute to this improvement. PEEP increases the functional residual capacity of the lung, which will improve both the overall and the regional ventilation of the lung, specifically converting zone 3 conditions to those of zone 2. PEEP probably reopens closed alveoli in pulmonary edema and improves oxygenation by translocating edema fluid from the closed alveoli to the interstitium and opening that alveolus for gas exchange.

Clinically, PEEP has little to no effect on oxygenation of patients with healthy lungs, but it can be quite efficacious in patients with ARDS, where it may allow adequate oxygenation with nontoxic levels of inspired oxygen. Recent studies evaluating the use of PEEP as a means of *preventing* ARDS were unimpressive.

PEEP is generally applied in a range of pressures from 2.5 cm H_2O to 20 cm H_2O. At the lower end of the spectrum, PEEP has minimal effect on the cardiovascular system, while at the upper end, profound hemodynamic compromise frequently occurs. Impaired venous return to the right atrium and ventricle owing to increased mean intrathoracic pressure (with PEEP) results in decreased preload and consequently lowered cardiac output.

A number of standards have been applied to optimize the use of PEEP in critically ill patients, including "best" PEEP, "optimal" PEEP, etc. "Best" PEEP is the level of PEEP that maximizes O_2 delivery to the tissues. A typical trial of increasing levels of PEEP will show increasing PaO_2 (and saturation on the steep, ascending portion of the oxyhemoglobin dissociation curve). As PEEP is increased, there will eventually be reduction of the cardiac output. An approximate formula for oxygen delivery to the tissues is

$$O_2 \text{ delivery (mL/min)} = 10 \text{ (dL/L) x cardiac output (L/min) x } [1.39 \text{ (mL } O_2/g \text{ Hgb) x Hgb (g/dL) x } SaO_2]$$

Increases in PaO_2 will, therefore, increase delivery readily when the SaO_2 is low, but minimally on the flat, upper part of the oxyhemoglobin dissociation curve. A

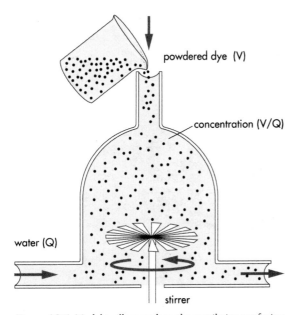

Figure 13-7 Model to illustrate how the ventilation-perfusion ratio determines the PO_2 in a lung unit. Powdered dye is added by ventilation at the rate *V* and removed by blood flow *Q* to represent the factors controlling alveolar PO_2. The concentration of dye is given by *V/Q*. (Reproduced from West JB. *Ventilation blood flow and gas exchange.* 3rd ed. Oxford: Blackwell, 1977.)

point will be reached where the balance between increasing saturation and decreasing cardiac output peaks at maximal O_2 delivery, which then declines with higher levels of PEEP. The point of optimal balance between cardiac output and oxygen saturation, and therefore of maximal oxygen delivery, is "best" PEEP.

Ventilation

Primary control of ventilation occurs in the pons and medulla. The pneumotaxic center and apneustic centers are found in the pons. They interact with the inspiratory and expiratory centers of the medulla and with the lungs via vagal afferents. The phrenic nerve is the efferent limb of the circuit. Control of respiration is quite complicated, poorly understood, and clearly involves different mechanisms in quiet spontaneous breathing, volitional breathing, and breathing during exercise. Recent research indicates that a complicated scheme of excitatory and inhibitory feedback loops modulate respiratory control under most conditions.

While the carotid body chemoreceptors are responsive to rises in CO_2, the primary response to elevations in CO_2 resides in the central medullary chemoreceptors. These receptors lie on the anterolateral surface of the medulla, and respond to rises in cerebrospinal fluid (CSF) P_{CO_2}, which cause a decrease in CSF pH. The direct mediator of the ventilatory response seems to be the CSF pH rather than P_{CO_2}. One reason for the hyperventilation seen with some intracranial lesions may be that CSF pH falls as a result of metabolic breakdown products from the lesion (i.e., subarachnoid blood) and stimulates hyperventilation. Similarly, after prolonged mechanical hyperventilation, some patients will develop a compensatory low CSF pH. When they are then allowed to breath spontaneously, they will continue to hyperventilate until their CSF pH rises to normal levels.

The relationship between the P_{CO_2} and the minute ventilation is linear over the range seen in most clinical settings, so that a doubling of the P_{CO_2} will result from halving the minute ventilation; and conversely, doubling the minute ventilation will halve the P_{CO_2}. This allows easy correction of disordered P_{CO_2} on a mechanical ventilator, from the relationship

$$\text{Minute ventilation}_a \times P_{{CO_2}a} = \text{Minute ventilation}_b \times P_{{CO_2}b}.$$

Mechanical Ventilators

Mechanical ventilators have historically ranged from the huge negative pressure ventilators known as iron lungs to the simple, positive-pressure, self-inflating "Ambu" bags found ubiquitously in the hospital environment. Positive-pressure ventilators have become increasingly sophisticated and expensive, and ventilator modalities have proliferated into a confusing array of choices, including **controlled ventilation, assist control ventilation, intermittent mandatory ventilation, pressure support ventilation, airway pressure release ventilation, mandatory minute volume, etc.** Each strategy represents an attempt to provide the patient with mechanical ventilatory support and differs in provisions for patient triggering, patient-controlled tidal volume, and minute ventilation. Most modern ventilators readily permit switching between modalities.

Despite sporadic attempts to demonstrate a "best" method for weaning from mechanical ventilation, most studies have shown that no strategy is significantly better than another. What follows is a succinct explanation of the most commonly used choices.

Controlled ventilation can be selected on many older ventilators but is what amounts to a default choice on newer ventilators. It represents passive ventilation, where the patient does not trigger a breath and does not determine the tidal volume or the minute ventilation. This exists, de facto, in paralyzed, brain dead, or hyperventilated patients (whose CO_2 is below their set threshold), regardless of the chosen modality: a head trauma victim who is being hyperventilated to a P_{CO_2} of 20 mm Hg with an intermittent mandatory ventilation rate of 20 breaths per minute is undergoing controlled ventilation.

Assist-control ventilation is more patient dependent in that, at respiratory rates greater than the **operator-determined** minimum, the patient triggers each breath with an inspiratory effort. Every breath is delivered with the operator-determined tidal volume. Weaning from assist-control ventilation is generally done with increasingly long periods without mechanical support, until the patient is independent of the machine.

Intermittent mandatory ventilation permits some spontaneous breaths of **patient-determined** volume. A preset minimum of a given number of breaths of predetermined tidal volume are chosen by the operator. Additional minute ventilation is patient dependent. Weaning is done by slowly reducing the number of preset mechanical breaths, thereby increasing the percentage of minute ventilation for which the patient is responsible.

Pressure support ventilation differs in being a pressure-cycled as opposed to a volume-cycled mode. Each inspiratory effort by the patient triggers the application of a preset pressure to the ventilator circuit. Depending on the compliance of the patient's thorax (lungs and chest wall), this pressure will result in the delivery of a greater or lesser tidal volume. The preset pressure is applied until the patient initiates exhalation. Patients are weaned by reducing the amount of pressure applied with each breath. Some patients find this more comfortable because of the ability to control the duration of inspiration and exhalation.

Weaning is the route from total ventilatory support to extubation. At the time that extubation is considered, "weaning parameters" become an issue. A variety of criteria have been proposed to support extubation, and they are often used in conjunction with a weaning "trial." A spontaneous minute ventilation of less than 10 liters per minute (that can be doubled voluntarily), a forced vital capacity greater than 15 cc/kg, and a negative inspiratory force greater than 20 cm H_2O are all useful criteria supporting extubation. Tests of adequate gas exchange include an A–a gradient less than 300 mm Hg, shunt of less than 10–20%, and a dead space/tidal volume ratio of less than 55–60%.

Pulmonary Function Tests

One of the most commonly used tests of pulmonary function is the **forced expiratory volume (FEV)**, which is most often expressed as the FEV_1, or the volume exhaled in the first second. FEV_1 can be used in conjunction with the **forced vital capacity (FVC)** to classify patients as having normal, obstructive, or restrictive patterns. Normal FVC in an adult is about 5–7 liters, and normal FEV_1 is 80% of that. In restrictive disease, the FEV_1 and the FVC are both reduced, but the ratio may be normal to slightly elevated. In obstructive disease, both the FEV_1 and the FVC are reduced, and the ratio is severely reduced to 30% or 40%. Another measure of expiratory flow is the $FEF_{25-75\%}$, which is the average flow rate measured over the middle portion of expiration. Flow volume curves are used to differentiate restrictive from obstructive disease in a visual display and can also be helpful in differentiating intrathoracic from extrathoracic obstruction.

Determination of lung volumes such as **total lung capacity (TLC)**, **functional residual capacity (FRC)**, and the **residual volume (RV)** all require the use of helium dilution or body plethysmography. The TLC is self-explanatory, while the FRC is the volume of gas remaining in the lung after normal expiration, and the RV is the gas remaining after maximal expiration. **Inspiratory reserve volume (IRV)** and **expiratory reserve volume (ERV)** are other frequently cited lung volumes (Figure 13-8).

The FRC is a major reservoir, second only to hemoglobin, for oxygen in the human body, and causes of decreased FRC will result in decreased oxygenation, particularly with increased demand or decreased supply. In order to understand this, one must understand the concept of the **closing capacity (CC)**, which is the lung volume at which airways begin to close, resulting in inadequate ventilation of distal alveoli.

Many factors may alter the relationship between the FRC and the CC, so that if the FRC falls below the CC, some airways close (causing microscopic atelectasis), and hypoxia develops. The FRC falls with obesity, upper abdominal surgery, ARDS, pulmonary edema, pregnancy, the supine position (as opposed to the erect position), and general anesthesia. FRC increases with obstructive lung disease and can be increased by the application of PEEP. The closing capacity increases with advancing age, smoking, chronic bronchitis, and pulmonary edema, and probably reflects the elasticity of the lungs. One obvious clinical correlate of the above relationships is that postoperative patients nursed in the supine position after upper abdominal surgery will be at great risk for the development of atelectasis, owing to a fall in their FRC below the closing capacity.

Other measurements which are used to assess pulmonary function include the **diffusing capacity**, the **maximum breathing capacity**, and **lung compliance**. The diffusing capacity is measured using carbon monoxide. Its utility is controversial, but it is used to follow diseases with thickened blood-gas interfaces, such as diffuse interstitial fibrosis, sarcoidosis, and asbestosis. The maximum breathing capacity is measured by having the patient breath as much air as possible in a 15-second period. It is relatively nonspecific but sensitive as a measure of gross inspiratory and expiratory reserve. **Pulmonary compliance** is defined as the volume change per unit of pressure change across the lung. This can be divided into lung compliance (reflecting the distensibility of the lung) and chest wall compliance. This is measured using a body plethysmography. Lung compliance decreases with pulmonary edema, ARDS,

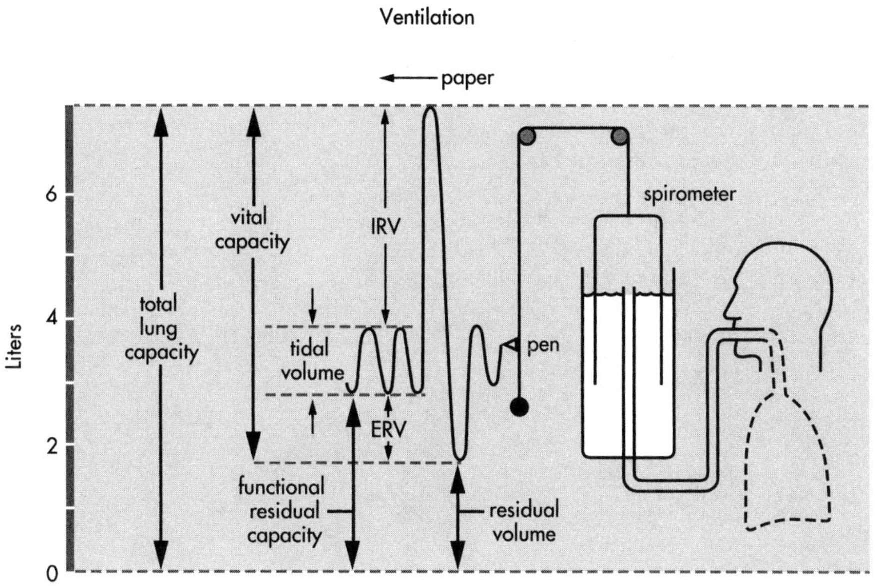

Ventilation

← paper

Figure 13-8 Lung volumes. Note that the functional residual capacity and residual volume cannot be measured with a spirometer. IRV, inspiratory reserve volume. ERV, expiratory reserve volume. (Reproduced from West JB. *Respiratory physiology—the essentials.* 3rd ed. Baltimore: Williams & Wilkins, 1985:13.)

pulmonary fibrosis, pulmonic consolidation, and pleural disease; and chest wall compliance falls with pathological conditions of the chest wall. Compliance will increase with emphysema, where loss of elastin reduces recoil, or in conditions leading to "flail" chest, such as multiple rib fractures or an unstable sternum.

Pulmonary function tests (PFTs) are performed preoperatively for two reasons: Patients at high risk for perioperative pulmonary complications, who are having nonpulmonary procedures, may have pulmonary function testing preoperatively to help formulate a plan for postoperative management. Patients who are scheduled for lung resection are at special risk, and are often evaluated with standard and specialized pulmonary function tests to evaluate the feasibility of tolerating the anticipated resection of lung tissue. Pulmonary function tests are frequently performed on patients with lung cancer complicated by chronic obstructive pulmonary disease (COPD). COPD increases the risk associated with lung resection. Tests that may be useful for assessing risk include spirometry with arterial blood gas analysis, split perfusion lung scanning, regional ventilation testing, exercise testing with measurement of maximal oxygen uptake, and right heart catheterization with measurement of pulmonary artery pressures.

Regional perfusion testing is done with Xe^{133} and the peak radioactivity of each lung is proportional to the degree of perfusion of each lung. With regional ventilation testing, the peak of radioactivity over each lung is proportional to the degree of ventilation. Balloon occlusion of a bronchus is infrequently performed but simulates the postoperative condition, permitting simulation of postoperative arterial blood gas or spirometry. Postoperative right heart function may be impaired in patients with COPD and can be tested with selective pulmonary artery occlusion of the lung segment to be resected. A significant rise in the mean pulmonary artery pressure indicates that the patient will be likely to develop respiratory or right heart failure postoperatively.

The following criteria are indicative of high risk for lung resection: an FVC less than 50% of predicted, an FEV_1 less than 50% of FVC, an FVC less than 2 liters, maximal voluntary ventilation less than 50% of predicted, a ratio of RV to TLC greater than 50%, or a diffusing capacity less than 50% of predicted. Findings consistent with operability are a mean pulmonary artery pressure on balloon occlusion and exercise less than 35 mm Hg, a systemic PaO_2 value on balloon occlusion and exercise greater than 45 mm Hg, or a predicted postpneumonectomy FEV_1 value greater than 0.8 liters.

Preoperative testing should be obtained on optimal medical therapy, and the testing strategy should be graduated, where more complicated or expensive tests are performed only if indicated by the patient's failure to pass easier tests.

A pragmatic approach and one taken by many physicians is to obtain an arterial blood gas analysis and routine pulmonary function tests on patients scheduled for lung resection and base further workup and extent of resection on the results of these tests.

Bibliography

American College of Physicians. Preoperative pulmonary function testing. *Ann Intern Med* 1990;112:793–794.

Nunn JF. *Applied respiratory physiology.* 3rd ed. London: Butterworths, 1987.

West JB. *Pulmonary pathophysiology—the essentials,* 3rd ed. Baltimore: Williams & Wilkins, 1985.

West JB. *Respiratory physiology—the essentials.* 3rd ed. Baltimore: Williams & Wilkins, 1985.

Zibrak JD, O'Donnell CR, Marton K. Indications for pulmonary function testing. *Ann Intern Med* 1990;112: 763–771.

14 ANESTHESIA

C. William Hanson III

The components of operative anesthesia include some combination of amnesia, analgesia, sedation, anxiolysis, paralysis, and unconsciousness. The maintenance of a quiet surgical field and cardiovascular stability are of foremost importance. These ends may be served in a given patient with local anesthesia, regional anesthesia, or general anesthesia. While a specific anesthetic approach will be indicated in some cases, patient or surgeon preference can be accommodated in many routine anesthetics.

The stages of anesthesia as described by one of the pioneers in the discipline, Guedel, were used in the era of ether and chloroform anesthesia. Clinical signs included pupillary size and position; respiratory rate, pattern, and depth; and airway reflexes. Stage 1 is the state of normal consciousness, with normal muscle tone and movements, normal pharyngeal reflexes, and pupillary signs. Stage 2 is the stage of excitement or disinhibition, when breathing becomes irregular, muscle tone is increased, and airway reflexes become hyperactive. It is the period in which the patient is most vulnerable to laryngospasm and vomiting. Stage 3 is the plane of surgical anesthesia, with regular, shallow respiration, blunted airway reflexes, and no response to surgical stimuli. The fourth stage is the stage of anesthetic overdose, and if unrecognized, is shortly followed by cardiovascular collapse and death.

Many of the clinical manifestations of the four stages described by Guedel's system are not seen with either inhalational or intravenous agents used today: Stage 2 is intentionally bypassed with high doses of intravenous induction agents such as thiopental, narcotics blunt airway reflexes and modify pupillary signs, and paralytic agents eliminate movement as reliable signs of inadequate surgical anesthesia.

Monitoring

Certain tools have become standard intraoperative monitors for virtually all anesthetics in most modern operating rooms. They include a noninvasive blood pressure monitor, the electrocardiogram (ECG), either a precordial or esophageal stethoscope, a patient temperature monitor, and, in many operating rooms, a pulse oximeter. The pulse oximeter, a noninvasive measure of arterial oxygen saturation, permits early diagnosis of hypoxia: the oxygen saturation drops below 95% at a PO_2 below 60 (see Figure 4-3).

Patients undergoing general anesthesia may breathe spontaneously or, if paralyzed, be placed on a ventilator. There are a variety of ventilator monitors and alarms built into most modern anesthesia machines. Respiratory rate and tidal volume monitors are universal. Pressure monitoring allows the detection of low circuit pressure (in the event of a disconnection from the ventilator) and high circuit pressure (kinking, mainstem bronchus intubation, etc.).

Some operating rooms may employ end-tidal capnometry or mass spectrometry as routine monitors during general anesthesia. Capnometry measures the level of CO_2 in the circuit, and is fundamentally useful as an indicator of endotracheal, as opposed to esophageal, intubation. With normal lungs, where end-tidal CO_2 is typically less than 5 torr below arterial CO_2, capnometry also serves as a reliable noninvasive measure of systemic P_{CO_2}. End-tidal capnometry and the interpretation of the waveform of exhaled CO_2 can give a great deal of information about the patient's cardiopulmonary interface: i.e., bronchospasm can be diagnosed from a delayed upstroke in the end-tidal capnogram

Mass spectrometry is used to measure the end-tidal concentration of oxygen, nitrogen, carbon dioxide, nitrous oxide, halothane, isoflurane, and enflurane, permitting real-time correlation between exhaled concentration of gases and anesthetic level.

An intra-arterial catheter may be chosen for frequent blood gas monitoring or "beat to beat" blood pressure monitoring where a narrow blood pressure range must be maintained (Table 14-1).

A central venous line may be used to monitor intravascular volume where left ventricular filling conditions can be presumed to correlate with central venous pressures (CVP); it may also be used to infuse vasoactive medications and aspirate air from or infuse volume into the central circulation (see Table 14-1).

The pulmonary arterial catheter (PAC) is preferred to the central venous line when there are any abnormalities of the tricuspid valve, right ventricle, pulmonary vasculature, mitral valve, or pericardium, i.e., conditions under which the pulmonary capillary occlusion or wedge pressure (PCWP) is a more reliable measure of the left ventricular end-diastolic volume (LVEDV) than the CVP (see Table 14-1). It is also felt by some to be a reliable early indicator of left ventricular ischemia. This presupposes that ischemia (and only ischemia) causes increases in PCWP owing to decreases in LV compliance. The use of the PCWP as an indicator of left ventricular preload (left ventricular end diastolic *volume),* relies on the assumption that there is a predictable proportional relationship among pulmonary artery diastolic, PCWP, left ventricular end-diastolic pressures, and LVEDV.

New technology has led to the development of continuous "on-line" arterial blood gas analysis and mixed venous oximetry with specially modified arterial and pulmonary arterial catheters. Some institutitions use continuous arterial blood gas analysis on cardiopulmonary bypass; others routinely monitor cardiac patients with mixed venous oximetry catheters.

The urinary catheter permits indirect evaluation of renal and splanchnic blood flow in patients with normal kidneys. Urine output of greater than 0.5 cc/kg/h is consistent with adequate renal blood flow in an adult. A catheter is typically used in any lengthy case or where impaired renal blood flow is of importance (i.e., abdominal aortic aneurysmectomy).

A twitch monitor is applied to the skin overlying a peripheral nerve to assess objectively the level of neuromuscular blockade when neuromuscular blocking agents are used. A train of four electrical stimuli (40–50 mA) is applied over 2 seconds (2 Hz), typically to the ulnar nerve where the adductor pollicis muscle (thumb apposition) is monitored for effect. With depolarizing drugs (succinylcholine), there is equal attenuation of all four twitch responses. When nondepolarizing drugs (pancuronium, vecuronium) are used, the train demonstrates "fade," with the last twitch smaller than the first. This is analogous to the "fatigue" seen on similar testing with myasthenic patients.

There are a number of more advanced monitors that are used with procedures that might affect the integrity of the central nervous system. Electroencephalographic (EEG) monitoring is used for carotid endarterectomy and by some centers for coronary artery or cardiac valvular surgery. Brainstem auditory evoked responses (BAERs) and visual evoked responses (VERs) are used to ensure the integrity of the affected neural pathways during neurosurgical procedures. Somatosensory evoked potentials (SSERs) are monitored with procedures on the spine or vascular supply to the spinal cord (i.e., thoracic aneurysmectomy). Monitoring may be done by the anesthesiologist or, more typically, by a dedicated technician.

There are also a number of new noninvasive and invasive monitors of cardiac performance. One device that has gained a great deal of recent attention is the trans-esophageal echocardiogram (TEE). Advocates of this technology espouse its real-time evaluation of left ventricular wall-motion and end-diastolic volume. It is used to detect air embolism, aortic dissection, valve malfunction, and myocardial ischemia as manifested by regional wall-motion abnormalities. It is currently employed primarily in the cardiac surgical suites, while weaning the patient from cardiopulmonary bypass.

Anesthetic Techniques

The spectrum of anesthetic techniques extends from infiltration with local anesthetic to the suspended ani-

TABLE 14-1. Intravascular Monitoring

Indications for Placement	Risks of Procedure
Arterial Line	
Cardiac surgery	Infection
Major vascular surgery	Thrombosis
Pulmonary resections	
Intracranial operations	
Major trauma procedures	
Major organ transplant (liver)	
Deliberate hypotension	
Deliberate hypothermia	
Patients having major surgery with:	
• significant pulmonary disease	
• significant cardiovascular disease	
• obesity	
Central Venous Lines	
Cardiac surgery	Bleeding
Surgery with large volume shifts	Infection
Potentially hypovolemic patients (i.e., bowel obstruction)	Carotid puncture
Shock	Pneumothorax
Massive trauma	Nerve damage
	Thoracic duct trauma (on left)
	Venous thrombosis
	Air embolization
	Venous or cardiac perforation
Pulmonary Artery Catheter	
General Surgery	
Major surgery in patients with heart disease	Those of central venous cannulation
Patients with significant coronary artery disease	*plus*
Septic surgical patients	Arrhythmias
Massive trauma	Pulmonary arterial rupture
Shock	Pulmonary infarction
Planned aortic clamping	Knotting
Severe pre-existing respiratory failure	Endocardial or valvular damage
Pre-existent pulmonary emboli	
Cirrhosis	
Liver transplant	
Cardiac Surgery	
Poor left ventricular function	
Recent infarction	
Valve replacement (on left side)	
Pulmonary hypertension	

mation of deep hypothermia, from hypnosis to barbiturate coma. Much of today's anesthesia involves "balanced" technique, which implies the use of relatively small doses of multiple drugs directed at the specific components of anesthesia. Epidural anesthesia might be used in combination with light general anesthesia, for example, when profound abdominal relaxation and anesthesia is required in a cardiomyopathy patient who would not tolerate deep, general systemic anesthesia. This stands in contrast to older, "pure" techniques, where high concentrations of fewer agents, i.e., ether and oxygen, were used to provide unconsciousness, analgesia and relaxation simultaneously. In balanced anesthesia, each drug and route of administration is selected for its profile of action and toxicity.

LOCAL ANESTHETICS

These agents are weakly basic molecules with a lipophilic end connected to a hydrophilic end by either an amide or ester link. They function by blocking the propagation of afferent and efferent nervous impulses— providing sensory anesthesia and motor paralysis, respectively. Local anesthetics inhibit the function of the sodium channel in the neural membrane and there-

by block the initiation and conduction of action potentials. The exact mechanism by which sodium channel function is blocked has not been elucidated.

All local anesthetics are characterized by their intermediate linkage structure as aminoesters or aminoamides (Figure 14-1). Certain generalizations can be made about these two groups based on the nature of the linkage. The ester linkage is metabolized by plasma cholinesterase, while local anesthetics with an amide linkage are metabolized hepatically. In general, the ester agents are shorter-acting than the amides, tend to be less toxic on a milligram per milligram basis, but have a higher incidence of "true" allergic reactions, based on a cross-sensitivity to para-aminobenzoic acid (PABA).

Local anesthetics are used topically, subcutaneously, and in a wide variety of perineural locations for major nerve block. The route and rate of administration,

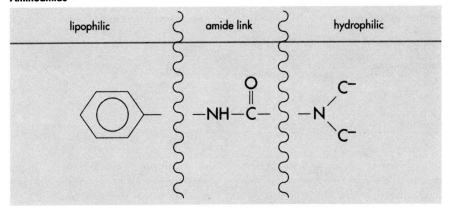

Figure 14-1. The two types of intermediate links of local anesthetics.

chemical nature of the drug, use of vasoconstrictors, total dose, and drug concentration will all have effects on the duration of action and safety of a given drug and block (Table 14-2).

Lidocaine

This is perhaps the most commonly used local anesthetic, having a wide margin of safety, a moderate duration of action, and intrinsic sedative and antiarrhythmic effects when given intravenously. It is an amide, diffuses well, and is used in a variety of concentrations for virtually all blocks.

Bupivacaine

Used slightly less often than lidocaine, this agent results in good sensory and motor blockade, generally lasting longer than lidocaine. It is more toxic than lidocaine owing to its ability to bind avidly and durably to cardiac sodium channels, resulting in conduction abnormalities, arrhythmias, and myocardial depression. It is an amide, diffuses poorly, and is used primarily for major nerve blocks.

Mepivacaine

This drug has a similar margin of safety, dose range, and slightly longer duration of action than lidocaine. It is an amide, diffuses well, and is used primarily for major nerve blocks.

Etidocaine

Etidocaine has a duration of action comparable to that of bupivacaine and is known for its ability to provide motor block out of proportion to its sensory block. It is an amide and is used relatively infrequently, primarily for epidural blocks.

Procaine

A very short acting ester, this drug has a very wide margin of safety, is rapidly metabolized by serum pseudocholinesterase, and is used primarily for local infiltration.

Cocaine

Because of its abuse potential, this drug has fallen into disfavor, although it is the prototypical local anesthetic. It has potent vasoconstrictive properties and spreads well. Its licit use is largely confined to topical mucosal application. It is a short-acting ester, with potent cerebral excitatory effects.

Tetracaine

This is the longest-acting ester and has a duration of action comparable to that of the amides. It is used topically and in spinal anesthesia, where its narrow hemodynamic margin of safety is of less consequence.

Toxicity

Other agents, such as chloroprocaine, prilocaine, benzocaine, cyclonine, dibucaine, etc., all have specific applications but tend to be used infrequently.

A major concern about the use of local anesthetics is their cardiovascular and central nervous system toxicity. Toxicity is mediated by changes in sodium conductance in the affected organs. Toxicity is frequently said to occur at a given dose for a given weight; yet, the fallacies of this statement are several: (1) Toxicity is primarily related to the blood level seen in an affected organ, so that only 10 mg of lidocaine in a cerebral artery may be toxic. (2) Systemic blood levels vary as a function of the rate of absorption from a site: drugs given for intercostal nerve block are absorbed much more rapidly than drugs given subcutaneously, and therefore while the two blocks may result in the same ultimate blood level for the same dose, the intercostal

---

TABLE 14-2. Local Anesthesics

Local Anesthetic	Duration	Use[a]
Aminoester		
Procaine	Short	l,m,s
Cocaine	Short	t
Tetracaine	Intermediate	t,s
Chloroprocaine	Short	l,m,e
Aminoamide		
Lidocaine	Intermediate	t,l,m,e,s
Bupivacaine	Long	l,m,e,s
Mepivacaine	Intermediate	l,m,e
Etidocaine	Long	l,m,e

[a]t, Topical; l, local; m, major nerve block; e, epidural; s, spinal.

nerve block will result in a higher peak concentration. (3) A patient in congestive heart failure weighing 80 kg will have a very different volume of distribution for lidocaine than a lean, 80-kg athlete, and therefore quite different blood levels for the same dose of drug.

Given these caveats, some generalizations can be made about cardiovascular and central nervous system (CNS) toxicity. Toxicity is dose related, with higher doses predictably causing more symptoms. Central nervous system symptoms tend to precede cardiovascular symptoms: five to ten times the convulsive dose of any local anesthetic is required to cause cardiovascular collapse. Measures to limit the total dose or the rate of uptake will tend to lessen toxicity; i.e., using lower concentrations and adding a vasoconstrictor are beneficial. The use of benzodiazepines, barbiturates, or inhalational anesthetics decrease CNS toxicity by raising the seizure threshold.

INHALATIONAL AGENTS

General endotracheal anesthesia generally implies some combination of oxygen with or without nitrous oxide and a volatile anesthetic, i.e., halothane, isoflurane, or enflurane. Ether, chloroform, and cyclopropane are of largely historical interest, while at least two new inhaled anesthetics are in clinical trials: sevoflurane and desflurane. It is not commonly recognized that under appropriate conditions (such as hyperbaric pressures), a wide variety of gases, including inert gases, can act as anesthetics. Nitrogen narcosis or "rapture of the deep" demonstrates nitrogen's ability to act as an anesthetic at high pressures.

The mechanism of action of anesthetic gases is not fully understood. There are a number of different theories, including depression of CNS synaptic transmission, derangement of normal CNS cell membrane architecture or function, and anesthetic–membrane protein interactions. Researchers have observed that anesthetic potency of gases corresponds to their lipid solubility (the Meyer-Overton rule), that high pressure (100–200 atm) reverses the anesthetic effects of some agents, possibly through the compression of expanded cell membranes, and that anesthetics cause increased fluidity of membranes.

The primary effector site of anesthetic gases is the CNS. The conduit for delivery of the gas to the CNS is the lung; and the standard measure of potency for inhaled anesthetics is arbitrarily defined as the minimum alveolar concentration (MAC) of a given gas at 1 atm that produces immobility in 50% of subjects exposed to a noxious stimulus. A number of extensions have been made to the concept of MAC, including MAC/AWAKE (the point at which response to verbal commands reappears), MAC/BAR (the concentration at which there is no sympathetic nervous system response to a noxious stimulus), and MIR (a comparable measure for intravenous anesthetics).

MAC has been criticized as a yardstick but remains useful as a means of comparing anesthetic effects between drugs, within a species and among species. For example, MAC is quite consistent across species; in other words, the ratio between the MAC of drug A compared to the MAC of drug B will remain the same across species. Similarly, within one species, a given dose of narcotic tends to reduce MAC by the same percentage regardless of the anesthetic gas studied.

MAC is expressed in terms of percentage of *1 atm,* so that the MAC of nitrous oxide, which is 105%, is unachievable at sea level but becomes reachable at more than 1 atm.

While MAC is measured at equilibrium between inspired and alveolar concentrations, the brain is the site of action of the agent, and it is only when the alveolus and the brain are at the same partial pressure that the term becomes of value. It is the factors governing the uptake of the agent from the alveolus and the distribution to the brain that determine the speed of onset of anesthesia.

A key to understanding the rate of uptake of a gas is an understanding of the distinction between **concentration** and **partial pressure** of a gas in solution, i.e., the concept of solubility. At equilibrium between the alveolus and the brain, the partial pressures of a gas will be the same in both locations. The concentration of gas A in the blood will be lower than that of gas B at the same partial pressure if gas A is less soluble in blood than gas B. Since it is the partial pressure not the concentration of a gas that determines MAC, less soluble gases are quicker in onset, attaining effective partial pressures at lower concentrations. Similarly, for a given gas, equilibration will take longer between alveolus and blood in states of higher cardiac output: the higher blood volume per unit time exposed to the alveolus results in greater uptake of agent and, therefore, lower alveolar partial pressure relative to inspired partial pressure.

With these concepts in mind, anesthetic uptake on induction can be understood as a cascade from the highest partial pressure in the inspired gas to the lowest

TABLE 14-3. Inhalational Anesthetics

Agent	MAC (%)	Adverse Effects
Nitrous oxide	105.0	Low solubility Rapid onset and offset
Halothane	0.8	Cardiac arrythmias Hepatitis Myocardial depression
Enflurane	1.7	May cause seizures at high doses Myocardial depression
Isoflurane	1.2	Coronary artery steal Myocardial depression (least) Tachycardia

in the CNS. Factors that will increase the speed of induction are high inspired partial pressure (called over-pressure), increased alveolar ventilation (which will quickly refresh the alveolar reservoir), decreased anesthetic solubility (with more rapid equilibration of partial pressures), decreased peripheral tissue uptake (with higher mixed venous partial pressures), and decreased cardiac output (which will also hasten equilibration).

During the maintenance phase of anesthesia, the inspired, alveolar, mixed venous, and brain partial pressures will have equilibrated. The speed of recovery from anesthesia will depend on many of these same factors in reverse, with the additional factor of the amount of anesthetic sequestered in the patient, which is a function of the duration of anesthesia and the tissue solubility of the anesthetic (more time and higher tissue solubility will result in longer time to arousal).

The ideal anesthetic gas would be very insoluble, nonpungent, and potent with minimal cardiovascular effects. The older gases (ether, chloroform) tended to be very soluble, while the disadvantages of current agents are their toxicities and depressant cardiovascular effects (Table 14-3).

Nitrous Oxide

This nonpungent gas is the least soluble of the agents currently in use; but it is not very potent, with a MAC of 105%. Its lack of potency results in its use as an adjuvant gas at relatively high partial pressures. A major

drawback is its ability to expand internal gas spaces. When used at 66%, it will equilibrate rapidly with and expand gas in closed spaces (inner ear, intestines, pneumothoraces) threefold.

Halothane

This is the oldest of the halogenated hydrocarbon gases. It is both more potent (MAC = 0.8%) and more soluble than nitrous oxide. Like all of the halogenated agents, it causes myocardial depression. It is also known to cause a variety of cardiac arrhythmias (atrial and ventricular), particularly in the presence of increased epinephrine levels. Its use has been limited in recent years because of concerns about halothane hepatitis, which is probably immune mediated, potentially fatal, and found more often in overweight females having upper abdominal procedures. Because "halothane hepatitis" is rarely seen in children, and halothane has a pleasant odor, its recent use in the United States has been primarily in anesthetizing children.

Enflurane

Less soluble than halothane, and less pungent than isoflurane, enflurane's use is limited primarily because it is somewhat more soluble than isoflurane. There are some concerns about its fluoride metabolite and the development of renal fluoride toxicity. It too is a myocardial depressant. Its MAC is 1.7%.

Isoflurane

The newest of the halogenated "potent agents," isoflurane is less of a myocardial depressant than its cousins, may cause a tachycardia, and may cause a coronary "steal" syndrome. It is quite pungent and poorly suited to mask induction of anesthesia. As a result of its low solubility relative to halothane and enflurane, it is quickest in onset and offset. Its MAC is 1.2%.

INTRAVENOUS ANESTHESIA

New drugs have become available in the last several years that make the concept of total intravenous anesthesia a realistic possibility. A variety of agents are used in intravenous anesthesia, including sedative-hypnotics, narcotics, and paralytics. The traditional use of these agents has been as ancillary components of inhalational anesthesia in a **balanced** technique; they have not been used for total intravenous anesthesia because no drug has been sufficiently potent, brief of action, and lacking in side effects when used as an infusion that it would serve that purpose (Table 14-4).

Barbiturates

These are the traditional agents for the intravenous induction of anesthesia and include thiopental, thiamylal, and methohexital. They are metabolized in the liver and then excreted in the urine. One of the desirable properties of these agents is their relative ease of titration. An intravenous bolus can be given in order to achieve therapeutic levels rapidly. Then, owing to rapid redistribution, the drug effect disappears. Unfortunately, after repeated doses, peripheral storage areas such as fatty tissue become saturated, and recovery from anesthesia slows.

Barbiturates probably act on CNS γ-aminobutyric acid (GABA) receptors. These are the most common inhibitory receptors in the CNS, and when stimulated, down-modulate nerve transmission. Many researchers feel that actions on the GABAergic receptors are common to all intravenous anesthetic agents.

Barbiturates depress the medullary and pontine respiratory centers and may cause profound respiratory depression when administered as a bolus. They also act as cardiovascular depressants and cause peripheral vasodilation and myocardial depression when given in excessive doses. Patients whose peripheral resistance or cardiac performance is already impaired are at greater risk. A beneficial effect of barbiturates is the reduction they induce in cerebral metabolism and oxygen consumption. They provide cerebral protection when administered to selected patients prior to cardiopulmonary bypass.

Benzodiazepines

These agents have been primarily used as anxiolytics in this country; but as with barbiturates, they are felt to have effects on GABAergic receptors and have been used as induction drugs. Diazepam is an oil-soluble, hepatically metabolized drug that has been rarely used since the advent of midazolam, a water-soluble benzodiazepine that is hepatically metabolized and has a short elimination half-life. In Europe, midazolam has been used more extensively as an induction agent because of its minimal cardiovascular effects in most patients.

Midazolam has also been used extensively as a seda-

TABLE 14-4. Intravenous Agents

Drug	Induction Dose[a]	Duration[b]	Unique Properties
Barbiturates			
Methohexital	1.0–1.5 mg/kg	Minutes	↓ ICP, ↑ HR
Thiopental	3.0–5.0 mg/kg	Minutes	↓ ICP
Benzodiazepines			
Diazepam	0.3–0.6 mg/kg	Hours	Slow onset
Midazolam	0.2–0.4 mg/kg	30–90 min	Profound amnestic
Narcotics			
Fentanyl	5.0–100 mg/kg	6–24 h	Stable BP, CO
Sufentanil	1.0–20 mg/kg	6–24 h	Stable BP, CO
Alfentanil	50–100 μg/kg	30–90 min	Stable BP, CO
Miscellaneous			
Etomidate	0.3 mg/kg	Minutes	↓ ICP, ↓ ACTH
Propofol	1.5–2.5 mg/kg	Minutes	↑ HR, ↓ SVR
Ketamine	1.0–2.0 mg/kg	15–60 min	Bronchodilator; ↑ HR, ↑ SVR

[a]To induce anesthesia as a sole agent in a healthy adult.
[b]Will vary considerably from patient to patient. Range represents usual clinically important duration of action.
BP, Blood pressure; HR, heart rate; ICP, intracranial pressures; SVR, systemic vascular resistance.

tive-hypnotic, with profound amnestic properties. It is used alone and in combination with narcotics for short procedures. It should be noted that when administered as an adjuvant, midazolam may have potent respiratory and cardiovascular depressive effects.

Narcotics

The first narcotic anesthetic was given to a dog by Percival Christopher Wren and Robert Boyle in the 17th century. The drug was tincture of opium. We now have an array of synthetic narcotics and have characterized several CNS opioid receptors. We know of endogenous opioids—enkephalins and endorphins—and have designed agonists, partial agonists, and antagonists.

Opioids are not sedative-hypnotics and do not seem to work by the GABAergic system. Their interaction with the opioid receptors of the brain and spinal cord mediate effects on perception of pain, mood, respiration, circulation, and the bowel and the urinary tract. They are hepatically metabolized. Variations in speed of onset and offset are due to differing lipid solubility (more lipid soluble, faster onset) and degrees of redistribution.

All of the narcotics are used as components of a variety of techniques: anesthesia with sedation; balanced inhalational and intravenous anesthesia; for postoperative pain management (e.g., with epidural narcotics); and as a part of narcotic-oxygen anesthesia for cardiac surgery. They are unable to provide total intravenous anesthesia both because of the respiratory depression induced and the potential for intraoperative awareness that exists even with profound doses.

The most commonly used narcotics are morphine and fentanyl. The latter is a synthetic agent with a short half-life, high potency, and minimal cardiovascular effects when administered alone.

Other Intravenous Anesthetics

There are a variety of other agents available or soon to be available as intravenous anesthetics. They include ketamine, which is used for dissociative anesthesia; etomidate, which acts on the GABA system; and propofol. The latter agent has just been released in this country after extensive testing in Europe. It may be the first agent suitable for total intravenous anesthesia. It is supplied in a suspension of lecithin, it is short-acting, and it leaves patients awake and alert at the conclusion of the anesthetic.

MUSCLE RELAXANTS

There are several ways in which to effect muscle relaxation in current anesthetic practice. The first is to abolish the motor signal at its source, the neuron. This can be done with deep inhalational anesthesia but requires levels of anesthesia that have effects on the cardiovascular system as well. A second method is to ablate the motor signal as it moves from the CNS to the muscle, as in spinal and epidural anesthesia. Pure muscle relaxants (depolarizers and nondepolarizers) act on the neuromuscular junction (Table 14-5).

TABLE 14-5. Neuromuscular Blockers

Agent	Loading Dose (mg/kg)	Duration[a]	Clearance	Autonomic Effects	Histamine Release
Depolarizing					
Succinylcholine	1.5–2.0	Minutes	Enzymatic	+Sympathetic +Vagal	–
Nondepolarizing					
Curare	0.6	90 min	Renal, hepatic	Sympatholytic	+++
Pancuronium	0.1	90 min	Renal	Vagolytic	–
Gallamine	3.5	120 min	Renal	Vagolytic	–
Metocurine	0.4	120 min	Renal	Sympatholytic	++
Vecuronium	0.1	60 min	Renal, hepatic	None	–
Atracurium	0.5	60 min	Enzymatic	None	+

[a]After administration of an intubating/loading dose.

The nerve signal is carried electrically down the axon to the nerve ending where packets of acetylcholine (ACh) are released. The ACh packet crosses the junction and binds to a receptor on the muscle cell at the motor end-plate (a group of receptors). A channel on the ACh-receptor package opens, allowing the passage of Na^+. The entry of Na^+ into the cell causes Ca^+-mediated muscular contraction.

Depolarizing muscle relaxants such as succinylcholine (or the rarely used decamethonium) react with the receptor at the same site as ACh, causing an initial depolarization (and fasciculation of the muscle). Since these drugs dissociate less readily from the receptor, prolonged depolarization results, causing neuromuscular block. Succinylcholine is very rapid in onset and offset. It is metabolized intravenously by plasma pseudocholinesterase. Precautions about its use result from the drug's ability to initiate malignant hyperthermia, cause massive (potentially fatal) K^+ release in denervated muscle or burns, or prolonged paralysis in patients lacking normal pseudocholinesterase.

Nondepolarizing drugs do not act at the ACh-binding site but, rather, at another part of the receptor, competitively inhibiting transmitter binding. Curare is the prototypical nondepolarizing agent. Pancuronium, vecuronium, atracurium, and several new agents all have varying half-lives, and there are new drugs with half-lives approaching that of succinylcholine.

There is a substantial safety margin with neuromuscular transmission, and 80% of receptors must be blocked before any degree of blockade is evident. Blockade is reversed with acetylcholinesterase inhibitors, which substantially raise the intrasynaptic concentration of ACh, putting ACh at a competitive advantage and allowing for displacement of the neuromuscular blocker.

REGIONAL ANESTHETICS

Regional anesthesia implies sensory and/or motor blockade of some region of the body with local anesthetic. The local anesthetic may be applied topically, subcutaneously, perineurally, or centrally. Regional blockade may be used as the sole form of anesthesia or as an adjunct to general anesthesia. The advantages of regional anesthesia include postoperative pain relief; the ability to avoid general anesthetics with myocardial depressant effects; and, in the awake patient, the opportunity to monitor central nervous system function during the operation.

The systemic implications of regional blockade may be significant with the more central nerve blocks. In addition to their sensory and motor effects, local anesthetics effect a chemical sympathectomy in the affected body region. This results in vasodilation and, when the block is proximal to the high thoracic cardiac accelerator nerves, bradycardia. The combination of bradycardia and peripheral pooling of blood can cause profound hypotension. Conversely, vasodilation may be a desirable method of enhancing blood flow during revascularization procedures.

Commonly used major nerve blocks include those of the brachial plexus, the sciatic and femoral nerves, the intercostal nerves, and the ilioinguinal nerve. The central axis blocks are the spinal, epidural, and caudal anesthetics. Spinal anesthesia is generally administered in a single injection into the subarachnoid space and therefore has a duration of action determined by the drug(s) and doses used. Epidural anesthetics are frequently administered through a catheter and can, therefore, be used over an extended period with repeated doses. Epidural opiates can be administered to extend analgesia into the postoperative period. Some studies have shown that epidural analgesia shortens postoperative hospital stays and limits respiratory complications.

Conclusions

Most anesthetics consist of combinations of drugs and techniques, and it is the judicious combination of techniques to minimize toxicity and maximize effect that characterizes well-performed anesthesia.

Bibliography

Barash PG, Cullen BF, Stoelting RK, eds. *Clinical anesthesia.* Philadelphia: Lippincott, 1989.
Dripps RD, Eckenhoff JE, Vandam LD, eds. *Introduction to anesthesia.* Philadelphia: WB Saunders, 1988.

Michael F. Beers

15 NONRESPIRATORY FUNCTIONS OF THE LUNG

The lung, although primarily an organ for gas exchange, also performs several important nonrespiratory tasks, mainly as a consequence of its physiologic interposition between the right and left sides of the circulation, its unique architecture, and the metabolic activities of the assorted cells that of which it is comprised.

The primary goal of this chapter is to review certain nonrespiratory functions of the lung as they relate to basic concepts of cellular physiology and integrative biology. The pertinent structure and cell biology of particular tissue elements of the lung will be reviewed. Details of individual cellular functions will then be integrated into discussions of the various nonrespiratory functions of the lung. Finally, selected problems emphasizing pathophysiology of nonrespiratory functions as related to specific pulmonary diseases will be examined. Discussions of diagnostic tests will appear throughout when they are illustrative of basic cellular function or dysfunction.

Anatomy and Cellular Function: Design and Structure of the Lung

From a functional viewpoint, lung tissue can be organized into four major units, each composed of various cell types arranged to perform specific tasks. These include the conducting airways, parenchyma, pulmonary defense system, and vasculature.

CONDUCTING AIRWAYS

The airways of the lung systematically branch dichotomously over an average of 23 generations, eventually ending in blind sacs. The basic morphology of the trachea, bronchi, and nonalveolated airways is similar (Figure 15-1). The walls of the airways are lined by a mucosal surface composed of a **pseudostratified, ciliated columnar epithelium** mosaically interspersed with **mucous-secreting goblet cells** and orifices leading to submucosal bronchial glands (both serous and mucous exocrine cells). Underlying this are supporting connective tissues (lamina propria) and a smooth muscle sleeve.

Ciliated Airway Epithelium

Like other epithelial surfaces, the airway mucosa serves as a physical barrier, regulates salt and water balance of airway secretions, and secretes specialized substances important to host defense efforts such as **mucus** and **immunoglobulins** (predominantly IgA). In addition,

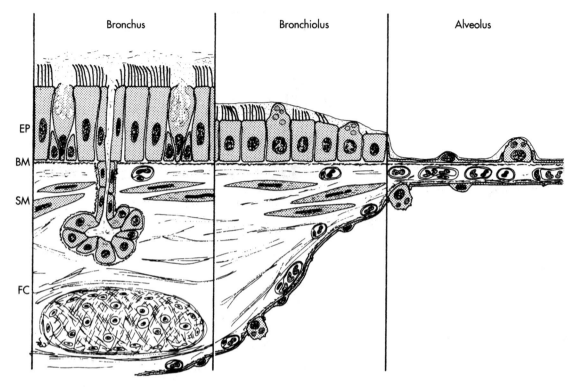

Figure 15-1 Airway wall structure at the three principal levels. The epithelial layer (EP) gradually becomes reduced from pseudostratified to cuboidal and then to squamous, but retains its organization as a mosaic of lining and secretory cells. The smooth muscle layer (SM) disappears in the alveoli. The fibrous coat (FC) contains cartilage only in bronchi and gradually becomes thinner as the alveolus is approached. BM, basement membrane. (Reproduced from Weibel ER, Taylor CR. Design and structure of the human lung. In Fishman AP, ed. *Pulmonary diseases and disorders.* New York: McGraw-Hill, 1988:14.)

each epithelial cell possesses a tuft of **kinocilia** at the apex that beat in a coordinated fashion, resulting in clearance of secreted mucus toward the oropharynx **(mucociliary escalator).** Toward the periphery, the epithelial layer gradually becomes thinner, the cells more cuboidal, and the cilia shorter.

Nonciliated Airway Cells

Interspersed throughout the airway mucosa, these cells are of several types:

Mucous (Goblet) and Serous Cells
These exocrinelike cells are arranged as submucosal gland-like structures in large airways or as single cells in smaller airways. Mucin, the product of the goblet cells, is highly viscous, consisting of acidic glycoproteins, and serves as a trap for inhaled particulates. Serous cells produce **lysozyme,** a small water-soluble peptide with antimicrobial properties.

Clara Cells
Though found in the terminal and respiratory bronchioles, the exact function of Clara cells is as yet unknown.

Endocrine Cells
In addition to ciliated and exocrine varieties, cells of neuroendocrine origin have been described within conducting airways. Called **Feyrter** or **Kulchitsky** cells, they store and metabolize biogenic amines, suggesting that these cells belong to the class of APUD (amine-precursor uptake and decarboxylation) cells.

LUNG PARENCHYMA (THE ALVEOLAR REGION)

At the end of the conducting airways lie the gas exchanging units of the lung, the alveoli. Nearly 75% of all cells of the lung comprise these basic structures of lung parenchyma. Figure 15-2 illustrates basic structural relationships within alveolar units.

In addition to type I epithelial cells that line the alveoli, the alveolar regions also contain: (1) Type II epithelial cells, (2) vascular endothelial cells, (3) interstitial cells, (4) alveolar macrophages, lymphocytes, and mast cells.

Alveolar Lining Cells

Type I Epithelial Cells

Rather simple in appearance and constituting only 8% of total lung cell number, these thin cells possess a large

surface area which lines the alveolar walls and serves to minimize the distance between the alveolar air spaces and the pulmonary capillaries. This structure facilitates gas exchange while maintaining an effective barrier between air and blood. Lacking significant subcellular organelles or mitochondria, these cells are felt to be relatively metabolically inactive.

Type II Epithelial Cells

In contrast, type II cells are small (9 μ), spherical pneumocytes also found lining the alveoli. Composing 60% of all alveolar epithelial cells (but only 4% of the surface area), these cells have five major functions: (1) synthesis

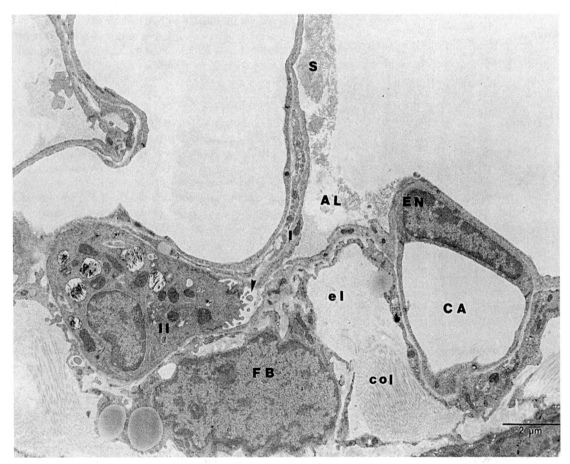

Figure 15-2 Electron micrograph of an alveolar unit. The alveolar space (AL), lined by type I cells (I) and type II cells (II), contains pulmonary surfactant (S) shown here as tubular myelin. Surfactant is actively secreted by a type II cell into a partially collapsed alveolar space (*arrow*). An endothelial cell (EN), adjacent to type I cell, forms a pulmonary capillary (CA). The alveolar interstitium contains collagen (col) and elastin (el) and a fibroblast (FB). (Courtesy of AB Fisher, MD, and Henry Shuman, PhD. Electron Micrograph Core Service at the Institute for Environmental Medicine, University of Pennsylvania School of Medicine, Philadelphia, PA.)

and secretion of pulmonary surfactant, (2) protection/ recovery from oxidant injury, (3) xenobiotic drug metabolism, (4) regulation of transepithelial water movement, and (5) replacement of damaged type I cells.

Interstitium

The interstitium of the lung can be loosely defined as the space between the vascular endothelium, airway epithelium, and pleural mesothelium. Composed both of cellular constituents and extracellular matrix (collagen, elastin, and proteoglycans), the pulmonary interstitium serves as a mechanically supportive structure (in part, responsible for the elastic properties of the lung) and establishes a lymphatic fluid space.

Fibroblasts
Normally quiescent and intercalated throughout the interstitium, these cells are responsible for the production and maintenance of collagen (chiefly type I collagen) and elastin. Abnormal regulation of this process may play a role in the development of pulmonary fibrotic patterns.

Tissue Macrophages
Primarily situated in perivascular and peribronchiolar sheaths and within interlobular septae, these large, irregular cells are functionally similar to the more widely studied alveolar macrophages (discussed below).

Miscellaneous Contractile Cells
Myofibroblasts, pericytes, and smooth muscle cells have been found in the interstitium.

CELLS OF THE PULMONARY DEFENSE SYSTEM

Alveolar Macrophages

These are large (10-15 μ), irregularly shaped phagocytic cells that are transiently attached to the alveolar epithelium by pseudopodia. These cells are derived from blood monocytes, settle in the pulmonary interstitial tissue, and migrate into the alveoli, becoming a partially self-replicating cell population.

Though they possess large numbers of phagosomes and lytic enzymes (e.g., lysozyme), macrophages should not be considered just scavenger phagocytes, for they have significant immunologic effector activity and secretory function as well. Macrophages are important

in the induction of specific T-lymphocyte responses (cell-mediated immunity) and for T-cell-dependent B-lymphocyte response to soluble antigens (humoral immunity). The importance of these interactions is underscored by the frequency, variety, and severity of lung infections in immunocompromised individuals.

Lymphocytes

Within the lung, lymphocytes are present both in the alveolar space as well as in subepithelial tissue layers of both the alveolar interstitium and the airways (as bronchus-associated lymphoid tissue within the lamina propria). Within the alveolar space, all subpopulations of T and B lymphocytes have been found. They are known to interact with alveolar macrophages in processing of airway antigens and thus are important in normal host defense; their dysfunction is implicated in a variety of immunological diseases.

Mast Cells

Measuring 20–30 μ in diameter and distinctly characterized by large numbers of cytoplasmic secretory granules, mast cells have been noted within the interstitium and occasionally the alveolar space. Metabolically, these cells have been shown to contain histamine, heparin, serotonin, slow-reacting substance (SRS, now known to be eicosanoids of the leukotriene family), and several proteolytic enzymes. Mast cells are key in anaphylactic and IgE-mediated responses in the lung.

Polymorphonuclear Leukocytes

Not normally found in the lung parenchyma of healthy individuals (but marginated in alveolar capillaries), these cells are readily recruitable for inflammatory responses. They are drawn to needed sites by chemotactic stimulati from macrophages and other cells.

PULMONARY VASCULATURE

From its origin at the base of the right ventricle, the course of the precapillary pulmonary vasculature roughly parallels that of the bronchial tree, ending in a dense, hexagonal-shaped network enveloping alveolar units with an average internal capillary diameter of 8 μ. Pulmonary veins draining the capillary bed are different in that they generally are separate from the airways.

The regulation of pulmonary blood flow and gas

exchange by pulmonary endothelium is discussed in other chapters. However, the pulmonary endothelium also performs a variety of physical and metabolic functions.

Estimated to be the most common type of cell in the lung (composing 35–40% of all parenchymal cells), the pulmonary vascular endothelial cell is a nonfenestrated variety joined by tight junctions. Although morphologically similar at all levels of the pulmonary vascular tree, endothelium in two regions of the lung should be distinguished: Alveolar capillary endothelium and endothelial cells lining the conducting vessels.

Within alveolar regions, endothelial cells are as thin as 0.1 μ with scanty cytoplasm, but they contain significant numbers of subcellular organelles (e.g., mitochondria, Golgi cells, etc.) concentrated in the perinuclear region. By the nature of their tight junctions, these cells serve as an important barrier for transepithelial water movement (limiting fluid accumulation in the alveolar interstitium) while still serving as an efficient gas-exchanging surface.

Endothelial cells of the pulmonary arteries and veins are thicker, and parts of their cytoplasm are more richly endowed with subcellular organelles. These cells are metabolically more active than their capillary counterparts. The surface contains microvilli that may be important in the tremendous absorptive capacities of the pulmonary vasculature reported for select compounds such as serotonin. These cells contain **angiotensin-converting enzyme (ACE)** and are important in the metabolism of many compounds, including angiotensin I, prostaglandins, serotonin, and other biogenic amines. Because the entire cardiac output traverses the lungs, this metabolic activity often assumes significant importance.

DIAGNOSTIC EVALUATION OF LUNG CELLS: BRONCHOALVEOLAR LAVAGE

The technique of **bronchoalveolar lavage (BAL)** allows direct assessment of many of the cellular constituents of the airways and alveolar spaces and is useful in the evaluation of many pulmonary diseases. With the aid of a fiberoptic bronchoscope, sterile buffered saline is infused through the working channel of a scope wedged in a third- or fourth-generation bronchus of a pulmonary segment in aliquots of 50–300 mL. After removal and pooling of aliquots, the fluid can be analyzed for protein content, differential cell count, and cytological staining.

Table 15.1. Cellular and Soluble Constituents in Bronchoalveolar Lavage Fluid[a]

Cells	
Macrophages	84 ± 1^b
Lymphocytes	11 ± 1^b
T cells	62 ± 2^c
Helper (T4)	46 ± 3^d
Suppressor (T8)	25 ± 2^d
B cells	5 ± 2^c
Neutrophils, eosinophils, basophils	$<1^b$

Soluble Factors	
IgG, IgA	+
IgM	−
C4, C3, factor B	+
C5	−

[a]All values are for normal nonsmokers; data are expressed as mean ± SD.

[b]Expressed as a percentage of total cells.

[c]Expressed as a percentage of lymphocytes; other lymphocyte types (e.g., null, NK) not expressed.

[d]Expressed as a percentage of T cells; other T-cell subtypes not expressed.

Data from Daniele RP, Elias JA, Epstein PE, Rossman MD. Bronchoalveolar lavage: role in pathogenesis, diagnosis, and management of interstitial lung disease. *Ann Intern Med* 1985;102:93–108.

The profile of respiratory cells and protein recovered by BAL in normal subjects appears in Table 15-1. Of note is that in healthy, nonsmoking individuals, macrophages are the predominant cell type. The profile is overwhelmingly reflective of the cellular constituents of the alveolar space (interstitial and vascular cells are not sampled) and it can be altered by a variety of infectious and inflammatory diseases, which will be discussed.

Nonrespiratory Functions of the Lung

PHYSICAL AND RELATED FUNCTIONS

The Lung as a Vascular Filter

The pulmonary capillary network receives the entire cardiac output and is strategically interposed between the systemic venous and arterial circulations. With an internal capillary diameter of 8 μ, it has the capacity to act as a physiological sieve, protecting vital systemic organs from harmful materials. Generally, particles smaller than the pulmonary capillary circulation will be trapped, although experimentally, larger particles up to 400 μ have been reported to traverse the circulation (most likely via direct arteriovenous shunts).

Sieving of Thromboemboli

Organized thrombus from the venous circulation (typically the lower extremities) is regularly trapped in the lungs. Autopsy studies have confirmed the presence of pulmonary thromboembolism in over 50% of all patients; however, most emboli tend to be small and result in no significant damage. The properties of the lung and its microcirculation as a physiological sieve can be utilized in the clinical assessment of the pulmonary circulation. When radiolabeled macroaggregated albumin (particle size = 10–30 μ) is injected intravenously, the circulating particles become trapped in the lung capillary bed in a distribution proportional to regional blood flow. Deposited particle profiles are imaged by gamma-camera detection of emitted energy. Thus, occlusion of a segmental or lobar pulmonary artery will produce a localizable anatomic defect owing to a paucity of labeled particles.

Physiologic Emboli

Other, less common substances trapped by the pulmonary microcirculation include (1) fat from the bone marrow of long bone fractures, (2) bone marrow fragments, (3) placental trophoblast in pregnant or postpartum females, and (4) tumor cells from distant primary tumor sites (which have a propensity to lodge at the periphery of the lower lobes).

Other Particulates

Injectable inert particulates such as talc or other pill fragments used by intravenous drug addicts can be trapped by, accumulate within, and even obliterate the pulmonary capillary bed via stimulation of granulomatous reactions.

Elimination of Volatile Substances

In addition to the normal exchange of respiratory gases (O_2 and CO_2), the lung is capable of excreting any nonrespiratory metabolite in the blood that is volatile at 37°C and permeable to the alveolar capillary membrane.

Expired acetone by diabetics in ketoacidosis and in fasting individuals, methylmercaptan (derived from methionine metabolism) recovered in cases of liver failure ("fetor hepaticus"), and ethanol (used in screening alcohol breathalyzer tests in automobile drivers) are three examples of volatiles that can be detected.

Filtration of Inhaled Particles

Inhaled air can contain a significant amount of particulate matter, which, in the lung, can have one of three fates, depending largely on particle size and/or shape. Very small particles (0.2–0.3 μ) remain suspended in air and are exhaled with the next breath. Large particles (>5 μ) usually impact on the mucoid surface of larger airways and are excreted via the mucociliary escalator. Intermediate particles (0.5–3.0 μ) may penetrate to the gas-exchange surface of the lower respiratory tract where alveolar macrophages phagocytize, then excrete them via the tracheobronchial tree.

Independent of size, gravity, or air flow, uniquely shaped particles such as asbestos fibers or silica may traverse large airways and impact on the epithelia of distal lung regions.

PULMONARY HOST DEFENSE MECHANISMS

Like the gastrointestinal tract, but distinct from other organ systems, the lung is relatively accessible to the outside world and is constantly assaulted by microbes, allergens, particles, and toxins from the ambient environment.

The first line of defense against most pulmonary infections are local defense mechanisms present in the oronasopharynx and large airways (immunoglobulins, mucociliary clearance, and cough). Despite the efficiency of this system in controlling the inspired load, microorganisms and particles from inspired air as well as aspirated secretions from colonized nasopharynges do reach air-exchange surfaces. However, distal airways and alveoli normally remain sterile owing, in large part, to an elaborate array of secondary defenses.

Table 15-2 summarizes mechanisms employed in pulmonary host defense and the impact of potential defects on lung health. Although the important steps are listed individually, there is an extraordinary amount of overlap and interaction between local defense-phagocytic mechanisms and humoral/cell-mediated immunity.

TABLE 15-2 Pulmonary Host Defenses

Host Mechanisms	Function	Described Defects	Impact and Potential Infection
Nasopharynx/Conducting Airways			
Mechanical barriers (larynx, cough)	Anatomic barrier for secretions	Bypassing barriers (tracheosto-my, endotracheal tube)	Aspiration of micro-organisms
Mucociliary clearance	Particle removal Particle entrapment	Abnormal cilia Abnormal mucous	Poor removal of secretions Excessive secretions
Local immunoglobulin secretion (IgA)	Coat mucosa	IgA deficiency	Recurrent sinopulmonary infection
		Breakdown by proteases	Abnormal colonization
Iron-containing proteins (transferrin, ferritin)	Inhibit bacterial growth	Iron deficiency	Increased bacterial colonization
Alveolar Region			
Immunoglobulins (IgG)	Opsonization	IgG$_2$/IgG$_4$ deficiency Acquired hypogamma-globulinemia	Sinopulmonary infections Pneumonia (encapsulated organisms)
Surfactant	Nonimmune opsonins	Decreased synthesis Acute lung injury	Loss of opsonization (macrophage) Alveolar Collapse
Alveolar macrophage	Phagocytosis	Immunosuppression (cell-mediated)	Poor killing of intracellular pathogens
Polymorphonuclear leukocytes	Phagocytosis and bacterial killing	Immunosuppression (absent) Defect in killing function Poor chemotaxis	Increased gram negative and fungal infections
Complement	Enhances opsonization	C$_3$ or C$_5$ deficiency	Increased infection
Immune Response (Augmenting Mechanisms)			
T cell	Cell-mediated immunity Enhance macrophage function	Immunosuppression (iatrogenic or AIDS)	Opportunistic infection
B cell	Humoral immunity	Immunosuppression	Increased infection with encapsulated organisms

METABOLIC FUNCTIONS OF THE LUNG

Surfactant and Phospholipid Metabolism

The lung is a true metabolic organ. It is involved in synthesis, storage, transformation, and degradation of a large variety of substances, many of which are unique to the lung.

Pulmonary **surfactant** is a lipid-protein complex found lining the alveolar surface whose physiological function is to lower surface tension at the air-liquid interface of the alveoli and to maintain the stability of alveolar units (prevent collapse) at low lung volumes. Surfactant is approximately 80% phospholipid, 10% other lipid, and 10% protein. The predominant phospholipid synthesized is **dipalmitoyl phosphatidyl-choline (DPPC)** and accounts for much of the surface activity; three surfactant-specific proteins (surfactant proteins A, B, and C) are essential for full physiologic and biophysical activity.

Figure 15-3 schematically depicts turnover pathways and potential control points for surfactant metabolism. **Alveolar type II cells** play a central role in surfactant metabolism. They synthesize, secrete, recycle, and degrade surfactant components. Alveolar macrophages also internalize phospholipid and may play an adjunctive role in alveolar clearance of surfactant.

The turnover of lung surfactant is rapid, with a half-life of less than 11 hours. In order to maintain normal alveolar levels, both synthesis and removal of surfactant must be regulated. Two diseases are illustrative of abnormal surfactant turnover. In **respiratory distress syndrome**, seen in premature neonates (less than 34 weeks gestation), the immature lung is incapable of manufacturing sufficient surfactant to maintain normal physiological function. **Pulmonary alveolar proteinosis** can

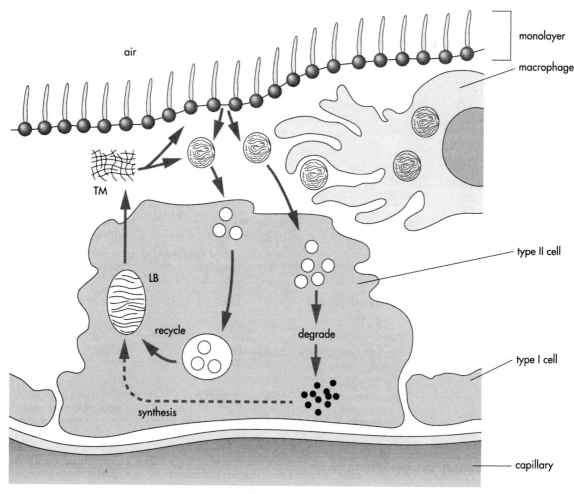

Figure 15-3 A schematic model for alveolar surfactant turnover and metabolism. Components of surfactant are synthesized in the type II cell and stored in lamellar bodies (LB), until they are secreted into the alveolar airspace. The secreted lamellar body contents can unwind to form tubular myelin (TM), which may be the precursor to the monomolecular surface film that is enriched in dipalmitoylphosphatidylcholine. The type II cell appears to play a major roll in surfactant clearance by internalizing lipids that may either be incorporated into lamellar bodies and eventually resecreted (recycled) or degraded, and the products removed from the surfactant pathway or reutilized for synthesis of new surfactant components. Alveolar macrophages probably phagocytose surfactant; the importance of the macrophage in surfactant clearance is unclear. The roles of other lung cells are also not known. (Reproduced from Wright JR, Hawgood S. Pulmonary surfactant metabolism. *Clinics Chest Med* 1989;10(1):87.)

result from abnormal accumulation of surfactant lipids and proteins within the alveolar space resulting from decreased removal of surfactant components.

Beyond surfactant phospholipid synthesis, the lungs also perform other types of lipid metabolic functions, including the de novo synthesis of fatty acids, esterfication of lipids, hydrolysis of lipid-ester bonds, oxidation of fatty acids, and conversion of arachadonic acid to eicosanoids (see Prostaglandin and Leukotriene Metabolism, below).

Serotonin Metabolism

Serotonin, also known as **5-hydroxytryptamine (5-HT)**, is a biogenic amine found chiefly in platlets and in endocrine cells of the gastrointestinal tract. Under normal conditions, 5-HT plasma levels are less than 10 ng/mL. It has been demonstrated in humans that 65% of a dose of 5-HT injected into the right atrium is removed from blood on one passage through the lungs and that the vascular endothelial cell is responsible for this clearance.

The uptake of serotonin by endothelial cells is a sodium- dependent, carrier-mediated, active transport process that requires intracellular energy. Thus, injury to the endothelial cell or any insult that inhibits cellular energy production (e.g., hypoxia) will affect serotonin transport.

Once internalized, 5-HT is rapidly metabolized by cytosolic monoamine oxidase and aldehyde dehydrogenase to yield **5-hydroxyindoleacetic acid (5-HIAA)**, an inactive compound.

Processing of Angiotensin (Angiotensin-Converting Enzyme)

Angiotensin II, a potent vasoconstrictor important in blood pressure regulation, is a peptide produced from the cleavage of its precursor peptide angiotensin I. **Angiotensin I** is secreted by the kidney in response to renin stimulation. The enzyme responsible for this conversion is **angiotensin-converting enzyme (ACE)**, found on pulmonary capillary endothelia. Angiotensin-converting enzyme is present in other tissues, but because of its strategic location and its large endothelial surface area, the lung vasculature plays a major role in angiotensin conversion.

Angiotensin-converting enzyme can be quantitated in blood and has been particularly useful in managing patients with sarcoidosis in whom serum levels often correlate with disease activity. Serum ACE levels are elevated in several other inflammatory diseases, including tuberculosis, leprosy, and diabetes.

Fibrinolysis

Because of its efficiency as a sieve, the lung is quite adept at trapping microthromboemboli. Without an effective mechanism for ridding itself of aggregated and clotted material, the pulmonary vasculature would slowly occlude. Endogenous fibrinolysis by the lung is important in maintaining "hemofluidity."

The details of blood coagulation and fibrinolysis are discussed in Chapter 5. The pulmonary capillary endothelium has been shown to be an important source for plasmin activator (responsible for converting plasminogen to plasmin) and thrombokinase (which converts prothrombin to thrombin). In addition, both mast cells and endothelial cells contain large amounts of heparin, which inhibits clot formation.

Histamine Metabolism

The lung is rich in histamine, predominantly contained in mast cells. Histamine is synthesized by the decarboxylation of the amino acid histidine and stored within cytoplasmic granules of the mast cell. Activation of mast cells results in degranulation and release of histamine. Histamine is inactivated by enzymatic degradation by monamine oxidase or N-methyl transferase.

The pulmonary effects attributed to histamine include bronchoconstriction via an effect on bronchial smooth muscle and mediation of the inflammatory response in anaphylactic shock.

Prostaglandin and Leukotriene (Eicosanoid) Metabolism

Eicosanoids are products derived from the complex metabolism of arachidonic acid. The principal classes of pulmonary arachidonic acid metabolites are cyclo-oxygenase-derived compounds (prostaglandins) and lipo-oxygenase-derived compounds (leukotrienes). An additional fatty acid metabolite, platelet-activating factor (PAF), is produced during cleavage of arachidonic acid from membrane lipids.

Like other tissues, the lung maintains a distinct profile of eicosanoid metabolism. As Table 15-3 demonstrates, different lung cells make different eicosanoid products. These compounds are often rapidly metabo-

TABLE 15-3. Role of Eicosanoids in Mediating Cellular and Physiological Responses in the Lung

Source	Eicosanoid(s)	Mediated Response	Role
Airway Cells	PGE_2	Alters bronchial smooth muscle tone	Asthma
	PGI_2	Alters bronchial smooth muscle tone	Asthma
		Produced during hyperinflation	V-Q matching
	PGD_2	Increases airway resistance	Asthma
Type II Cells	PGI_2, PGE_2, TXB_2	Unknown	??
	LTB_4, LTC_4		
Vascular Endothelium	PGI_2	Vasodilation/blood flow regulation	Released by shear stress
	PAF	Vasodilation	??
	LTC_4	Vasoconstriction	Released by hypoxia
Other Lung Cells	PAF (mast cell)	Vasodilation	??
	Thromboxane (platelets)		
Exogenously Administered			
Inhalation	LTC_4	Increases mucous secretion	Acts on mucous cells
	LTD_4	Increases cilia beating	Acts on ciliated cells
Intravenous	LTD_4, TXA_2	Vasoconstriction	??
	PGF_2, PGE_1	Vasodilation	??

LT, leukotriene; TX, thromboxane; PG, prostaglandin; PAF, platelet activating factor.

lized, making exact quantitation of concentration, localization of target tissue, and determination of biologic effect of endogenously synthesized eicosanoids difficult.

Much of our understanding of function is derived from observations using exogenously administered substrate. Regardless of the complexity of this system, eicosanoids play important roles in membrane permeability, modulation of smooth muscle tone, cell to cell communication, inflammation, and cell growth. Both the airways and the pulmonary circulation respond to administered eicosanoids. Membrane damage in lung injury, stretching of tissues during vascular shearing, and airway inflammation are recognized stimuli for lung eicosanoid release.

Pathophysiology of Nonrespiratory Functions in Lung Disease

In addition to mediation of normal lung functions, derangements in nonrespiratory functions can produce a variety of pulmonary disease states. Complex interactions between functions can produce a mosaic of pathophysiological mechanisms. The following selected examples illustrate these interactions.

PHYSICAL AND RELATED FUNCTIONS GONE AWRY

Pulmonary Thromboembolism

The sieving of microemboli by the pulmonary vasculature usually occurs without incident. The embolic occlusion of a large (segmental or lobar) pulmonary artery is less subtle, and the range of clinical manifestations includes hypoxemia, hemodynamic disturbances (shock or cardiac arrest), and airway obstruction. The pathophysiologic derangement induced by a pulmonary embolism is out of proportion to that anticipated from a localized occlusion of a pulmonary artery. It appears to represent vascular obstruction plus a secondary train of complicating events mediated by alterations in other nonrespiratory lung functions. Regional hypoxia and the release of serotonin (either from platelets or damaged vascular endothelium) cause vasoconstriction and resultant pulmonary hypertension. The role of other vasoactive mediators is currently uncertain. Bronchoconstriction can be prevented by the administration of heparin (a known inhibitor of mast cell degranulation), suggesting that **histamine** contributes to secondary manifestations of pulmonary embolism. Whether other modulators of bronchial smooth muscle tone are involved (e.g., eicosanoids) is unclear.

Fat Embolism

Long bone fractures may produce a lung injury characterized by hypoxia, disseminated diffuse lung infiltrates, and pulmonary edema. This delayed sequela of embolization of fat from a fracture seems out of proportion to the severity of the initial event. Microemboli of neutral fat released from bone marrow cause acute obstruction of pulmonary capillaries. Local lipase activity then releases free fatty acids, which evoke an inflammatory response, resulting in a diffuse **vasculitis** and a **capillary leak syndrome**.

Particulate Inhalation and Occupational Lung Disease: Asbestos

Asbestosis, a diffuse parenchymal lung disease, is representive of a family of inhalational pulmonary diseases in which inhaled particulates traverse the primary defense system present in large airways. It is characterized by the development of pulmonary fibrosis, restrictive pulmonary function, and pleural disease, and is the end result of a cascade of events in the lung following chronic inhalational exposure to asbestos fibers.

Used in a wide variety of insulating and fireproofing applications, asbestos particles are large, but unlike spherical particles of the same size, they possess unique aerodyanamic properties owing to their cylindrical shape. When inhaled, they are carried deep into the tracheobronchial tree, impacting at branch points of respiratory bronchioles, bypassing the ciliated epithelium of large airways.

Alveolar macrophages, migrating up from the alveoli, ingest the particles and become activated. The release of cytokines and chemoattractants by macrophages then recruits neutrophils to the site and increases the local inflammatory response through protease and oxidant release. The pattern of parenchymal lung injury may be indistinguishable from that of idiopathic pulmonary fibrosis (IPF), as reflected by the neutrophil-predominant cell profiles of BAL specimens in both disorders.

Cigarette Smoke

Pyrolysis of tobacco is an incomplete combustive process and gives rise to a complex mixture of particulates, noxious gases, and aromatic compounds (including carbon monoxide, nitric oxide, tar, benzopyrene, volatile hydrocarbons, nitrosamines). In addition to its carcinogenic potential, tobacco smoke has been shown to alter other lung functions. Best characterized is its effect on mucociliary clearance. Tracheal epithelial cilia exposed to smoke beat at a decreased frequency. Smoke promotes mucosal gland hypertrophy and hypersecretion of mucus. One consequence of poor mucous clearance is an increased potential for pulmonary infection.

Smoking also promotes an enhanced inflammatory response within the alveolar mileu. BAL of smokers reveals an increase in total cell counts as well as a relative increase in the number of macrophages and neutrophils. Cigarette smoke stimulates macrophages to release neutrophil chemoattractant factor. Proteases released from the neutophils, accompanied by inactivation of α_1-antitrypsin, a potent antiprotease, results in a proliferative inflammatory cell response accompanied by a protease-antiprotease imbalance. Chronic exposures can induce significant lung destruction, resulting in emphysema or chronic bronchitis.

Oxidant Injury and Lung Repair

Exposure to high oxygen concentrations results in damage to the alveolar epithelium. Although type I cells are susceptible to oxidant injury and die from exposure, alveolar type II cells seem more resistant to such damage. The cellular basis for antioxidant defenses of type II cells seems to be the presence of high intracellular levels of antioxidants such as ascorbate (vitamin C) and glutathione. Type II cells are involved in the repair of alveolar architecture resulting from oxidant damage to the less well equipped type I cell. After exposure to 90% O_2, type II cells show mitotic figures and increased DNA synthesis. Type I cells, incapable of division, die and are replaced by replication and transformation of cuboidal, surfactant-secreting type II cells into flattened, squamouslike cells. This pattern has also been noted following N_2 exposure and in many lung injury models, suggesting that proliferation and dedifferentiation of type II cells is an important mechanism of lung repair.

ALTERATIONS IN PULMONARY HOST DEFENSE: INFECTION IN IMMUNOCOMPROMISED PATIENTS

Pulmonary infection in healthy adults is rare unless mitigating circumstances intervene such as exposure to particularly virulent organisms. In contrast, whether congenital, acquired, or iatrogenic, defects in local pulmonary defenses will produce specific patterns of opportunistic infections. Table 15-4 outlines pulmonary infections associated with major host defects. The pathophysiologic basis for defects seen in certain patients is discussed below.

Transplant Patient (Solid Organ)

Modern organ transplantation techniques employ powerful immunosuppressive agents to prevent rejection. In particular, cyclosporine, corticosteroids, and antithymocyte globulin alter normal T-lymphocyte function and profoundly affect normal macrophage-lymphocyte interactions. The result is an iatrogenic reduction in cell-mediated immunity and a propensity for viral and fungal infection.

AIDS Patient

Infection with the human immunodeficiency virus (HIV) results in an acquired defect in cell-mediated immunity. This appears to be due to HIV-induced destruction of the CD4+ T-helper cell population. The resulting cellular immune defect includes decreased helper-suppressor cell ratio, lymphopenia, and cutaneous anergy. The most common pulmonary infections in this group are *pneumocystis carinii, cytomegalovirus,* and tuberculosis.

Multiple Myeloma

This disorder, characterized by proliferation of monoclonal B-cell clones, is representative of impairment of antibody formation. The lack of adequate immunoglobulin results in poor opsonization of encapsulated organisms and accounts for the increased frequency of infection with *Pneumococcus* and *Haemophilus influenzae.*

Leukemic Patient (Myelogenous)

Both the intrinsic nature of myeloproliferative disorders and the consequences of aggressive chemotherapy decrease the number of functional granulocytes. Infection with staph species, gram-negative bacilli, and aspergillus are more common in this group.

ALTERATIONS IN IMMUNE FUNCTION: INTERSTITIAL LUNG DISEASE

Just as suppression of pulmonary immune function can produce opportunities for infection, inappropriate amplification of those responses can result in abnorm-

TABLE 15-4. Pulmonary Infections in the Immunocompromised Host

Host Defense Defect	Disease	Pulmonary Infection
Abnormal mucous	Cystic fibrosis	*Pseudomonas* species *Staphylococcus aureus* Influenza
Depressed cell-mediated immunity	Solid organ transplant AIDS Corticosteroids (high dose) Lymphoma	Tuberculosis, herpes viruses *Pneumocystis carinii, Toxoplasmosis gondi,* *cytomegalovirus, Cryptococcus*
Impaired antibody formation	Multiple myeloma B cell lymphoma Lymphocytic leukemia Congenital hypogammaglobulinemia	*Streptococcus.pneumonia* *Hemophilus influenza*
Neutropenia	Post chemotherapy Myeloproliferative disorders	Gram negative bacteria *Aspergillus* species *Staphylococcus* species

ally accelerated patterns of lung inflammation. The lung has a relatively restricted response to injury. The two basic patterns of lung injury in interstitial lung disease, as assessed by bronchoalveolar lavage, are lymphocyte predominant and neutrophil predominant. Interstitial lung diseases that illustrate the major injury patterns of alveolar lung inflammation are sarcoidosis and idiopathic pulmonary fibrosis.

Sarcoidosis

Representative of a lymphocyte-predominant disorder, sarcoid is a multisystem granulomatous disorder presenting most frequently with bilateral hilar lymphadenopathy, diffuse interstitial lung disease, and skin or occular disease. This disorder is characterized by an enhancement of cellular immune response, although the triggering antigen has not been identified.

In the lung, BAL demonstrates increased lymphocyte counts. Studies of T-cell subsets have revealed increases in T-helper cells and decreases in T-suppressor cells. An intense interaction of T cells and macrophages mediated through a network of newly described cytokines, including interleukin 1 and interleukin 2, is thought to produce the characteristic noncaseating granulomas seen in tissue biopsies.

Increased serum ACE levels appear to originate from the epithelioid cells of the granulomas; this measurement can be used to assess the degree of disease activity and to follow treatment response.

Idiopathic Pulmonary Fibrosis (Fibrosing Alveolitis)

IPF is an interstitial lung disease in which other known causes of fibrosis have been excluded. The diagnosis is confirmed by lung biopsy. In contrast to sarcoid, IPF is characterized by a neutrophil predominant alveolitis and the presence of neutral proteases in lavage fluid. Less is known regarding specific cell-to-cell interactions, but it appears that neutrophil protease activity and possibly oxygen free radicals play a role in lung tissue destruction.

Acknowledgments *The author would like to thank Alfred P. Fishman, M.D., for his inspiration and critical review of this manuscript, and Susan Gregory, M.D., for helpful suggestions in its preparation.*

Bibliography

Daniele RP, Elias JA, Epstein PE, Rossman MD. Bronchoalveolar lavage: role in pathogenesis, diagnosis, and management of interstitial lung disease. *Ann Intern Med* 1985;102:93–108.

Heinemann HO, Fishman AP. Nonrespiratory functions of the mammalian lung. *Physiol Rev* 1969;49:1–47.

Hyers TM, ed. Pulmonary embolism and hypertension. *Clin Chest Med* 5(3):1984: 383–554.

Johns CJ. Sarcoidosis. In Fishman AP, ed. *Pulmonary diseases and disorders.* New York: McGraw-Hill, 1988:619-645.

Reynolds HY: Host defense impairments that may lead to respiratory infections. *Clin Chest Med* 8:339–358 1987.

Staub NC, Albertine KH. The structure of the lungs relative to their principal function. In Nadel J, Murray J, eds. *Respiratory medicine.* Philadelphia: WB Saunders, 1988: 13–36.

Voelkel NF, Stenmark KR, Wescott JY, Chang SW. Lung eicosanoid metabolism. *Clin Chest Med* 1989;10(1):95-107.

Weibel ER. Lung cell biology. In Fishman AP, Fisher AB, eds. *Handbook of physiology, Section 3: the respiratory system, vol 1: circulation and nonrespiratory functions.* Bethesda, MD: American Physiological Association, 1984:47–91.

Wright JR, Hawgood S. Pulmonary surfactant metabolism. *Clin Chest Med* 1989;10:83-95.

Michael L. Nance

16 MOTILITY OF THE GASTROINTESTINAL TRACT

Motility of the gastrointestinal tract is a complex, highly integrated function that allows movement of intraluminal contents. Motility is affected by anatomic, neural, and hormonal factors. The motile state of the gastrointestinal tract, in turn, affects regulation of other gut functions such as secretion and absorption.

Motility begins with the oral ingestion of food, which is propelled into the esophagus by movements of the tongue against the palate, and ends with the passage of stool past the rectum and anal sphincters.

Discussion of motility based on a regional approach will begin with the esophagus.

Esophagus

ANATOMY

The esophagus can be divided into three functional zones: **upper esophageal sphincter (UES)**, **esophageal body**, and **lower esophageal sphincter (LES)**. The average adult esophagus is a muscular tube 20 cm in length, lined with squamous epithelium and composed of both striated and smooth muscle fibers. The UES and upper portions of the esophageal body are composed of striated muscle. The bulk of the esophageal body and LES are composed of smooth muscle. The UES is approximately 2–4.5 cm in length and is formed from the horizontal fibers of the inferior pharyngeal constrictor muscles, of which the cricopharyngeus is the lowest. The esophageal body has an outer longitudinal and inner circular muscle layer. The LES is a functionally, but not anatomically, distinct zone of high pressure, approximately 2–4 cm in length, at the esophagogastric junction.

REGULATION

The esophagus has both intrinsic and extrinsic innervation. The intrinsic, or enteric, system is the continuum of that which extends from the esophagus to the anus and is composed of two interconnected plexuses, the **myenteric (Auerbach's)** and **submucosal (Meissner's)**. Cholinergic, noradrenergic, and nonadrenergic, noncholinergic (NANC) fibers are present. Extrinsic innervation of the esophagus is derived from the somatic, sympathetic, and parasympathetic nervous systems. The striated muscle is innervated by somatic motor fibers via the vagus nerve. The parasympathetics of the cervical esophagus travel via the recurrent laryngeal nerves. Those of the distal esophagus travel via thoracic vagal fibers. Most parasympathetic fibers are cholinergic; peptides may also act a neurotransmitters, but their role is unclear. Parasympathetic stimulation causes esophageal muscle contraction, although it causes relaxation of the LES. Sympathetic fibers to the esophageal body travel via the superior and inferior cervical ganglia and ganglia of the thoracic sympathetic chain; fibers to the LES travel via the greater splanchnic nerve. Sympathetic fibers act on the myenteric plexus to modulate rather than direct motor input.

PATTERNS OF CONTRACTION

The UES is tonically closed at rest. With each inspiration there is excitatory parasympathetic discharge to the UES to prevent air entry into the esophagus. Other excitatory stimulants of UES tone are slow esophageal distension, acid contents, gagging, and the Valsalva maneuver. Tone is decreased with sudden esophageal distension, belching, or vomiting.

When a swallow is initiated, tonic excitatory discharge to the UES decreases, resulting in relaxation. Elevation and forward movement of the cricoid cartilage assists in opening the UES. Peristalsis continues down through the esophageal body with a maximum pressure of 150 mm Hg. A peristaltic wave takes about 6-8 seconds to proceed through the esophagus with an average velocity of 3 to 4 cm/s. The peristaltic wave traverses both striated and smooth muscle segments of the esophagus. Afferent fibers from the esophagus may affect the central control mechanism, altering the force and velocity of contraction in the striated and smooth muscle segments.

The mechanisms responsible for production, propagation, and regulation of peristaltic waves are still controversial. Both central and local intramural mechanisms have been suggested. It is clear, however, that the central and local mechanisms produce a highly integrated response, most likely through excitatory cholinergic neurons. Other local and central outputs generated in response to sensory feedback (intraluminal distension, intramural contraction) act to shape the integrated message.

At rest, the LES is closed. A tonic pressure of 20 mm Hg is maintained through a combination of intrisic myogenic and excitatory neural mechanisms. The neural component is based on acetylcholine-mediated vagal excitatory fibers. The LES tone increases with beta blockers, suggesting there is underlying adrenergic inhibitory tone as well. LES tone fluctuates every 1.5 to 2 hours with the **migrating motor complex (MMC,** discussed below). Sensation of an ingested meal or an increase in intraabdominal pressure causes an increase in LES tone, probably via vagal afferent pathways. Swallowing acts to decrease LES pressure within 1.5–2.5 seconds. The lowered pressure is maintained for 6–8 seconds as the peristaltic wave traverses the esophageal body. This relaxation is most likely due to a combination of cessation of tonic excitatory input and active inhibition of the muscle. Relaxation is followed by a rise to a pressure above resting for 7–10 seconds (Figure 16-1A).

Primary esophageal peristalsis is induced by swallowing and requires intact extrinsic nervous input. Secondary peristalsis, in response to muscle distension, is mediated by intrinsic mechanisms.

MOTILITY DISORDERS

Gastroesophageal incompetence is a failure of the LES to contract adequately, leading to reflux. Achalasia is characterized by an amotile esophageal body with a nonrelaxing LES, causing a clinical picture of esophageal obstruction and regurgitation. Diffuse esophageal spasm is a poorly understood condition characterized by intermittent, discoordinated painful contractions throughout the smooth muscle and LES components of the esophagus. There are many esophageal dysmotility syndromes secondary to systemic disease states such as scleroderma and amyloidosis, and the neurotrophic diseases, such as amyotrophic lateral sclerosis, diabetes, and stroke. Motility disorders are best illustrated through manometric studies (Figure 16-B,C).

Stomach

ANATOMY

The stomach is composed of four layers: mucosal, submucosal, muscular, and serosal. The muscular layer is composed of three distinct muscle layers: an outer longitudinal layer, continuous with the longitudinal layers

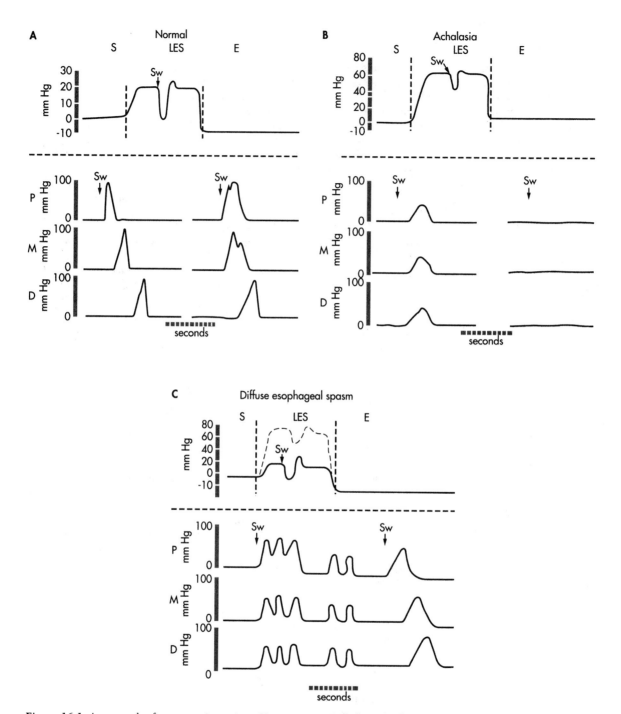

Figure 16-1 An example of manometric tracings. *Upper tracings:* Pull-through of catheter from stomach (S), across lower esophageal sphincter (LES), to esophagus (E). Relaxation of LES evaluated during a swallow (Sw). *Lower tracings:* Catheter placed in esophagus with openings 5 cm apart at proximal (P), middle (M), and distal (D) sites. The response to two wet swallows is shown. **A,** Normal esophagus. **B,** Achalasia. **C,** Diffuse esophageal spasm; normal and abnormal patterns represent the intermittent nature of this problem. (Reproduced from Nelson JB, Castell DO. Esophageal motility disorders. *Disease of the Month* 1988;34(6)297–389. Yearbook Medical Publishers.)

of the esophagus and duodenum, with fibers predominantly in the distal two thirds of the stomach along the greater and lesser curves; a median circular layer; and an inner oblique layer, which is most prominent proximally along the lesser curve. The stomach terminates in the **pylorus**, which is composed of thickened bundles from the circular layer and fibers from the longitudinal layer. Contraction of the circular fibers leads to closure of the pylorus, whereas contraction of the longitudinal bands will open the pylorus.

REGULATION

Neural control of gastric motility is mediated intrinsically as well as by extrinsic sympathetic and parasympathetic innervation. The sympathetics originate in the thoracic ganglia and travel via splanchnic nerves to the celiac plexus and on to the stomach. Parasympathetics are carried via the anterior vagus, which gives off a branch to the liver and the posterior vagus, which gives off a branch to the celiac ganglion.

PATTERNS OF CONTRACTION

For the purpose of understanding motility, the stomach can be divided into two areas: an oral (or proximal) one third and a (caudad) or distal two thirds. The oral region is tonic and does not exhibit peristaltic activity. Contractions in this area are prolonged and produce elevations in pressure that last up to 6 minutes. Motility in this region is primarily concerned with accommodation and regulation of intragastric pressure, which is accomplished via vagal reflexes. Receptive relaxation in response to oral stimulation or esophageal distension produces a reduction in intragastric pressure. Gastric accommodation, which occurs in response to increased gastric volume and prevents large changes in intragastric pressure, is vagally mediated as well. These reflexes are mediated through vagal efferents via a nonadrenergic, noncholinergic messenger, most likely vasoactive intestinal polypeptide (VIP).

Contractions in the caudad region are primarily high in intensity and short in duration. Contractions typically begin in the mid-stomach and move distally, increasing in force and velocity. These contractions last 2–20 seconds and occur three to five times per minute. Contractions occur as a result of action potentials generated by pacesetter potentials or spontaneous, episodic depolarizations of the smooth muscle cells. These pacesetter potentials originate along the gastric curvatures and are propagated distally. Spread occurs more rapidly along the greater curvature than along the lesser curvature, allowing the contraction waves to reach the pylorus simultaneously. Not all pacesetter potentials are followed by action potentials. The duodenum has a pacesetter mechanism as well with a frequency somewhat greater than that of the stomach. The slower gastric potentials are conducted across the pylorus to the duodenal bulb, allowing for gastroduodenal coordination.

As the contraction moves distally, the gastric contents are pushed forward. The peristaltic wave, however, progresses faster than the gastric contents and eventually overtakes them. This results in the phenomenon of retropulsion, which acts to mix and digest the gastric contents thoroughly. Not all of the gastric contents are retropulsed back into the stomach with the peristaltic wave, allowing for some gastric emptying to occur with each peristaltic wave.

The rate of gastric emptying is highly regulated via inhibitory feedback mechanisms. The degree of inhibition varies with the chemical and physical composition of the contents entering the small bowel. This regulation is mediated by receptors sensitive to changes in the osmotic pressure and chemical nature (i.e., pH, concentration) of the gastric effluent. Other modulators of gastric emptying that are less well understood are neural and hormonal (e.g., cholecystokinin) in nature.

The pacesetter potentials occur in the fed and nonfed state. During the fasting or interdigestive state an additional contractile pattern exists, the **migrating motor complex (MMC)**. Approximately every 90 minutes an MMC originates in the stomach and travels to the terminal ileum, usually over a period of 90 minutes. As the complex is propagated distally, the velocity diminishes. The MMC has four overlapping phases. Phase I is characterized by a decrease in the number of pacesetter potentials, of which only a small proportion continue as action potentials. Phase II is associated with an increase in the incidence and intensity of action potentials. During phase III nearly all action potentials are of maximal amplitude and duration. These action potentials produce particularly forceful contractions. Phase IV is characterized by a rapid decrease in the incidence and intensity of action potentials. Regulation of the MMC is most likely dependent on vagal tone. Vagal output associated with feeding interrupts the cycle, which is then superseded by a pattern similar to phase II with intermittent but relatively frequent action potentials that last as long as food remains in the stomach.

MOTILITY DISORDERS

Isolated dysmotility syndromes of the stomach are unusual. More commonly, the motility is altered as part of a complex of findings. Gastroparesis occurs in response to local conditions such as a gastric ulcer and generalized conditions such as diabetes, amyloidosis, and hypothyroidism. Motility is diminished after surgical vagotomy. The nature of postoperative paralytic gastric ileus is poorly understood, but self-limited. An increase in gastric motility may be associated with conditions such as duodenal ulcers, Zollinger-Ellison syndrome, hyperthyroidism, and others.

Gallbladder and Biliary Tract

ANATOMY

The gallbladder has a muscularis layer composed of interlacing smooth muscle cells. Longitudinal fibers course the length of the gallbladder; however, the circular fibers form a more prominent layer throughout the gallbladder. The sphincter of Oddi is a discrete, 5- to 15-mm-long muscular portion of the distal common bile duct at its junction with the duodenum.

REGULATION

The gallbladder contracts in response to cholinergic stimuli, principally thorough vagal parasympathetics that travel via the hepatic branches of the anterior vagal trunk. Cholinergic input also plays an important role in bowel reflexes, such as antral and duodenal distention, which result in gallbladder contraction. Additional evidence of the importance of vagal input is the postvagotomy state, characterized by biliary stasis. The gallbladder also responds, to a lesser extent, to sympathetic neural inputs that originate in the celiac plexus. Both α- and β-receptors have been identified. The excitatory α-receptors appear to be masked by the inhibitory β-receptors. The sympathetic effect can only be demonstrated in the stimulated gallbladder. Evidence also exists for a nonadrenergic, noncholinergic (NANC) neuron, which may contribute to the overall inhibitory tone. It has been suggested that VIP acts as the neurotransmitter for these neurons.

While cholecystokinin (CCK) is the most potent stimulant of gallbladder contraction, other hormones and peptides have also been shown to produce the same effect. Gastrin is structurally similar to CCK and has been shown in some studies to cause gallbladder contraction. Debate exists as to whether the contraction noted is physiologic or purely pharmacologic. Secretin, which is routinely released along with CCK, has been shown to augment the action of CCK. It alone, however, does not stimulate the gallbladder to contract. Vasoactive intestinal polypeptide, a neuropeptide, will decrease the basal gallbladder motor activity as well as blunt the CCK-induced contraction. More recently discovered peptides, such as peptide YY and pancreatic polypeptide, are still under investigation but may have some modulatory effect on gallbladder contraction.

In addition to contraction of the gallbladder, transmission of bile into the duodenum requires relaxation of the sphincter of Oddi. Cholecystokinin has been implicated as a hormonal mediator of sphincter relaxation, allowing flow of bile through the sphincter. The sphincter is also supplied with both sympathetic and parasympathetic nerves. An increase in vagal tone, as with feeding, is associated with a decrease in sphincter tone.

PATTERNS OF CONTRACTION

Gallbladder motility has two distinctive phases, the interdigestive and digestive phases. During the interdigestive phase the gallbladder is not completely at rest as was once thought. The gallbladder is transiently and cyclically contracting during phase II of the MMC. Thus delivery of bile into the duodenum during the interdigestive phase is due to active contraction of the gallbladder independent of changes in sphincter tone. Contraction must overcome resting sphincter tone of 10–30 mm Hg. The neural and hormonal control mechanisms of gallbladder contraction in the interdigestive phase have not been clearly delineated. Motilin probably plays at least a contributory role in contraction as its serum level rises during phase II of the MMC and experimental infusion of this hormone produces active contraction of the gallbladder. The function of interdigestive gallbladder contraction is unclear but probably serves to reduce cholesterol precipitation and the accumulation of debris.

During the digestive phase, the gallbladder contracts in response to feeding and CCK; normally within 1 to 2 minutes of presentation of the stimulus. Simultaneously, the resting tone of the sphincter of Oddi is reduced. Continuous infusion of CCK, as noted in experimental models, produces a greater evacuation of the gallbladder than a bolus of CCK. Continuous infusion of CCK, which simulates the fed state, leads to 50–75% emptying of the gallbladder over a 30- to 45-minute period. The relationship of volume and composition of meals to the levels of CCK in the circulation is not well understood.

MOTILITY DISORDERS

Primary motility disorders of the gallbladder are uncommon. Biliary stasis, however, occurs in the postvagotomy state and may predispose to cholelithiasis and subsequent cholecystitis. It is unclear whether this stasis is due to decreased gallbladder tone or increased sphincter tone. Biliary dyskinesia, characterized by severe, episodic abdominal pain, results from an elevated tone in the sphincter of Oddi. This condition may be a cause for postcholecystectomy pain and occurs independent of cholelithiasis.

Small Bowel

ANATOMY

The adult small bowel varies in length from 5 to 7 m. Like the stomach the small bowel is composed of four histologic layers. The muscularis propria is composed of an inner circular and an outer longitudinal layer. Both layers are important in movement of intestinal contents. The specific roles and degree to which each layer is involved with propulsion of intraluminal contents is unclear. However, the circular layer is felt to be most important in aboral movement.

REGULATION

Control of muscular contractions is multifactorial. Both intrinsic and extrinsic neural stimuli as well as hormones influence the contractile pattern. The intrinsic neural system affects contraction via local reflexes, such as the **intestinointestinal reflex,** in which local distension leads to inhibition of contraction; this is a spinal reflex mediated through sympathetic, but independent of parasympathetic, pathways. The extrinsic system (parasympathetic via vagus and sympathetic via splanchnics and celiac and superior mesenteric ganglia) allows central regulation of intestinal motility and the integration of intestinal motility with body physiology. Hormones (e.g., CCK, secretin) alter the contractile pattern through local effects on the smooth muscle cells.

PATTERNS OF CONTRACTION

Important in the movement of bowel contents is the temporal relation of the contractions that are produced in the small bowel. Sequential contractions of the bowel from oral to aboral produce the characteristic peristaltic wave. Local contraction of the bowel will force intraluminal contents in both directions, and it is the state of the adjacent bowel that then determines the degree of aboral movement of the food bolus.

The small bowel responds to the migrating motor complex. The MMC produces coordinated sequential contractions in the aboral direction. The MMC usually, but not always, originates in the stomach, and most of the complexes are transmitted the entire length of the small intestine. This pattern exists predominantly in the fasted state and is replaced with a seemingly random pattern after feeding, which is influenced by both neural and hormonal input. Contractions that occur in the fed state resemble phase II of the MMC and are propulsive. In addition to the MMC, the individual smooth muscle cells have a basal rhythm or **slow waves**, independent of the MMC. Some of these slow wave depolarizations lead to regional action potentials and localized contractions. The frequency of depolarization with subsequent contraction varies along the length of the small intestine; with the frequency decreasing progressively in the aboral direction.

MOTILITY DISORDERS

Motility disorders of the small bowel are principally those of hypomotility. Most common is the postoperative paralytic ileus, which is usually benign and self-limited. A vast array of motility disorders, which present with a picture of pseudo-obstruction can occur. Except for rare primary or familial syndromes, abnormal motility is most often due to systemic disease. Systemic disease acts at various levels to cause small bowel dysmotility. It may affect the musculature or nervous or endocrine responses.

Colon and Rectum

ANATOMY

The colon is typically 1.5 m in length and is composed of inner circular and outer longitudinal muscle layers. These layers differ somewhat from those of the stomach and small bowel. The outer longitudinal layer is a continuous layer, consisting primarily of three bundles of muscle fibers, the **taenia,** with only a thinner layer between these bundles. The circular layer also is continuous, with regularly spread tight bands of muscle fibers forming the **haustrae.** The longitudinal layer becomes uniformly thick at the rectum, eventually merging with the external anal sphincter. The circular layer becomes the internal anal sphincter.

REGULATION

Like the other portions of the gastrointestinal tract, the colon has both intrinsic and extrinsic innervation. Intrinsic innervation is based primarily on the myenteric plexus. Extrinsic innervation consists of sympathetic and parasympathetic inputs. The sympathetics innervating the proximal colon pass through the superior mesenteric ganglion and those innervating the distal colon pass through the inferior mesenteric ganglion. The rectal sympathetics are from the hypogastric plexus. Parasympathetics to the proximal colon are carried via the vagus; distally they are carried via the pelvic nerves.

PATTERNS OF CONTRACTION

The colon has no MMC. Contractions appear more random in nature. In the proximal colon contractions are disorganized and do not produce effective propulsive forces. Rather, the proximal colon acts to mix the contents, allowing for maximal exposure to the mucosal surface with attendant absorption of water. Propulsive forces do occur during a phase called the **mass movement.** Mass movements occur one to three times daily. Their stimulus is poorly understood. During mass movement, phase-independent local contractions cease and an organized contraction acts to move lumenal contents aborally. The distal colon, in addition to random contractions, also has a higher frequency of organized segmental contractions. These contractions act to slow the forward movement of the luminal contents. As in the proximal colon, most propulsion occurs during the mass movement.

The rectum is usually empty. Segmental contractions of the rectum, at a rate slightly faster than the sigmoid colon, slow the influx of material. When the rectum does fill, the distention initiates the **rectosphincteric reflex,** which ultimately causes a decrease in internal anal sphincter tone. Voluntary control of the external anal sphincter, via somatic efferents, allows defecation to occur when desirable. Maneuvers to increase intraabdominal pressure and lower the floor of the pelvis aid in evacuation of the rectum. Reflexive relaxation of the internal anal sphincter is transient. In the absence of defecation, accommodation of the rectal vault can occur, terminating the rectosphincteric reflex. Distention by additional fecal matter will reinitiate this cycle.

MOTILITY DISORDERS

The causes and symptoms of colonic motility disorders are similar to those seen in the small intestine. Additionally, a symptom complex of irritable colon syndrome has been described. These patients manifest recurrent painful constipation or painless diarrhea. Patients with constipation demonstrate more colonic segmental contractions that deter forward movement of contents and allow excess absorption of water. Patients with diarrhea have fewer segmental contractions and thus more rapid transit. Colonic diverticulae may be related to an increase in segmental contractions. Hirschsprung's disease is a congenital motility disorder characterized by the absence of ganglion cells in the myenteric plexus. The involved bowel may include any length from only the anus to the entire colon but is always contiguous, and starts at the anus. This entity usually presents with chronic constipation early in life.

Bibliography

Christensen J. Motility of the colon. In Johnson LR, ed. *Physiology of the gastrointestinal tract, Vol I.* Philadelphia: WB Saunders, 1987:665.

Code CF, Marlett JA. The interdigestive myoelectric complex of the stomach and small bowel of dogs. *J Physiol* 1975;246:289.

Diament NE. Physiology of esophageal motor function. *Gastroenterol Clin North Am* 1989;18(2):425.

Haubrich WS. Irritable bowel syndrome. In Berk JE, ed. *Gastroenterology, Vol IV*. Philadelphia: WB Saunders, 1985: 2425.

Jeffers LJ. Motility disorders of the biliary tract. In Berk JE, ed. *Gastroenterology, Vol VI*. Philadelphia: WB Saunders, 1985:3782.

Meyer JH. Motility of the stomach and gastroduodenal junction. In Johnson LR, ed. *Physiology of the gastrointestinal tract, Vol I*. Philadelphia: WB Saunders, 1987: 613.

Roth JLA. Post-cholecystectomy syndrome. In Berk JE, ed. *Gastroenterology, Vol VI*. Philadelphia: WB Saunders, 1985:3815.

Rowan C, Gonella J. Extrinsic control of digestive tract motility. In Johnson LR, ed. *Physiology of the gastrointestinal tract, Vol I*. Philadelphia: WB Saunders, 1987:507.

Ryan JP. Motility of the gallbladder and biliary tree. In Johnson LR, ed. *Physiology of the gastrointestinal tract, Vol I*. Philadelphia: WB Saunders, 1987:695.

Snape WJ Jr. Pathophysiology of colonic motility disorders. In Berk JE, ed. *Gastroenterology, Vol IV*. Philadelphia: WB Saunders, 1985:2407.

Summers RW, Johlin FC. The pathophysiology, evaluation and management of motility disorders of the biliary tract. *Gastroenterol Clin North Am* 1989;18(2)425.

Weisbrodt NW. Motility of the small intestine. In Johnson LR, ed. *Physiology of the gastrointestinal tract, Vol I*. Philadelphia: WB Saunders, 1987:631.

Linda S. Callans

17 GASTROINTESTINAL EXOCRINE FUNCTION

This chapter will focus on the exocrine function of the salivary glands, the stomach, the biliary tract, and the pancreas. The nature of each glandular secretion and the cellular mechanisms of secretion and its regulation will be discussed with attention to the glandular response to meals. Understanding the normal physiology adds insight into the pathophysiology, diagnosis, and treatment of various disease processes involving gut exocrine function.

Salivary Glands

Saliva is secreted in the oropharynx, where it mixes with food to begin the digestive process. The **parotid glands** secrete a serous type of saliva containing ptyalin (an α-amylase), while the **sublingual and buccal glands** secrete a mucous type containing mucin for lubricating purposes. The **submaxillary glands** secrete both serous and mucous saliva.

The salivary glands are composed of acini, which secrete ptyalin or mucin (depending on the gland type), and ducts, which alter the electrolyte composition. In the ducts, bicarbonate ions are actively secreted while a Na^+-K^+ ATPase pump facilitates the active resorption of sodium in exchange for potassium. Thus, saliva has a relatively high bicarbonate and potassium concentration and a low sodium concentration. The final electrolyte composition, however, is determined to a certain degree by the rate of acinar secretion; at high flow rates there is minimal modification of the electrolyte concentrations within the ducts.

Salivary secretion is controlled by the salivatory nuclei in the brain via parasympathetic nerves. These nuclei receive taste and tactile signals from the tongue and oropharynx as well as more subjective input from the appetite centers and the higher cortex. Stimulation affects the volume as well as the type of saliva secreted.

The Stomach

The stomach serves as a reservoir in which food is mechanically churned and passed into the small bowel in metered amounts via the pylorus. The food particles are also mixed thoroughly with pepsin (a proteolytic enzyme) and gastric acid. Acidification of food in the stomach not only aids in the digestive process by providing the proper pH environment (pH 1.5–5) for enzyme activation, but also plays a protective role in creating a bacterial barrier. The surface mucous cells secrete a thin layer of alkaline mucous that is essential in the protection of the gastric mucosa from injury resulting from high acid concentrations.

GASTRIC ACID PRODUCTION AND SECRETION

The fundus of the stomach is the site of acid production as well as pepsin and intrinsic factor secretion. The antrum not only provides the propulsive force of the stomach but also contains the gastrin-secreting cells (G cells) that play a major role in the control of acid secretion.

The **fundic or oxyntic glands** are composed of mucous neck cells, chief cells that secrete pepsin, and parietal cells that secrete hydrochloric acid and intrinsic factor (Figure 17-1). **Chief cells** secrete pepsin in the form of an inactive precursor, pepsinogen, which is then hydrolyzed and activated in the acid environment of the stomach.

The **parietal cell** is specially suited to acid production. Energy for acid secretion is provided by numerous basal mitochondria. A complex system of intracellular membranes allows HCl to be secreted safely sequestered away from the cytoplasm. Hydrochloric acid is actively secreted against a steep chemical gradient by the action of an H^+-K^+ ATPase **(the proton pump)** bound to these intracellular membranes. During active secretion the tubular membranes coalesce into larger cannaliculi that open into the glandular lumen and release a concentrated acid solution with a pH of 0.8.

Control of Acid Secretion

Hydrochloric acid secretion is controlled on the cellular level by the binding and activation or inactivation of various receptors on the basal membrane of the parietal cell (Figure 17-2). **Muscarinic receptors (M1)** bind acetylcholine (ACh), **gastrin receptors** bind gastrin, and **H2 receptors** bind histamine. Both ACh and gastrin receptors produce a rise in intracellular calcium through the intermediary inositoltriphosphate. Inositoltriphosphate mobilizes intracellular stores of calcium from the rough endoplasmic reticulum; an influx of extracellular calcium through membrane channels may also occur. H2 receptors, on the other hand, activate adenylate cyclase, resulting in a rise in cyclic AMP (cAMP). Calcium and cAMP serve as second messengers by activating cytoplasmic protein kinases that ultimately activate the H^+-K^+ adenosine triphospha-

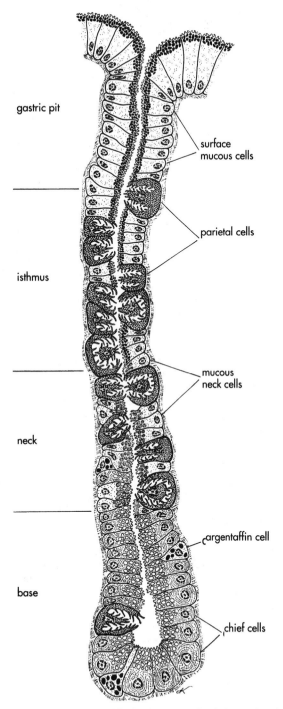

Figure 17-1 Structure of a fundic gastric gland. (Reproduced from Ito S, Winchester RJ. The fine structure of the gastric mucosa in the bat. *J Cell Biol* 1963;16:543.)

gastric pit

surface mucous cells

isthmus

parietal cells

mucous neck cells

neck

base

argentaffin cell

chief cells

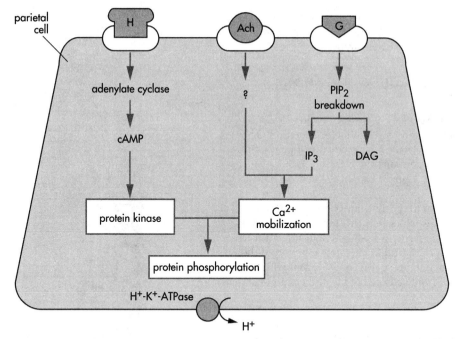

Figure 17-2 Cellular mechanism of acid secretion. H, Histamine; G, gastrin; DAG, diacylglycerol. PIP, Phosphoinositoldiphosphate; IP_3, inositol triphosphate. (Reproduced from Debas HT, Mulholland MW. Drug therapy in peptic ulcer disease. *Curr Probl Surg* 1989;26(1):14.)

tase (ATPase) pump. Thus, the proton pump is the final common pathway to acid secretion stimulated by ACh, gastrin, and histamine.

Gastric acid secretion is controlled by neural, hormonal, and paracrine pathways (Figure 17-3). The **neural pathway** is mediated by the vagal release of ACh in response to the thought, site, smell, and taste of food. **Hormonal control** of gastric acid secretion is effected by gastrin, a peptide hormone produced and secreted by the G cells in the antral glands. Gastrin is released in response to antral distension, rising gastric pH, and various ingested substances or parially digested proteins that serve as potent secretagogues in the antrum. The **paracrine influences** are primarily mediated by locally released histamine from both mast cells and other paracrine cells in the fundic glands. The factors controlling histamine release have not yet been clarified.

Inhibition of gastric secretion occurs by several mechanisms. Obviously vagotomy or inhibition of vagal input decreases acid secretion by eliminating the stimulation of parietal cells by acetylcholine. Gastrin secretion and therefore gastric acid secretion is inhibited by **somatostatin,** a peptide hormone secreted by the

fundic mucosa and pancreatic D cells. Somatostatin also has a direct inhibitory effect on the parietal cell. Acid in the duodenum stimulates **secretin** release which inhibits gastrin-dependent acid secretion. Fat in the duodenum also inhibits gastric secretion, perhaps owing to **gastric inhibitory peptide (GIP)** or **neurotensin** release; **cholecystokinin (CCK)** may also play a role. Several other peptide hormones, such as enteroglucagon, bombesin, and peptide YY, also play a role in the inhibition of acid secretion.

Negative feedback inhibition of acid production occurs as low gastric luminal pH's inhibit gastrin release, leading to decreased acid secretion. As less acid is secreted, the luminal pH rises and more gastrin is released, which in turn stimulates acid secretion.

Various drugs interact with parietal cells at the cellular level, blocking the secretion of hydrochloric acid. For example, the **H2 blockers** cimetidine and ranitidine bind the H2 receptors and block the stimulation of HCl secretion by histamine. **Omeprazole** selectively inactivates the H+-K+ ATPase, thereby blocking the final step in acid production and effectively turning off acid secretion.

REGULATION OF ACID

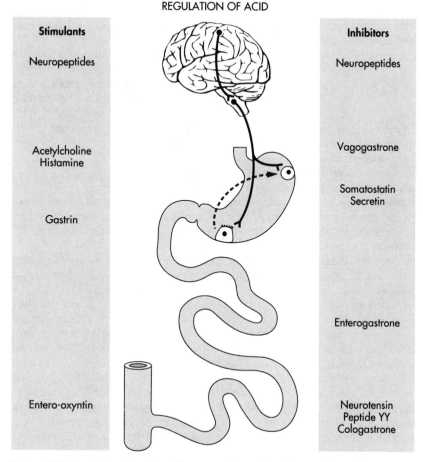

Figure 17-3 Regulation of gastric acid secretion. (Reproduced from Debas HT, Mulholland MW. Drug therapy in peptic ulcer disease. *Curr Probl Surg* 1989;26(1):10.)

Phases of Gastric Acid Secretion

Four phases of acid secretion have been described: the **interdigestive phase**, the **cephalic phase**, the **gastric phase**, and the **intestinal phase.**

Hydrochloric acid is normally secreted from the fundic glands at a basal rate between 2 and 5 mEq per hour during the **interdigestive phase.** Basal acid output is attributed to resting vagal tone and exhibits a diurnal variation with a peak around midnight and a low at 7 A.M.

The **cephalic phase** is mediated by the vagus nerve and is initiated by the thought, site, smell, or taste of food. Vagal discharges release ACh, which acts directly on the parietal cell (the M1 receptors) as well as on the antral G cells. This vagal enhancement of gastrin release

further induces acid production. Additionally, somatostatin release is suppressed by the vagus, thereby removing some of the baseline inhibition of acid secretion.

The **gastric phase** of acid secretion is mediated by local nerve reflexes and the release of gastrin. Antral distension, increases in pH form the buffering effect of food, and the presence of specific foods are sensed by stretch receptors and chemoreceptors in the stomach wall, which in turn stimulate the G cells to release gastrin. Gastrin then stimulates the parietal cell and acid secretion rises in response to food in the stomach.

The **intestinal phase** is less clearly understood. The contribution of the intestinal phase to gastric secretion is minimal, accounting for perhaps 5% of the maximal acid output. The main stimulus is thought to be due to gastrin produced in small amounts by the duodenum in response to distension and various secretagogues in the duodenum. Other peptide hormones may play a minor role.

DISORDERS OF GASTRIC ACID SECRETION

Ulcer disease of the duodenum has a definite association with acid hypersecretion, although not all patients with duodenal ulcer demonstrate hyperacidity. Medical and surgical treatment of ulcer disease is based on an understanding of the physiology and mechanisms of acid secretion. Effective medical intervention may include antacids to neutralize intraluminal acid; H2 blockers, which bind the H2 receptors on parietal cells, preventing histamine-stimulated acid secretion; omeprazole, which inactivates the H^+-K^+ ATPase pump, thereby blocking the final step in acid secretion; and surface coating agents (e.g., sucralfate).

The surgical treatment of ulcer disease consists of vagotomy (truncal, selective, or highly selective) with or without a drainage procedure. Denervation of the stomach eliminates acetylcholine stimulation of the G cells and parietal cells, thereby reducing acid secretion. The basal acid output is lower, and the cephalic phase of acid secretion is absent. Antrectomy may be combined with vagotomy, thus removing the G cell mass and the gastrin-stimulated component of acid secretion.

Recurrent ulceration or **marginal ulcers** after surgery for ulcer disease may occur in the setting of incomplete vagotomy, retained antrum, or gastrinoma. Obviously, incomplete vagotomy will result in persistent stimulation of the parietal cells by vagal discharges and the potential for recurrent disease. In the case of retained antrum, an island of antral tissue is sequestered in the duodenal stump after incomplete antrectomy. While gastrin secretion from the antral G cells is normally subject to negative feedback inhibition by gastric acid, the retained cells are continuously bathed in alkaline bile and pancreatic juice in the duodenum, and therefore secrete high levels of gastrin constantly. Fundic parietal cells are thus continuously stimulated by gastrin, resulting in acid hypersecretion and ulceration.

Hypergastrinemia and subsequent acid hypersecretion and ulcer diathesis are also characteristic of the **Zollinger-Ellison syndrome.** This syndrome is caused by non-β cell islet tumors of the pancreas that secrete gastrin. The autonomous secretion of gastrin results in very high gastrin levels and elevated basal acid outputs.

These patients also have abnormal responses to provocative tests with calcium and secretin, as discussed in the next section.

Gastric ulcers, in contrast to duodenal ulcers, are not associated with acid hypersecretion. Instead they may result from a primary injury to the gastric mucosa, rendering it more susceptible to damage from the stomach's acid environment. Medications or reflux of bile and pancreatic juice through the pylorus may contribute to the primary mucosal injury.

EVALUATION OF GASTRIC SECRETION

Most tests of gastric secretion involve sampling of the gastric contents via a nasogastric tube with evaluation of the volume of secretion as well as the concentration of hydrochloric acid secreted. **Basal acid output** in normal patients (and many patients with peptic ulcer disease) ranges from 2 to 5 mEq/h, while the basal acid output is greater than 15 mEq/h in over half the patients with Zollinger-Ellison syndrome. **Maximal acid output** is measured after infusion of histamine or pentagastrin and is reflective of parietal cell mass. The normal range for maximal acid output is 30–40 mEq/h. In patients with Zollinger-Ellison syndrome, the ratio of basal acid output to maximal acid output is high (usually greater than 0.6), reflecting the high basal rate of secretion.

Serum gastrin levels are also useful in the diagnosis of Zollinger-Ellison syndrome. Gastrin levels are normally less than 150 pg/mL, while many patients with Zollinger-Ellison syndrome have levels greater than 1000 pg/mL. Provocative tests with calcium or secretin infusion can identify patients with Zollinger-Ellison syndrome whose gastrin levels are only moderately elevated. In patients with gastrinoma, both calcium and secretin stimulate gastrin secretion. On the other hand, gastrin levels in normal patients or patients with hypergastrinemia owing to retained antrum will change little after calcium infusion, and actually fall after secretin infusion (secretin normally inhibits gastrin secretion).

The Biliary Tract

Bile functions as an emulsifier, facilitating the digestion, solubilization, and absorption of fats and lipid-soluble vitamins. Bile is also the primary route for solubilization and excretion of cholesterol. Bile is formed by the hepatocyte and secreted into the bile cannaliculi, which drain into the bile ducts. Water and electrolyte composition is then altered by the ductal eptihelium. From the common hepatic ducts bile can drain directly into the duodenum via the common bile duct and ampulla of Vater, or be stored and concentrated in the gallbladder in preparation for the next meal.

COMPOSITION OF BILE

Bile is primarily composed of bile acids, cholesterol, phospholipids, and bilirubin, with the addition of various proteins, water, and electrolytes. **Primary bile acids** (cholate and chenodeoxycholate) represent 80%

of bile acids in gallbladder bile, with secondary bile acids making up the remainder. Primary bile acids are synthesized in the hepatocyte from cholesterol and then recycled through the enterohepatic circulation. **Secondary bile acids** are produced from primary bile acids by bacterial dehydroxylation in the intestinal lumen. Deoxycholate accounts for most of the recycled secondary bile acids, whereas lithocholic acid is primarily excreted in the stool after sulfation in the liver.

Bile acids are conserved through the **enterohepatic circulation** (Figure 17-4). After absorption from the intestine, bile acids are recycled back to the liver via the portal venous system, absorbed by the hepatocyte, and

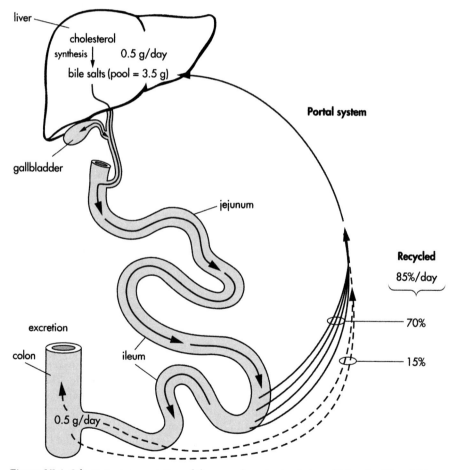

Figure 17-4 Schematic representation of the enterohepatic circulation of bile salts. The *solid lines* entering the portal system represent conjugated bile salts absorbed via ileal transport. The *broken lines* represent deconjugated bile salts resulting from bacterial action. (Reproduced from Tyor MP, Garbutt JT, Lack L. Metabolism and transport of bile salts in the intestine. *Am J Med* 1986;51:620.)

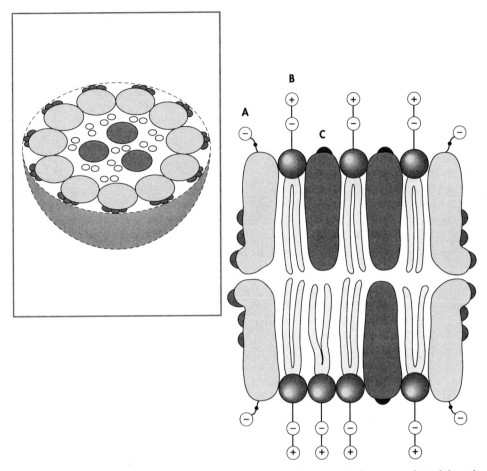

Figure 17-5 Structure of a micelle (provisional). Cross section, *left;* longitudinal section, *right.* **A,** bile acid; **B,** lecithin; **C,** cholesterol. The polar portions of each molecule face outward in contact with the surrounding water, and the nonpolar portions face inward, creating a lipid interior. (Reproduced from Soloway RD. Gallstone disease. In Brooks FP, ed. *Gastrointestinal pathophysiology.* New York: Oxford University Press, 1974:177.)

resecreted into the bile. Absorption from the intestine occurs by two mechanisms. **Conjugated bile acids** are absorbed in the terminal ileum by a specific receptor-mediated active transport system driven by a Na^+-K^+ ATPase. **Bile acids deconjugated** by intestinal bacteria (free bile acids) can be absorbed by passive nonionic diffusion, mainly in the colon, but also in parts of the small bowel. **Sulfated bile acids** are polar substances that cannot be absorbed by the gut and are excreted in stool. Approximately 70% of the bile acids absorbed from the intestine are conjugated and 15% are deconju-

gated. Only about 15% of the bile acid pool is newly synthesized each day to replace that lost in the stool.

Phospholipids (mainly **lecithin**) and **cholesterol** are the other main components of bile. These water-insoluble molecules are solubilized by bile acids in the form of **mixed micelles** (Figure 17-5). Strongly polar bile acids form micelles with the hydrophilic tails outward, interacting with the aqueous environment and the nonionized heads toward the center, creating a nonpolar environment in which lecithin and cholesterol can be dissolved. The solubility of cholesterol depends on

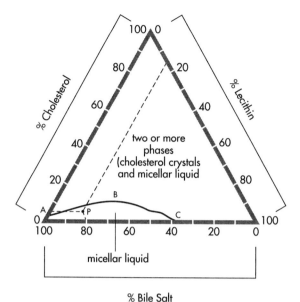

Figure 17-6 Method for presenting three major components of bile (bile salts, lecithin, and cholesterol) on triangular coordinates. Each component expressed as percentage mole of total bile salt, lecithin, and cholesterol. *Line ABC* represents maximum solubility of cholesterol in varying mixtures of bile salt and lecithin. *Point P* represents bile composition containing 5% cholesterol, 15% lecithin, and 80% bile salt and falls within the zone of a single phase of micellar liquid. Bile having a composition falling above line would contain excess cholesterol in either supersaturated or precipitated form (crystals or liquid crystals). (Reproduced from Redinger RN, Small DM. Bile composition, bile salt metabolism, and gallstones. *Arch Intern Med* 1972;130:620.)

the amounts of lecithin and bile acids present (Figure 17-6). Changing the relative concentrations of the bile lipids may lead to supersaturation of cholesterol and subsequent precipitation with stone formation.

Bilirubin, the breakdown product of heme, is solubilized and excreted in bile. Unconjugated bilirubin is taken up by carrier-mediated transport into the hepatocyte, where it is bound by cytoplasmic proteins (proteins Y and Z), conjugated with glucuronide, and secreted into the bile. Bacteria in the gut reduce bilirubin to **urobilinogens,** which are mainly excreted with the feces. Some urobilinogen is absorbed from the gut and then excreted by the kidney. A fraction of urobilinogen is oxidized to **urobilin,** which gives stool its brown color.

In addition to the three bile lipids and bilirubin,

hepatic bile formed at the cannalicular membrane contains various proteins. These include lipoproteins, glycoproteins, immunoglobulins, and small amounts of amylase, among others. The electrolyte and water content is altered by the ductal epithelium and gallbladder mucosa as discussed in the next section.

FORMATION OF BILE—CELLULAR MECHANISM

Hepatic bile formation is not completely understood. At the cellular level, hepatocytes have specialized membranes that interface with hepatic sinusoidal blood on some surfaces, while forming part of the bile cannalicular wall on another (Figure 17-7). Bile acids are either

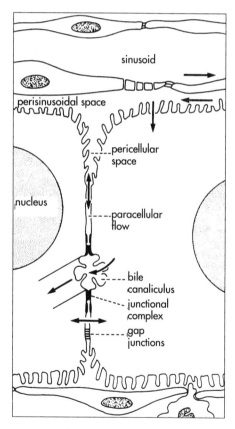

Figure 17-7 Spatial relationships of hepatocytes, sinusoids, and bile canaliculi. (Reproduced from Arias IM, et al., eds. *The liver: biology and pathobiology.* New York: Raven Press, 1988:5.)

absorbed from the sinusoids (the enterohepatic circulation) or synthesized de novo from cholesterol within the hepatocyte. **Bile acid absorption** is thought to occur via a carrier-mediated facilitated transport system. A Na$^+$-K$^+$ ATPase pump in the membrane sets up a chemical gradient by actively pumping sodium out of the cell. Bile acid transport is then coupled to sodium, which flows into the cell down the chemical gradient. Once inside the cell, bile acids are conjugated with either glycine or taurine and then secreted into the canaliculus in the form of micelles. It is postulated that lecithin and cholesterol, components of the cannalicular membrane, are then leached out of the membrane by the bile acids to form mixed micelles (see Figure 17-5). The mixed micelles within the cannaliculi increase the luminal osmotic pressure, and water follows passively into the lumen.

Both **bile-acid-dependent** and **bile-acid-independent** mechanisms of bile secretion are thought to exist. As described above, the hepatic secretion of bile lipids and water is highly dependent on the secretion of bile acids. Bile-acid-independent secretion also occurs at the level of the canaliculus. This component of bile secretion is presumably based on electrochemical gradients established by sodium pumps, resulting in the transport of electrolytes and water into the canaliculus. The ductal epithelium further contributes to the bile-acid-independent secretion by secreting a bicarbonate-rich solution in response to secretin.

Bile is modified not only in its passage through the ducts, but also in the **gallbladder** through the absorption of water and other molecules. Bile stored in the gallbladder is maximally concentrated within 4 hours, with 90% of the water absorbed across the mucosal epithelium. This absorption of isosmotic fluid occurs by passive diffusion of solute across the luminal membrane down an electrochemical gradient established by active transport of sodium out of the cell at the lateral membrane. Larger molecules, such as bilirubin, lecithin, and bile acids, are also absorbed in small amounts, probably in a receptor-mediated fashion. Finally bile is acidified in the gallbladder to a final pH of 7.0.

In summary, bile is formed by secretion of bile lipids (bile acids, cholesterol, and lecithin), bilirubin, and proteins by the hepatocyte, with modification of the water and electrolyte composition and pH at the level of the canaliculus, the bile ducts, and the gallbladder. Minimal changes in the bile lipid composition may occur by absorption in the gallbladder, depending on the duration of bile storage and the integrity of the mucosa. These changes may affect cholesterol solubility and play a role in the pathogenesis of cholesterol gallstones.

FACTORS DETERMINING BILE COMPOSITION

Bile composition can be altered by changing the rate of bile acid secretion as well as the types of bile acids secreted (primary or secondary); by varying the amount of cholesterol secreted into bile; and by modifying the water and electrolyte content of bile.

Bile acid synthesis and secretion is highly dependent on the **size of the bile acid pool** and the **rate of recirculation** of the bile acids back to the liver; the larger the pool or the more rapid the recirculation, the higher the rate of bile acid secretion. Since bile acid concentration is one of the main determinants of bile cholesterol solubility, factors that increase bile acid secretion will improve cholesterol solubility, while factors decreasing bile acid secretion will decrease cholesterol solubility.

Reduction of the bile acid pool markedly reduces bile acid secretion. For example, during a fast (even overnight) much of the bile acid pool is sequestered in the gallbladder, thus decreasing the circulating pool, while cholesterol secretion is minimally affected. Hepatic bile then becomes increasingly saturated with cholesterol. In addition, the gallbladder bile composition is altered by prolonged storage in the gallbladder, since bile acids, lecithin, and bilirubin as well as water and electrolytes can be absorbed by the mucosa.

Diet plays an important role in bile composition, mainly by affecting cholesterol excretion. High caloric intake results in increased cholesterol levels in bile, while decreased cholesterol intake reduces the cholesterol in bile. Obesity in general is associated with higher bile cholesterol secretion and a higher incidence of cholesterol gallstones.

Aside from decreasing dietary cholesterol intake, vegetarian or bran diets may help to desaturate bile by indirectly increasing the use of cholesterol for bile acid synthesis, thereby decreasing its secretion into bile. This effect is based on a complex negative-feedback inhibition of de novo bile acid and cholesterol synthesis by the recirculating bile acids. In the absence of animal fats or in the presence of bran, colonic bacteria have decreased ability to form secondary bile acids. Since deoxycholate, a secondary bile acid, normally inhibits chenodeoxycholate synthesis, reduction of the secondary bile acid results in increased primary bile acid synthesis from cholesterol and decreased cholesterol excretion into bile.

CONTROL OF BILE SECRETION

Two major hormones control the secretion of bile in reponse to meals: **cholecystokinin-pancreozymin (CCK-PZ)** and **secretin.**

The main stimulus for gallbladder contraction is provided by **CCK-PZ,** which is released by the intestinal mucosa in response to fats and partially digested proteins. Thus bile excretion is timed appropriately to aid in the solubilization and digestion of fatty foods. **Vagal stimulation** during the cephalic phase of gastric secretion also causes weak contraction of the gallbladder in response to a meal.

The hormone **secretin** influences bile secretion by stimulating the ductal epithelium to secrete a watery solution rich in bicarbonate. Secretin is released in response to acidification of the duodenal mucosa by gastric chyme. Thus secretin facilitates alkalinization of the duodenal contents by altering the bile electrolyte composition, in addition to stimulating the flow of alkaline pancreatic secretion.

DISORDERS OF THE BILIARY SYSTEM

The major disorders of the biliary tract are related to abnormalities in the lipid composition of bile or the interruption of the enterohepatic circulation. This section will focus on the pathophysiology of gallstone formation, biliary obstruction, and abnormalities in ileal absorption of bile acids.

The formation of **cholesterol gallstones** is thought to be related to abnormalities of bile composition, resulting in supersaturated or "lithogenic" bile. As depicted in Figure 17-6, the solubility of cholesterol depends on the relative concentrations of cholesterol, bile acids, and lecithin. With alterations in bile composition (mainly an increase in cholesterol, or a decrease in bile acids or lecithin in the bile), bile becomes supersaturated and microscopic cholesterol crystals form. These crystals (or other solids in bile such as calcium bilirubinate or bacteria) serve as seeds for further precipitation and eventually macroscopic stones are formed. This nucleation process is a key step, since many patients may have supersaturated bile without gallstones.

Although surgery remains the treatment of choice for gallstones, gallstone dissolution has met with some success. Cholesterol saturation may be reduced by the ingestion of bile acids such as chenodeoxycholate or ursodeoxycholate, which increase the bile acid pool as well as decrease biliary cholesterol secretion. Successful dissolution of cholesterol stones occurs in selected patients after prolonged use of oral bile acids alone or following extracorporeal shock wave lithotripsy. Alternatively, cholesterol stones may be more directly dissolved by infusion of various solutions through a percutaneous catheter (mono-octanoin or methyl tert-butyl ether, for example).

Biliary tract obstruction may be caused by stones, stricture, or tumor. The clinical presentation of biliary obstruction illustrates the underlying pathophysiology. Common bile duct obstruction produces intrahepatic cholestasis and eventual mixing of bile and blood as the cannaliculi rupture into the adjacent sinusoids. Jaundice with conjugated hyperbilirubinemia results. Bile acids circulating through the blood are deposited in the skin, causing pruritis. Steatorrhea and malabsorption may develop with long-standing obstruction, since no bile acids are available for fat absorption. Acholic stools result from the absence of bilirubin (and therefore urobilin) in the intestine, and there is no urobilinogen detectable in the urine. In the case of chronic cystic duct obstruction, hydrops of the gallbladder develops as the bilirubin pigments and bile acids are absorbed by the gallbladder mucosa, leaving a clear, watery fluid.

Interruption of the enterohepatic circulation owing to impaired bile acid absorption can occur with diffuse ileal diseases such as Crohn's disease, radiation enteritis, or amyloidosis. Nonabsorbed free bile acids are mucosal irritants, producing a severe secretory diarrhea or cholerheic enteropathy. As the bile acid pool decreases as a result of wasting in the stool, fat absorption is impaired and steatorrhea may ensue. Furthermore, decreased bile acid recirculation and secretion into bile may result in supersaturation of bile and predispose to cholesterol gallstone formation. The liver adapts to the decreased bile acid pool, however, by increasing primary bile acid synthesis; and cholesterol, the metabolic precursor, is subsequently reduced, eventually desaturating the bile.

Ileal resection or bypass produces effects similar to diffuse ileal diseases and may be complicated by fat and bile acid malabsorption with steatorrhea and cholerheic enteropathy. Distal ileal bypass, however, has been described as a surgical treatment for hypercholesterolemia and hypertriglyceridemia. The site of cholesterol and bile acid absorption is bypassed, resulting in higher excretion into stool. Cholesterol utilization rises as primary bile acid synthesis is stimulated to replete the bile acid pool, and serum cholesterol levels may fall as much as 40%.

Bacterial overgrowth, or **blind loop syndrome,** is another cause of fat malabsorption resulting from impaired bile acid function. The deconjugated pool of bile acids is markedly increased by the action of the intestinal bacteria. These deconjuagated bile acids are inefficiently absorbed by passive diffusion in the ileum, fat absorption is impaired, and bile acids are lost in the stool decreasing the total bile acid pool.

Cholestyramine, a bile acid binder, can limit the diarrhea associated with bile acid malabsorption. It may also be helpful in reducing the pruritis associated with skin bile acid deposition in patients with biliary obstruction. Further, cholestyramine has been used to lower serum cholesterol levels since hepatic synthesis of bile acids from cholesterol is increased to compensate for bile acids lost in the stool bound to the resin.

EVALUATION OF THE BILIARY TRACT

Diagnosis of biliary disease is based on evaluation of the anatomy and function of the biliary tract. Ultrasound is useful in defining the size ot the ducts as well as the presence of gallstones. Acute inflammation may be suggested by a thickened gallbladder wall or fluid around the gallbladder.

Nuclear isotope scans provide information about function as well as anatomy. Technetium-99m-labeled derivatives of iminodiacetic acid are injected intravenously, taken up by the hepatocyte, and excreted in the bile. In a normal study, the liver and the gallbladder are visualized and there is flow into the duodenum in a timely fashion. Hepatocellular dysfunction will interfere with hepatocyte uptake. Cystic duct obstruction, as seen in acute cholecystitis, results in nonvisualization of the gallbladder. Common duct obstruction prevents flow into the intestine.

Biliary tract obstruction is associated with abnormal **serum liver function tests.** Specifically, the conjugated bilirubin, γ-glutamyl transferase, and alkaline phosphatase are elevated. This pattern contrasts with the unconjugated hyperbilirubinemia seen with hemolysis or the elevation of aspartate transaminase and alanine transaminase seen with primary hepatocellular disease. Urine urobilinogen will be absent in complete biliary obstruction since its excretion is dependent on the conversion of bilirubin to urobilinogen in the gut. Simple cholecystitis may demonstrate no abnormalities of serum liver function studies, because cystic duct obstruction alone does not impair biliary excretion.

Bile composition can be directly evaluated after placement of a nasoduodenal tube or cannulation of the ampulla of Vater. Infusion of cholecystokinin-pancreozymin (CCK-PZ) produces contraction of the gallbladder and excretion of bile, which can be aspirated and analyzed for the presence of cholesterol crystals. Cholecystokinin-pancreozymin infusion can also be used as a provocative test to reproduce a patient's symptoms in cases of biliary dyskinesia.

The **bile salt breath test** can be used to identify patients with malabsorption caused by bacterial overgrowth. With bacterial overgrowth there is increased deconjugation of bile acids in the intestine, resulting in poor bile acid absorption and fat malabsorption. The bile salt breath test consists of ingesting ^{14}C-glycinecholate, which is deconjugated by the bacteria in the intestine. The radiolabeled glycine is absorbed and metabolized, and ultimately $^{14}CO_2$ is excreted and can be measured in the breath.

The Pancreas

The pancreas is made up of tubuloalveolar exocrine glands interspersed with endocrine islets. The exocrine glands drain into a series of ducts. A division of function exists between the acinar cells and the ductal cells of the tubuloalveolar glands. The **acinar cells** are responsible for the production and secretion of many of the digestive proteins, including proteases (mainly trypsin and chymotrypsin), amylase, lipase, and nucleases. The **ductal epithelium,** on the other hand, secretes a bicarbonate-rich watery solution that serves to alkalinize the duodenal contents.

Pancreatic enzymes are synthesized in the acinar cells as inactive precursors (proenzymes) in the rough endoplasmic reticulum, processed through the Golgi apparatus, and stored in vesicles or zymogen granules. Secretion occurs by fusion of the zymogen granules with the apical membrane and exocytosis. The proenzymes are later activated by enterokinase in the duodenum. Prior to release into the duodenum, however, the water and **electrolyte composition** of the pancreatic secretion is altered by the ductal epithelium. Bicarbonate is actively secreted in the proximal ducts and then exchanged for chloride in the distal ducts (Figure 17-8). The final electrolyte composition depends on the flow

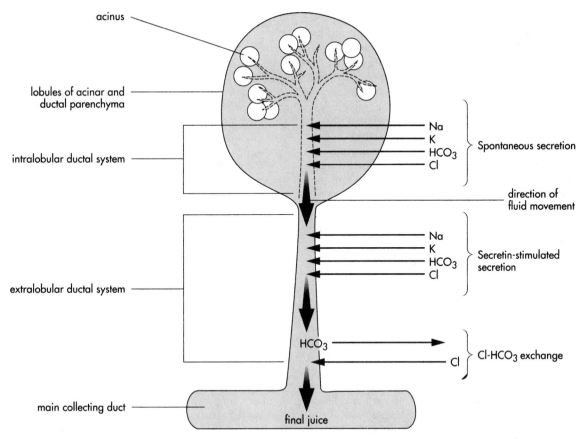

Figure 17-8 Schematic representation of pancreatic electrolyte secretion at the whole tissue level. The separation of spontaneous electrolyte and protein secretion in the intralobular ducts indicates functionally distinct and not necessarily spatially distinct processes. (Reproduced from Swanson CH, Solomon AK. A micropuncture investigation of the whole tissue mechanism of electrolyte secretion by in vitro rabbit pancreas. *J Gen Physiol* 1973;62:426.)

rate. At rapid rates, there is little time for bicarbonate-chloride exchange, and the final bicarbonate concentration is quite high (135 mEq/L).

Pancreatic secretion is controlled by secretin, CCK-PZ, and ACh, as discussed in the next chapter. These molecules bind to specific receptors on the ductal epithelial and acinar cell membranes. Secretin activates adenylate cyclase, causing a rise in intracellular cAMP, which in turn activates cytoplasmic protein kinases. Alternatively, calcium is the second messenger for the CCK-PZ and ACh stimulation of acinar cells. The CCK-PZ- and ACh-receptor complex mediates the formation of inositol triphosphate, which releases calcium from intracellular organelles. The rise in intracellular calcium activates various protein kinases, which ultimately result in exocytosis of zymogen granules at the apical cell membrane.

CONTROL OF PANCREATIC SECRETION

Pancreatic secretion is subject to both hormonal and neural control. **Cholecystokinin-pancreozymin** and **secretin** are the major hormones stimulating pancreatic secretion, although **gastrin** and other peptides such as neurotensin and vasoactive intestinal peptide also play a role. **Neural input** from the vagal release of ACh as well as local neural reflexes (also through ACh) act directly on the acinar and ductal cells to stimulate secretion. Inhibition of pancreatic secretion mainly occurs by attenuation of the above stimuli, but **somatostatin** and perhaps pancreatic polypeptide also inhibit pancreatic secretion. Further, trypsin and chymotrypsin in the intestine exert a negative feedback inhibition of further enzyme release through unclear mechanisms.

As with gastric acid secretion, there are three phases of pancreatic secretion in response to a meal. The **cephalic phase** is mediated by the vagus nerve, which not only stimulates the acinar cells directly but also stimulates antral gastrin release, which enhances pancreatic secretion. The **gastric phase** is based on the release of gastrin as well as local and vagovagal reflexes in response to antral distension. The **intestinal phase** is mediated by secretin and CCK-PZ. **Secretin** is released in response to acidification of the duodenum and acts to increase secretion of the bicarbonate-rich solution from the ductal epithelial cells. Cholecystokinin-pancreozymin is released in response to fats and partially digested proteins in the duodenum and primarily stimulates the acinar cell secretion of the digestive enzymes.

DISORDERS OF PANCREATIC FUNCTION

Acute pancreatitis results from the inappropriate activation of pancreatic enzymes and autodigestion of pancreatic and peripancreatic tissues precipitated by any one of a number of factors. Normally three protective mechanisms exist to prevent enzyme activation. First, the enzymes are secreted as inactive precursors to be activated by enterokinases in the duodenum. Second, protease inhibitors are secreted by the acinar cells and mix with the proenzymes in the pancreatic duct. Third, the sphincter of Oddi prevents reflux of duodenal contents into the pancreatic duct, avoiding early activation of pancreatic enzymes.

These protective mechanisms may be overcome by various factors such as endotoxins or exotoxins, ischemia, trauma, and viruses. Pancreatic duct obstruction may play a role. The common channel theory proposes that bile reflux into the pancreatic duct is the initiating event in proenzyme activation in gallstone pancreatitis. Activation of proteases eventually leads to the activation of other enzymes such as lipases, amylases, nucleases, and collagenases, resulting in autodigestion and elevation of various enzymes in the serum and urine.

Unlike acute pancreatitis, **chronic pancreatitis** is associated with permanent loss of glandular function owing to progressive fibrosis. Pancreatic insufficiency with loss of exocrine function results in maldigestion of fats and proteins, malabsorption, and severe malnutrition. Oral pancreatic enzyme replacement may relieve the steatorrhea by improving digestion and absorption of fats and allow for some weight gain.

EVALUATION OF PANCREATIC FUNCTION

Serum levels of pancreatic enzymes are often elevated in the setting of acute pancreatitis, though the degree of elevation does not seem to correlate with the severity of the attack. Serum amylase and lipase are most commonly used clinically to identify acute pancreatitis, although other enzymes may also be elevated. The urinary amylase-creatinine ratio may be a more sensitive indicator of pancreatitic inflammation.

The malabsorption associated with pancreatic insufficiency is mainly due to the maldigestion of fats in the absence of pancreatic lipase. The diagnosis of steatorrhea can be made by examination of the stool with Sudan stain and quantification of 72-hour fecal fats.

The **Lundh test meal** provides another measure of pancreatic function. A standardized test meal of fats, carbohydrate, and protein is given that results in the endogenous release of CCK-PZ and stimulation of pancreatic secretion. Intraduodenal trypsin concentrations can then be measured to assess the adequacy of pancreatic function. Duodenal contents can also be analyzed after stimulation with exogenous secretin or CCK.

The **bentiromide test** of pancreatic exocrine function involves the measurement of para-aminobenzoic acid in the urine. A synthetic peptide, benzoyl-tyrolyl-*p*-aminobenzoate, is administered orally that is then cleaved by chymotrypsin, releasing para-aminobenzoic acid, which is absorbed and excreted in the urine.

Bibliography

Aronchick CA, Brooks FP. Anatomy and physiology of the biliary tract. In Berk JE, ed. *Bockus Gastroenterology.* 4th ed. Philadelphia: WB Saunders, 1985:3449–3485.

Brooks FP. Physiology of the exocrine pancreas. In Berk JE, ed. *Bockus gastroenterology.* 4th ed. Philadelphia: WB Saunders, 1985:3844–3876.

Debas, Haile T, Mulholland MW. Drug therapy in peptic ulcer disease. *Curr Probl Surg* 1989;26(1):1.

Guyton AC. *Textbook of medical physiology.* 7th ed. Philadelphia: WB Saunders, 1986:770–786.

Mansbach CM II, Grundy SM. Bile acid and cholesterol homeostasis. In Berk JE, ed. *Bockus gastroenterology.* 4th ed. Philadelphia: WB Saunders, 1985:1567–1596.

Small DM. Pathogenesis of cholesterol stones In Berk JE, ed. *Bockus gastroenterology.* 4th ed. Philadelphia: WB Saunders, 1985:3499–3508.

Wolfe MM, Soll AH. The physiology of gastric acid secretion. *N Engl J Med* 1988;319(26):1707–1715.

Kathleen J. Reilly

18 ENDOCRINE FUNCTION OF THE GASTROINTESTINAL TRACT

The Amine Precursor Uptake and Decarboxylation (APUD) Cell Theory
The Brain-Gut Axis
Mechanism of Secretion and Receptor Interaction
Individual Gastrointestinal Hormones
   Gastrin
   Cholecystokinin
   Secretin
   Gastric Inhibitory Peptide
   Enteroglucagon
   Somatostatin
   Neurotensin
   Motilin
   Peptide YY
Enteric Neuropeptides
   Vasoactive Intestinal Peptide
   Bombesin and Gastrin-Releasing Peptide
   Substance P
   Serotonin
   Neuropeptide Y
   Opioid Peptides/Enkephalins
Pancreatic Hormones
   Insulin
   Glucagon
   Pancreatic Polypeptide

The gastrointestinal tract is the most complex of endocrine organs. Its effector cells are located diffusely throughout the digestive tract and it lacks discrete glandular components, making this system difficult to classify and study. However, the diffuse nature of the system does not change its essential function: that is, the production of chemical messengers to execute vital communication between cells. An additional difficulty

in classification of gastrointestinal hormones is that control of gut peptides is not always classically "endocrine" in nature; neurocrine and paracrine regulation are frequently involved as well. These properties cannot be completely separated, as some peptides are known to have more than one mechanism of action.

A **hormone** is conventionally defined as a chemical transmitter synthesized by endocrine cells, often grouped together into ductless glands, and secreted into the blood for transport to distant sites where it acts on the internal metabolism of another cell or group of cells. The term **paracrine** is used to indicate hormonelike action of a chemical messenger that is produced by an endocrine cell but that is released into the interstitium to act on cells located close to the cells in which it is synthesized, not requiring blood transport. Because the chemical messenger does not enter the bloodstream it is not technically a hormone, but paracrine function may be considered local hormone action. **Neurocrine** function includes neurosecretory cells located in the central and peripheral nervous system that produce a chemical substance that is transported along the nerve axon and released from nerve endings. The transmitter may then act via crossing a synaptic gap (neurocrine proper), by entering the circulation (neuroendocrine), or by diffusion through the interstitium (neuroparacrine). Neurocrine function cannot be separated from classical endocrine function in the gut, as will be described later.

The contribution of paracrine and neurocrine factors in cellular communication may indicate that traditional methods of evaluation of endocrine function, primarily measurement of peripheral hormone levels by venous blood sampling, may be inadequate to evaluate not only effective hormone concentration, but also hormonal action on target cells. Rather, receptor antagonist and specific antiserum studies will be necessary to quantify activity and assess regulation on a cellular level.

This chapter will discuss the major recognized hormones of the gastrointestinal system. There will be a description of the structure of each hormone as it is functionally relevant, the stimuli for and mechanisms of secretion, actions of that hormone, and finally pathophysiology associated with each hormone.

The Amine-Precursor Uptake and Decarboxylation (APUD) Cell Theory

Cells with unique staining properties were described by histologists in the mid-1800s and called acidophilic, basophilic, osmiophilic, or chromaffin cells (by analogy to adrenal chromaffin cells). When the silver-reducing power of these cells was recognized, they were then grouped as **argentaffin cells.** One product contained in the secretory granules of argentaffin and chromaffin cells was identified as **5-hydroxytryptamine (serotonin).**

In 1966, Pearse first used the **APUD** concept to group this series of cells, with common histologic and chemical features, that functioned in the synthesis and secretion of gut mediators. The acronym APUD was employed to describe the unifying characteristics of these cells; the letter A refers to their (inconstant) content of endogenous **a**mines; P and U to their potential for preferential **u**ptake of the amino acid **p**recursors of the two fluorogenic amines, dopamine and 5-hydroxytryptamine; and the letter D, to the **d**ecarboxylation of these amines. Some authors added an S to the end to indicate the **s**torage function of these cells as well.

Although the term APUD describes the amine-handling function of these cells, their common ultrastructural features and cytochemical properties are what led to their amalgamation as a group. These cell features are the presence of specific, characteristic cytoplasmic granules; a high content of esterases or cholinesterases; and high levels of α-glycerophosphate dehydrogenase.

The APUD series has been revised and expanded and now is described as having a central division, consisting of cells of the pituitary (**melanocyte-stimulating hormone [MSH]** and **adrenocorticotropic hormone [ACTH]**-producing cells), pineal gland and hypothala-

mus, and a peripheral division, including the **gastroenteropancreatic (GEP)** system, endocrine cells of the lung, melanoblasts of the skin, adrenal chromaffin cells, thyroid C cells, parathyroid cells, carotid body type I cells, and cells of the urogenital tract. Included within this classification are approximately 40 amines and peptides.

Defects in the APUD cell concept do exist. Both endodermal and neuroectodermal origins of gut endocrine-paracrine cells have been considered, and the embryonal origin of the APUD cells has been the source of much controversy. While some APUD cells do appear to have neural crest or neuroectodermal embryonic origins, it is clear that several, i.e., antral G cells, do not. Conversely, some endodermally derived cells found in the gastrointestinal tract *are* capable of uptake and processing of bioamine precursors. Also, not all hormone-producing cells are capable of amine precursor uptake and decarboxylation.

The Brain-Gut Axis

In addition to a common embryologic origin of neural and endocrine tissues, a functional link was discovered when substance P, a peptide first isolated from the brain, was pinpointed to nerves and endocrine cells of the gut. Thus was recognized the first of many hormones and peptides that are found and presumably function in both the nervous and endocrine systems and together compose the so-called brain-gut axis. Other familiar hormones in this group include **neurotensin, serotonin, enkephalin, somatostatin, cholecystokinin (CCK), gastrin,** and **vasoactive intestinal peptide (VIP).** These peptides and bioamines each appear to have distinct pharmacology and physiology, which differ with each target tissue. How this distinction and selectivity for target tissues is maintained, except for the exclusion properties of the blood-brain barrier, is not yet clear.

Mechanism of Secretion and Receptor Interaction

Classically, a hormone produced by one cell is secreted into the bloodstream and causes action or regulation of a cell distant from its parent cell. Hormone receptors in general are proteins or glycoproteins located on the cell membrane of target cells that are able to bind the hormone and, in so doing, convey an intracellular message or action.

Throughout the body two distinct intracellular messenger systems have been identified—namely, the **cyclic adenosine monophosphate (cAMP)** and **calcium/cyclic guanosine monophosphate (Ca/cGMP)** systems. Those gastrointestinal hormones known to work via cAMP include glucagon, secretin, VIP, and **gastric inhibitory peptide (GIP)**. Hormone binding to the cell membrane activates the enzyme adenylate cyclase, which, in the presence of magnesium, converts ATP to cAMP, which, in turn, binds to a protein kinase, thereby activating it. The protein kinase, then, in the presence of calcium and ATP, phosphorylates any of a variety of intracellular enzymes, appropriately activating or inactivating them and thereby altering cell function. The hormones gastrin and CCK are thought to act via stimulation of both release of intracellular calcium and influx of extracellular calcium. The calcium may cause altered enzyme activity itself or may cause accumulation of cGMP, which will lead to altered cellular phosphoinositol metabolism and thereby convey a cellular message. Many hormones, including insulin and somatostatin, are not known to work through secondary messengers but have widespread effects on ion movement, glucose transport, and enzyme activation and also on DNA, RNA, and protein synthesis.

Individual Gastrointestinal Hormones (Table 18-1)

GASTRIN

One of the earliest identified endocrine cells of the gut was the gastrin-producing **G cell,** found primarily in the gastric antrum and sparsely distributed in the duodenum. The G cell is easily identified in the glands of the antral mucosa as a medium-sized ovoid or pear-shaped cell with hormone-containing vesicular granules located at the base, close to the blood supply.

Chemically, gastrin is a peptide that exists in one of several forms. Because the carboxyl-terminal pentapeptide sequence is identical with that of CCK, gastrin can activate CCK receptors (i.e., those for gallbladder con-

traction) and CCK can activate gastrin receptors (i.e., those for acid secretion). However, each peptide has its most potent effects at its own receptor.

Gastrin release is induced by the presence of peptides, amino acids, or calcium in the gastric lumen, and by antral distension. Intraluminal (but not intravenous) phenylalanine and tryptophan are the amino acids that most strongly stimulate gastrin release. Vagal stimulation causes gastrin secretion. β-Adrenergic stimulation also induces gastrin release that may be reduced by administration of a beta blocker. **Bombesin,** also known as **gastrin-releasing peptide (GRP),** is another neural stimulant of gastrin secretion. Gastrin release is inhibited by acidification of gastric contents to a pH below 3, by somatostatin, and by topical administration of certain prostaglandins.

Actions

The primary action of gastrin is stimulation of **gastric acid secretion.** Gastrin causes increased mucosal blood flow to the acid-producing areas of the stomach and increased secretion of **pepsinogen** (which may in fact be secondary to the increased luminal acidity). **Histamine, acetylcholine,** and gastrin interact to determine overall gastric acid secretion. Interruption of cephalic-vagal mechanisms, i.e., by vagotomy or anticholinergic medication, will decrease the response of acid-producing cells to gastrin. Histamine (H2) blockers have a similar effect, reducing histamine-stimulated acid production.

Lesser effects of gastrin include mild stimulation of antral motility, stimulation of pancreatic enzyme secretion, and increased secretion of intrinsic factor. Gastrin has an important trophic effect, particularly on the acid-secreting mucosa of the stomach. Gastrin stimulates DNA, RNA, and protein synthesis in the small intestine, colon, and oxyntic gland area of the stomach, but not in the esophagus or gastric antrum. A small trophic effect is exerted on the pancreas, but it is considered minor in comparison to that of CCK. The trophic effects of gastrin are inhibited by secretin and VIP. It is interesting that gastrin-secreting tumors lead to hypertrophy and hyperplasia of the acid-secreting mucosa of the stomach but lesser sustained elevations of gastrin (i.e., postvagotomy) do not produce similar hyperplasia.

There has been much debate over the role of gastrin on **lower esophageal sphincter (LES)** tone. Gastrin has been thought to increase LES pressure, at least at

Table 18-1. Gastrointestinal Hormones

Hormone	Major Site of Secretion	Major Stimulants of Secretion	Primary Actions
Gastrin	Antrum Duodenum	Peptides, AA's, C²⁺, antral distension, vagal and adrenergic	Stimulates gastric acid and pepsinogen secretion Stimulates gastric mucosal growth
CCK	Duodenum Jejunum [Ileum]	Fat components Peptides Amino acids	Pancreatic endocrine and exocrine stimulation With secretin, stimulates pancreatic alkaline secretion Gallbladder contraction Sphincter of Oddi relaxation Inhibits gastric emptying
Secretin	Duodenum Jejunum [Ileum]	Luminal acidity Fatty acids	With CCK, stimulates alkaline pancreatic secretion Pancreatic insulin secretion Increased volume and alkalinity of bile Inhibits gastric acid secretion
GIP	Duodenum Jejunum	Glucose Fat and protein Adrenergic stimulation	Inhibits gastric acid and pepsin secretion Enhances pancreatic insulin release in response to hyperglycemia
Entero-glucagon	Small bowel (esp. terminal ileum)	Intraluminal, glucose, fat	May compete with pancreatic glucagon ?
Somatostatin	Pancreatic islets (D cells) Pylorus Duodenum	*Pancreas:* glucose, amino acids, CCK *Gut:* fat, protein, acid	Inhibits release of most GI hormones Inhibits gastric acid secretion Inhibits small intestinal water and electrolyte secretion Inhibits secretion of pancreatic hormones
Neurotensin	Ileum Rest of GI tract	Fat components	Unknown; possible inhibition of gastric secretion and emptying; may alter intestinal motility pattern
Motilin	Duodenum Jejunum	?Nervous stimulation	Stimulates upper GI tract motility May initiate the migrating motor complex
Peptide YY	Terminal ileum Colon Rectum	Fatty acids, ?CCK Bile	Inhibits autonomic neurotransmission to the GI tract (probably β-adrenergic) Inhibits pancreatic bicarbonate secretion Inhibits contraction of the gallbladder

CCK, Cholecystokinin; GIP, gastric inhibitory peptide.

supraphysiologic levels; its regulatory role on LES pressure under normal conditions remains controversial.

Pathophysiology

Hypersecretion of gastrin is most commonly due to the presence of a **gastrinoma,** as in **Zollinger-Ellison syndrome (ZES).** Retained antral mucosa after antrectomy and Billroth II gastrojejunostomy also causes basal acid hypersecretion and hyperplasia of acid-secreting mucosa. Primary G-cell hyperplasia and hypergastrinemia is found in patients with a hyposecretory or achlorhydric state owing to atrophic gastritis or after vagotomy. Less common causes include pyloric stenosis, gastric outlet obstruction, and short-bowel syndrome. Hypergastrinemia frequently causes severe peptic ulcer disease and diarrhea. Deficiency of gastrin-producing cells has not been reported.

The Zollinger-Ellison syndrome describes patients with a triad of gastric acid hypersecretion, ulcer diathesis refractory to conventional medical and surgical therapy, and a gastrin-producing tumor. Diarrhea (33%) and hypokalemia are also frequently present. The tumors are usually multiple (70%) and occur most commonly in the pancreas, less frequently in the upper duodenum or antrum, and very rarely in other sites. Although there are no gastrin-producing cells in the pancreas, the cells of pancreatic gastrinomas frequently resemble gastric G cells. Others believe that the pancreatic D cell (see below, Somatostatin) is the most likely source of gastrin production in pancreatic gastrinomas. Gastrinomas may produce other hormones, including pancreatic polypeptide, insulin, and ACTH.

The diagnosis of ZES is made by demonstrating basal acid secretion of more than 10 to 15 mEq/h and hypergastrinemia. Thirty percent of patients also have associated endocrine disorders, including insulinoma, hyperparathyroidism, pituitary tumor, or adrenal adenoma. Radiologically, enlarged gastric mucosal folds are observed, one or more ulcers are identified, and there is usually increased gastric and intestinal fluid content. Fasting hypergastrinemia is diagnostic but is actually found in only 50% of patients. A variety of provocative tests are used in diagnosis of ZES, but none alone is diagnostic.

CHOLECYSTOKININ

Cholecystokinin is produced by **I cells** found in the duodenum and jejunum, and less commonly in the ileum. It was originally isolated as a 33 amino acid peptide, but it has many naturally occurring molecular forms. High concentrations of various forms of CCK peptides in the cerebral cortex have also been demonstrated. The I cell consists of granules that are solid, less vesicular than those found in G cells, and nonreactive with silver stains. These cells are identified immunohistochemically with antibodies directed against the non-C-terminal portion of the molecule (the portion that is distinct from the gastrin molecule). Cholecystokinin contains a sulfated tyrosyl at position 7; desulfation produces a peptide that has the biological activity of gastrin.

Fat components in the small intestinal lumen are the most potent stimulants of CCK release. A fatty acid chain length of at least nine carbons is the minimum necessary for stimulation; triglycerides cause no stimulation unless they become hydrolyzed to monoglycerides. Micelle formation from fatty acids with bile acids markedly enhances release. Peptides and essential amino acids both cause release of CCK, but undigested proteins have a minimal effect. Tryptophan and phenylalanine elicit the strongest amino-acid-stimulated response. Cholecystokinin secretion appears to be independent of vagal stimulation; however, vagal stimulation or vagotomy will alter the effect of CCK on its target tissues, namely, the gallbladder and pancreas.

Actions

Cholecystokinin is a major stimulant of pancreatic **enzyme secretion.** Cholecystokinin also stimulates pancreatic **endocrine secretion** (insulin and glucagon) and potentiates the primary effect of secretin in stimulating pancreatic water and bicarbonate secretion. The mechanism of secretion is via alteration of intracellular calcium movement, cGMP levels, and phosphoinositol metabolism. Cholecystokinin has a trophic effect on the pancreas and in combination with secretin produces dramatic increases in pancreatic weight, DNA, RNA, and protein content.

Cholecystokinin acts on gastrointestinal smooth muscle. It is a potent regulator of biliary smooth muscle, affecting **gallbladder contraction** and **relaxation of the sphincter of Oddi.** This effect on the gallbladder is 100 times as strong as that of pentagastrin and most likely a direct one, as it is not inhibited by atropine or other neuromuscular blockers.

Cholecystokinin causes relaxation of the LES and has been shown in vitro to antagonize a constricting action of gastrin at this site. Cholecystokinin also affects gastrointestinal motility, inhibiting gastric emptying of liquids and, experimentally, increasing small intestinal transit time, possibly by disruption of the migrating motor complex (see Chapter 16). Cholecystokinin inhibits stimulated gastric acid secretion and is one of the candidate **enterogastrones,** substances believed to be responsible for fat-induced inhibition of gastric acid secretion.

Cholecystokinin-8 has been postulated as a mediator of the sensation of satiety when food is present in the stomach or small intestine. Since CCK is found also in the brain and cerebrospinal fluid and does not cross the blood-brain barrier readily, CCK of central origin may have a role in regulation of behavior and food intake.

Serum levels of CCK have been found to be unchanged after gastric surgery for morbid obesity.

Pathophysiology

Impaired CCK release has been documented in patients with upper small intestinal celiac disease that corrects with treatment of the condition. No documented CCK-secreting tumors are known.

SECRETIN

Secretin is composed of 27 amino acids arranged in a helical pattern. Structurally, it shares remarkable similarities with VIP, GIP, and pancreatic glucagon. Secretin is produced by **S cells** found throughout the small intestine, especially concentrated in the duodenum and jejunum. S cells contain small polymorphic granules and are argyrophilic, in contrast to CCK-containing I cells. No secretin has been demonstrated in pancreatic extracts. Secretin activity has been detected in brain preparations.

The most potent stimulant for secretion of secretin is **intraluminal acid.** Secretin is released when the duodenal pH drops below 4.5. To a lesser degree, fatty acids will affect its release. Secretin is not stimulated by vagal impulses, and vagotomy has no effect on secretin responses.

Actions

Secretin stimulates the pancreas to secrete large volumes of alkalotic pancreatic fluid. When given alone it causes only minimal pancreatic enzyme secretion, but, with CCK, the combined effects on both pancreatic enzyme and bicarbonate secretion are more than doubled. This additive effect is likely a result of stimulating different mechanisms of secretion; whereas CCK function is mediated by the Ca/cGMP system, secretin utilizes cAMP as its intracellular messenger.

Despite the fact that secretin is not released in response to intraduodenal glucose, it does stimulate pancreatic insulin secretion and enhances the insulin response to glucose. The insulin response to secretin is directly proportional to the basal insulin concentration. The effects of secretin on insulin secretion are not altered by surgical vagotomy, atropine, or beta blockade with propranolol.

Secretin increases biliary bicarbonate, chloride, and water secretion, as well as biliary volume, and decreases the concentration of bile salts. It appears to act directly on the bile ducts. Secretin stimulates the secretion of pepsin into the gastric lumen while inhibiting gastric acid secretion. Secretin antagonizes the effects of gastrin; and in patients with hypergastrinemia owing to atrophic gastritis or isolated retained antrum, secretin acts to decrease serum gastrin levels. Secretin has been nicknamed "nature's antacid," because almost all of its actions decrease the amount of acid in the duodenum. Secretin also promotes pepsinogen secretion by chief cells.

Other effects of secretin include slowing of gastric emptying and upper intestinal motor activity, relaxation of lower esophageal sphincter pressure, and a mild diuresis.

Pathophysiology

No cases of isolated secretin production by tumor have been reported; however, there has been one case in which a pancreatic tumor produced five different hormones, including secretin.

GASTRIC INHIBITORY PEPTIDE

Gastric inhibitory peptide (GIP) producing **K cells** are found in the human duodenum and jejunum and are ultrastructurally unique, containing large granules that show a targetlike pattern on silver staining. Gastric inhibitory peptide is a linear peptide containing 43 amino acid residues.

Stimulants for GIP release include intraduodenal (but not intravenous) carbohydrate, fat, and protein. Interestingly, specific amino acids, including leucine, lysine, isoleucine, histidine, arginine, and threonine cause GIP release, whereas phenylalanine, tryptophan, and valine, which are known to cause release of gastrin, CCK, and pancreatic polypeptide, have no effect on GIP release. GIP secretion does not appear to be affected by vagal innervation, but β-adrenergic stimulation may cause release. GIP secretion in response to a meal may be regulated by other gastrointestinal and pancreatic hormones. For example, exogenous glucagon decreases fasting serum GIP concentrations and also markedly inhibits the response to a test meal in humans.

Actions

Gastric inhibitory peptide has two major physiologic functions: inhibition of gastric secretion and enhancement of insulin release in the presence of hyperglycemia. As its name suggests, GIP is a strong inhibitor of pentagastrin-stimulated acid and pepsin secretion and a somewhat less potent inhibitor of histamine-stimulated gastric secretion. In addition, GIP inhibits water and electrolyte absorption in the small bowel.

Glucose stimulates endogenous GIP secretion. GIP, in turn, enhances endogenous insulin release in the presence of hyperglycemia. It is possible that GIP may account for the increased glucose excretion and enhanced insulin responses obtained during intestinal absorption of glucose as compared with intravenous administration of glucose, and some would prefer the term "glucose-dependent insulinotropic peptide" rather than "gastric inhibitory peptide." Put simply, GIP release is stimulated by nutrients in the intestine and, in turn, in the presence of hyperglycemia, plays a role in regulation of pancreatic insulin secretion.

Pathophysiology

In patients with chronically elevated GIP levels, chronic watery diarrhea has been reported. In addition, enhanced GIP secretion to glucose or fat stimulation has been described in patients with diabetes mellitus, obesity, chronic pancreatitis, and duodenal ulcer.

ENTEROGLUCAGON

The finding that total pancreatectomy in dogs did not eliminate the presence of immunoreactive glucagon from the circulation began a search for the source of molecules with glucagonlike activity. This group consists of a variety of peptides that together are known as enteroglucagon, and many authors prefer the term **glucagonlike immunoreactivity.**

Immunochemical staining characteristics have identified the **L cell,** found throughout the small and large intestine, as the source of enteroglucagon. The concentration of nonpancreatic glucagon immunoreactivity is highest in the terminal ileum and colon.

Oral administration of glucose inhibits release of pancreatic glucagon but actually stimulates intestinal enteroglucagon secretion. In addition, experimental administration of fat into the duodenum leads to an increase in both pancreatic glucagon and enteroglucagon, whereas instillation of fat into the distal small bowel leads to an increase only of enteroglucagon.

Actions

The biological actions of extrapancreatic glucagon are not clear; however, radioimmunoassays have shown that enteroglucagon may compete with pancreatic glucagon at the receptor level. The actions of pancreatic glucagon, including glycogenolysis, lipolysis, gluconeogenesis, and ketogenesis have not yet been found to be attributable to nonpancreatic glucagon substrates, and further investigation is warranted.

Pathophysiology

One case report exists of a patient with an endocrine tumor in the kidney that produced enteroglucagon. Pathologically, the patient had hyperplasia of intestinal villi, slowed transit time, and minimal fat malabsorption. These abnormalities corrected after tumor resection. No deficiency states have been identified.

SOMATOSTATIN

Somatostatin is secreted as a 116 amino acid precursor known as **prosomatostatin** that is processed to two physiologically active peptides of 14 and 28 amino acids each. Somatostatin has been identified in nerves and cell bodies in the central and the peripheral nervous systems. In the gastrointestinal tract, somatostatin is secreted by endocrine D, or δ **cells,** throughout the gut; they are most dense in the pylorus, duodenum, and **pancreatic islets.** D cells are ultrastructurally unique in possessing dendriticlike cell processes that lie in close contact with blood vessels and other cells, particularly gastric G and parietal cells and pancreatic β (see below, Insulin) cells. The morphology and wide distribution of D cells is functionally important since somatostatin is thought to have a paracrine (local modulatory) function, as well as significant effects on endocrine and exocrine secretions in the gastrointestinal tract.

In animal studies, somatostatin release is stimulated by intraluminal infusion of fat, protein, acid, and sucrose. The source of this somatostatin does not appear to be the gastric antrum, as antrectomy does not alter stimulated plasma levels. The mechanism of secretion may involve endogenous opioids, as secretory responses are blunted by naloxone. Highest values of somatostatin are found in the interdigestive period. Augmented release has been found in humans during insulin hypoglycemia, an effect abolished by vagotomy. Pancreatectomy does not diminish baseline or stimulated plasma somatostatin levels.

Actions

Somatostatin has a wide variety of effects on the gastrointestinal tract, including **inhibition of release of several peptide hormones and antagonism of their peripheral effects,** as well as influences on gut motility and absorption. In the brain, somatostatin inhibits release of **growth hormone** and **thyroid-stimulating hormone** from the pituitary.

In the stomach, somatostatin plays a role in regulation of gastric acid production. Experimentally, it is released in response to duodenal acidification and acts to inhibit gastric acid release. Intravenous somatostatin inhibits the gastric acid response to gastrin and to cholinergic stimulation, but has little influence on histamine-induced secretion. In addition, somatostatin causes inhibition of basal, food-stimulated, and neurally stimulated gastrin release and markedly decreases serum gastrin levels in gastrin-producing tumors.

Although most evidence indicates that somatostatin acts humorally on the stomach, i.e., via inhibition of gastrin secretion and parietal cell response, direct local action of somatostatin on parietal cells has also been postulated. Support for this concept is evident from the proximity of the cell processes of D cells to parietal cells. When somatostatin antiserum is infused in an isolated gastric preparation, acid production increases markedly.

Somatostatin inhibits absorption of amino acids in the small intestine. In addition, it blocks glucagon-induced jejunal water and electrolyte secretion. The latter effect may account for its therapeutic use in diarrheal states.

Somatostatin inhibits the release of most known gastrointestinal hormones. A tonic role for suppression of pituitary and gut hormones, but not pancreatic hormones, is suggested by the observation that somatostatin antiserum administration leads to increases in growth hormones and glucagonlike immunoreactivity, but not insulin or pancreatic glucagon.

Somatostatin is secreted by D cells of pancreatic islets in the same forms found in the gut. It inhibits the secretion of insulin, glucagon, and pancreatic polypeptide. The secretion of pancreatic somatostatin is stimulated by several of the same stimuli that increase insulin secretion, i.e., glucose and amino acids, particularly arginine and leucine. In addition, CCK infusion stimulates pancreatic somatostatin release. Somatostatin binds directly to the secretory vesicles containing insulin. The degree of inhibition of insulin secretion is directly proportional to the number of islet receptors bound by somatostatin that, in turn, is proportional to the degree of insulin stimulation. This feedback system is ideal, because insulin release is directly coupled to a mechanism for its inhibition without requiring an intermediate messenger. It appears that alteration in somatostatin receptor binding, rather than local or systemic concentrations, is most important in regulation of insulin secretion.

Pathophysiology

D cell tumors of the pancreas are known as **somatostatinomas** and clinically are characterized by diabetes mellitus, maldigestion with diarrhea and steatorrhea, cholelithiasis, and hypochlorhydria. These tumors are rare and slow-growing, but highly malignant. They are found most frequently in the head of the pancreas and are infrequently correctly diagnosed preoperatively. In many cases, the tumors also have associated pancreatic polypeptide cell hyperplasia, which may be responsible for some of the clinical manifestations. Diagnosis is usually made histologically, as tumor cells contain a characteristic granule considered diagnostic. Preoperative venous blood sampling will reveal high levels of somatostatin.

SMS 201-995 is a synthetic octapeptide analog of somatostatin synthesized from native somatostatin. It has been used to reduce hormonally mediated diarrheas and to inhibit the release of hormones from gastrointestinal endocrine tumors, including insulinoma, glucagonoma, gastrinoma, and adult onset nesidioblastosis. It has been found to decrease circulating levels of the ectopically produced hormones by greater than 50%. It has also been proposed for use in postgastrectomy "dumping syndromes," possibly slowing gastrointestinal transit time. It is ineffective in antagonizing diarrhea in cholera-induced intestinal secretion and currently, it is not considered useful in the treatment of diarrhea that is not hormonally mediated. Somatostatin analog is also often effective in decreasing the fluid output of enterocutaneous and pancreatic fistulas, allowing them to close more rapidly and more often spontaneously than with bowel rest alone.

NEUROTENSIN

Neurotensin exists as a tridecapeptide found in identical forms in both brain and gut. The C-terminal region appears to be central in the determination of biologic activity. Neurotensin-secreting **N cells** are found in highest concentration in the ileal mucosa, with fewer numbers in the jejunum, stomach, duodenum, and colon.

Ingestion of a mixed meal results in elevation of neurotensin immunoreactivity, with fat being the strongest stimulant. A minimum fatty acid chain length of four carbons is necessary for a response, and intravenous fat does not elevate plasma neurotensin activity.

Actions

No physiologic role for neurotensin is known. One of the most likely roles for neurotensin is as an **enterogastrone,** mediating inhibition of gastric acid secretion and/or emptying after fat ingestion. It has been shown to inhibit pentagastrin-stimulated gastric acid and pepsin secretion and appears to inhibit gastric motor activity. Neurotensin increases intestinal fluid secretion, augments intestinal blood flow, stimulates glycogenolysis and glucagon release, and inhibits insulin release. It stimulates secretion of growth hormone, ACTH, luteinizing hormone, and follicle-stimulating hormone and causes mast cell histamine release. Whether any of these effects are physiologically significant is still unclear.

Pathophysiology

Neurotensin is found in several gastrointestinal and pulmonary tumors, almost always in association with another peptide, and thus when a patient's symptoms are relieved by tumor resection, it has been difficult to ascribe the presence of specific symptoms to neurotensin.

MOTILIN

Motilin is a 22 amino acid peptide isolated from the upper small intestine. The motilin **M** cell is characterized ultrastructurally by small, round, solid granules and microfilaments. Motilin release occurs in the **fasting state,** often corresponding with the onset of the interdigestive myoelectric complex in the duodenum. Acidification of the duodenum produces elevation of plasma motilin, as does fat ingestion. Vagal cholinergic neural pathways may regulate motilin release.

Actions

Motilin acts on smooth muscle of the upper gastrointestinal tract to stimulate motility. There is a strong positive correlation between cyclic increases in plasma motilin levels and initiation of the **interdigestive myoelectric complex.** Motilin initiates myoelectric complexes in the antroduodenal region that are propagated distally in the small intestine.

Motilin causes strong contraction of the LES in the fasting, but not the fed, state. The effect that can be inhibited by atropine and hexamethonium, suggesting a neural mechanism of action. Motilin increases the rate of gastric emptying of liquid, but not solid meals, an effect blocked by vagotomy. Motilin has no known effect on pancreatic secretion but does increase electrical activity of the gallbladder and sphincter of Oddi during the interdigestive period. Central nervous system effects of motilin include excitation of corticospinal neurons, stimulation of feeding, and growth hormone stimulation.

PEPTIDE YY

Peptide YY is a 36 amino acid peptide structurally similar to **pancreatic polypeptide.** The name, peptide YY, is derived from the fact that both the amino- and carboxyl-terminal residues are tyrosine (abbreviated Y). Peptide YY is most prominent in the terminal ileum, rectum, and colon.

Peptide YY is released 10–30 minutes after a mixed meal or intraduodenal administration of bile or fatty acids. Peptide YY release may stem from neural or endocrine signals in the proximal small intestine. Cholecystokinin may be a humoral releasing factor for peptide YY release. Severing neural pathways to the distal bowel has no effect on peptide YY secretion.

Actions

Peptide YY inhibits autonomic neurotransmission in the gastrointestinal tract, possibly by inhibition of β-adrenergic transmission. It halts the migration of interdigestive contractions in the stomach in the fasting, but not the fed, state. It causes inhibition of pancreatic bicarbonate secretion and contraction of the gallbladder.

Exogenously administered peptide YY prolongs small bowel transit time and decreases fluid loss in VIP-induced diarrhea. Exogenous peptide YY also causes inhibition of pancreatic protein secretion at low doses and at high doses will also inhibit pancreatic bicarbonate and gastric acid secretion. This action may prove to be therapeutically useful in patients with gastric and pancreatic fistulas, as well as diarrheal states.

Enteric Neuropeptides

Parasympathetic and sympathetic nervous stimulation have long been known to modulate gastrointestinal function via the classic neurotransmitters acetylcholine and norepinephrine. More recently it has become evident that noncholinergic, nonadrenergic neurotransmitters have actions on the gut that cannot be inhibited by classic cholinergic and adrenergic blockers. In addition, unique nerve endings containing vesicles similar to those found in gut endocrine cells have been recognized within the myenteric nerve plexus.

The enteric neuropeptides (Table 18-2) are a diverse group of molecules with hormonal and paracrine functions, as well as nervous system transmitter function. Peptide synthesis occurs in the neuron cell body, and those destined for secretion are packaged into granules and transported down the axons, where they are stored in the nerve terminals until release.

There is difficulty discriminating between the roles of these neuropeptides as hormones or neurotransmitters. All are present elsewhere in the body in either neurons or endocrine cells. Neuropeptides released from

Table 18-2. Enteric Neuropeptides

Hormone	Major Site of Secretion	Major Stimulants of Secretion	Primary Actions
VIP	Small bowel Colon Gallbladder Pancreas Sphincter	Acid, fat, ethanol Sympathetic stimulation inhibits GI nervous stimulation (possibly nicotinic-receptor mediated)	Increases intestinal, pancreatic, and biliary secretion Relaxes GI smooth muscle Splanchnic vasodilitation
Bombesin/GRP	Gastric antrum and fundus	Vagal stimulation	Excitatory effects on motility and secretion Evokes release of other gut peptides, especially gastrin
Substance P	Gut nerves and endocrine cells	Increased intraluminal pressure	Smooth muscle contraction ?Peristaltic reflex
Serotonin	Pylorus Small bowel Large bowel	Nervous stimulation	Smooth muscle contraction
Neuropeptide Y	Pancreatic neurons	Nervous stimulation	Uncertain actions on distal ileum and colon ?Role in insulin release Inhibits acetylcholine and norepinephrine release May have role in regulation of insulin release
Opioids/enkephalins	Myenteric plexus	Unknown	Depresses acetylcholine release on gut muscle; slows transit time Inhibits pancreatic secretion Enhances electrolyte absorption

GRP, Gastrin-releasing peptide; VIP, vasoactive intestinal polypeptide.

nerve endings may have local paracrine effects or may act hormonally at distant sites after delivery into the circulation. The cellular mechanisms of action are similar to that of other hormones, i.e., binding to cell surface receptors causing changes in calcium flux, intracellular nucleotide levels, and changes in the phosphatidylinositol system.

The peptides now classified as "neuropeptides" include substance P, serotonin, VIP, bombesin–GRP, and the opioids. Some investigators also include somatostatin, CCK, and neurotensin along with newer members **neuropeptide Y** and galanin.

VASOACTIVE INTESTINAL PEPTIDE

Vasoactive intestinal peptide is a 28-residue member of a family of four peptides with remarkably similar amino acid composition, including secretin, glucagon, and GIP. Thus far the existence of specialized endocrine VIP cells distinct from A (see below, Glucagon), K, L, or S cells has not been proven. Vasoactive intestinal peptide was first thought to be located in gut endocrinelike cells, but more recent data point to a purely neural localization in the gut. Vasoactive intestinal peptide is also distributed throughout the brain, peripheral nervous system, and urogenital tract. Vasoactive intestinal polypeptide densely populates the nerve fibers and cell bodies throughout the small bowel, the colon, the gallbladder wall, and the pancreas. It is especially abundant in the gastrointestinal sphincters, including the lower esophageal sphincter, pylorus, sphincter of Oddi, and the openings of the ureters, urethra, and vas deferens. Vasoactive intestinal peptide-containing cell bodies and nerve fibers are found in the celiac, superior mesenteric, and sympathetic ganglia, and VIP-like immunoreactivity has been found in neuroblastomas and astrocytomas.

Electrical nervous stimulation of the pancreas and gastrointestinal tract cause release of VIP. Neither atropine nor β-adrenergic blocking agents inhibit VIP release caused by vagal stimulation, but the response is blocked by hexamethonium, implicating postsynaptic nicotinic receptor mediation. Splanchnic (sympathetic) stimulation inhibits vagally induced VIP release, possibly via vasoconstriction, impairing delivery into the venous system. Ingestion of a meal in humans does not cause a significant increase in peripheral concentrations of VIP, but intraduodenal instillation of acid, fat, and ethanol causes serum VIP levels to rise.

Actions

Vasoactive intestinal peptide affects many aspects of gastrointestinal function, including intestinal secretion, motility and blood flow, gastric and biliary secretion, pancreatic endocrine and exocrine function, and liver metabolism. Many of these actions are those of its related peptides, secretin and GIP, and some of their physiologic effects may indeed occur via VIP receptors.

Vasoactive intestinal peptide markedly increases intestinal secretion. In the jejunum, VIP has been shown to cause a decrease in water and sodium absorption and an increase in water and electrolyte secretion. Vasoactive intestinal peptide resembles cholera toxin and prostaglandin E_1 in its ability to stimulate adenylate cyclase and cAMP production in intestinal epithelial cells. This stimulation of cAMP production and intestinal secretion can be blocked by somatostatin.

Vasoactive intestinal peptide fibers innervate gastrointestinal circular smooth muscle, causing relaxation. Esophageal distension releases VIP, which in turn causes gastric relaxation. There is also considerable evidence that VIP physiologically mediates relaxation of smooth muscle in blood vessels and thus may be responsible for vasodilatation of gastrointestinal mucosal blood supply.

Vasoactive intestinal peptide is a partial agonist for pancreatic exocrine secretion and may actually mediate the pancreatic responses to vagal stimulation.

Pathophysiology

VIPoma is an islet cell tumor that clinically produces a syndrome of intractable watery diarrhea, hypokalemia and achlorhydria (**WDHA** or **Verner-Morrison** syndrome). Symptoms include massive volumes of tea-colored diarrhea, hypokalemia with serum levels usually below 3 mEq/L, basal gastric hypochlorhydria, or achlorhydria that fails to respond to histamine stimulation, glucose intolerance, hypercalcemia, flushing, an atonic gallbladder, and psychosis. Other clinical derangements frequently result from the severe metabolic abnormalities.

Diagnosis is made by clinical symptomatology, elevated serum VIP levels (present in most, but not all patients), and positive reaction to VIP antiserum. Several cases have been described with all the clinical manifestations of the Verner-Morrison syndrome and a pancreatic tumor, but normal VIP levels and high pancreatic polypeptide levels. In contrast, pancreatic tumors productive of pancreatic polypeptide exist without the WDHA syndrome. Vasoactive intestinal peptide-producing tumors associated with diarrhea are not limited to the pancreas but may also be seen with ganglioneuroma, ganglioneuroblastoma, medullary thyroid carcinoma, pheochromocytoma, or bronchogenic carcinoma. In addition, hypersecretion of several gut secretory products, gastrin, calcitonin, serotonin, prostaglandins, and substance P may produce similar diarrheogenic syndromes.

BOMBESIN AND GASTRIN-RELEASING PEPTIDE

The terms **bombesin** and **gastrin-releasing peptide (GRP)** describe a group of biologically active neuropeptides that are found in both the brain and the gastrointestinal tract and share a common C-terminal sequence. Bombesin is released from the gastric antrum and fundus in response to vagal stimulation. Bombesin receptors have been identified on pancreatic acinar cells and cellular action is conveyed via the Ca/cGMP intracellular mechanism.

Actions

Bombesin has excitatory effects on motility and secretion. This group of peptides likely elicits release of other gut peptides, including GIP, pancreatic polypeptide, insulin, glucagon, and somatostatin, and these may account for many of its postulated effects. Bombesin has been proven to release gastrin and it appears that bombesin/GRP peptides elicit vagally evoked gastrin secretion that is not blocked by atropine. Few other actions of bombesin are known, but it may cause release of substance P from canine colon, increasing contractility in the colonic muscularis mucosa.

SUBSTANCE P

Substance P was the first gut neuropeptide to be discovered. It contains 11 amino acids and is found throughout the brain and spinal cord, in gut nerves and mucosal endocrine cells. There is debate as to whether the majority of plasma substance P is of neuronal or mucosal cellular origin. It has been suggested that histamine release may play a role in some of the effects of substance P, as receptors for the peptide are present on mast cells.

Actions

Substance P causes contraction of gastrointestinal smooth muscle. Its effects on smooth muscle are manifested directly on the gut myocytes as well as indirectly by evoking activity in cholinergic myenteric pathways. Substance P is released as a result of increased intraluminal pressure and distension and elicits the peristaltic reflex.

Pathophysiology

There are no pathophysiologic states of isolated substance P secretory abnormalities. Substance P is secreted by some carcinoid tumors.

SEROTONIN

Serotonin (**5-hydroxytryptamine; 5-HT**) is secreted by argentaffin or *enterochromaffin cells* of the gastrointestinal tract. In addition, 5-HT can be detected histochemically in mast cells, thyroid cells, pancreatic B cells, and enterochromaffin cells in the pulmonary system. Enterochromaffin cells are found mostly in the mucosa of the pylorus and in the small and large intestine, with relatively few in the mucosa of the gastric fundus, pancreas and biliary tract. Enterochromaffin cells, although grossly the same, display ultrastructural differences in each type of gastrointestinal mucosa.

Actions

Serotonin acts on nerve cells and/or smooth muscle cells to cause contraction. Evidence exists that serotonin may be an important neurotransmitter in gut motility, mediating excitatory postsynaptic potentials in myenteric plexus neurons. In addition, serotonin may exert some of its effects by releasing acetylcholine.

Pathophysiology

Enterochromaffin cell tumors, in particular carcinoid tumors, release large amounts of serotonin and substance P into the circulation. Carcinoids are tumors that may have their origin in many organs, including breast, lung, liver, gallbladder, thymus, or ovary; but they are most common in the gastrointestinal tract. They may be found anywhere, from mouth to anus, but most commonly in the appendix (35%), small bowel (25%), rectum and rectosigmoid (12%), colon (7%), esophagus and stomach (1%), lungs and bronchi (14%), and other sites (5%). Multiple primaries are not uncommon (occurring in up to 30% of cases) and when present are usually all in the small intestine.

Carcinoid tumors arise from enterochromaffin cells of the gut and frequently are argyrophilic, staining strongly with silver salts. They may secrete a variety of hormones and bioamines, including histamine, serotonin, 5-HT, ACTH, kallikrein, and prostaglandins. Appendiceal carcinoids are usually small (1–2 cm) nodules and rarely metastasize (0.2%). In contrast, extra-appendiceal carcinoids in the gastrointestinal tract are submucosal lesions that are usually less than 3 cm in diameter but may become much larger. The overlying mucosa may be intact, making diagnosis difficult.

The size of the tumor correlates with prognosis; most small bowel carcinoids larger than 2 cm and colonic carcinoids larger than 5 cm are associated with metastases. Appendiceal carcinoids are usually asymptomatic; those in other parts of the gastrointestinal tract may be silent for a long period of time but may eventually produce a set of symptoms known as the **carcinoid syndrome.** Serotonin (5-HT) is the major product of the tumor and its metastases; 98% of 5-HT is degraded on first pass through the hepatic and pulmonary circulations to 5-hydroxyindoleacetic acid **(5-HIAA).** Typically the syndrome is seen in patients with extensive liver metastases or in tumors whose venous drainage bypasses the portal system, thus eliminating hepatic deamination of secretory products (i.e., tumors of the lung or ovary). Only 5–10% of patients with gastrointestinal carcinoids develop carcinoid syndrome. This syndrome consists of vasomotor disturbances, primarily skin flushing; hypermotility of the intestine resulting in episodic watery diarrhea, nausea, and vomiting; bronchospasm, leading to dyspnea and wheezing; right-sided cardiac involvement with valvular thickening and endocardial fibrosis leading to stenosis; and hepatomegaly secondary to hepatic metastases.

Diagnosis is made by the identification of 5-HIAA in the urine. Important in the diagnosis of carcinoid is the fact that it is frequently associated with other malignancies (15% with appendix, 10% with rectal, and 30%

with small intestinal). More than one-half of the concurrent carcinomas occur in the gastrointestinal tract.

Serotonin has also been implicated as a mediator of postgastrectomy dumping and other hypermotility syndromes.

NEUROPEPTIDE Y

Neuropeptide Y is a 36 amino acid peptide that shares structural homology with peptide YY and pancreatic polypeptide. Whereas pancreatic polypeptide's site of action is the endocrine pancreas, and peptide YY acts on the distal ileum and colon, neuropeptide Y immunoreactivity has been detected only in the peripheral and central nervous system. It is present in highest concentrations in nerve fibers in the adrenal medulla and pancreas.

Its actions are unknown, but it has been found to inhibit both acetylcholine and norepinephrine release, and it may have a role in the autonomic regulation of insulin release.

OPIOID PEPTIDES/ENKEPHALINS

The endogenous opiates in the gastrointestinal tract consist of several small peptides derived from two precursors, **proenkephalin** and **prodynorphin**, both derived from a single genome. The extent of their functions is not yet known, although direct evidence exists that enkephalins are synthesized in the myenteric plexus. At least three different binding sites have been identified in the gut (μ, δ, and κ), but there may be others (ε, σ) as in the central nervous system.

Actions

Much of what is known about opioid release comes from antagonism studies with naloxone. Opioids appear to depress acetylcholine release on electrical stimulation of gut muscle, with obvious widespread effects.

The therapeutic value of opiate alkaloids in slowing intestinal transit has long been appreciated in the treatment of diarrhea. Opiates have important antisecretory effects, enhancing electrolyte absorption, probably by actions on the submucosal neuronal plexus. Opiates inhibit pancreatic secretion but have inconsistent effects on gastric acid secretion.

Pancreatic Hormones

The pancreas produces at least four peptides with hormonal activity crucial to gastrointestinal function: insulin, glucagon, somatostatin, and pancreatic polypeptide (Table 18-3). Pancreatic somatostatin secretion was discussed above.

INSULIN

Insulin is a polypeptide consisting of two chains, α and β, linked by disulfide bridges. It is produced in **B, or β cells** in the pancreatic islets of Langerhans. B cells are generally located centrally within the islets and contain rounded vesicles. Insulin is synthesized and transported through the endoplasmic reticulum as **pre–pro-insulin,** which is then modified and folded to form **pro-insulin,** which in turn is cleaved within the secretory vesicle to form insulin. Secreted insulin is attached to a 31 amino acid polypeptide known as the **C (connecting) peptide.** Levels of this peptide can be measured and used

as an index of pancreatic B-cell function in patients receiving exogenous insulin.

Insulin secretion is complex, involving a variety of stimulatory and inhibitory factors. Appropriate secretion requires adequate concentrations of calcium and potassium. The major stimulant for insulin secretion is elevated blood glucose (usually greater than 100 mg/dL), which is sensed directly by the pancreas. The response of insulin secretion to hyperglycemia is biphasic, with an initial rapid rise in insulin levels, followed by a second prolonged response. There is evidence that the initial release of insulin is due to release of intracellular calcium stores, whereas later effects are due to inflow of extracellular calcium into the B cells.

Catecholamines have a dual effect on insulin secretion; they inhibit secretion via α-adrenergic receptors and stimulate β-receptor action. The net effect is usually inhibition of insulin secretion by catecholamines. Stimuli that increase intracellular cAMP levels increase insulin secretion, probably by effects on intracellular calcium levels. These stimuli include β-adrenergic agonists, glucagon, and phosphodiesterase inhibitors (i.e., theophylline). Vagal stimulation of pancreatic islets in-

Table 18-3. Pancreatic Hormones

Hormone	Major Site of Secretion	Major Stimulants of Secretion	Primary Actions
Insulin	B, or β, islet cells	Elevated blood glucose Inhibited by catecholamines Vagal stimulation Glucagon, secretin, CCK, gastrin, GIP	Facilitates glucose uptake by muscle, fat, and white blood cells Increases muscle and hepatic glycogen synthesis Decreases gluconeogenesis Increases lipid synthesis, decreases lipolysis Increases protein synthesis Causes potassium entry into cells
Glucagon	A, or α, islet cells	Stimulated by sympathetic (β-adrenergic) stimulation, starvation, protein meals, hormones Inhibited by glucose, insulin, fatty acids, ketones, α-adrenergic agonists, somatostatin	Gluconeogenesis, glycogenolysis, lipolysis, ketogenesis
Somatostatin		*(See Table 18-1)*	
Pancreatic polypeptide	Pancreatic islets	Protein intake, cholinergic stimulation	Inhibition of pancreatic exocrine secretion

CCK, Cholecystokinin; GIP, gastric inhibitory peptide.

creases insulin secretion. Sympathetic stimulation of the pancreas inhibits secretion. Autonomic innervation of the pancreas is not necessary for plasma glucose regulation. Indeed, the denervated, transplanted pancreas regulates glucose homeostasis normally.

Glucagon, secretin, CCK, gastrin, and GIP all appear to stimulate insulin secretion. GIP, however, appears to be the most potent stimulant to insulin secretion in the presence of hyperglycemia and is believed to act by increasing cAMP level in the B cells. Insulin secretion is inhibited by a number of drugs, including thiazide diuretics and diazoxide.

Actions

Insulin facilitates glucose uptake, primarily in muscle cells, white blood cells, and adipose tissue. It does not cause glucose entry into red blood cells, cells of the brain, kidney, or gastrointestinal mucosa. It increases muscle glycogen synthesis and decreases the release of muscle glucogenic amino acids. Insulin decreases hepatic glucose output, owing to decreased gluconeogenesis and increased glycogen synthesis, and increases hepatic lipid synthesis. It activates lipoprotein lipase and increases triglyceride deposition in adipose tissue.

Insulin increases protein synthesis in ribosomes of muscle and liver cells and decreases muscle protein catabolism. This effect may be partially due to protein sparing in the presence of adequate intracellular glucose concentrations.

Insulin is important in cellular electrolyte balance. It causes potassium to enter cells. Insulin increases the activity of Na,K-ATPase in cell membranes, and in addition transports hydrogen ions (H^+) out of cells in exchange for sodium (Na^+).

Pathophysiology

The clinical syndrome resulting from insulin deficiency is **diabetes mellitus.** In diabetes, numerous biochemical abnormalities are present that result in elevated extracellular blood glucose levels with diminished intracellular glucose concentration. These effects occur most dramatically after a meal and are a consequence of both decreased peripheral glucose utilization caused by impaired glucose entry into cells and increased hepatic glucose production owing to failure of insulin inhibition of gluconeogenesis.

Broadly, diabetes mellitus is characterized by hyperglycemia, glycosuria (because the renal capacity for glucose resorption is exceeded), ketosis, acidosis, polyuria (resulting from osmotic diuresis), polydipsia (owing to resultant dehydration), and polyphagia (from urinary caloric loss). Low intracellular glucose concentration means that energy requirements must be met by mobilization of fat and protein stores. A result of fat metabolism is ketosis.

In diabetes mellitus, there is decreased amino acid entry into muscle cells and increased hepatic amino acid consumption for gluconeogenesis. There is also an increase in amino acid catabolism and diminished muscle protein synthesis, with resultant negative effects on growth and development.

Abnormalities in fat metabolism in diabetes are due to increased lipolysis, production of ketone bodies, and decreased cellular synthesis of fatty acids and triglycerides from glucose. Uncontrolled diabetes can be extremely dangerous with overwhelming ketone production, resulting in acidosis and eventual coma.

Insulin Excess

Insulinomas, or functional B cell tumors of the pancreas, are the most common of the islet cell tumors. In approximately 2% of patients, the tumor may be extrapancreatic, usually adjacent to the pancreas. Most are solitary and benign and are found in any part of the pancreas; approximately 5% are malignant. These tumors secrete insulin and pro-insulin into the plasma at uncontrolled rates. The characteristic clinical triad **(Whipple's triad)** consists of hypoglycemic episodes with serum glucose <50 mg/dL; symptoms of confusion, obtundation, and loss of consciousness that are temporally related to fasting or exercise; and rapid relief of the attacks with administration of oral or parenteral glucose. Patients are usually obese, as a result of overeating to relieve symptoms of hypoglycemia. In chronic cases, polyneuropathy, muscular atrophy, and psychiatric disturbances may occur. Some patients have only mild hypoglycemia and never become symptomatic. Insulinomas may be part of Wermer's syndrome **(MEN I)** and there may be a familial pattern to the occurrence of insulinomas.

Clinically, demonstration of normal or elevated plasma insulin levels after an overnight fast is useful in diagnosis. In addition, high levels of proinsulin and C-peptide are often present. Surreptitious insulin administration can be excluded by comparing insulin levels with C-peptide levels.

Nesidioblastosis is a syndrome in children less than 2 years old, with persistent hyperinsulinism beginning in the first few weeks of life associated with persistent hyperplasia and neoformation of islet cells, particularly B cells.

GLUCAGON

Glucagon is a large linear polypeptide. True glucagon and **glicentin,** a larger molecule with some glucagon activity, are found in the gastrointestinal mucosa, as well as in the **A,** or **α cells** of the pancreatic islets of Langerhans.

Various factors affect pancreatic glucagon secretion. Secretion is increased by β-adrenergic stimulation, protein meals, glucogenic amino acids, starvation, and various hormones. Secretion is inhibited by glucose, insulin, fatty acids, and ketones, α-adrenergic agonists, and somatostatin.

Actions

Glucagon causes gluconeogenesis, glycogenolysis, lipolysis, and ketogenesis. It raises blood glucose by stimulating adenylate cyclase in hepatic cells, leading to breakdown of hepatic glycogen, although it does not cause glycogen breakdown in muscle. Glucagon increases ketogenesis and hepatic gluconeogenesis from amino acids. Miscellaneous effects include stimulation of growth hormone, insulin, and pancreatic somatostatin secretion, and positive cardiac inotropy.

Pathophysiology

Glucagonomas are rare tumors of pancreatic A cells, which produce a clinical syndrome of mild diabetes mellitus; erythematous, migratory, necrotizing skin lesions; and anemia in the presence of high serum glucagon levels. Most glucagonomas are malignant and some produce glicentin as well. Other characteristics of this syndrome include hypoaminoacidemia, a relatively high incidence of thromboembolic complications, alopecia, hyperpigmentation, glossitis or stomatitis, ungual dystrophy, weight loss, and occasionally neurologic and/or psychiatric disturbances.

PANCREATIC POLYPEPTIDE

Pancreatic polypeptide (PP) is a 36 amino acid linear peptide. Pancreatic islet cells, structurally similar but immunohistochemically distinct from D cells, are the site for production and storage of pancreatic polypeptide; plasma levels are undetectable after total pancreatectomy. Pancreatic polypeptide-containing cells exist in islets as well as being scattered throughout the parenchyma, but are most abundant in tissue in proximity to the duodenum.

Pancreatic polypeptide release is stimulated by protein intake and cholinergic stimulation. Intravenous infusion of amino acids produces a significant but much smaller response. Pentagastrin administration causes rapid rises in plasma levels, whereas somatostatin administration can abolish its response to meals. Ingestion of glucose produces a small initial increase in pancreatic polypeptide levels, followed 3–6 hours later by a larger increase when blood glucose is decreased. Intravenous insulin causes a large increase in PP during the time of maximal hypoglycemia. Vagal cholinergic mechanisms are important in the regulation of PP release. The PP response to insulin hypoglycemia is abolished by prior atropine administration.

Actions

The most dramatic action of PP is inhibition of pancreatic exocrine secretion. Pancreatic polypeptide inhibits both basal and stimulated pancreatic protein and bicarbonate secretion. The inhibition is more marked in the presence of intraduodenal protein. Pancreatic polypeptide also relaxes the gallbladder and stimulates choledochal tone. It is also a very weak stimulant of basal gastric acid secretion, independent of vagal effects.

The role of PP in regulation of digestion and metabolism is not clearly established. Pancreatic polypeptide may modulate the pancreatic secretory response to feeding, and in addition, may modulate biliary and intestinal motility, possibly by altering motilin release.

Pathophysiology

Pancreatic polypeptide may be produced by islet cell tumors and often is produced with another peptide, particularly VIP. Elevated PP is common in patients with gastrinoma and insulinoma, and levels may fail to correct after tumor resection. Plasma PP levels are increased in patients with diabetes mellitus, especially type I, and levels correlate with severity of the diabetes. A defect in PP release has been identified in patients with Prader-Willi obesity syndrome.

Bibliography

Bloodworth JMB, Jr, ed. *Endocrine pathology*. Baltimore: Williams & Wilkins, 1982.

Essman WB, ed. *Hormonal actions in non-endocrine systems* Jamaica, NY: Spectrum Publications, 1983.

Fedorak RN, Allen SL. Effect of somatostatin analog (SMS 201-995) on *in vivo* intestinal fluid transport in rats. A limited systemic effect. *Dig Dis Sci* 1989;34:567–572.

Friesen SR, ed. *Surgical endocrinology: clinical syndromes*. Philadelphia: JB Lippincott, 1978.

Ganong WF. *Review of medical physiology*. 12th ed. Los Altos, CA: Lange Medical Publications, 1985.

Glaser B, Shapiro B, Glowniak J, Fajans SS, Vinik AI. Effect of secretin on the normal and pathological beta cell. *J Clin Endocrinol Metab 1988;* 66:1138–43.

Greeley GH Jr, Jeng YJ, Gomez G, Hashimoto T, Hill FL, Kern K, Kurosky T, Chuo HF, Thompson JC. Evidence for regulation of peptide YY release in the proximal gut. *Endocrinology* 1989;124:1438–43.

Greeley GH Jr, Lluis F, Gomez G, Ishizuka J, Holland B, Thompson JC. Peptide YY antagonizes beta adrenergic stimulated release of insulin in dogs. *Am J Physiol* 1988;254: E531–E537.

Hopman WPM, Wolberink RGJ, Lamers CBJ, Van Tongeren JHM. Treatment of the dumping syndrome with the somatostatin analogue SMS 201-995. *Ann Surg 1988;207: 155–59.*

Johnson LR, ed. *Gastrointestinal physiology*, 3rd ed. St Louis: Mosby, 1985.

Johnson LR, Christensen J, Grossman MI, Jacobson ED, Schultz SG, eds. *Physiology of the gastrointestinal tract, Vol I.* New York: Raven Press, 1981.

Keele CA, Neil E, Joels N, eds. *Samson Wright's applied physiology.* Oxford: Oxford University Press, 1982.

Kellum JM, Kuemmerl JF, O'Dorisio TM, Rayford P, Martin D, Engle K, Eolf L, Sugarman HJ. Gastrointestinal hormone responses to meals before and after gastric bypass and vertical banded gastroplasty. *Ann Surg* 1990;211:763–71.

Robbins SL, Cotran RS, Kumar V, eds. *Pathologic basis of disease.* 3rd ed. Philadelphia: WB Saunders, 1984.

Woltering EA, Mozell EJ, O'Dorisio TM, Fletcher WS, Howe B. Suppression of primary and secondary peptides with somatostatin analog in the therapy of functional endocrine tumors. *Surg Gynecol Obstet* 1988;167:453–62.

Michael L. Nance and Edward B. Savage

19 DIGESTION AND ABSORPTION IN THE GASTROINTESTINAL TRACT

Absorption of water, electrolytes, and nutrients via the gastrointestinal tract is the primary means by which the body obtains fuel. The absorptive process is dependent on other gastrointestinal (GI) functions, such as secretion, digestion, and motility, that will affect the rate and form in which nutrients are available for assimilation.

Absorptive capabilities vary throughout the GI tract and can be affected by local or systemic disease processes to produce characteristic malabsorptive syndromes.

Anatomic Considerations

The GI tract is uniquely adapted to maximize its absorptive capacity. The majority of absorption takes place in the small intestine and colon. The stomach has less absorptive capacity owing to the paucity of villi and leaky intercellular junctions, which are abundant in the small bowel and colon. The small bowel has several anatomic features that enhance its absorptive capacity. Mucosal folds or **valvulae conniventes** increase the surface area threefold. These folds are most prominent in the duodenum and jejunum. Mucosal projections, called villi, occur throughout the small bowel and further increase the surface area by a factor of ten. Finally, a brush border of microvilli located on the cells increases the surface area an additional 20 times. Cumulatively, these anatomic features act to increase the absorptive surface area 600-fold for a total area of approximately 250 m^2. Because of this enormous capacity, the small bowel accounts for 80–90% of fluid absorption. The colon, with similar anatomic features provides a significant additional absorptive surface.

Transport Mechanisms

Absorption of elements from the GI tract is dependent on specific cellular mechanisms that transport molecules across the intestinal mucosa. Many of these mechanisms require energy expenditure by the cell (active); others occur freely (passive). Two major categories of transport mechanisms exist: **paracellular** and **transcellular**. Paracellular transport occurs via leaky intercellular junctions that allow passage of molecules down an electrochemical gradient without the expenditure of energy. The resistance to movement across these channels increases as one progresses from the proximal small bowel to the distal colon. Paracellular transport is the primary pathway for transport of water. Transcellular transport is often an "active" or energy-dependent process that moves molecules, via carrier proteins, into the cell from an area of low concentration to an area of higher concentration. Transcellular transport can also be "**facilitated**" (i.e., passive, down a concentration gradient, facilitated by carrier molecules).

Absorption of Fluids and Electrolytes

WATER

In addition to that ingested, significant amounts of water and solutes are secreted into the GI tract (see Table 3-1). Nearly 98% of intraluminal water is absorbed by the GI tract. The majority is absorbed in the jejunum (60%); the remainder in the ileum (25%) and colon (15%). The efficiency of absorption, however, is greatest in the colon, which absorbs approximately 87% of that delivered to it. Water is transported primarily via paracellular mechanisms as an isotonic fluid, traveling with various solutes. To a lesser extent, water is absorbed via a transcellular pathway in conjunction with the active transport of solutes or ions.

SODIUM

Like water, nearly 98% (all but 4 mEq) of intraluminal sodium is absorbed on a daily basis. The jejunum is the major site of sodium absorption. The ileum and colon also contribute, but to a lesser extent. Unlike water, most sodium is transported via active transcellular mechanisms. A smaller portion of sodium is transported passively. Active transport of sodium is a two-step process involving carrier-mediated transport into the cell from the luminal side, followed by transport into the blood and interstitium by the Na^+,K^+-ATPase pump located on the basal membrane. Several carrier mechanisms exist

for movement of sodium into the cell: (1) One mechanism involves cation exchange of Na^+ for H^+ along with the anion exchange of HCO_3^- for Cl^-, with a net electrically neutral flux of NaCl into the cell. (2) Intraluminal monosaccharides and amino acids are absorbed with sodium via a common carrier in the brush border. (3) High intraluminal concentrations of monosaccharides promotes passive reabsorption of sodium and water.

POTASSIUM

Potassium is absorbed predominantly in the jejunum by passive diffusion along an electrical gradient and with the flow of water. Potassium is actively excreted in the colon. All but about 10 mEq/day of potassium is absorbed.

CHLORIDE

Chloride is absorbed by both active and passive mechanisms. The predominant pathway is passive and in conjunction with the absorption of sodium (either active or passive). To a lesser extent, the ileum and colon can absorb chloride by an active chloride/bicarbonate exchange. In the normal state, all but 2 mEq/day are absorbed.

BICARBONATE

Bicarbonate is usually secreted by active mechanisms into the ileum and colon. This HCO_3^- binds with H^+ to form H_2CO_3 and subsequently CO_2 and H_2O. This CO_2 is transported back into mucosal cells where it can bind with OH^- to re-form HCO_3^-.

Absorption of Vitamins and Minerals

CALCIUM

Calcium is absorbed via an active, carrier protein-mediated mechanism. Absorption is greatest in the duodenum but also occurs in the jejunum and ileum. On average 1 g of calcium is consumed and 200–300 mg of calcium is secreted into the GI tract each day. Forty percent of the calcium in this pool is absorbed. Calcium absorption is regulated by vitamin D and parathyroid hormone. Parathyroid hormone stimulates production of the active form of vitamin D, which in turn stimulates synthesis of the carrier protein responsible for calcium absorption.

IRON

Iron is primarily absorbed in the duodenum. **Elemental iron** is absorbed by the mucosal cells bound to small molecules such as sugars and amino acids. **Heme iron** is absorbed directly and released from the heme within the cell. The rate of uptake varies with the needs of the body, usually about 10% of the dietary intake. The iron is subsequently released into the blood and bound to **transferrin.**

ASCORBIC ACID

Absorption of ascorbic acid (**vitamin C**) occurs in the ileum by active transport coupled to sodium. This is promoted by the transmembrane sodium electrochemical gradient. To maintain the gradient, sodium is extruded from the cell into the blood stream by an energy-dependent Na^+,K^+-ATPase. The ascorbic acid passively diffuses from the cell into the bloodstream.

COBALAMIN

Cobalamin (**vitamin B_{12}**) is absorbed by active transport linked to glycoprotein carrier molecules, most notably **intrinsic factor.** Intrinsic factor is secreted by gastric mucosa, and absorption of cobalamin requires gastric acid secretion. Absorption occurs in the distal portion of the ileum. A small amount can be absorbed throughout the small intestine by passive means but only when administered in pharmacologic doses.

FOLATE

Absorption of folate occurs in conjunction with sodium by active transport. The proximal jejunum is the predominant site of absorption. Passive diffusion of folate into the cell is observed only when pharmacologic dietary supplement doses are given. Once inside the cell, folate is transported down a simple diffusion gradient into the bloodstream.

BIOTIN

Biotin absorption probably occurs as a result of sodium-linked active transport, most notably in the proximal small intestine.

THIAMINE

Thiamine (**vitamin B_1**) is actively absorbed from the intestinal lumen via a carrier protein. Absorption occurs predominantly in the duodenum and to a lesser extent in the jejunum and ileum. Passive diffusion may also occur if dietary supplements are given.

VITAMIN B_6

While not well understood, the mechanism for vitamin B_6 absorption is most likely passive diffusion. The proximal small bowel appears to be the predominant site of absorption.

NIACIN, PANTOTHENATE, AND RIBOFLAVIN

Absorption of these vitamins is incompletely understood, but most evidence points to a passive diffusion pathway.

Absorption of Fats, Proteins, and Carbohydrates

Most fats, carbohydrates, and proteins are presented to the intestinal tract in forms that are too bulky to be absorbed. Digestion, both mechanical and chemical, is usually necessary prior to absorption.

FATS

Fat absorption is a complex, multistep process. Fats include triglycerides, cholesterol, phospholipids, and long chain fatty acids. Gastric peristaltic activity in conjunction with **lingual lipase** (secreted by glands on the back of the tongue) initiates the process of fat breakdown and emulsification. Of the fat components, only short chain fatty acids are absorbed in the stomach. The majority of fats are presented to the duodenum, where they stimulate secretion of pancreatic lipase, pancreatic carboxylester hydrolase, and phospholipase A_2. **Pancreatic lipase** hydrolyzes triglycerides to 2-monoglyceride and fatty acid. **Pancreatic carboxylester hydrolase** also catalyzes the hydrolysis of many lipids. **Phospholipase A_2** catalyzes the hydrolysis of phospholipid. Bicarbonate in pancreatic juice aides solublization by ionizing fatty acids. The end products of these processes, fatty acids, 2-monoacylglycerol and lysophospholipids, form aggregates with bile salts called **micelles** (see Figure 17-5). Bile acids (especially those in the conjugated form) are **amphipathic**, having both hydrophobic and hydrophilic regions. In micelle form, the bile acids orient themselves with the hydrophilic portions outward, allowing interaction with the aqueous environment. The hydrophobic portions are oriented inward, where they can harbor hydrophobic lipids.

Absorption of free lipids is limited by the cell membrane itself and an unstirred water layer that exists over the brush border. The mixed micelle, with its hydrophilic outer surface, is able to diffuse passively through this water layer. Once through the unstirred water layer, the micelle dissociates, releasing the lipid byproducts. Transmission across the cell membrane is variable and dependent on the permeability coefficients of the individual lipids. Once inside the cell, the lipid components reorganize to form **chylomicrons** (lipoproteins containing nonpolar lipids, sterols, fat-soluble vitamins, phospholipid, and protein) that are subsequently transported out of the cell into the blood.

Medium chain fatty acids deserve special mention because they can be absorbed in the absence of pancreatic lipase and bile.

PROTEINS

Proteins are broken down into their constituent amino acids and peptides by the enzymes of the GI tract. This begins in the acidic **environment** of the stomach (pH < 5), which converts pepsinogen to pepsin. **Pepsin** cleaves the peptide bonds between aromatic amino acids. Once in the alkaline environment of the small intestine, pepsin activity ceases. Here, **enterokinase**, secreted by the intestinal mucosa, activates the pancreatic enzyme **trypsin** from its precursor trypsinogen. Trypsin then activates the pancreatic enzymes **chymotrypsin, elastase**, and **carboxypeptidases A** and **B** from their precursors. These enzymes break down protein to free amino acids and oligopeptides (predominantly dipeptides, tripeptides, and tetrapeptides). Most digestion takes place in the jejunum, but intact protein can reach the ileum. Absorption of amino acids, dipeptides, and tripeptides occurs via active, carrier-mediated transport systems. The amino acid carrier systems are driven by the transmembrane sodium gradient. An additional sodium-independent, facilitated diffusion pathway has

been demonstrated but is of lesser importance. Molecules larger than tripeptides must undergo further digestion by **peptide hydrolase enzymes** at the level of the brush border prior to absorption.

The rate of absorption varies among the amino acids and is dependent on chemical structure. Branched chain amino acids are absorbed most rapidly; neutral amino acids are more readily absorbed than charged amino acids. After absorption into the cell, further transport into the portal circulation occurs by poorly understood mechanisms.

Protein malabsorption can occur with global pancreatic insufficiency, selective deficiency of digestive enzymes, and mucosal abnormalities.

CARBOHYDRATES

Carbohydrates ingested in the normal diet include monosaccharides and polysaccharides (e.g., starches). Only monosaccharides can be absorbed by the GI mucosa. Gastrointestinal enzymes act to digest polysaccharides to oligosaccharides, disaccharides, and the usable monosaccharides. Digestion begins with **salivary amylase** and continues with **pancreatic amylase,** which break the 1,4 bonds of amylose. Further digestion is carried out by brush-border-associated **disaccharidases** (e.g., **sucrase, glucoamylase** (maltase), **lactase**). Certain carbohydrate bonds cannot be broken down by available enzymes. Carbohydrate moieties composed of these molecular linkages are called **fiber** and include **cellulose** and **pectin.**

The brush border is poorly permeable to water-soluble monosaccharides. Glucose and galactose are absorbed by **active transport** mechanisms that are dependent on the sodium gradient and electrical potential of the cell membrane. This permits the transport of these monosaccharides against a steep concentration gradient. In contrast, fructose is absorbed by **facilitated diffusion** and cannot be absorbed against a concentration gradient. Less is known about transport across the basal membrane into the blood, but it appears to be a sodium-independent event mediated by a basolateral exit pump.

Carbohydrates are not absorbed in the colon. However, bacterial fermentation can yield products absorbable by the colon. These include fatty acids (C1–4), alcohols, and gases. Absorption of these breakdown products of monosaccharides functions to reduce luminal osmoles, promoting colonic water reabsorption.

Carbohydrate malabsorption can result from many

mechanisms. Although no appreciable digestion occurs in the stomach, the stomach meters the delivery of carbohydrate to the small intestine. Rapid delivery to the small intestine can cause malabsorption. Pancreatic insufficiency reduces the efficacy of carbohydrate digestion. Deficiency of brush border disaccharidases can occur secondary to mucosal abnormalities or as a result of primary enzyme deficiency. Finally, monosaccharide absorption can be affected by mucosal injury or abnormality.

Absorption of Bile Salts

The conjugated bile acid pool averages 3.5 g in the adult. This pool circulates approximately six times per day (see Figure 17-4). Approximately 500 mg are lost in the feces each day. The majority of bile acids are absorbed in the terminal ileum, most likely via sodium-limited transport mechanisms. Other areas of the GI tract are able partially to assume bile acid reabsorption in the absence of the ileum, but an overall decrease in the circulating bile salt pool usually occurs. When significant, this results in reduced fat absorption and excess delivery of bile salts to the colon, which can lead to diarrhea and steatorrhea.

Special Considerations

GALLBLADDER ABSORPTION

The gallbladder has the ability to absorb water and solutes. By means of this mechanism, the gallbladder concentrates the bile. The gallbladder absorbs sodium and chloride by active cotransport mechanisms and water absorption follows passively. The gallbladder is also capable of absorbing some sugar molecules and amino acids by sodium-limited transport mechanisms.

DRUG ABSORPTION

Oral drug preparations are absorbed from the GI tract by both active and passive mechanisms. The majority of absorption occurs by passive means in the proximal small intestine. Many factors affect the rate of absorption, including pharmacologic characteristics of the drug (e.g., rate of dissolution) and local conditions (e.g., pH, intestinal transit time). Perturbations of the local conditions can affect the rate of drug absorption. Food, for example, alters the intestinal milieu via enzymatic stimulation and motility changes. Disease states that affect the absorptive surface (e.g., amyloidosis, sprue) can also alter drug bioavailability. The presence of other drugs may alter absorption (e.g., antacids alter the pH; antibiotics alter the microflora).

MALABSORPTION

Malabsorptive syndromes are common. They can occur because the GI tract is unable to process raw materials (i.e., digestive abnormalities), cannot transport molecules across the mucosal cell membrane, or cannot assimilate materials once absorbed. Syndromes may be inherited or acquired, local or diffuse processes, and may involve one or many of the nutrient components.

Diarrhea can cause malabsorption. Bacterial or virally mediated diarrhea produces a hypermotile state in the GI tract that limits the time of exposure of the luminal contents to the absorptive surfaces. As a result, excess fluid and electrolytes are lost in the feces. Malabsorption syndromes can also cause diarrhea. Failure to absorb certain nutrients results in an excessive intraluminal osmolar load, which causes a requisite amount of water to be retained as well. Excess fluid and nutrients are lost in the feces.

Short bowel syndrome occurs in patients undergoing major intestinal resection following mesenteric vascular catastrophes or repeated resections for chronic progressive diseases such as Crohn's disease. Loss of the jejunum is better tolerated than loss of either the duodenum or distal ileum. The small bowel can gradually adapt through mucosal hyperplasia to restore some absorptive capacity. After loss of the terminal ileum, however, adaptive measures cannot completely compensate to normalize bile acid and cobalamin absorption. Loss of excessive bile acids in turn impairs absorption of lipids, fat-soluble vitamins, and drugs, and may predispose to cholelithiasis. If the extent of bowel lost exceeds the capacity to adapt, malnutrition and vitamin deficiency will develop. Loss of the large bowel is associated with fluid and electrolyte abnormalities, the severity of which is dependent on the length lost. The small intestine gradually adapts to overcome the fluid and electrolyte losses that characterize the postcolectomy state.

Bibliography

Adibi SA. Protein assimilation. In Berk JE, et al., eds. *Gastroenterology, vol III.* Philadelphia: WB Saunders, 1985:1530.

Armstrong WM. Cellular mechanisms of ion transport in the small intestine. In Johnson LR, ed. *Physiology of the gastrointestinal tract, vol II.* New York: Raven Press, 1987:1251.

Borgstrom B. Fat assimilation. In Berk JE, et al., eds. *Gastroenterology, vol III.* Philadelphia: WB Saunders, 1985:1510.

Guyton AC. *Textbook of medical physiology.* Philadelphia: WB Saunders, 1986:787.

Kalser MH. Absorption of cobalamin (vitamin B12), folate, and other water-soluble vitamins. In Berk JE, et al., eds. *Gastroenterology, vol III.* Philadelphia: WB Saunders, 1985:1553.

Kalser MH. Water and mineral transport. In Berk JE, et al., eds. *Gastroenterology, vol III.* Philadelphia: WB Saunders, 1985:1538.

Levitt MD. Carbohydrate assimilation. In Berk JE, et al, eds. *Gastroenterology, vol III.* Philadelphia: WB Saunders, 1985:1520.

Mansbach CM, Grundy SM. Bile acid and cholesterol homeostasis. In Berk JE, et al., eds. *Gastroenterology, vol III.* Philadelphia: WB Saunders, 1985:1567.

Powell DW. Intestinal water and electrolyte transport. In Johnson LR, ed. *Physiology of the gastrointestinal tract, vol II.* New York: Raven Press, 1987:1267.

Rogers AI, Corbett FS. Intestinal drug absorption. In Berk JE et al., eds: *Gastroenterology, vol III.* Philadelphia: WB Saunders, 1985:1597.

Rose RC: Absorptive functions of the gallbladder. In Johnson LR, ed. *Physiology of the gastrointestinal tract, vol II.* New York: Raven Press, 1987:1455.

Rose RC. Intestinal absorption of water-soluble vitamins. In Johnson LR, ed. *Physiology of the gastrointestinal tract, vol II.* New York: Raven Press, 1987:1581.

Shiau Y. Lipid digestion and absorption. In Johnson LR, ed. *Physiology of the gastrointestinal tract, vol II.* New York: Raven Press, 1987:1527.

Stevens BR, Kamnitz JD, Wright EM. Intestinal transport of amino acids and sugars: advances using membrane vesicles. *Ann Rev Physiol* 1984;46:417.

Weser E, Urban E. The short bowel syndrome. In Berk JE, et al., eds. *Gastroenterology, vol II.* Philadelphia: WB Saunders, 1985:1792.

20 BASIC CONCEPTS OF IMMUNOLOGY

James F. Markmann

Immune Organs
Immune Cells and Mediators
  Antigen-Specific and Nonspecific Immune Cells
  Antigen-Presenting Cells
  Natural Killer Cells
  Lymphokines
  B Lymphocytes
  Anti-Idiotypic Antibodies
  T Lymphocytes
  Major Histocompatibility Complex Antigens
Typical Immune Response
Monoclonal Antibodies

The immune system is composed of a complex network of cells and cellular products primarily designed to defend an individual from potentially harmful microbiological invaders. To accomplish this task, the immune system must be capable of specific recognition and elimination of a vast array of pathogenic intracellular and extracellular organisms such as viruses, bacteria, fungi, and parasites. Implicit in the immunologic recognition of an object as foreign is the capacity to discriminate "self" structures from non-self determinants carried by the pathogen.

Immunosurveillance, a secondary function of the immune system, is the defense of the organism from endogenously generated threats to survival in the form of malignant cells. Although less well defined than the immune response to microorganisms, it is now clear that the immune system can modify significantly the progression of malignant tissues.

This chapter will review the cellular machinery and mechanisms employed in the basic cellular immune response. Subsequent chapters will apply these concepts to the two areas of surgery most heavily influenced by immunobiology: transplantation and oncology.

Immune Organs

The immune organs can be divided into primary and secondary lymphoid tissues. The primary lymphoid organs include the bone marrow and thymus, which serve as a self-perpetuating source of immune precursor cells and as a site for their maturation. During fetal development the yolk sac, and later fetal liver, fulfill these duties. Secondary immune organs, which house mature, functional lymphoid cells, include the lymph nodes, spleen, and Peyer's patches of the gastrointestinal tract. Primary and secondary organs consist of locally derived cells that make up the framework of the tissues. These structural cells in some cases may also contribute to the maturation and differentiation of lymphocytes that reside in, or pass through, a particular organ. For example, the epithelial cells of the thymic stroma participate in the education of developing T lymphocytes.

Both primary and secondary organs are ultimately populated with bone-marrow-derived immune cells such as B lymphocytes, T lymphocytes, and antigen-presenting cells (macrophages and dendritic cells). It is these bone-marrow-derived cells that actively participate in an immune response.

Specific regions within each lymphoid organ may preferentially house different lymphocyte subsets. Lymphocytes enter lymph nodes after transgressing specialized vessels called high endothelial venules that express lymphocyte homing receptors. B lymphocytes then localize in primary follicles surrounded by a paracortical region rich in T cells. During an immune response, proliferating B cells form expanding germinal centers.

The spleen houses cells of both erythroid and lymphoid lineage. The former are concentrated in the red pulp; the latter, in the white pulp. Cellular entry into the spleen, unlike the lymph node, is not receptor specific and therefore makes the spleen well suited for its blood-filtering function. Splenic T cells are found in highest concentration in the periarteriolar lymphocyte sheaths. Aggregates of B lymphocytes are found in the adjacent primary follicles and germinal centers.

Immune Cells and Mediators

ANTIGEN-SPECIFIC AND -NONSPECIFIC IMMUNE CELLS

The immune system is conveniently divided into antigen-specific and nonspecific components. Only two immune cell types, B lymphocytes and T lymphocytes, are able to recognize foreign antigen specifically. This ability to selectively bind to unique foreign structures or antigen derives from the antigen-specific receptors used by the two cell types. Antigen-nonspecific immune cells include antigen-presenting cells (APC), such as macrophages and dendritic cells (DC), natural killer (NK) cells, and lymphokine-activated killer (LAK) cells. Most of the secreted immune mediators, called cytokines or lymphokines, do not act in an antigen-specific manner. The actions of the antigen-nonspecific components of the immune system are tightly regulated by antigen-specific cells, especially T cells of the CD4 subset.

Immune cells are routinely distinguished by characteristic cell surface proteins or markers defined and identified by experimental exposure to monoclonal antibodies. Many of these phenotypic markers have ultimately been shown to be proteins important in the characteristic function of the cell type. Some commonly used markers for the major immune cell populations are listed with their known functions in Table 20-1.

ANTIGEN-PRESENTING CELLS

Cells capable of taking up foreign antigens and presenting them to T lymphocytes in a form that T cells can

TABLE 20-1. Characteristic Phenotypes of Immune Cells

Cell Type	Cell Surface Markers	Marker Function
T Lymphocyte	T-cell receptor	Composite MHC/antigen binding
	CD3	T-cell-receptor expression T-cell transmembrane signaling of activation
	CD2	T-cell activation signalling by alternate pathway
	IL-2 receptor	IL-2 binding T-cell activation and proliferation
	CD4	Binds class II; restricts antigen recognition to class-II associated antigens
	CD8	Binds class I; restricts antigen recognition to class-I associated antigens
B Lymphocyte	Surface immunoglobulin	Antigen binding Cellular activation
	Class II	Class II restricted antigen presentation to CD4+ cells
Macrophages	Class II MAC-1	Class II restricted antigen presentation to CD4+ cells C3b receptor
NK cells	CD16	Fc receptor for Ig binding
	IL-2 receptor	IL-2 binding Cellular activation

MHC, major histocompatibility complex; NK, natural killer cell.

recognize are termed APCs. Since T cells can be stimulated only by antigen presented by an APC, APCs play a pivotal role in initiating an immune response. To execute this duty, an APC must be able to carry out four important functions. First, APCs must be able to ingest foreign antigens. This may consist of simple endocytosis or may entail specific recognition of antigen via cell surface receptors. Second, following antigen uptake, an APC must process or enzymatically degrade antigen into small peptide fragments. This process is dependent on intracellular organelles such as lysosomes, which contain proteolytic enzymes capable of protein breakdown. Third, peptides of the correct size are delivered through the appropriate intracellular pathway to bind to major histocompatibility complex (MHC) class II molecules (see below) expressed by APCs. Antigen bound to class II is then exported to be re-expressed on the cell surface. Bound to class II on the APCs surface, antigen is then in a form that can trigger class II-restricted T cells bearing the correct antigen-specific receptor. Finally, an APC must produce soluble lymphokines such as interluekin-1 (IL-1) during the process of antigen presentation. T cells bear cell surface receptors for IL-1 molecules. IL-1 binding is requisite for T-cell activation. Only when a T cell encounters the appropriate foreign antigen–class II MHC complex presented by an APC, which also delivers the needed soluble lymphokine, will a primary immune response be initiated.

The four steps—antigen uptake, processing, association with MHC class II antigen, and lymphokine signal delivery—are carried out mainly by three immune cells: macrophages, dendritic cells, and B lymphocytes. These cells also each possess specialized characteristics for efficient antigen presentation. Macrophages, for example, are known for their phagocytic activity and thus are ideal for antigen uptake. In addition they are well equipped for degradation of engulfed proteins via phagosome-lysosome interaction. Dendritic cells, on the other hand, while possessing less phagocytic activity than macrophages, have a very high density of class II antigen expression and, because of their dendritic processes, a large surface area for T-cell interaction. Dendritic cells are the most potent subset of APCs and are thought by some to be the predominant, if not sole, stimulators of a primary immune response.

B lymphocytes are unique APCs in their capacity for **specific** antigen uptake. As will be discussed in greater detail below, B cells utilize surface-bound immunoglobulin (antibody) as their antigen-specific receptor.

Antigen bound by this receptor can be internalized, processed, and presented on the cell surface in association with B-lymphocyte class II MHC antigens. By means of this strategy, B cells can selectively present the relevant antigen (i.e., the antigen for which they have receptor specificity) to T cells that are specific for antigenic determinants present in the same protein. In this way, T cells and B cells bearing receptor specificity for the same antigen can be brought into proximity during an immune response, thus allowing T cells to deliver lymphokine signals necessary for B-cell activation and differentiation. It is unclear whether the T cell that recognizes antigen presented by a B cell must first be activated by the same antigen presented on another APC such as a dendritic cell.

NATURAL KILLER CELLS

Natural killer cells are lymphocytes found in greatest concentration in spleen and peripheral blood. Natural killer cells are neither T cells nor B cells. Natural killer cells are defined by their spontaneous ability to lyse certain tumor cell targets in vitro. Unlike cytolytic T lymphocytes (CD8+), no presensitization to the tumor target is required. In addition, NK-mediated killing is not dependent on MHC antigen expression by the target cell. The lymphokines γ-interferon (IFN) and IL-2 produced by CD4+ T cells can significantly augment the tumorcidal activity of NK cells. Following exposure to IL-2 under the appropriate in vitro conditions, NK cells may differentiate into LAK cells. Lymphokine-activated killer cells cells are more potent effectors of tumor cell lysis in vitro and are cytotoxic to a broader range of tumor targets than are NK cells.

LYMPHOKINES

Lymphokines are soluble mediators, secreted by lymphocytes, that provide a means of intercellular communication. The signals carried by lymphokines are not antigen specific but are only active on cells bearing the relevant lymphokine receptor. Frequently lymphokines can be produced by more than one cell type or can exert multiple effects on multiple cells.

Recent advances in molecular biology have lead to an explosion in the characterization of new lymphokines. More than ten interleukins have been described. The best-studied lymphokines, their main cell source, cellular targets, and major biologic actions are listed in Table 20-2.

TABLE 20-2. Lymphokines

Lymphokine	Cell Source	Cell Target	Major Biologic Effect
IL-1	Macrophage	T cells B cells	T-cell coactivation factor B-cell development Fever, anorexia Enhances lymphokine production (IL-2, IL-4, IL-6)
IL-2	T cells	T cells B cells NK cells	Autocrine/paracrine stimulator of T-cell growth and differentiation Regulation of immunoglobulin synthesis NK activation
IL-3	T cells	Lymphohematopoetic precursor cells	Stimulation of multiple cell lineages
IL-4	T cells	B cells	Co-stimulator of B-cell growth Immunoglobulin regulation
IL-5	T cells	B cells	Stimulation of B-cell growth and immunoglobulin synthesis
IL-6	T cells Macrophages	T cells B cells	B-cell differentiation Hybridoma growth Fever
TNF	Macrophages	T cells B cells	Tumor cell lysis Fever Cachexia
α/β-IFN	Macrophages T cells Fibroblasts	Nonlymphoid cells Macrophages	Antiviral effects Macrophage activation Augments MHC antigen expression Increases natural killer cell activity
γ-IFN	T cells	Macrophages T cells Nonlymphoid cells	Macrophage activation Enhanced natural killer cell activity Increased MHC antigen expression Antiviral activity

IFN, Interferon; IL, interleukin; MHC, major histocompatibility complex; NK, natural killer cell; TNF, tumor necrosis factor.

B LYMPHOCYTES

B cells are bone-marrow-derived cells whose primary function is the production and secretion of immunoglobulins (Ig). B cells first undergo differentiation in the bone marrow and do not require passage through the thymus for their development. Mature B cells reside in the secondary lymphoid organs with high concentrations in the spleen and the Peyer's patches of the gastrointestinal tract.

B cells provide one of the immune system's two arms of antigen-specific responsiveness. The cell-surface antigen receptor used by B cells is membrane-bound immunoglobulin. Antigen binding by cell-surface antibody is the primary trigger for B-cell proliferation, differentiation, and antibody secretion. Soluble mediators such as IL-2 and IL-4 provided by T-helper cells are necessary for B-cell maturation. These lymphokine signals are delivered during the recognition of antigen by T cells presented by B cells.

The antibody molecule synthesized by B cells can mediate the neutralization of antigen and antigen-bearing organisms by opsonization and clearance by the reticuloendothelial system or by activation of the complement cascade (Figure 20-1). Antibodies can also bind NK cells and macrophages via their Fc receptors (see below). This endows NK cells and macrophages with antigen specificity and gives rise to antibody-dependent cell-mediated cytotoxicity (ADCC). In their simplest form antibodies are composed of four polypeptides, two identical heavy (H) chains and two identical light (L) chains (Figure 20-2). Both H and L chains contain constant-region and variable-region domains. Antibody-constant regions of the H chain endow antibody classes with their characteristic effector functions.

Five major classes of antibody exist—IgD, IgM, IgG,

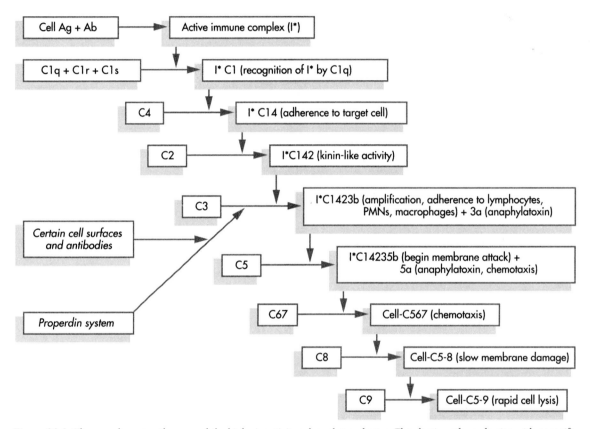

Figure 20-1 The complement pathways and the biologic activity released at each step. The classic pathway begins with a specific antigen-antibody reaction. The properdin pathway is triggered by a more nonspecific interaction between cell surfaces and the molecules that make up the properdine systems. Both pathways, however, converge at the C3 step, where most of the biologic activity associated with complement activation begins. Amplification also occurs at several steps but it is greatest at C3. The subseqent steps lead to the molecular condensation on the target cell surface, which ultimately results in membrane damage and lysis. There are several other important consequences of complement activation. The presence of these molecules on the target cell surface makes them adherent to other cells. Macrophages, platelets, polymorphonuclear leukocytes, and lymphocytes adhere and increase the damage to the graft cells. The steps through C5 are largely enzymatic in nature; the C3 and C5 components, for example, are split during activation, releasing chemotactic and vasoactive (anaphylatoxins) molecules. Attachment of the C5b molecule to the cell begins the condensation ending in membrane damage; this seems to occur away from the immune complex. Interaction of the C6 and C7 components results, additionally, in the release of another chemotactic factor. The activation of the complement pathway, therefore, contributes to many of the features seen in allograft rejection; cellular infiltrates, adherent PMNs and platelets, thrombosed vessels, interstitial edema, and cellular damage. (Reproduced from Schwarz SI, Shires GT, Spencer FC. *Principles of surgery.* 5th ed. New York: McGraw-Hill, 1989:398.)

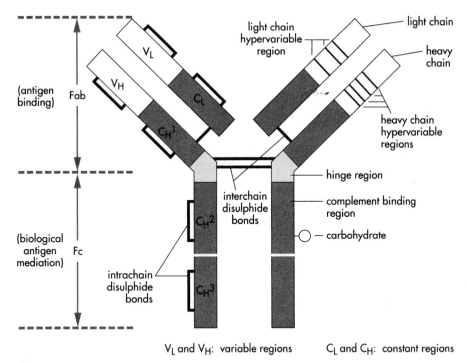

Figure 20-2 Topology and functional architecture of the IgG molecule. (Reproduced from Wasserman RL, Capra JD. Immunoglobulins. In: Horowitz MI, Pigman W, eds. *The glycoconjugates.* New York: Academic Press, 1977:323–348.)

IgA, and IgE. IgD is found on the surface of immature B cells and is thought to be important in cell activation signals. IgM is also found on the surface of B cells. In the serum IgM is found in a pentameric form and for this reason is very high in avidity. IgM is produced early in a primary immune response and is excellent at complement fixation. IgG accounts for 90% of serum Ig and after binding antigen activates complement. IgG is the only immunoglobulin that readily crosses the placenta. Fc receptor binding of IgG may arm NK cells for ADCC. IgA is important in mucosal immunity. IgA monomers dimerize following addition of a joining peptide. To be secreted across mucosal surfaces a secretory component must also be present on the IgA dimer. IgA is secreted in clostrom and provides some degree of intestinal immunity for the fetus. IgE binds mast cells and basophils via IgE specific Fc receptors. Antigenic triggering of IgE during an allergic response leads to release of vasoactive mediators, including histamine and leukotrines.

Following association of H and L chain pairs, the variable region of these molecules produces two identical antigen-binding regions. Since an individual cell and

its progeny can each express only a single H-chain variable region and a single L-chain variable region, the antigen-binding capability of B cells is monoclonal. In other words, all antibodies produced by a given B cell, either expressed on its surface or secreted extracellularly, are capable of binding only a single, or a few closely related, antigen molecules.

A result of the monoclonality of antibody production by B cells is that to achieve a sufficiently diverse antigen-binding repertoire, an enormous panel of B lymphocytes, each with a distinct antigen-binding specificity, is required. It has been estimated that up to 10^8 different antibody molecules are likely needed for effective immunity. It would be inefficient to produce these by encoding each of the 10^8 individually in germline DNA. Instead, a strategy of combinatorial component assembly is used to generate antibody diversity.

First, the binding region for antigen is formed by an interaction of two polypeptide chains, the H and L chains. To obtain 10^8 unique binding sites employing two proteins would require only 10^4 of each encoded in DNA if they were randomly associated to form pairs.

Since the variable-region segment of each chain is composed of subsegments called variable (V), joining (J), and in the H chain, diversity (D)-creating segments, multiple unique binding sites can be derived from a single DNA segment. For example, 10^4 different heavy chain variable regions could be generated using only 100 V, 10 J, and 10 D segments randomly selected and combined. Thus by applying this simple strategy, an extensive repertoire of immunoglobulin is possible with an economy of DNA usage. Two additional mechanisms are employed by B cells to increase antibody diversity further. First, in a process termed N-region diversity, by rearrangement of the D segment with the V segment in the heavy chain locus there is some random addition of amino acids to the amino-terminus of the D segment. Second, following antigenic stimulation of B cells, the immunoglobulin molecule may undergo mutation, altering the variable domain. Mutation in this region occurs at a rate up to 10^5 times that expected in the usual somatic mutation at other DNA loci. Mutation leading to antibodies with better "fit" or higher affinity for the relevant antigen will be selected preferentially during the progression of an immune response. This process, termed "affinity maturation," causes antibody affinity for antigen to be greater late in an immune response than shortly after the response begins.

Genetic rearrangement not only allows the immune system to produce antigens with a diverse spectrum of antigen-binding ability, but also permits the full repertoire to be transferred to antibody classes with different effector functions. In a process termed class switch, the heavy chain variable region composed of associated V, D, and J segments can be linked to the gene segments encoding any of the constant-region domains. Thus, a response initially with a predominance of IgM antibodies may later switch to mostly IgG. Antigen-binding regions utilized by IgM-producing B cells can later be found on B cells expressing IgG molecules. Regulation of heavy chain switch likely involves T-cell regulation. T-cell-derived lymphokine signals delivered during the immune responses have been shown to influence heavy chain switch.

ANTI-IDIOTYPIC ANTIBODIES

To generate a repertoire of 10^8 distinct antigen-binding conformations, immunoglobulins must themselves carry unique amino acid sequences in the variable domain. These sequences, called idiotypes, if carried by an antibody present in sufficient quantity, may themselves be antigenic and potentially recognizable by other antibodies. For example, during the course of an immune response to a virus, if an immunoglobulin produced by a clone of B cells reaches a high enough titer, other antibodies called anti-idiotypic antibodies that have specificity for unique determinants on the binding region of the original antibody, may be induced. It has been postulated that anti-idiotypic antibodies regulate an immune response by blocking the binding of the original antibody to antigen. In theory, anti-idiotypic antibodies themselves may induce other antibodies (anti-anti-idiotypic), giving rise to a network of immune regulation. Anti-idiotypic antibodies may assume clinical relevance upon administration of monoclonal antibodies for immunotherapy. Administration of OKT3 antibody to immunosuppressed transplant recipients may be met with generation of anti-idiotypic antibodies that limit its efficacy.

T LYMPHOCYTES

T cells, like B cells, are derived from precursors found in the bone marrow. Unlike B cells, however, T-cell differentiation is dependent on and takes place within the thymus. Two important events take place during intrathymic T cell maturation: (1) deletion of autoreactive T-cell clones and (2) selection for T cells that can recognize antigen when bound to self-MHC molecules.

T cells are defined by the membrane-bound T-cell receptor (TCR), which is similar in some respects to B-cell immunoglobulin (Figure 20-3). Like immunoglobulin, it is monoclonally expressed on the cell surface, but unlike antibody, its major functions are carried out at the cell surface, not in secreted form. When bone-marrow-derived T-cell precursors enter the thymus, they lack the TCR and the subset markers CD4 and CD8. Not until the TCR is expressed can the positive and negative selection steps mentioned above take place.

The TCR has a spectrum of intrinsic affinity for MHC molecules. It is necessary therefore to eliminate cells that generate receptors having a binding affinity high enough to be potentially autoreactive to self-MHC or to self-antigen bound to self-MHC. Deletion of autoreactive clones takes place by an undetermined mechanism that depends on T-cell interaction with thymic APCs expressing self-MHC molecules or self-MHC molecules complexed with other self-antigens.

In the second step of intrathymic development, T cells that express receptors potentially able to recognize foreign antigen bound to self-MHC molecules receive a

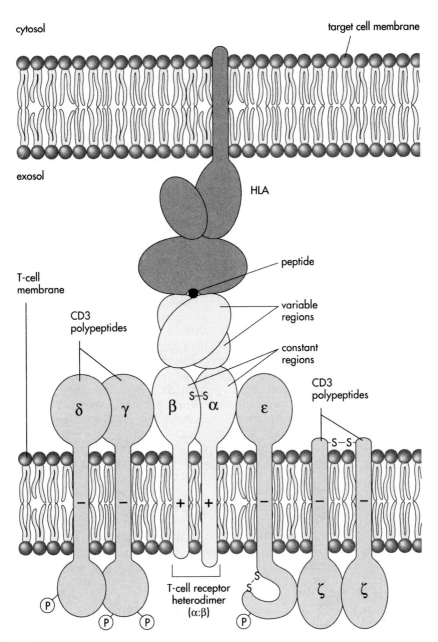

cytosol

target cell membrane

exosol

HLA

T-cell membrane

CD3 polypeptides

peptide

variable regions

constant regions

CD3 polypeptides

δ γ β S–S α ε

S–S

− − + + − − −

P

P P

S–S

ζ ζ

T-cell receptor heterodimer (α:β)

P

Figure 20-3 Interaction of HLA and the T-cell-receptor complex. The α-and β-polypeptide chains of the T-cell receptor form a heterodimer linked by a disulfide bond (S–S) and anchored in the T-cell membrane. The heterodimer recognizes and binds to peptide associated with an HLA molecule on the surface of a presenting cell. The nonpolymorphic CD3 polypeptides (designated γ, δ, ε, and ζ) are assembled together with the T-cell-antigen receptor, and are probably involved in signal transduction. P denotes phosphorylation site. (Reproduced from Krensky AM, Weiss A, Crabtree G, Davis MM, Pasham P. T-lymphocyte-antigen interactions in transplant rejection. *N Engl J Med* February: 1990;322:510–517.)

positive differentiation signal, are expanded, and are allowed to populate the peripheral immune tissues. The precise details of this step remain obscure. The net result observed, however, is that the mature T-cell population can preferentially respond to antigen when present in the context of self-MHC molecules. Following intrathymic maturation, T cells populate all secondary lymphoid organs, with the highest concentration in the lymph nodes.

As a population, T cells have the capacity, via the TCR, to bind specifically a vast array of antigens comparable in diversity to that seen with B cells. The antigen-binding portion of the TCR is composed of two polypeptides. In most T cells, α- and β-chains make up the TCR. In a less well studied subset, a second form of TCR is expressed composed of γ- and δ-chains. Each chain has variable-region and constant-region domains. When associated in their functional form on the T-cell surface, the variable regions assume a conformation capable of antigen binding.

Diversity in the TCR variable-region domains is accomplished in T cells by genetic mechanisms similar to those employed in B cells. The receptor binding site is a composite of two polypeptide chains. The variable domain of each chain is the product of multiple separately encoded subsegments linked together by genetic rearrangement. A number of V and J segments are encoded at the α-loci; and V, D, and J segments are present in the β-chain loci. The random selection of a single V, D, and J segment for each chain and N-region diversity provides the extensive repertoire required for antigen binding.

Interestingly, T cells apparently do not rely on somatic mutation of their antigen receptor to increase receptor diversity, as occurs in B cells. This may be in part to ensure that autoreactive cells are not generated by changes in receptor binding following receptor selection during development in the thymus.

While the TCR is similar to the receptor used by B cells, it is significantly more complex both structurally and functionally. In addition to the α- and β-chains of the TCR, a number of other T-cell surface proteins contribute to antigen binding by T cells. One group of proteins, termed CD3, is strongly associated with the antigen-specific TCR. CD3 is a complex of proteins present in all cells bearing a functional TCR and is thought to be required for TCR expression on the cell surface. Its major role may be transduction of the activation signal from the TCR to the T-cell cytoplasm following antigen binding. Because of its intimate relationship with

the TCR, CD3 has effectively been used as a target for immunosuppression. Monoclonal antibodies such as OKT3 that specifically bind a protein within the T_3 complex have proven to be potent immunosuppressive agents.

Additional T-cell surface molecules such LFA-1 and CD2 also assist T-cell antigen recognition. They may serve to stabilize the interaction of the TCR with antigen/MHC. In addition, the molecules that define the two major T-cell subsets CD4 and CD8 participate in stabilizing the TCR during recognition of antigen.

The TCR is designed to recognize antigen only when the antigen is bound to either class I or class II MHC molecules. This may function to focus T-cell immunity to intracellular pathogens such as viruses while antibody secreted by B cells deals with antigen free in the body's fluids. Two major subsets of T cells exist: CD4+ T cells, which bind antigen only when presented in the context of class II MHC molecules (T_4 subset), and CD8+ T cells, which bind antigen only when presented in the context of class I MHC molecules (T_8 subset). CD4+ and CD8+ T cells have traditionally been termed the T-helper and T-cytotoxic subsets. This distinction is oversimplified in that each subset defined phenotypically has the potential for either helper or cytotoxic function. The correlation of phenotype with MHC-restricting element, either class I or class II, is more consistent and biologically relevant.

CD4+ T cells, because of their preference for antigen recognition when associated with class II, are relegated to activation by cells that are class II positive, namely, APCs. For this reason CD4+ T cells serve a predominant role in the early steps of an immune response. Their interaction with an APC bearing the appropriate antigen triggers proliferation, differentiation, and production of a set of soluble mediators termed lymphokines that act as both autocrine and paracrine mediators. The CD4+ subset can be segregated further into TH1 and TH2 cells, depending on the specific lymphokines produced. TH1 cells produce IL-2, γ-IFN, and lymphotoxin, and most likely participate in cytotoxic T-lymphocyte (CTL) generation. TH2 cells produce IL-4 and IL-5 and may primarily function in B-lymphocyte activation.

The second major T-cell subset contains CD8+ cells. Antigenic recognition by CD8+ cells occurs only when the antigen is presented in association with class I MHC molecules. The fact that class I molecules are expressed by all nucleated cells in humans implies that CD8+ cells can potentially interact with almost any cell in the body. Since a major function of CD8+ cells is to lyse virally infected cells, the ubiquitous distribution of class I ensures that all cells are susceptible to the CTL effector arm of the cellular immune response.

MAJOR HISTOCOMPATIBILITY COMPLEX ANTIGENS

MHC antigens are cell-surface glyoproteins that were first identified by Snell, who observed that grafts exchanged between inbred lines of mice were rejected most vigorously if the donor and recipient differed at the MHC locus. In man three classes of MHC antigens exist. Class I and class II antigens have as their primary function the regulation of the immune response. Class III proteins are a miscellaneous group of molecules and include the 21-hydroxylase enzyme and some of the components of the complement cascade. The significance of the location of class III genes within the MHC is not known.

The most striking characteristic of class I and class II MHC antigens is their high degree of sequence polymorphism. At each genetic loci multiple alleles may exist. The precise role of class I and class II antigens in the immune response and the reason for their extensive polymorphism has become clear only in recent years. The first insight in this area came in 1976 when Doherty and Zinkernagel found that self-type MHC structures were needed for successful recognition of antigen by host lymphocytes. This requirement has been termed MHC restriction.

Subsequent early work demonstrating that the ability to respond to individual protein antigens was correlated with expression of specific MHC alleles and that certain autoimmune diseases were associated with expression of a particular MHC antigen lead to labeling MHC genes as immune response genes. It is now understood that the central role of the MHC in immune responsiveness derives from the fact that T cells require a composite structure of foreign antigen complexed with an MHC molecule to become activated.

Class I and class II MHC gene products serve principally as semiselective receptors for antigen. Their main function is to serve as a scaffolding for presentation of antigen to the TCR. Class I antigens are expressed on all nucleated cells and present antigen only to CD8+ T cells. Class II antigens are expressed only by APCs and present antigen selectively to CD4+ T cells. (The roles of class I and class II antigen are discussed in more detail in Chapter 21.)

Class I molecules have in their external domain a "groove" capable of holding a small peptide 10 to 15 amino acids in length. An analogous region may exist in class II structure. It is speculated that proteins taken up by an APC are degraded in such a way that some of the resulting fragments are capable of binding to class II. Evidence suggests that a hierarchy of peptide binding affinities may exist and that MHC alleles may have varying capacities to bind a particular peptide. This fact may explain the high degree of polymorphism found in MHC molecules. If only a single MHC molecule existed it is possible that by chance some peptides might be incapable of MHC binding and therefore could escape immune recognition.

Typical Immune Response

A primary immune response begins when antigenic material is introduced into the body. A number of routes of antigen entry are possible and in part determine the outcome of the response. In general, however, the body is designed to handle antigenic challenge in almost all tissues. The few tissues that are fully incapable of an immune response are termed immunologically privileged sites. These include the anterior chamber of the eye, the testes, and the central nervous system within the blood-brain barrier. Antigen introduced into these locations is immunologically inert. This has been attributed to the absence of efferent lymphatic drainage from these tissues. Certain tissues, especially those exposed to the external environment, are equipped for antigen handling. Blood-borne antigen is cleared by the spleen, whereas antigen entering the extravascular tissue is transported via afferent lymphatics either in free form or more likely after ingestion by APCs to local lymphoid tissue (lymph nodes, Peyer's patches, etc.).

An immune response is initiated when an antigen is processed and presented by an APC in the context of class II antigens (Figure 20-4). Presentation of the antigen activates a CD4+ class II restricted T-cell with a TCR specific for the antigen coupled to self-class II. Simultaneous with the antigen triggering of the TCR, the APC supplies a second signal in the form of soluble lymphokines. IL-1 is the best studied of these molecules, but other lymphokines, such as IL-6, may also participate.

The signaling between the T cell and APC is not unidirectional. Lymphokines made by T cells like γ-IFN can significantly influence the activity of APCs. γ-IFN,

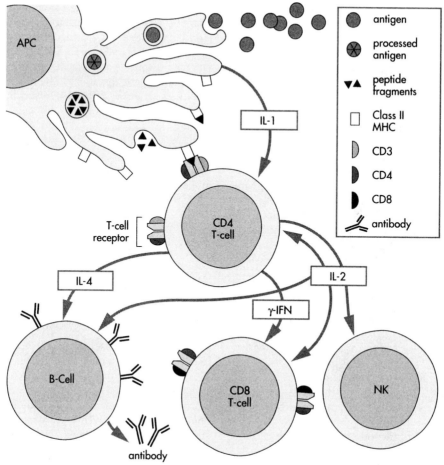

Figure 20-4 The imune response antigen is phagocytosed by an antigen-presenting cell and processed into peptide fragments. These fragments associate with class II MHC antigens and are presented on the APC's surface. Antigen-specific T cells (CD4) are then activated via their TCR (with associated T_3 complex and T_4 molecules). An accessory signal provided by the APC (such as IL-1) is necessary for T-cell activation. Activated T cells produce a panel of lymphokines, including IL-2, IL-4, and γ-interferon. Factors released by CD4 T cells are required for activation of immune effector cells (B cells, CD8 T cells, and NK cells).

also called macrophage-activating factor, increases macrophage activity in a variety of ways, including the enhancement of MHC class II antigen and Fc receptor expression.

The activation of the CD4+ T cell is a key regulatory step in the response. Upon activation, CD4+ cells produce the lymphokine IL-2. IL-2 can act as both an autocrine and paracrine mediator. IL-2 binding by T-cell IL-2 receptors triggers proliferation and differentiation of antigen-activated T cells.

Activation of CD4+ cells may enlist participation of

many other immune effector cells. As mentioned, γ-IFN secreted by CD4+ cells augments macrophage activity. It may also enhance the immunogenicity of target tissues by increasing MHC antigen expression. IL-2, IL-4, IL-5, and IL-6 secreted by CD4+ T cells are necessary for B-cell activation and Ig secretion. B cells and T cells cooperating in response to antigen can be brought together by B-cell presentation of antigen to T cells. Immunoglobulin secreted by B cells can damage pathogens directly by complement activation or can bind to antigenic determinants (opsinization), facilitating clearance by the reticuloendothelial system. Immunoglobulin can also bind other immune cells via Fc receptors. Mast cells, basophils, NK cells, and macrophages bind Ig as a part of their immune effector function.

Development of cytolytic activity by CD8+ T cells is also influenced by CD4+ cells. After recognition of antigen in a class I restricted manner, CD8+ cells require IL-2 and other differentiation factors produced by CD4+ cells to mature into CTLs. Once generated, CTLs have the ability to lyse cells expressing the proper antigen in the context of class I MHC antigen.

IL-2 and γ-IFN produced by CD4+ cells are known to augment the activity of NK cells. Development of LAK cells from NK cells is dependent on IL-2. Both NK cells and LAK cells exhibit tumoricidal activity (see Chapter 23). The mechanism by which LAK and NK cells recognize target cells is undetermined. It clearly differs from target recognition by T cells in that MHC structures are not required. Natural killer cells and macrophages can bind Ig via Fc receptors, thus permitting ADCC.

Monoclonal Antibodies

Monoclonal antibody technology takes advantage of the exquisite specificity of a single antibody manufactured in large amounts. This technology has had an impact on nearly every area of modern biology. Monoclonal antibodies are produced by immortalization of a B-lymphocyte population that has within it a high frequency of B cells specific for an antigen of interest. Immortalization is brought about by the fusion of B cells with a lymphoid tumor line, usually of B-cell origin but one that does not itself secrete antibody. Successful fusion generates lines of cells that divide autonomously and indefinitely but that are capable of production and secretion of an antibody identical with that of the B cell originally fused. Following screening for fusions with the desired specificity, a near permanent and inexhaustible source of a antibody is obtained by growing the cell line in vitro and harvesting the material secreted.

Bibliography

Bjorkman PJ, et al. Structure of the human class I histocompatibility antigen, HLA-A2. *Nature* 1987;329:506–512.

Braciale TJ, et al. Antigen presentation pathways of class I and class II MHC-restricted T lymphocytes. *Immunol Rev* 1987; 98:95–114.

Buus S, Sette A, Grey HM. The interaction between protein-derived immunogenic peptides and IA. *Immunol Rev* 1987; 98:115–141.

Klein J. *The natural history of the major histocompatibility complex.* New York: Wiley, 1986.

Paul WE. *Fundamental immunology.* 2nd ed. New York: Raven Press, 1989.

Rosenberg SA. Adoptive immunotherapy for cancer. *Sci Am* 1990;262:62–69.

Unanue ER. Antigen presenting function of the macrophage. *Ann Rev Immunol* 1984;2:395–428.

Unanue ER. The regulatory role of macrophages in antigenic stimulation. Part two: Symbiotic relationship between lymphocytes and macrophages. *Adv Immunol* 1981;31:1–136.

Zinkernagel RM, Doherty PC. Immunological surveillance against altered self components by sensitized T lymphocyte in lymphocytic choriomeningitis. *Nature* 1974;251: 547–548.

Zinkernagel RM, Doherty, PC. MHC restricted cytotoxic T cells: studies on the biologic role of polymorphic major transplantation antigen in determining T cell restriction specificity. *Adv Immunol* 1979;27:51–177.

James F. Markmann

21 IMMUNOBIOLOGY OF TRANSPLANTATION

The fields of immunology and transplantation have been intimately intertwined throughout their histories. Early transplant work provided many insights into fundamental immune mechanisms, and today important advances in clinical transplantation usually find their origin in basic immunology.

The prime impediment to transplantation is the immunologic barrier to engraftment. When tissues are transplanted from one organism to another, an immune response, similar in many respects to the response to foreign microbiological invaders described in the previous chapter, consistently ensues if the donor and recipient are not genetically identical. Grafts transplanted between genetically identical donor-recipient pairs are termed **isografts**. Grafts between nonidentical members of the same species are termed **allografts**; grafts between different species, **xenografts**. A graft taken from and returned to the same individual is called an **autograft**.

Donor-Recipient Interactions

The magnitude of an allograft response correlates well with the degree of antigenic disparity between donor and recipient. Antigenic disparity means that antigens present on donor cells are not expressed by the recipient. For example, in a given hypothetical donor-recipient pair, one expressing only "a" antigens and the other expressing "a" and "b" antigens, graft rejection can be expected after transplanting "ab" grafts into "a" recipients but not "a" grafts into "ab" recipients. This rejection is due to the recognition by "a" recipients of foreign "b" determinants or antigens expressed by "ab" donor cells.

The converse reaction—the recognition of host antigens by lymphoid cells of a graft—is termed a graft-versus-host (GVH) response and occurs only under special circumstances. The grafted tissue must include immunocompetent lymphoid cells, such as bone marrow grafts or grafts of small intestine. In addition, the recipient must be immunologically suppressed to prevent destruction of the donor lymphoid cells by those of the recipient.

Graft Antigens

MAJOR ANTIGENS

Early work in transplantation identified a single genetic locus responsible for a uniquely strong rejection response. Antigens encoded by this region are termed major histocompatibility (MHC) antigens. Major histocompatibility antigens constitute the main stimulus evoking allograft rejection. This property of MHC antigens can be attributed to three distinguishing characteristics. First, MHC antigens are ubiquitously distributed; all nucleated cells express class I antigens. Class II antigens are expressed only on antigen-presenting cells (APCs)—B cells, macrophages, and dendritic cells. However, APCs are dispersed throughout the body in both the lymphoid and nonlymphoid organs. Thus, all commonly grafted tissues express both class I and class II antigens.

Second, MHC antigens are highly polymorphic. MHC polymorphism virtually guarantees that a pair of individuals randomly selected from the population will differ at multiple MHC loci. Even among siblings in a family only about one in four will inherit the same alleles.

Finally, perhaps the most important reason MHC antigens play such a prominent role in graft rejection stems from their function in T-cell antigen recognition. The antigen-specific receptor utilized by T cells is designed to respond to antigens when they are associated with self-MHC molecules. A by-product of this characteristic is that foreign MHC molecules, which are similar in structure to self-MHC molecules, perhaps with peptide antigens bound to them, are potent triggers of T-cell activation. This was first clearly demonstrated by the finding that whereas only a small number of clones of T cells respond to a given protein or nominal antigen presented in the context of self-MHC, up to a few percent of the entire T-cell population may become activated when confronted with APCs bearing foreign MHC molecules.

MINOR ANTIGENS

In addition to MHC antigens, a diverse group of minor histocompatibility antigens also exist. Although the precise number is unknown, estimates from animal studies suggest that from 40 to more than 100 minor antigens are possible. Like MHC antigens, minor antigens can prompt graft rejection, though the response is slower. An example of a minor antigen is the mouse H-Y antigen. H-Y expression is determined by the Y chromosome and is therefore present only in males. H-Y disparity can lead to the rejection of male grafts by females of the same inbred strain of mice. As with other minor antigens, an antibody response to the antigen is difficult to demonstrate. Of even greater difficulty has been the isolation and characterization of individual minor antigen protein molecules.

The recognition of minor antigens by T lymphocytes is thought to occur in an MHC-restricted manner. It seems likely that any cellular protein with sequence polymorphism is a potential minor antigen and consequently a trigger for graft rejection. Thus, minor antigens are likely derived from a diverse group of proteins serving general housekeeping functions for cells and, unlike MHC antigens, are only indirectly related to the immune system. If this is the case, minor antigens may only appear on the cell surface following degradation and association with MHC during the intracellular journey of MHC to the cell surface. This might explain the difficulty in the characterization and isolation of minor antigen proteins.

THE HUMAN LEUKOCYTE ANTIGEN COMPLEX

In the human, the MHC is also termed the HLA (human leukocyte antigen) complex and is located on chromosone 6. It contains three class I loci—HLA-A, -B, and -C; and three class II families—HLA-DR, -DQ, and -DP. Multiple alleles exist for each locus. In all, more than 70 class I and 30 class II alleles have been identified.

In clinical transplantation, tissues are usually identified by the alleles present at the HLA-A, -B, and -D loci. The inheritance of MHC alleles occurs in a group known as a haplotype (in the absence of intra-MHC crossover during germ-cell production). Thus each parent can contribute either of its two haplotypes encoded by the MHC on their pair of chromosome 6. For example, given the two hypothetical parental genotypes, four possible offspring combinations are possible (Table 21-1).

TABLE 21.1. Genetics of MHC Antigens

Maternal HLA Haplotype	Potential Progeny
A1–B5–DR1	A1–B5–DR1
A2–B7–DR2	A9–B8–DR3
	A1–B5–DR1
	A10–B12–DR4
Paternal HLA Haplotype	
A9–B8–DR3	A2–B7–DR2
A10–B12–DR4	A9–B8–DR3
	A2–B7–DR2
	A10–B12–DR4

Thus a given sibling will have a one in four chance of MHC identity with another sibling (two-haplotype match), a one in two chance of a one-haplotype match, and a one in four chance of being completely MHC discordant (zero-haplotype match). In addition, each child will share at least one haplotype with each parent.

A number of techniques have been employed to detect polymorphism in MHC antigens. Initially, serum from multiparous females was used in leukoagglutation assays. Since most lymphocytes express only class I antigens, the antigens detected with sera were predominantly class I molecules. As a result, class I antigens were originally termed serologically determined antigens. Today monoclonal antibodies have been generated that detect determinants on both class I and class II structures and can be used along with complement to identify reactive cells.

A second approach takes advantage of the finding that lympohcytes from two MHC-incompatible individuals mixed together in vitro will mount an immune response to each other. The magnitude of the response can be evaluated by determining the rate of cell division. If the mitotic activity of one of the two populations is impaired, either pharmacologically or by irradiation, a one-way mixed-lymphocyte reaction results. Proliferation of the population with unaltered mitotic capacity in this setting can be detected by incorporation of radiolabeled markers into newly synthesized DNA during cell division. The rate of proliferation provides an indication of antigens present on the APCs of the stimulator population and not present in the responder population. Thus, this in vitro response parallels the allograft response in which donor antigens (in this case stimulator) are recognized by recipient (or responder) lymphocytes. Genetic-mapping studies have identified disparity at the MHC class II locus (but not class I locus) as the stimulus for responder cell activation and proliferation in this assay. CD4+ T cells have been found to be the major subset of responding cells, and class II+ APCs, especially dendritic cells, the major constituent of the stimulator population inducing activation.

More recently molecular biology has provided specific molecular probes and sequencing technology, allowing detection of subtle differences in MHC genes and the proteins they encode. However, unlike the techniques discussed above, antigenic differences detected by this method are not necessarily immunologically relevant.

Immunological Mechanisms of Graft Rejection

TYPES OF GRAFT REJECTION

Allograft rejection can occur with a spectrum of severity and tempo. The most rapid form is termed **hyperacute rejection.** With hyperacute rejection preformed recipient antibodies target the vascular endothelium of the transplanted tissue. Antibodies specific for MHC antigens, blood group antigens, and others can mediate this process. Only vascularized grafts, such as kidney or heart grafts, are immediately vulnerable to this mechanism. Skin grafts and other nonvascularized grafts, which require a period of time for their blood supply to become contiguous with that of the recipient, are initially invulnerable. Actual graft destruction produced by preformed antibody is dependent on activation of the complement cascade and other vasoactive mediators that destroy the integrity of graft vessels or lead to thrombosis. Immunosuppressive agents have not been identified to prevent or halt this process effectively. It generally can be avoided, however, by pretransplant donor-recipient cross-matching. The contribution of antibody to other forms of graft rejection is disputed but at most probably plays a minor role.

The most frequently observed form of rejection is termed **acute rejection.** It is first observed about 1 week after transplantation. Acute rejection is characterized by a progressive lymphocytic infiltration of the graft and is thought to be a T-cell-dependent event. Foreign MHC antigens expressed by graft cells are the major stimulus for acute rejection, though it can also be induced by minor histocompatibility antigens. T-cell involvement in the response is supported by its susceptibility to commonly used immunosuppressive agents, including antilymphocyte globulin (ALG) and the monoclonal anti-T-cell antibody OKT3.

Both CD4+ and CD8+ T cells have the potential to damage a foreign graft. The exact contribution of each T-cell subset apparently depends on the antigenic disparity between donor and recipient. Helper function, in the form of lymphokine production, and cytotoxic activity, can be supplied by either CD4+ or CD8+ cells, depending on the particular antigen involved. However, both a population with helper function and a population with cytotoxic function are required for T-cell-mediated rejection. Absence of either population can result in an ineffective or indolent rejection.

Accelerated rejection is similar to acute rejection in character but with more rapid onset. Accelerated rejection occurs in recipients previously sensitized to donor-type antigens and is an example of an anamnestic or secondary immune response.

Chronic graft rejection can occur months to years after transplantation. The mononuclear cell infiltrate is generally less intense than that observed in acute rejection. Graft fibrosis and vascular changes may predominate histologically. The precise immune mediators effecting chronic graft damage are not known. Both antibody-mediated and cell-mediated components may exist.

MECHANISMS OF GRAFT REJECTION

An allograft presents the host with a complex array of cells and cellular antigens as targets of immunity. While many of the details of the response are unknown, a coherent model of T-cell-mediated graft rejection can be derived from a knowledge of physiologic T-cell function. It is well accepted that T-cell activation by foreign antigen, including foreign MHC molecules, is dependent on specialized class II MHC-bearing antigen-presenting cells. In theory, during graft rejection, APCs could be supplied either by the host or by a population of passenger leukocytes carried along with the graft.

Foreign class II antigens present on graft APCs, such as dendritic cells, provide the most potent stimulus for activation of CD4+ host leukocytes. This encounter most likely occurs in local lymph nodes but might also take place within the graft itself. CD4+ T-cell activation results in lymphokine production and permits involvement of multiple immune effector mechanisms. NK cells, B lymphocytes, macrophages, and cytotoxic T cells have all been identified as graft-infiltrating cells. While participation of non-T cells in graft rejection almost certainly occurs, without T-cell involvement acute graft rejection will not take place.

The "**passenger leukocyte hypothesis**" is based on the premise that only graft APCs are immunologically relevant, and therefore deletion of this population from the graft prior to transplantation should promote graft survival. Considerable experimental evidence obtained from the study of endocrine grafts supports this contention. Application of this strategy to more complex vascularized organ grafts has been less successful.

Antirejection Strategies

DECREASED GRAFT IMMUNOGENICITY

A number of attempts have been made to identify and nullify the graft-related promotors of rejection. As mentioned above, in experimental endocrine grafts, graft immunogenicity can be significantly reduced by elimination or inactivation of graft APCs prior to transplantation. This can be accomplished (1) by treatment with anti-class II MHC antibody and complement, (2) by maintaining the tissue in vitro for a period prior to grafting to allow selective attrition of the lymphoid cells, and (3) by exposure of the graft to ultraviolet irradiation, a treatment known to render APCs nonfunctional. Although conceptually sound, this strategy has not yet been successfully applied to clinical transplantation.

HISTOCOMPATIBILITY MATCHING OF DONOR AND RECIPIENT

Considering the importance of foreign MHC molecules in promoting allograft rejection, a logical approach is to choose donors concordant for recipient MHC alleles. The most commonly used method of tissue typing for MHC antigens employs banks of defined antisera directed against specific HLA alleles. Donor and recipient peripheral blood lymphocytes are individually mixed with anti-HLA sera in the presence of complement. Cell lysis is indicative of a positive reaction and the presence of a given allele.

In addition to MHC typing, with rare exceptions donor and recipient must be ABO blood group compatible. The presence of preformed antibodies against ABO antigens can result in rapid graft loss.

Finally, a cross-match or lymphotoxicity assay is performed. In this test recipient serum is incubated with donor lymphocytes in the presence of complement. Lysis of donor cells is an indication of preformed recipient antibodies against donor antigens.

All allografts require ABO compatibility. The need for HLA matching and cross-matching varies with the type of organ transplanted. Specific organ requirements and related graft survival rates are detailed in Table 21-2.

To avoid antigenic incompatibility, the ideal donor-recipient combination is identical twins. In this case, graft rejection cannot occur, since not only are MHC antigens shared but also minor histoincompatibilities

TABLE 21-2. Pretransplant Evaluation and Expected Graft Survival

Organ Graft	Pretransplant Requirements	Subgroups	Approximate 1-Year Graft Survival (%)[a]
Kidney	ABO compatibility Crossmatch negative HLA match preferred	HLA identical sib 1-haplotype match Cadaver donor	95 90 80
Liver	ABO compatibility		70
Pancreas	ABO compatibility Crossmatch negative HLA match preferred		65
Heart	ABO compatibility	With cyclosporine Without cyclosporine	80 55

[a]Graft and patient survival vary significantly dependent on multiple factors including transplant center. The data presented are representative approximations.
HLA, Human leukocyte antigen.

do not exist. If there is no identical twin, HLA typing of family members can identify donors whose organs will have the best probability of survival in the recipient. When grafts are exchanged between siblings, complete MHC identity occurs only 25% of the time. In general, a strong correlation exists between the extent of MHC compatibility and graft survival between related individuals. The benefit derived from HLA matching is less dramatic using cadaveric donors. This may be due in part to the extensive minor antigen incompatibility encountered using unrelated donors. With the advent of more effective immunosuppressive agents, the increased survival derived from HLA matching is less evident.

RECIPIENT IMMUNOSUPPRESSION

The ability to suppress the recipient's immune system and hence its response to a foreign graft has been the mainstay of antirejection therapy in clinical transplantation. The precise immunosuppressive regimen employed not only varies among transplant centers because of personal preference but also is constantly evolving as new information and newer agents become available. Before the introduction of cyclosporine, the combination of azathioprine and corticosteroids was widely used. The addition of cyclosporine to form a "three-drug regimen" has permitted improved success with a reduction in the requirement for azathioprine and corticosteroids. An unyielding requirement thus far in the field of transplantation is the need for lifelong im-

munosuppression. Unlike many models of allografting in experimental animals, it has not been possible to achieve a stable graft-host relationship in humans without chronic immunosuppression.

Corticosteroids

Steroid therapy currently holds a prominent place in transplantation. Despite the absence of a clear understanding of their mechanism of action, steroids have been found to be efficacious in preventing graft rejection and the treatment of rejection episodes already in progress. Steroids function by binding to intracellular receptors, forming a molecular complex that posesses DNA binding capabilities. In lymphocytes this has been shown to result in inhibition of DNA and RNA synthesis.

Steroids have a number of well-documented immunologic effects. At sufficient doses steroids may be lymphocytolytic, though it is unlikely this is their predominant effect in vivo. Steroids are known to have antimacrophage properties. Production of interleukin-1 (IL-1), an important cofactor for T-cell activation, is blocked by corticosteroids. Chemotaxis by macrophages is also reduced. In general, steroid therapy exerts a nonspecific antiinflammatory effect and, like other immunosuppressants, predisposes the host to opportunistic infections.

The other side effects from steroid administration are those expected from physiological corticosteroid excess. Hypertension, obesity, peptic ulcer disease, hyperglycemia, and avascular necrosis of bone are all common with chronic steroid administration.

Azathioprine

Azathioprine is a purine analog that is the most widely employed antiproliferative agent in organ transplantation. Antiproliferative agents have in common their ability to inhibit lymphocyte mitosis. Included in this group are alkylating agents, radiation, and antimetabolites.

Antimetabolites such as azathioprine inhibit lymphocyte proliferation by substituting for cellular compounds, leading to an inhibition of or interference with a required biosynthetic pathway. In the case of azathioprine, the drug is converted by the liver to 6-mercaptopurine. After the addition of ribose-5-phosphate, 6-mercaptopurine ribonucleotide has structural similarity to inosine monophosphate. Production of DNA and RNA is inhibited by blocking conversion of inosine monophosphate to the essential purines adenosine and guanine.

The side effects produced by azathioprine are directly related to its desired biological effects. Most importantly, severe bone marrow suppression can occur, leading to profound leukopenia. Hepatic toxicity is another common side effect.

Many other antiproliferative agents have been tried in organ transplantation with varying degrees of success. Alkylating agents, such as nitrogen mustard and cyclophosphamide, and folic acid antagonists, such as methotrexate, while highly immmunosuppressive, have been found to be too toxic for the chronic immunosuppression required for organ transplantation. Similarly, radiation therapy, while a potent immunosuppressant, has not yet found an established place in clinical organ transplantation.

Polyclonal and Monoclonal Antibody Preparations

Immunosuppression with antibodies directed against T-lymphocyte determinants can be either polyclonal or monoclonal in specificity. The first antibody successfully employed was antilymphocyte globulin (ALG). Antilymphocyte globulin is produced by injection of animals such as horses or rabbits with human lymphocytes. The immune response generated in the host animal will result in production of antibodies directed against human lymphocyte determinants. Serum harvested from an injected animal is purified in a process that includes adsorption with platelets and red blood cells in an attempt to minimize contaminating antibodies directed toward erythrocyte and thrombocyte products. Since the antibodies generated are polyclonal and reactive to many antigenic determinants, they exert a broad and nonspecific immunosuppressive action when administered to humans.

A refinement of this approach is the use of monoclonal antibodies. In this case, a clone of an antibody specific for a single lymphocyte determinant can be produced using techniques described in the previous chapter. The most successful example is the monoclonal antibody OKT3, which is a mouse antibody specific for a component of the T3 complex on human T cells. Administration of OKT3 exerts a profound immunosuppressive effect by its ability selectively to compromise T-cell function.

Since both polyclonal and monoclonal antibodies are produced in xenogenic animals, the antibodies themselves are potentially antigenic to human recipients. An immunoglobulin response can be generated to foreign determinants on both the constant and variable regions of the administered antibody. The immune response generated against monoclonal antibodies appears to be more complete and limiting than the response against polyclonal serum. For this reason, OKT3 use is often restricted to a one- to two-week course. The effect of OKT3 can be monitored by examining recipients for the presence of T3-bearing lymphocytes. Successful OKT3 therapy should lead to a prompt and dramatic reduction in the T3-positive lymphocyte populations in peripheral blood.

The side effects of antisera or monoclonal antibody administration are variable. Nonspecific symptoms, such as fever, chills and nausea, are common, especially with initial dosing.

A number of other monoclonal agents are under investigation. Antibody directed at IL-2 receptors has shown some efficacy in initial clinical trials. This agent has the theoretical advantage of only reacting with activated T cells, since only activated T cells express a high level of IL-2 receptors. With this strategy, it may be possible selectively to target immune cells activated to graft antigens.

Monoclonal antibodies specific for T-cell subsets have proven efficacious in experimental animals. Antibody specific for the CD4 molecules appears especially promising. CD4+ T cells are known to be regulatory cells essential in almost every arm of the cellular immune response and provide an attractive target for immunosuppression in humans.

Cyclosporine A

Cyclosporine A is a fungal lipophilic endecapeptide that has been found to have potent immunosuppressive activity without generalized myelotoxicity. In experimental animal systems cyclosporine has been shown to inhibit T-cell-dependent antibody production, delayed-type hypersensitivity reactions, antigen- and protein-driven T-cell proliferation, and cytotoxic T-lymphocyte generation in vitro; graft-versus-host disease; several forms of autoimmune disease; and allograft rejection. The clinical performance of cyclosporine in organ transplantation has been equally impressive. The use of cyclosporine has lead to a dramatic improvement in the survival of most organ allografts. Its use in heart, liver, pancreas, and lung transplantation has helped to transform these procedures into clinically acceptable therapies.

Cyclosporine's mode of action is incompletely defined but appears to focus on the T lymphocyte. Cyclosporine inhibits T-cell activation. It does not alter T-cell binding of antigen nor the transmembrane antigen activation signal mediated by the CD3-complex. The immunosuppressive effect occurs after the calcium influx occurring with T-cell activation. The earliest step in the activation cascade known to be inhibited by cyclosporin is the transcription of mRNA encoding a panel of lymphokines, including IL-2 and γ-interferon. The mechanism of inhibition is unclear. Cyclosporine is lipophillic and can pass through cell membranes and bind intracellular receptor molecules. Cyclosporine has been found to bind intracellular calmodulin, a molecule important in intracellular calcium-mediated signaling. Cyclosporine also binds cyclophillin, a protein that binds cyclosporine and it analogs, in proportion to their immunosuppressive activity but that has undefined regulatory activities. An attractive but unproven hypothesis is that cyclosporine binds to an intracellular receptor that has DNA-binding capacity or the ability to alter the activity of regulatory proteins and leads to the inhibition of lymphokine gene transcription.

Cyclosporine has a number of toxic effects both related and unrelated to its desired immunosuppressive action. Similar to other immunosuppressive agents, cyclosporine predisposes those treated to infectious complications. Interestingly the use of cyclosporine with prednisone compared to the traditional regimen of aza-thioprine and prednisone was associated with an overall reduction in the incidence of opportunistic infections.

The other side effects of cyclosporine administration include hypertrichosis, gingival hypertrophy, hypertension, hyperglycemia, and hepatotoxicity. Clinically, the most significant and limiting side effect is nephrotoxicity. Cyclosporine nephrotoxicity occurs with a spectrum of severity and possibly through a variety of mechanisms. In kidney transplantation, when the recipient's creatinine rises, it is difficult to determine whether cyclosporine toxicity or graft rejection is to blame. A reduction in cyclosporine dosing is usually necessary.

FK506

FK506 is the newest immunosuppressive agent with documented clinical efficacy. FK506 is a macrolide antibiotic that has structural similarity to the drug rapamycin. FK506, like cyclosporine, is lipid soluble and binds to an intracellular receptor that is similar to that bound by cyclosporine.

FK506 apparently exerts its immunosuppressant affect in T cells after the early transmembrane activation signaling, but before transcription of the genes for lymphokine expression. Production of IL-2, IL-3, IL-4, TNF, γ-IFN and granulocyte macrophage colony-stimulating factor have also been found to be blocked by treatment with FK506 before T-cell activation. While cyclosporine may exert similar effects, it does so at drug levels many times higher than that required by FK506.

Preliminary clinical trials of FK506 have demonstrated its efficacy when used as the prime immunosuppressive agent after transplantation. Initial attempts to combine FK506 with cyclosporine caused significant elevation in blood cyclosporine levels and toxicity. Since then FK506 has shown success when used along with steroids in attempts to rescue liver grafts undergoing rejection resistant to conventional treatment. The short-term side effects of FK506 appear to be similar to those of cyclosporine A. The long-term efficacy and side effects are not yet known.

Bibliography

Auchincloss HA, Sachs DH. Transplantation and graft rejection. In: Paul WE, ed. *Fundamental immunology*. 2nd ed. New York: Raven Press, 1990:889–923.

Bach FH, Sachs DH. Transplantation immunology. *N Engl J Med* 1987;317(8):489–492.

Barker CF, Naji A, Dafoe DC, Perloff LJP. Renal transplantation. In: Sabiston D, ed. *Textbook of surgery.* Philadelphia: WB Saunders, 1991:374–393.

Kahan BD. Drug therapy: Cyclosporine. *New Engl J Med* 1989;321(25):1725–1738.

Klein J, ed. Allograft rejection. In *Natural history of the major histocompatibility complex.* New York: Wiley, 1986, chap 6.

Krensky AM, Weiss A, Crabtree G, Davis MM, Parham P. T-lymphocyte-antigen interaction in transplant rejection. *N Engl J Med* 1990;322(8):505–517.

Rosenberg A, Mizuochi T, Singer A. Analysis of T cell subsets in rejection of KB mutant skin allografts differing at class I MHC. *Nature* 1986;332:829–831.

Simmons RL, Miglior RJ, Smith CR, Reemtsma K, Najarian S. Transplantation. In: Schwartz SI, ed. *Principles of surgery.* 5th ed. New York: McGraw-Hill, 1989:387–458.

Soulillou JP, Cantarovich D, Le-Mauff B, Giral M, Robillard N, Hourmant M, Hirn M, Jacques Y. Randomized controlled trial of a monoclonal antibody against the interleukin-2 receptor (33B3.1) as compared with rabbit anti-thymocyte globulin for prophylaxis against rejection of renal allografts *N Engl J Med* 1990;322(17):1175–1182.

Terasaki PI. In: *Clinical transplants 1988.* Los Angeles, CA: UCLA Tissue Typing Laboratory, 1988.

David L. Bartlett

22 TUMOR BIOLOGY

As with most disease entities, it is no longer adequate to discuss cancer at the level of the organism. Much is now known at the cellular, subcellular, and molecular levels that has relevance to the clinical disease. A basic understanding of the biology of cancer is essential in order to determine such critical factors as prognosis, diagnosis, treatment, and prevention. Accurate histologic diagnosis and DNA ploidy, for instance, may have as much prognostic relevance in breast cancer as clinical axillary node status. Similarly, an understanding of tumor heterogeneity has resulted in more effective chemotherapeutic combinations and multimodal treatments. The purpose of this chapter is to review clinically important aspects of tumor biology in a discussion of the basic science of neoplasia. It should serve as an up-to-date reference for mechanisms of carcinogenesis, cell proliferation, and tumor metastasis. It will also review important aspects of tumor metabolism and host-tumor interactions. Tumor immunology is discussed in the next chapter.

It is important to realize that cancer is not a single disease process. Each tumor should be thought of as a unique entity with its own biology and its own, original therapeutic regimen. It should be remembered that the hosts are heterogenous, the tumors are heterogenous, and the cells are heterogenous within each tumor. Treatments will have to vary from case to case.

Characteristics of Malignancy

The word *tumor* is synonymous with *neoplasia*, which is a general term for any abnormal new growth of tissue. Neoplasias can be either benign or malignant in character. This chapter will focus on malignant neoplasias, but the difference between benign and malignant growths is not always obvious. There is actually a continuous spectrum from clearly benign tumors to extremely malignant tumors. There are characteristics of each that help differentiate between the two. In general, benign tumors are well circumscribed and surrounded by a capsule of connective tissue. They do not invade into surrounding structures and do not metastasize. Surgical resection is usually curative, so benign tumors do not usually influence life expectancy. Malignant tumors are characterized by excessive, uncoordinated, autonomous growth; a tendency toward **anaplasia** (undifferentiated cells that have lost resemblance to their normal counterparts) and **aneuploidy** (abnormal chromosomal complement); and most importantly, the ability to invade surrounding tissue and to metastasize to distant sites.

Normal cells undergo differentiation from a multipotent stem cell to a mature, functional adult cell that is eventually no longer able to undergo cell division. These cells have a finite life span. In addition, these normal cells respond to external stimuli. For example, contact inhibition limits cell division when a critical cell density is achieved. In addition, cells adapt to available nutritional substrates such that their proliferation can be stalled. It was once thought that a process of dedifferentiation accompanied tumor growth. Instead, tumor cells become arrested at different stages of differentiation, and are often quite undifferentiated or anaplastic.

They no longer respond to external stimuli regulating growth and proliferation, and do not usually mature to functional forms. Their proliferation is considered autonomous.

As part of their unregulated, uncoordinated growth, tumor cell proliferation becomes "sloppy." Tumors have many abnormal mitoses and chromosomal irregularities, and significant cellular disarray. Abnormal mitotic figures include **chromatin bridges, chromosome lagging,** and **multiple spindle apparatuses** within a single cell. The vast majority of tumors have a high incidence of aneuploidy. This can be measured using flow cytometric techniques. Routine histologic examination reveals an increased nuclear-to-cytoplasmic ratio. The aggressiveness of the tumor often correlates with the degree of aneuploidy. Structural chromosome abnormalities are also common and include **deletions, translocations,** and **inversions.** Perhaps the most common of these is the Philadelphia chromosome, seen in chronic myelogenous leukemia. This represents a (22,9) translocation. There is, in general, more heterochromatin, or repressed, nonfunctional portions of the genome in tumor cells, compared to euchromatin, representing actively transcribing portions.

The final characteristic to be discussed is the ability of malignant tumors to invade surrounding tissue and metastasize. This is undoubtedly the most important characteristic of malignancy and is the central theme around which we base the diagnosis and surgical treatment of cancer. If there were a way to prevent invasion and metastasis, all cancers would be curable.

Mechanisms of Tumorigenesis

In general, human tumors should be thought of as arising from a single, transformed cell. It is known experimentally that transplantation of a single, malignant cell can result in a tumor that can kill the host. Cell marker studies of human tumors have established monoclonality among all cells in the tumor, with the conclusion that most tumors have a **unicellular origin.** This does not imply that the cells are homogenous. Genetic and epigenetic instability result in a heterogenous population of cells. Nevertheless, the origin of a tumor is most often a single cell. Lesions tend to progress from cellular **atypia,** to **dysplasia,** then **carcinoma in situ,** and finally frank cancer. It should not be inferred that each tumor cell in a neoplasm progresses through these stages. Rather, a single cell is transformed within a dysplastic lesion and gives rise to all other cells within that tumor. In rare cases, where genetic predisposition or overwhelming carcinogen exposure results in multiple cells having a predisposition to malignant transformation, a tumor of multicellular origin may occur.

Mechanisms of carcinogenesis are as varied as the tumors themselves, but a few generalizations are possible. It is still accepted that the majority of tumors arise from a single, **"initiated"** cell, that, after a latent period of variable length, undergoes **"promotion"** resulting in a tumor (Figure 22-1). Initiation can occur via chemical, physical, biologic, or heritable means. Initiation is irreversible. Initiated cells can die or be killed, but they cannot revert to normal. Initiation must occur prior to promotion for a tumor to result. In contrast to promotion, a single exposure can result in initiation. Carcinogens and mutagens are considered initators.

Promoters, on the other hand, are agents that alter the expression of genetic information without reacting directly with the gene. These may be hormones, drugs, or other biologic stimuli that affect regulatory mechanisms within the cell. They often require prolonged exposure and may be reversible. These agents are not considered carcinogens and are not mutagenic. In simplified terms, after a mutation has been initiated, the promoter stimulates expression of that mutation. Some agents can act as both initiators and promoters and are termed **"complete carcinogens."**

Carcinogenesis occurs through many mechanisms. Chemicals act as carcinogens by forming reactive electrophilic intermediates that bind to DNA to form covalent adducts. These adducts then cause miscoding. The resultant damage can either be repaired by cellular enzymes or passed on to progeny cells through DNA replication. Once passed on, the lesion is permanent, and the cell is considered "initiated." Table 22-1 lists a variety of agents which have been associated with neoplasms based on epidemiologic studies. Most of these are considered carcinogens.

Another form of carcinogenesis is termed physical carcinogenesis. This term refers to direct physical damage by ionizing radiation and ultraviolet radiation. Energy in ionizing radiation causes splitting of water molecules within cells, releasing free radicals, which can damage DNA. The radiation can also cause direct damage to DNA bases and cause the sugar-phosphate backbone of the DNA strand to break. Ultraviolet radiation does not contain enough energy to ionize molecules, but it does put them in a short-lived, excited

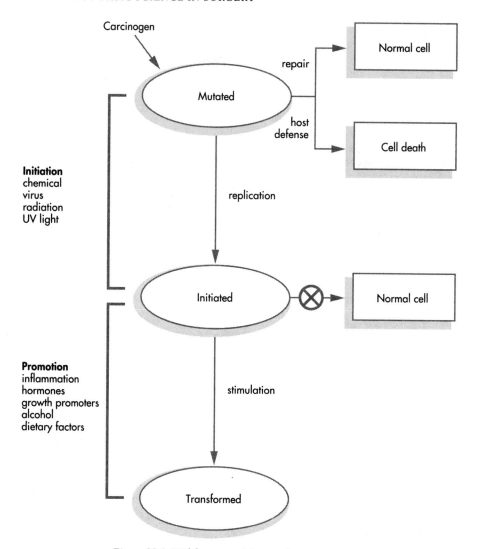

Figure 22-1 Widely accepted theory of carcinogenesis.

state—making them chemically reactive. Most research has concentrated on the formation of pyrimidine dimers as a result of UV radiation. These dimers appear to have a role in "initiation" of the cell.

Viral carcinogenesis has been studied for many decades. Some human tumors are now believed to be directly caused by viral transformation. These include hepatocellular carcinoma (hepatitis B virus), papillomas and cervical cancer (human papilloma virus), and Burkitt's lymphoma and nasopharyngeal carcinoma (Epstein-Barr herpes virus). There is also evidence that retroviruses cause adult T-lymphocyte leukemia.

Vaccines against these viruses have the potential to prevent occurrence of these tumors. Understanding the mechanisms of viral oncogenesis requires an understanding of **oncogenes** and **protooncogenes.** Protooncogenes are normal, human gene sequences that encode for proteins essential to normal growth regulation of cells. Protooncogenes can be converted to oncogenes by mutation, rearrangement, or incorporation into a viral genome. Oncogenes then contribute directly to the malignant transformation of the host cell.

Through numerous generations of viral infections, many protooncogenes have been incorporated into viral

TABLE 22-1. Some Examples of Chemicals Considered to Be Carcinogens

Agent	Tumor
Cultural	
Alcohol	Oropharynx, esophagus, liver, larynx
Cigarette smoke	Oropharynx, larynx, lung, esophagus, bladder
Aflatoxins	Liver
Industrial	
Vinyl chloride	Liver (angiosarcoma)
Benzene	Leukemia
Bis(chloromethyl) ether	Lung
Soots, oils, and tars	Skin, lung, bladder, GI
Aromatic amines	Bladder
Medical	
Alkylating agents	Bladder, leukemia
Estrogens	Liver
Diethylstilbesterol	Vagina
Azathioprine	Lymphoma, skin
Anabolic steroids	Liver

genomes. Once incorporated into the virus, they no longer have their normal, regulatory capability, and upon **transfection** of their genome, they are able to transform normal cells. This new gene fragment within the virus is known as a viral oncogene. DNA viruses incorporate their genome directly into host cells, while RNA retroviruses incorporate a DNA copy of their RNA. In addition to direct transfection with an oncogene, viruses can transform cells by indirectly activating cellular protooncogenes. A simplified example would be for the virus to insert an unregulated promoter adjacent to a cellular protooncogene, resulting in its unregulated transcription and transformation of the cell.

Another mechanism for carcinogenesis involves a genetic predisposition for certain types of tumors. Examples of this include familial polyposis coli, xeroderma pigmentosum, retinoblastoma, Wilms' tumor, Bloom's syndrome, Fanconi's anemia, and ataxia telangiectasia. Table 22-2 summarizes these entities. The mechanisms of tumorigenesis vary. In some, such as retinoblastoma and Wilms' tumor, a precise chromosomal location for gene mutation leading to a tumor has been identified. Many other tumors, such as breast cancers, have a distinct heritable predilection, but no specific mutations have been found. It may be that all

cancers have heritable subgroups that have not yet been identified.

Tumor Cell Kinetics and Proliferation

An understanding of tumor growth and cell kinetics is important to many aspects of oncology. Tumor doubling time and cell-cycle duration, for instance, have significance with regard to prognosis and response to chemotherapy. The **cell cycle** (see Figure 1-3) represents the stages through which each cell progresses on its way to forming two daughter cells. Techniques such as the percent-labeled mitosis curve can measure the duration of the cell cycle. This is very accurate for determining the rate of proliferation of a tumor. Flow cytometric analysis utilizes fluorescent DNA stains to determine the quantity of DNA present in each cell of a population. The quantity of DNA corresponds to a phase of the cell cycle. A 2n quantity corresponds to G1, 4n corresponds to G2 and M, and those cells between 2n and 4n are in the S-phase. The number of cells in **S-phase** at a given time correlates with proliferation. This is the parameter that is used to estimate prognosis. Chemotherapeutic regimens that require actively dividing cells for their effect will theoretically have better results against tumors with a large S-phase population.

Tumor growth is determined by cell proliferation. In general, cell proliferation is in direct porportion to the number of cells present in the population. This results in constant doubling times and **exponential growth.** A tumor will seem to grow faster as it gets larger, but the doubling time is actually constant. Tumor growth or doubling time can be calculated using the following equation: $V = V_o \exp(0.693/T_d)$, where V_o is the tumor volume at time $t = 0$, and T_d is the tumor doubling time. At very large sizes the growth curve levels off. A significant amount of cell loss also occurs, from such factors as unsuccessful mitosis, cell shedding, metastasis, and cell death owing to starvation. Cells greater than 150 ʋm from nutrient capillaries die from inadequate nutrition. It is probably this cell loss that accounts for the leveling off of the growth curve at large volumes.

Figure 22-2 represents a hypothetical growth curve for a human tumor. Approximately 30–33 doublings occurred before the tumor reached a clinically detectable size of 1–10 g. Only a few more doublings will

TABLE 22-2. Hereditary Cancerous and Precancerous Disorders

Disorder	Predominant Tumors
Autosomal Dominant Inheritance	
Retinoblastoma	Retinoblastoma, sarcomas—orbital (following radiation) and at remote sites
Neurofibromatosis	Neurogenic sarcoma, acoustic neuroma, pheochromocytoma
Familial polyposis coli	Colonic cancer, adenomatous polyps
Gardner's syndrome	Colonic cancer, adenomatous polyps, osteomas
Peutz-Jeghers syndrome	Controversial whether predisposes to colonic cancer
Hereditary multiple endocrine neoplasia syndrome—type I (MEN I)	Tumors of pituitary gland, parathyroid gland, and pancreatic islet cells
Multiple endocrine neoplasia syndrome—type II (MEN II)	Medullary carcinoma of thyroid, pheochromocytoma, and parathyroid disease
Cutaneous malignant melanoma	Cutaneous malignant melanoma, other cancers
Von Hippel-Lindau disease	Hemangioblastoma of cerebellum, hypernephroma, and pheochromocytoma
Cancer—family syndrome	Adenocarcinomas (primarily of colon and endometrium)
Breast cancer in association with other malignant neoplasms	Breast cancer, sarcoma, leukemia, and brain tumor
Autosomal Recessive Inheritance	
Xeroderma pigmentosum	Basal and squamous cell carcinoma of skin, malignant melanoma
Fanconi's anemia	Leukemia and lymphoma
Bloom's syndrome	Acute leukemia, various carcinomas
Ataxia telangiectasia	Acute leukemia, lymphoma, and possibly gastric cancer
Turcot's syndrome	Colonic polyps, cancer, and brain tumors

Reproduced from Robbins SL, Cotran RS, Kumar V. *Pathologic basis of disease.* 3rd ed. Philadelphia: WB Saunders, 1984:264.

result in the death of the host. Assuming an average doubling time of 2 months, this represents the progression of this tumor for 5 years prior to clinical detection. This accounts for the occurrence of metastatic disease prior to diagnosis. This also exemplifies the difficulty in determining carcinogenic etiologies of tumors. Carcinogenic transformation generally occurs many years prior to the detection of a tumor.

Normal cell growth and proliferation appear to be regulated by external or exogenous growth factors. Many such factors specific for certain tissues have been described. Examples include **insulinlike growth factors,** specific for liver, adipose, and muscle cells; **epidermal growth factors** and **transforming growth factor,** specific for epidermal cells, fibroblasts, and epithelial cells; and **platelet-derived growth factors,** specific for fibroblasts, smooth muscle cells, and glial cells. These factors are polypeptides that are extremely active biologically. They seem to act in a paracrine or endocrine manner. They bind to specific receptors that transfer a signal through the membrane to the cytoplasm. The signal is then transferred, via second messengers, to the nucleus, where DNA synthesis is initiated.

It is easy to see how aberrations in this process could lead to malignant transformation. Some tumor cells have been found to synthesize their own peptide growth factors as well as the receptor for that factor. A process of self-stimulation occurs, resulting in autonomous growth, no longer regulated by the environment. The cell is thus malignant. Cells may also be

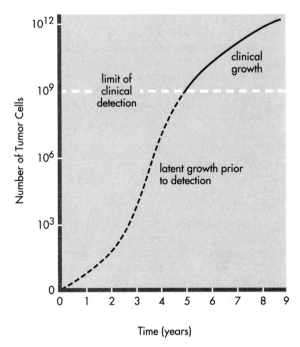

Figure 22-2 Hypothetical growth curve for a human tumor. Note the long latent period prior to clinical detection. (Reproduced from Tannock IF, Hill RP. *The basic science of oncology*. New York: Pergamon Press, 1987:143.)

TABLE 22-3. Examples of Oncogenes Classified by Function

Tyrosine-specific protein kinase	*src, abl, fes*
Protein kinase/ growth factor receptor-related	*erb-B, fms*
Growth factor related	*sis, Blym*
GTP binding (GTPase)	*ras* family
Nuclear ± DNA binding	*myc* family, *myb, fos*

Reproduced from Moosa AR, Robson MC, Schimpff SC. *Comprehensive textbook of oncology*. Baltimore: Williams & Wilkins, 1986:40.

membrane receptor for epidermal growth factor. Of note, the epidermal growth factor receptor has been found to have tyrosine kinase activity in its cytoplasmic end that acts to transmit the signal to the cytoplasm. In addition, src and fes oncogenes encode for cytoplasmic proteins with tyrosine protein kinase activity, and ras oncogenes encode for GTP- binding proteins. Finally, myc, myb, fos, and others encode for nuclear proteins that in the normal cell function directly to control cell proliferation and cell maturation. Oncogenes are discussed further in Chapter 23.

To date, only about 10% of human tumors have been found to involve oncogene activation, but this may change as more are discovered. Knowledge of the mechanisms of normal cell proliferation and differentiation has provided insight into mechanisms of cell transformation. Ultimately, very specific therapy may be directed at different steps along these pathways.

Invasion and Metastasis

The most important characteristics of malignancy are the tumor's ability to invade surrounding structures and to metastasize to different organs. A variety of mechanisms to explain these properties have been proposed. Specific treatment modalities directed at these mechanisms have been employed in experimental models with some success. Tumors vary in their propensity to invade and metastasize. In general, the less differentiated, anaplastic tumors with higher rates of mitosis and aneuploidy are more aggressive.

In order for a tumor cell to invade surrounding tissues, it must lose its own cell attachments, degrade the normal surrounding interstitial matrix, and be capable of moving into new areas. Simple, uncontrolled division

transformed by an increased sensitivity to normally occurring growth factors. This may manifest as a result of an increased number of surface receptors or increased affinity of existing receptors. These mechanisms have been shown to be operative in human squamous cell cancer of the head and neck. Another possibility is an abnormal amplification of the signal triggered by normal ligand-receptor interaction. This could occur in the cytoplasm via abnormal protein kinase activity or abnormal guanosine triphosphate (GTP)-binding proteins that activate the second messenger, adenylate cyclase. Also, aberrant nuclear proteins that receive the normal message could lead directly to abnormal DNA synthesis and cell proliferation.

It is interesting now to review protooncogenes and their products, which when overexpressed or mutated can transform cells. Protooncogene products have been found that function at each step of the pathway of growth factor stimulation (Table 22-3). For example, the sis oncogene product is homologous to the β chain of platelet-derived growth factor, and the erb-B oncogene encodes for a protein homologous to the cell is not enough to cause invasion. Benign tumors undergo uncontrolled, autonomous growth, but this simply results in a mass effect, pushing surrounding structures away, with secondary encapsulation. Malignant cells, on the other hand, lose cellular attachments and acquire the ability to digest basement membranes and connective tissue. They can then actively invade surrounding structures and metastasize.

Probably as a result of poor differentiation, malignant cells seem to lose their mechanical cell junctions that hold the cells together. They also lose receptors for compounds such as fibronectin, vitronectin, laminin, and collagen that are important in adhesion to the extracellular matrix. This is one of many prerequisites for invasion. Although free of attachments, cell invasion remains impeded by dense basement membrane and connective tissue.

It has been well documented that proteolytic enzymes secreted by or in response to malignant cells are responsible for the degradation of the extracellular matrix seen in malignant invasion. **Plasminogen activator** levels have been found to be increased in malignant tissues. These enzymes, which convert plasminogen to plasmin, can degrade a variety of tissue proteins. Levels of **cathepsins,** especially cathepsin B, and **collagenases,** particularly type IV collagenase, have also been shown to be increased in malignant tissue. Other proteinases associated with malignant invasion include proteoglycanase and elastase. Production of some of these enzymes may be related to protooncogene activation. Attempts to inhibit these enzymes have had limited success in preventing metastasis in animal models.

Once interstitial barriers are digested and cells are free of attachments, they must be able to move into surrounding tissue. Passive pressure from the expanding mass promotes this, but it has also been shown that some tumor cells have the capability to form pseudopods, allowing active motility.

Thus, the ability to metastasize requires completion of a cascade of events. A cell must first *lose existing attachments* and *invade* the vascular system. It must then be able to *survive in the circulation, arrest at a new site, extravasate* into the new tissue, and *establish growth* in that tissue. This process overall is quite inefficient. Far fewer than 1% of cells that enter the circulation actually form a metastatic nodule.

The ability to survive in circulation depends on a variety of factors. Cells may die owing to mechanical stress in small vessels, poor nutrition, or oxygen toxicity. Most importantly, the cells must evade the host immune system. A variety of effectors, including specific T lymphocytes, macrophages, and NK cells, can destroy circulating tumor cells. Cells successfully metastasize either by resisting these effectors or by overwhelming the system by their large numbers.

Once the cells have survived the circulation phase, they must arrest and extravasate into a new tissue location. The arrest of tumor cells depends on interaction with platelets and leukocytes, thrombus formation, and tumor embolization. Once lodged, the cells must attach to the capillary endothelial cells or basement membrane, digest, and move through the vessel wall. Tumor cells in vitro have been shown to extend pseudopods as a means of moving through capillary membranes. They may also follow leukocytes through the wall.

After relocating in a new organ parenchyma, metastatic cells must be capable of proliferating. The contribution of the "soil" to the ability of tumor cells to proliferate is controversial and under active investigation. It is quite possible that a lack of necessary growth factors or the presence of inhibitory factors may prevent the formation of a metastasis by some tumors in certain tissues. The **"soil and seed" hypothesis** was proposed by Paget in 1889 to explain the propensity for some tumors to metastasize to specific organs. Experimentally, this hypothesis has been verified by the identification of organ-specific metastasizing tumors, whose cells selectively localize in certain organs regardless of the site of inoculation.

Another important factor determining sites of metastasis is based on hemodynamic considerations. Organs with capillary beds receiving a large amount of blood flow from the tumor will be the most likely organs for metastasis to appear. Tumors with portal venous drainage tend to have hepatic metastases, while those draining systemically tend to have pulmonary metastases.

Thus, a combination of the number of cells delivered to an organ and the cell's ability to proliferate within that tissue probably determines metastatic incidence within that organ.

Distant metastatases may disseminate via hematogenous and/or lymphatic routes. Although some tumors have a predilection for lymphatic or hematogenous spread, the mechanisms are similar, and the two systems are widely interconnected. Therefore, the presence of lymph node metastases has some predictive value for the presence of distant hematogenous metastases.

The property of **tumor cell heterogeneity** is important in the discussion of metastasis. The genetic instability present in malignant tumors results in the generation of many different phenotypic cell clones within each tumor. Despite the fact that all cells in a tumor develop from a single clone, there is a wide variation in phenotypic properties such as antigenicity, response to chemotherapy, and the ability to metastasize. If a tumor is digested and subclones grown in vitro and reinoculated, the new tumors will range from a non-metastasizing tumor to a highly metastatic variant. In addition, immunogenicity and chemotherapeutic sensitivity will vary dramatically. Thus, chemotherapy and immunotherapy will most likely select for unresponsive phenotypes that will then proliferate and kill the host. Regimens employing multiple modalities with different mechanisms of action will have the highest likelihood of eliminating all subclones.

Laboratory Diagnosis

Differentiating benign from malignant tumors and determining the tissue and cell of origin of metastatic lesions can be quite challenging. A combination of clinical and gross anatomical characteristics, histologic appearance, and a variety of other modalities, such as immunohistochemistry, are used to make an accurate diagnosis.

Gross characteristics of malignant and benign tissues have previously been discussed. Benign tumors are almost always well encapsulated and mobile whereas malignant tumors have irregular borders, no distinct capsule, and evidence of gross invasion into surrounding structures which "fixes" them to those structures. Gross evidence of local lymph node metastasis confirms the diagnosis of malignancy. On histologic examination, characteristics of differentiation and mitosis are important. In general, all benign tumors should be well differentiated—resembling normal, mature cells of the tissue of origin. Malignant tumors tend to have large numbers of mitotic figures. The number of mitoses correlates with the aggressiveness of the tumor. More important than the absolute number of mitoses is the presence of atypical and bizarre mitotic figures, which are very characteristic of malignancy.

Poorly differentiated and aneuploid tumor cells have other distinguishing characteristics. The cells and their nuclei tend to be **pleomorphic** with a wide variety of shapes and sizes. The nuclear-to-cytoplasmic ratio is increased, approaching 1:1, as opposed to the normal 1:4 or 1:6. The nuclei are **hyperchromatic,** containing an abundance of DNA, which tends to stain darkly. Cellular orientation is disturbed. For example, cells that normally appear in glandular formations are in disarray. Malignant tumors also have less connective tissue and may have central areas of necrosis. Ultrastructural features such as nuclear chromatin, endoplasmic reticulum, ribosomes, and mitochondria will often be simplified, decreased, or otherwise abnormal. These characteristics can be appreciated with electron microscopy.

Cytoskeletal structures tend to be conserved even in cells that are quite undifferentiated. The cytoskeleton consists of microfilaments, microtubules, and intermediate-sized filaments. At least five types of intermediate filaments have been identified that are specific for certain cell types. These include neurofilaments, cytokeratin, desmin, glial filaments, and vimentin. A combination of electron microscopic examination and specific staining using antibody techniques (immunofluorescence or immunoperoxidase methods) can identify these filaments and help in determing the histogenetic origin of tumors. For example, cytokeratin is specific for epithelial and mesothelial tumors; desmin is specific for muscle cells; and neurofilaments are specific for neural cells.

Tumors are both graded and staged. **Staging** is a clinical entity based on the size of the primary lesions, its extent of spread to regional lymph nodes, and the presence of distant metastasis. **Grading** is based on cytologic examination. Specifically, grading depends on cell differentiation and the number of mitoses. The specific grades differ among neoplasms. In general, tumors are classified as grades I through IV, grade I being well differentiated with few mitoses, and grade IV being anaplastic with many mitoses (e.g., greater than ten mitoses per ten high-power fields for malignant retroperitoneal sarcoma). Grades and stages are used prognostically, and are important for determining what therapy is appropriate.

In many cases, for screening purposes and ease of collecting samples, cytologic specimens are obtained. Cytologic methods were first described by Papanicolaou in 1928 and have been most useful in screening for cervical and endometrial tumors. They are also useful for diagnosing thyroid nodules, breast cysts, and many other tumors accessible for aspiration. The specimen consists of individual cells and occasionally clumps of cells. Accurate diagnosis is difficult and is subject to sampling error. It is also dependent on the skill of the pathologist. The cells are usually classified as follows: class I, normal; class II, few atypical cells; class III, dysplasia; class IV, carcinoma in situ; class V, cancer. While lesions tend to progress from simple atypia, to dysplasia, to frank cancer, this does not imply that all tumor cells go through each of these stages. However, a highly dysplastic lesion has an increased incidence of a tumor forming within it (transformation of a single cell), and these lesions should be followed closely.

Specific **tumor markers** are helpful in accurately determining morphologic diagnoses of tumors. Accurate diagnosis is important, since very specific chemotherapeutic and radiotherapeutic protocols are used for given morphologies. In addition, tumor markers shed into the circulation provide a means to screen for tumors and follow for recurrence. The presence of specific tumor markers also provides the potential for future improvements in diagnostic accuracy (e.g., radiolabeled antibodies) and therapeutic specificity (antitumor agents bound to monoclonal antibodies). The sensitivity and specificity of tumor markers vary significantly and should be taken into account when determining their usefulness for screening populations or establishing diagnoses. Table 22-4 summarizes some of the important tumor markers. Of note, the tumor-associated antigen CA-125 has been useful clinically in monitoring treatment of ovarian cancer and may have a broader role in its management.

Tumor markers can be classified according to type. **Oncofetal proteins** such as carcinoembryonic antigen and α-fetoprotein are present during embryonic or fetal life, and for some reason reappear with certain malignancies. **Hormones** may be markers for tumors from tissues that normally produce that hormone, such as human chorionic gonadotropin in tumors of the placenta. They may also mark the growth of some nonen-

TABLE 22-4. Common Tumor Markers

Markers	Tumors
Immunologic	
E Rosettes	Leukemia/lymphoma T cells
Monoclonal antibodies	Leukemia/lymphoma T and B cells
Specific heavy-chain immunoglobulins	Leukemia/lymphoma B cells
κ-, λ-light chains	Leukemia/lymphoma B cells
Tumor-Associated Antigens	
Carcinoembryonic antigen	Colonic, pancreatic, bronchogenic, gastric, and breast carcinomas and other forms of cancer
α-Fetoprotein	Hepatocellular carcinoma, germ cell tumors (principally yolk-sac and endodermal sinus derivatives)
Pancreatic oncofetal antigen	Pancreatic, bronchogenic, and gastric carcinomas and others
CA 125	Ovarian cancer
CA 19-9	Pancreatic cancer
CA 15-3	Breast cancer
Tissue polypeptide antigen	Colorectal, breast, prostate, bladder, bronchogenic, carcinomas, and seminoma
Prostate-specific antigen	Prostate cancer
Hormones	
Human chorionic gonadotropin	Choriocarcinoma, hydatidiform mole, seminoma, embryonal and teratocarcinoma, and others
Human placental lactogen	Trophoblastic neoplasms
Calcitonin	Thyroid medullary carcinoma
Ectopic hormones	*See Table 22-5*
Serum Enzymes	
Acid phosphatase, tartrate-inhibitable	Prostatic carcinoma
Galactosyltransferase II	Pancreatic, gastric, and breast carcinomas

Adapted from Robbins SL, Cotran RS, Kumar V. *Pathologic basis of disease.* 3rd ed. Philadelphia: WB Saunders, 1984:267.

docrine tumors that are ectopic producers of a specific hormone. A classic example is the production of ACTH from small-cell carcinoma of the lung. The mechanism is not clear, but it involves expression of otherwise repressed portions of the genome.

Enzymes may also act as markers if released from tumors whose parent tissue normally produces this enzyme. When cell proliferation and cell turnover is high, these enzymes are released into the circulation. Acid phosphatase levels, for example, are markedly elevated in patients with prostate cancer.

Immunoglobulins may also serve as tumor markers. They are released by such tumors as multiple myeloma and B-cell lymphomas. Tumor-associated antigens may also be quite useful, as discussed above. Monoclonal antibodies directed against these antigens may direct radioisotopes for diagnostic imaging or antitumor agents for therapy. (Refer to Chapter 23 for a complete discussion of tumor-associated antigens.)

Host-Tumor Interactions

A tumor has a variety of effects on the host, most of which are detrimental and ultimately fatal. The tumor can be thought of as a parasite that drains the host of energy. It proliferates and invades normal structures and secretes substances that may have systemic effects. In reality, it is more complicated than a simple parasite-host relationship. The host has a variety of defenses that impact on the tumor. The most important are the immune response and immunosurveillance, which is discussed in Chapter 23.

Host dietary factors may also influence tumor growth. A protein-depleted diet can inhibit tumor growth, while hyperalimentation may stimulate it. It has been speculated that the anorexia associated with cancer may be a defense mechanism by which the host deprives the tumor of required nutrients. The host may also enhance the growth of tumors by supplying necessary growth factors or hormones to the tumor. It is well known that some forms of breast cancer require circulating estrogen for growth, such that surgical sterilization can sometimes cause tumor regression. A thorough understanding of host-tumor interaction may lead to improved modalities for treatment and palliation.

Some obvious consequences of tumor growth include organ dysfunction secondary to growth and invasion of the primary tumor. The tumor may ultimately destroy the organ from which it arises through mass effect and destruction by invasion. In addition, it can cause secondary local complications such as bowel obstruction, bleeding, and infection (a result of perforation or ulceration into a nonsterile field). Late in the course, the tumor may have an immunosuppressive effect on the host. This may be secondary to nutritional deficiencies or a stress response to the tumor. Thus, the host is more susceptible to infection and sepsis.

Nutritional consequences of tumor growth are quite complicated. First, the tumor acts as a parasite, draining energy and structural substrates that would otherwise be utilized by the host. However, this alone does not adequately explain the wasted state of the host. In addition, the tumor may affect the host's hormonal system and cause the production of cytokines (e.g., tumor necrosis factor). These effects along with other factors result in what is known as cancer cachexia. **Cachexia** is a syndrome of severe wasting, malaise, anorexia, and progressive weakness that accompanies tumor growth. It does not necessarily correlate with tumor bulk, location, or type, and different mechanisms probably contribute to the syndrome in different malignancies.

Tumor cells tend to be quite primitive in their metabolism. They tend to rely on glycolysis for energy and often produce lactate. They do not adapt well to the starved state, and while the rest of the host may have adapted to the use of fatty acids and ketones for energy, the tumor will continue to utilize glucose at a rapid rate. The host liver is then burdened by the need to convert lactate to glucose to supply the tumor with substrate. The presence of a tumor induces a decrease in the insulin to glucagon ratio and causes a peripheral resistance to insulin. The tumor also utilizes a large amount of amino acids, both as energy substrates and for proteins necessary for rapid proliferation. The tumor acts as a nitrogen trap. While the host progressively loses its nitrogen stores and undergoes muscle wasting, the tumor continues to grow and incorporate nitrogen. In addition to all the direct metabolic consequences of the tumor, a state of anorexia is induced. A variety of mechanisms for this have been proposed, but no universal cause has been recognized. This starved state compounds the nutritional problems of the host.

Another host-tumor interaction is the paraneoplastic syndrome. **Paraneoplastic syndromes** are symptom complexes related to tumors that cannot be readily explained by local factors of tumor growth and invasion. The most commonly recognized of these is probably ectopic hormone production from tumors such as oat cell

TABLE 22-5. Paraneoplastic Syndromes

Syndrome	Hormone	Tumor Type
Syndromes Associated with Ectopic Hormone Production		
Cushing's syndrome	ACTH	Oat-cell, thymoma, islet-cell tumors of pancreas, bronchial carcinoids of lung, medullary carcinoma of thyroid
Inappropriate ADH	ADH	Oat-cell, other tumors of lung, duodenum, pancreas, thymoma, lymphosarcoma
Gynecomastia	Gonadotropin	Lung carcinoma, rarely tumors of liver, adrenal, dysgerminoma of ovary
Hyperparathyroidism	PTH	Kidney, lung (squamous), pancreatic, and ovarian tumors
Hyperpigmentation	MSH	Oat-cell, lung tumors
Hyperthyroidism	TSH	Choriocarcinoma, hydatidiform mole, embryonal carcinoma of testis
Hypoglycemia	Insulinlike activity	Retroperitoneal and liver tumors
Hypocalcemia	Calcitonin	Medullary carcinoma of thyroid, breast carcinoma, oat-cell
Aplastic anemia	?	Thymomas
Erythrocytosis	Erythropoietin	Cerebellar hemangioma, renal cell, liver, and uterine tumors
Other Effects of Neoplasms on the Host		

Muscle and joint disturbances
  Polyarthritis (usually mild)
  Polymyositis (over age 40: 20% have occult cancer)
		Ovarian, uterine, breast, stomach, lung

Hypertrophic osteoarthropathy		Lung, esophagus, colon

Neuropathies (often seen with myopathies)
  Central
    Cerebellar degeneration
    Cerebral demyelination
  Peripheral
    Pure sensory, lower motor neuron, mixed
		Oat-cell, lung, breast, ovarian, lymphoma

Multiple thromboses		Pancreatic, other types of cancer
Nephrosis (lipoid nephrosis and membranous glomerulitis)		Occult neoplasm in elderly patients
Acanthosis nigricans		Adenocarcinoma lymphoma
Cachexia, loss of taste		Various types
Disseminated intravascular coagulation		Mucinous adenocarcinomas

Reproduced from Petersdorf et al., eds. *Harrison's principles of internal medicine.* 10th ed. New York: McGraw-Hill, 1983:760.
ADH, Antidiuretic hormone; PTH, parathyroid hormone; MSH, melanocyte-stimulating hormone; TSH, thyroid-stimulating hormone.

carcinoma of the lung. Table 22-5 summarizes some of the important paraneoplastic syndromes. In addition to endocrine-related paraneoplastic syndromes, there are nerve and muscle syndromes, which can mimic polymyositis or myasthenia; dermatologic disorders, such as acanthosis nigricans; and vascular and hematologic changes, such as Trousseau's phenomenon or disseminated intravascular coagulation. The mechanisms for these syndromes have not been worked out.

Endocrinopathies are probably the most common of

the paraneoplastic syndromes. They result from ectopic hormone production by cells that are not of endocrine origin. In many cases, the cells involved are part of the amine precursor uptake and decarboxylation system. These are specialized neurosecretory cells that are widely distributed throughout the body during embryogenesis. Some examples include oat-cell carcinomas of the lung, anaplastic carcinomas of the pancreas and gastrointestinal tract, and carcinoids. Common hormones produced include ACTH, antidiuretic hormone, and parathyroid hormone.

Bibliography

Azar HA. *Pathology of human neoplasms, an atlas of diagnostic electron microscopy and immunohistochemistry.* New York: Raven Press, 1988.

DeVita VT Jr, Hellman S, Rosenberg SA. *Cancer, principles and practice of oncology.* Philadelphia: JB Lippincott, 1985: 3–124,

Franks LM, Teich N. *Introduction to the cellular and molecular biology of cancer.* New York: Oxford University Press, 1986.

Klavins JV. *Tumor markers: clinical and laboratory studies.* New York: Alan R. Liss, 1985.

McKenna RJ, Murphy GP. *Fundamentals of surgical oncology.* New York: Macmillan, 1986:40–74.

Moossa AR, Robson MC, Schimpff SC. *Comprehensive textbook of oncology.* Baltimore: Williams & Wilkins, 1986:3–56, 187–198.

Petersdorf RG, Adams RD, Braunwald E, Isselbacher KJ, Martin JB, Wilson JD. *Harrison's principles of internal medicine.* 10th ed. New York: McGraw-Hill, 1983:751–764.

Pimentel E. *Oncogenes.* 2nd ed. Boca Raton, FL: CRC Press, 1989, vol 1.

Pitot HC. *Fundamentals of oncology.* 3rd ed. New York: Marcel Dekker, 1986.

Robbins SL, Cotran RS, Kumar V. *Pathologic basis of disease.* 3rd ed. Philadelphia: WB Saunders, 1984:214–272.

Tannock IF, Hill RP. *The basic science of oncology.* New York: Pergamon Press, 1987.

Michael D. Lieberman and Jonathon Freeman

23 TUMOR IMMUNOBIOLOGY

The concept that tumors express structures that can elicit a host response was first proposed more than a century ago by Paul Ehrlich. As our knowledge of the immune system subsequently increased, the hope arose that tumors would perhaps express unique structures (antigens) as a result of their tumor state. This would imply that such a **tumor-specific antigen** could be treated by manipulating the host immune response or by wholesale pharmacologic treatment of the tumor using new classes of immunologic agents.

However, the reality of such a tumor-specific antigen is still unproven. There are no known examples of any tumor that characteristically expresses a unique antigen that remains necessary for the tumor state. This is not to say that immunologic approaches to cancer are a failure. On the contrary, the last 50 years have marked an incredible expansion of our knowledge of how tumors arise, their unique characteristics, and how they may be treated. Although useful antigens completely *specific* for tumors remain elusive, their are a wide variety of antigens that are *associated* with a variety of tumors. Our increased knowledge of these antigens combined with a better understanding of the immune system has lead to

new approaches to treating cancer. These approaches necessarily take advantage of unique antigenic properties of the target tumor but differ widely in their effector mechanisms.

Tumor Antigens

Following Ehrlich, it was nearly 50 years before anyone proposed that tumors contain antigens capable of eliciting an immune response. In 1943, Gross demonstrated that inbred mice inoculated with a small amount of a chemically induced sarcoma derived from the same strain of mice failed to develop tumors when subsequently reinjected with the same tumor, compared to noninoculated control mice who did develop tumors.

Foley, in 1953, refined this model to show that this same type of tumor, induced by methylcholanthrine (MCA), had a unique antigen not shared by other, spontaneous tumors or by normal host tissues from the same strain.

In 1957, Prehn and Main broadened these studies to show that these MCA-induced tumors, transplanted to the same strain, evoked a specific, cell-mediated response, whereas skin grafts transferred between the same animals did not. The antigens unique to the tumor were termed tumor-specific transplantation antigens.

Although the MCA-induced tumor was an important model for demonstrating the host immune response to a tumor, it was recognized from the beginning to be different from spontaneous tumors. What was not known at that time was the variety of other mechanisms that could lead to cancer. In addition to mutagenic chemicals, we now know that tumors may be caused by such diverse processes as ultraviolet radiation, viral infection, abnormal genetic events, and mutation of various cellular enzymes. Although initially antigens were identified only for chemically induced tumors such as MCA, subsequent investigation has revealed that unique antigens may result from virtually any of these neoplastic processes.

Alteration of gene expression may represent a final common pathway to all neoplasia. How tumor antigens relate to this pathway, or pathways, is a vital question that remains to be answered. In general, an antigen associated with a tumor does not imply causation; that is, the antigen may be a marker for a tumor without being sufficient or necessary for the neoplastic process. Although this is a disadvantage in the sense that manipulation of such an antigen may not alter the neoplastic phenotype, the antigen may still be useful as a unique target for directing therapy.

An ideal tumor antigen, from a therapeutic point of view, would elicit a strong immune response; would be expressed only in neoplastic tissue (and not in either unrelated host tissue or nonneoplastic tissue of the same type); and, with therapeutic manipulation, would stimulate cure of the tumor. To date, no antigen has been found that has all these features. However, a number of antigens have some of these qualities.

Tumor antigens may be grouped into families according to specific features that presumably result from common properties associated with various common oncogenic processes. This classification helps highlight possible advantages and disadvantages to various therapeutic approaches. What follows is a discussion of five families of tumor-associated antigens: oncogene-associated tumor antigens, virus-associated tumor antigens, organ-specific tumor antigens, tumor antigen resulting from aberrant glycosylation, and oncofetal tumor antigens. Each family is explained briefly and then is followed by a summary of the possible clinical applications that are especially promising, or problematic, for each class. (Some of these antigens are reviewed in Table 22-4.)

ONCOGENE-ASSOCIATED TUMOR ANTIGENS

Proteins encoded by oncogenes are a large family of tumor-associated antigens. Oncogenes were first discovered in retroviruses as the DNA sufficient to cause tumors in infected hosts. In 1976, Bishop and Varmus made the discovery that one particular oncogene, src, is present in a closely related form in humans as part of our normal genetic makeup. Subsequently, many more examples of these normal counterparts, termed proto-oncogenes, were discovered. The obvious questions raised by these discoveries were what function the proto-oncogenes play in normal cells, and how the changes that create oncogenes from proto-oncogenes lead to neoplasia.

One of the most important aspects of oncogene proteins is their location in the cell. Some, such as the c-myc protein, are in the nucleus, while others, such as the ras protein, are in the cytoplasm. Although both these oncogene proteins may be identified in vitro by antibodies, the cells expressing these genes must be treated to allow the antibody to penetrate. In order to detect an oncogene protein in intact cells, the oncogene must encode a protein that is excreted or expressed on the cell surface. In fact, there are many examples of such oncogenes.

One example in particular is that of c-erbB-2—a tumor antigen that is especially promising as a possible therapeutic target. C-erbB-2 is closely related to a group of oncogenes that function as growth factor receptors. That is, they respond to specific signals from outside the cell and stimulate the cell to grow and divide. C-erbB-2 and its protein product, p185, have been found in abnormally high levels in a variety of human malignancies, including adenocarcinoma of the breast, colon, and pancreas. In murine models using the rat analog of C-erbB-2, termed neu, in vivo treatment with antibody specific to p185 protein has cured mice with tumors that express high levels of the neu protein.

One of the potential advantages of directing therapy at an oncogene antigen such as p185 (the neu protein) is that manipulation of the antigen itself may be sufficient to reverse tumor growth. Merely binding antibody to transformed cells in culture causes them to revert to normal, and treating mice with intravenous injection of antibody specific for p185 can cure the mice of tumors caused by the neu gene. Another advantage of directing therapy at oncogene-associated antigens is that their expression is normally limited to fairly low levels in a limited number of tissues; or in other words, they are fairly specific to the tumors with which they are associated.

These findings are very promising for developing possible human therapies, and more work is required to identify which human tumors may be amenable to such treatment. Although many of the oncogenes encode tumor antigens that are promising as targets for therapy, more must be learned about the specific function of oncogenes, their role in development, and the factors that control their expression.

VIRUS-ASSOCIATED TUMOR ANTIGENS

Antigens expressed as a result of viral infection represent a second major class of tumor antigens. In particular, some viruses are known to be associated with various malignancies, and antigens expressed by these viruses are therefore markers of infection and possible targets for therapy. Examples of such viruses include hepatitis B, associated with hepatocellular carcinoma, herpes simplex virus, associated with cervical cancer, and Epstein-Barr virus, associated with Burkitt's and other lymphomas.

Unfortunately, there are several theoretical problems with viral tumor antigens. First, they often infect more than one cell type, and thus they are not specific to the tumor. Second, the antigen expressed on the cell surface may not be important for tumorigenesis, so that direct manipulation may not be effective in controlling the neoplasia.

However, these viral antigens have proven useful in several ways. Testing for infection helps determine the risk of developing associated malignancy. In addition, hepatitis B virus antigen has been useful for developing a vaccine, which prevents infection and thus presumedly obviates the risk of associated malignancy. In the case of herpes simplex virus, knowledge of the association between infection and cervical cancer has stimulated efforts to increase public awareness for the need to take prophylactic measures to avoid infection.

ORGAN-SPECIFIC TUMOR ANTIGENS

In an attempt to overcome some of the problems of antigen specificity, many investigators have examined particular organs in search of unique antigens. A comparison of the differences between normal and neoplastic tissue can allow the identification of **organ-specific tumor antigens.** Because these antigens are often identified with unique antibodies, they hold great promise for treating various malignancies. In particular, malignant melanoma and tumors of the breast and prostate have a number of tumor antigens that are promising for both diagnosis and treatment. Nearly every organ has been investigated to some extent, with numerous candidate antigens identified in tissues including the pancreas, ovary, glial cells, lung, kidney, and hematopoetic lines.

Unfortunately, merely identifying an antigen specific to a tissue reveals nothing of its function. Therefore, manipulation of the antigen may not have any observable effect. This is related to the problem of antigen heterogeneity, or "antigen drift," in which small changes occur in the antigen from one cell generation to the next, sometimes even within the same region of a given tumor. A given antibody may recognize one form of an antigen but not recognize the related variant. Despite their name, these organ-specific antigens often are not completely specific. Antigens characteristic of neoplasms in one tissue may be expressed normally in other cell types, and antigens unique to a tissue type may not distinguish malignant from normal.

TUMOR ANTIGEN RESULTING FROM ABERRANT GLYCOSYLATION

Glycosylation of cellular structures, including membrane proteins, is often important for normal control and processing of these molecules. In the case of membrane proteins involved with important cell-surface signaling, alteration of these molecules may lead to the development of neoplasia. A variety of cellular enzymes exist that normally modify the glycosylation pattern of a number of surface proteins. Although the significance of these changes is not completely understood, mutations in these modifying enzymes may lead to altered cell growth.

This group of antigens is important because it represents another way in which mutation may give rise to cancer. These molecules expressed on the cell surface may be unique to a given tumor, thus providing a potential ideal target for immunologic attack. However, their importance is largely theoretical at present and will remain so until more is learned about the mechanisms of glycosylation and its relationship to control of cell functions.

ONCOFETAL TUMOR ANTIGENS

Carcinoembryonic antigen (CEA) and α-fetoprotein (α-FP) are the two most common examples of what are known as **oncofetal proteins.** As their name implies, they are expressed normally on various cells during fetal development but also occur in various adult malignancies. Although little is known of their function, it seems likely that they act similarly to oncogenes by controlling growth and differentiation. Like organ-specific antigens, they may be important in differentiation into mature tissue types.

Carcinoembryonic antigen and α-FP have particular clinical importance because, unlike most other tumor antigens, they are secreted and may be measured in the peripheral blood. Their drawbacks are that they appear neither unique to nor always present with any particular tumor. Carcinoembryonic antigen, although primarily found in tumors of the colon, is also occasionally elevated in tumors of the lung, pancreas, breast, and stomach. It may also be elevated in nonmalignant conditions, including pancreatitis, ulcerative colitis, and alcohol abuse. Because of this lack of specificity, its use is limited to detection of tumor recurrence in cases where previously elevated levels of CEA fall following successful resection of a secreting tumor.

Similarly, α-FP is a common marker of hepatoma and testicular teratoblastoma. In addition, it is a marker used prenatally to identify possible developmental defects, including anencephaly and open neural tube defects. However, as with CEA, α-FP is not completely specific for these conditions and is used to complement the diagnostic process or for monitoring therapy.

Antitumor Effector Mechanisms

Antitumor effector mechanisms can be broadly categorized into **antigen-specific** or **antigen-independent** mechanisms. In the first category, tumor-associated antigens are recognized as foreign by the host cellular immune system. The tumor cell expressing tumor antigens is recognized and processed by class II major histocompatibility complex (MHC) gene-restricted antigen-presenting cells (macrophages and dendritic cells). This complex of macrophage and tumor-associated antigen, in association with macrophage-elaborated cytokines such as interleukin-1 and interleukin-6, induce activation of an antigen-specific population of T-helper lymphocytes. Activated T-helper cells also produce cytokines, such as interleukin-2 (IL-2), which facilitate the clonal expansion of antigen-specific cytotoxic T lymphocytes. Cytotoxic T lymphocytes express the CD3 antigen and mediate antigen-specific recognition via the α/β T-cell antigen receptor in association with class I MHC gene product. Once recognized, the tumor cell is destroyed by the cytotoxic T lymphocytes through pore-forming proteins, perforins, and toxic soluble mediators, such as tumor necrosis factor and lymphotoxin. The important characteristics of cytotoxic T lymphocytes are their thymic dependence, antigen specificity, and restriction of cytotoxic function by major histocompatability complex antigens. Cytotoxic T lymphocytes exhibit oncolytic activity primarily to highly immunogenic tumors, which unfortunately are rare among human cancers.

Antigen-independent antitumor effector mechanisms are not dependent on MHC restriction or immunologic memory for tumor-associated antigen. **Natural killer (NK)** cells, identified morphologically as large granular lymphocytes, are the predominant effector cells mediating this natural immune defense mechanism. These cells appear to be a distinct population of lymphoid cells derived from null lymphocytes that express some T-cell markers early in differentiation and later acquire markers also present on macrophages and neutrophils. These lymphocytes represent 10% to 15% of peripheral blood lymphocytes and have been identified in liver, lung, lymph node, and spleen. NK cells have the capacity primarily to recognize and lyse a wide variety of cultured tumor cell lines in vitro and in vivo. However, the process of NK cell recognition of tumor cells remains elusive.

Experimental and clinical data support the role of NK cells in host resistance to neoplasia. Mice depleted of NK cells with anti-NK serum have markedly increased numbers of metastases in experimental tumor models. Conversely, enhancement of NK cytotoxicity with interleukin-2 or γ-interferon significantly diminishes the growth of primary tumors and the number of metastases in mouse tumor models. Patients with low NK function, for example, in the Chediak-Higashi syndrome, have an increased incidence of lymphoproliferative malignancies. Thus, a role for NK cells in antitumor surveillance has been postulated.

Recent studies have described a population of lymphocytes, most likely derived from NK cells and non-MHC-restricted T-cells, that upon exposure to IL-2 are transformed into **lymphokine-activated killer (LAK)** cells with potent cytolytic capabilities for neoplastic cells but not normal host tissues. Clinical trials utilizing IL-2 plus LAK cell immunotherapy in patients with metastatic melanoma or renal cell carcinoma resulted in a 10% complete and 20% partial regression rate.

Macrophages are another population of immunocytes that mediate natural cytotoxic properties. Macrophages can lyse tumor cells directly by the release of cytocidal lysosomal enzymes and through a form of antibody-dependent cellular cytotoxicity. Antibody-dependent cellular cytotoxicity is a mechanism of effector cell lysis in which tumor cell targets sensitized by specific antibodies are lysed by Fc receptor-bearing nonsensitized effector cells. Macrophages have Fc receptors that can bind to and destroy antibody-coated tumor cells. Antibody-dependent cellular cytotoxicity is also mediated by killer cells, derived from null lymphocytes, that express Fc receptors. Indirectly, macrophages may participate in tumor cell killing by their production of interferons, tumor necrosis factor, complement components, and arachidonic acid metabolites. Circumstantial evidence for an important role for macrophages in host antitumor defense is indicated by their accumulation at sites of spontaneous tumor regression.

Humoral-mediated immune effector mechanisms include both antigen-specific and -nonspecific components. Antibodies produced by plasma cells exhibit specificity for tumor-associated antigen. Once the antibody binds to the tumor cell, nonspecific lysis of the neoplastic cells occurs through complement or antibody-dependent cellular cytotoxicity mediated by macrophages or killer cells. Cytokines released by immunocytes can mediate tumor toxicity by direct cidal effects or indirectly by recruitment of other inflammatory immunocytes.

Immunotherapy

Immunotherapy is broadly defined into active and passive. The goal of active immunotherapy is to induce in the host a state of immune responsiveness to the malignancy. Passive immunotherapy directly transfers to the host biologically active agents with innate antitumor properties. Furthermore, both active and passive immunotherapies can be subdivided into techniques that generate a response that is specific or nonspecific for tumor-associated antigen. The complex immune responses and interrelationships set into motion by these therapies account for the limitation in strictly applying this classification system.

The success of immunotherapy in animal tumor model systems and promising results of patient trials utilizing active nonspecific immunostimulants including BCG or allogeneic vaccines fueled initial enthusiasm for biological response modifier therapy in the 1960s and 1970s. During the past decade, increased interest in immunotherapy has been propagated by the development of cloned recombinant human gene products (e.g., interferons, interleukins, tumor necrosis factor), improved mass cell culture techniques, and hybridoma technology, which has generated murine monoclonal antibodies directed against tumor-associated antigens.

ACTIVE IMMUNOTHERAPY

Central to the concept of active immunotherapy is the assumption that tumor-associated antigens exist on the malignant cell and, under certain circumstances, are recognizable by the host. Attempts to increase the host's immune response to specific tumor-associated antigens have included the use of autologous vaccines, hybrids of human tumor cells fused with xenogeneic tumor immunogens, and monoclonal tumor anti-idiotypic antibodies. Utilization of autologous vaccines has been applied most successfully to patients with colorectal cancer. Patients with Dukes' B2 and C colon cancer were randomized to receive immunization with irradiated autologous tumor cells plus BCG or no postoperative treatment. The vaccinated group had significantly less mortality and tumor recurrence than the control group. Importantly, the vaccinated patients demonstrated a delayed-type hypersensitivity response to their autologous tumor, indicating immunization. However, the majority of human trials with tumor vaccines have been less impressive in their results. A variety of explanations have been proposed for the difficulty in tumor immunization: (1) expression of tumor-associated antigens on normal tissues, resulting in tolerance to that antigen; (2) tumor heterogeneity; (3) ability of tumor cells to down-regulate MHC expression; and (4) tumor cell production of soluble factors that interfere with or suppress the action of immunocytes.

Active nonspecific immunostimulants broadly consist of four groups of substances: **biologic, chemical, chemotherapeutic,** and **cytokines.** Biological agents are derived from microorganisms including BCG, *Cornyebacterium parvum,* and OK432. These micro-organisms activate neutrophils, macrophages, NK cells, and lymphocytes. Clinical studies involving patients with melanoma and bladder malignancies have reported impressive local tumoricidal effects with intralesional or intravesicular BCG. Recently, the chemical immunomodulator levamisole has been shown to be synergistic with 5-fluorouracil in the adjuvant therapy of colorectal cancer. Conventional chemotherapeutic agents such as cyclophosphamide also modulate immune responsiveness. Low-dose cyclophosphamide synergizes with cytokine therapy in murine tumor models through an inhibition of T-suppressor cell function. Clinical trials are presently in progress.

The use of a variety of natural and recombinant cytokines has highlighted the recent resurgence of nonspecific active immune modulation in cancer therapy. Cytokines with potential therapeutic efficacy include the interferons, interleukins (Nos. 2, 4, and 6), tumor necrosis factor, and natural killer cell-stimulating factor.

The **interferons** are a family of proteins secreted by lymphocytes, monocytes, and fibroblasts with significant tumoricidal properties. Anticancer effects of interferons include enhancement of NK and monocyte cytotoxicity, induction or augmentation of expression of MHC antigens on tumor cells, making them more susceptible to elimination, and a direct antiproliferative effect on neoplastic cells. Clinical responses have occurred in 10–15% of patients with renal cell carcinoma, melanoma, myeloma, and Kaposi's sarcoma; 40–50% with lymphomas; and 80–90% of patients with hairy cell leukemia and chronic myelogenous leukemia.

Interleukin-2, produced by T lymphocytes, has been widely investigated as a potent active immune modulator. IL-2 induces the proliferation of cells bearing IL-2 receptors and enhances the cytotoxic capabilites of natural killer cells and T-lymphocytes. Lymphocytes incubated with IL-2 develop a capacity to lyse cultured and fresh tumor cells in vitro. The systemic administration of IL-2 to tumor-bearing mice mediates the regression of established pulmonary, hepatic, and subcutaneous metastases. Clinical trials utilizing high-dose IL-2 immunotherapy have demonstrated therapeutic response rates in patients with metastatic melanoma, renal cell carcinoma, and colorectal carcinoma.

PASSIVE IMMUNOTHERAPY

Passive immunotherapy includes the use of immunologic reagents such as monoclonal antibodies or adoptive transfer of cells to mediate direct antitumor response without requiring a host response. Similar to active immunotherapy, passive immunotherapy may be **specific** (e.g., **monoclonal antibodies, tumor-infiltrating lymphocytes**) or **nonspecific** (e.g., **LAK cells, activated macrophages, tumor necrosis factor**).

Monoclonal antibodies are specific for an antigen, can be produced in large quantities by hybridoma technology and can be conjugated to radioactive isotopes, chemotherapeutic drugs, and toxins. Furthermore, the Fc portion of the monoclonal antibody bound to tumor cells may bind complement or tumoricidal monocytes or killer cells, resulting in tumor cell destruction. Limited clinical success with monoclonal antibodies has been reported in patients with T- and B-cell lymphomas, gastrointestinal carcinomas, melanoma, and neuroblastoma. Future applications of monoclonal antibody technology utlizing the concept of anti-idiotypic networks may dramatically improve clinical results.

The adoptive transfer of tumor-infiltrating lymphocytes (TILs) represents another important example of passive specific immunotherapy. TILs are a population of lymphocytes isolated from growing tumors that are cultured and expanded in low doses of IL-2 in vitro. TILs have been isolated from most human tumors, demonstrate MHC-restricted lysis of tumor, and can be 50 to 100 times more potent than LAK cells in experimental tumor models. In a clinical trial, 11 of 20 patients treated with TILs had an objective remission. The specificity of TIL provides positive evidence that at least some patients manifest an immune reaction to their cancers.

The prototype for passive nonspecific immunotherapy resides with the systemic infusion of LAK cells derived from host lymphoid cells treated with high-dose IL-2 in vitro. Unlike the cell lysis mediated by antigen-specific cytotoxic T-lymphocytes, which recognize nominal antigen in association with major MHC determinants, the lytic action of LAK cells is non-MHC-restricted. LAK activity is mediated by a heterogenous population of cells that may be CD3 (T-cell receptor) positive or negative and CD16 (Fc receptor) positive. Functionally, LAK have the capacity to lyse a wide variety of fresh human tumor targets. A prospective randomized trial comparing high-dose IL-2 with high-dose IL-2 plus LAK therapy in patients with cancer reveal that both treatments can produce partial and complete responses, although the incidence of complete responses is higher when LAK cells are concomitantly administered with IL-2.

Summary

Despite the wide array of antigens that may now be identified with various tumors and potential host antitumor effector mechanisms, problems remain in utilizing them effectively for treatment. Although immunotherapeutic-induced regression of tumor growth may be accomplished in animal models, results in clinical trials have been less successful. The central problem with tumor immunotherapy most likely resides in the failure of tumor cells to express unique antigens, and the capacity of malignant cells effectively to evade host antitumor effector immunocytes through antigenic modulaton and by mechanical, suppressor, and toleragenic mechanisms. Despite these problems, investigation of tumor antigens and antitumor effector mechanisms has enormous benefit in the understanding of the process of tumor growth, as well as for the development of new approaches for diagnosis and treatment of cancer.

Bibliography

Brown VI, Hetrick JE, Greene MI. Adaptive and non-adaptive immunity to tumors. In press.

Brown VI, Hetrick JE, Greene MI. Tumor antigens and the immune response. In: Mitchell MS, ed. *The Biomodulation of cancer.* Elmsford, NY: Pergamon Press, in press.

Foon FA. Biologic response modifiers: The new immunotherapy. *Cancer Res* 1989;49:1621–1639, .

Hoover HC, Surdyke MG, Dangel RB, et al. Prospectively randomized trial of adjuvant active specific immunotherapy for human colorectal cancer. *Cancer* 1985;55:1236.

Rosenberg SA, Longo DL, Lotze MT. Principles and applications of biologic therapy. In: DeVita VT, Hellman S, Rosenberg SA, eds. *Cancer principles and practice of oncology.* 3rd ed. Philadelphia: JB Lippincott, 1989:301–347.

Rosenberg SA, Lotze MT, Yang JC, Aebersold PM, Linehan WM, Seipp CA, White DE. Experience with the use of high dose interleukin-2 in the treatment of 652 cancer patients. *Ann Surg* 1989; 210:474–485.

Rosenberg SA, Packard BS, Aebersold PM. Immunotherapy of patients with metastatic melanoma using tumor infiltrating lymphocytes and interleukin-2. Preliminary report. *N Engl J Med* 1988;319:1676–1680.

Alex C. Cech

24 PRINCIPLES OF RADIATION THERAPY AND CHEMOTHERAPY

Radiation and chemotherapy are different treatment modalities that complement each other as well as surgery in the treatment of neoplasia. Simply stated, the goal of these modalities is to destroy all tumor cells primarily or residual tumor cells after surgery. When this is not possible, both therapies are also employed to palliate the symptoms of incurable disease. A third use of radiation and chemotherapy is to treat tumors preoperatively to improve the chance of effecting a cure at the time of surgery. In each of these roles, radiation and chemotherapy should ideally restrict damage to the neoplastic cells, leaving surrounding normal tissue unharmed.

Radiation Therapy

The aim of radiation therapy is to cause a **selective cytotoxic effect** on the tumor cells with minimal structural or functional damage to surrounding normal tissues. Unfortunately, in clinical practice this is rarely realized, and one must accept some damage to normal tissues when eradicating tumors. The degree of selectivity depends on the variable sensitivity of various tissues, both normal and neoplastic, to the damaging effects of radiation. An additional factor is the ability to focus the radiation most intensely on the tumor, sparing the normal tissues.

Radiation beams used in clinical practice are primarily of two types: (1) **particulate**, most commonly electron, but also proton, neutron, and others; and (2) **electromagnetic**, consisting of γ-rays, produced in atomic nuclei, and x-rays, produced outside the nucleus. The distinction between these groups is blurred since beams of subatomic particles have certain wavelike characteristics, and electromagnetic radiation has characteristics of beams of separate quanta, or packets of energy. The particulate nature of electromagnetic (EM) radiation is demonstrated by the individual counts of radiation recorded by a Geiger counter, which senses EM radiation. Particle beams are produced in accelerators or by the emission of particles during the decay of unstable atoms. γ-rays are produced when an unstable nucleus like cobalt 60 decays to a more stable configuration. X-rays are produced whenever charged particles accelerate or decelerate, or electrons shift between the electron shells of an atom. X-rays can be produced in tubes where high voltage is used to accelerate electrons between filaments: as they strike the target filament they produce "braking radiation."

Electromagnetic beams are grouped according to energies. Relatively low energy radiation (10–125 keV) is called **superficial voltage radiation** and is most useful for diagnostic imaging. **Orthovoltage** (125–400 keV) and **supravoltage** (>400 keV) are used in radiation therapy.

ENERGY ABSORPTION

The effects of radiation on tissue depends on the absorption of its energy. Energy absorbed is measured in **Gray (Gy) units** (1 Gy equals 1 J/kg of tissue). One rad equals 1 centigray (cGy). Radiation is absorbed by different mechanisms for EM radiation and particle beams. The common end result is the production of excited or ionized molecules and the breakage of chemical bonds. Electrons occupy energy levels or shells around an atomic nucleus. Energy input can raise an electron to a higher energy shell, termed excitation, or can completely eject an electron from the atom, termed ionization. An ionizing event releases a large amount of energy, approximately 33 eV. This is sufficient energy to break a chemical bond. For example, breakage of a carbon-carbon double bond requires 4.9 eV.

Absorption of EM radiation occurs by one of three mechanisms: (1) the **photoelectric effect**, (2) the **Compton effect**, or (3) **pair production** (Figure 24-1).The photoelectric effect is primarily responsible for the absorption of low-voltage radiation, i.e., **10–125 KeV**. The incident photon is completely absorbed by the target atom. This excess energy is then released by ejecting a tightly bound electron from the K or L electron shells. This electron, called a photoelectron, then goes on to excite nearby atoms. The degree of absorption is proportional to the atomic number of the target atom to the third power (Z^3). This explains the greater absorption of bone relative to soft tissue.

The Compton effect involves free or loosely bound electrons. It is the primary mode of absorption of radiation in the 100-keV to 10-MeV range, and is the dominant mechanism of action of therapeutic radiation. The incident photon is only partially absorbed. The photon's energy is transferred to an electron, called a Compton or recoil electron, and a secondary or scatter photon. The Compton electron can go on to ionize sur-

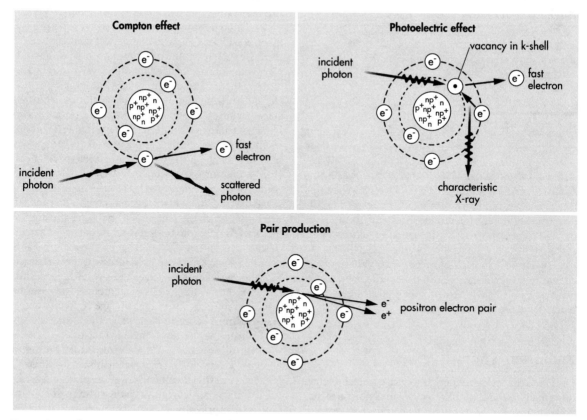

Figure 24-1 Three mechanisms of absorption of electromagnetic radiation. (Reproduced from Moss WT, Cox JD, eds. *Radiation oncology—rationale, technique, results.* St. Louis: CV Mosby, 1989:3.)

rounding atoms. The degree of absorption is proportional to the electron density of the target and not the atomic number.

Finally, EM radiation can be absorbed with the production of positron-electron pairs. An incident photon interacts with the electric field of an atom's nucleus and is completely absorbed. A pair of particles, an electron and positron, are formed, each receiving one-half of the photon's energy. The minimum energy required is the combined energy of a positron and an electron, 1.02 MeV. Absorption increases with increasing energy and is not clinically significant for beams less than 10 MeV. Absorption is also proportional to the atomic number of the target atom.

Particles, on the other hand, interact through collisions and the resultant transfer of kinetic energy. A large particle slows as it passes through tissue, gradually transferring energy to the surrounding atoms. As a particle slows, it spends more time near potentially ionizable atoms and the likelihood of collision increases. This creates a peak of energy transfer over a short distance at a particular tissue depth, called the **Bragg peak.** This characteristic allows a particle beam to be focused. The Bragg peak varies for particles of different mass and velocity.

RELATIVE BIOLOGICAL EFFECT

Radiation beams can be described by the amount of the ionization they cause. Some beams, like x-rays, are considered sparsely ionizing since they travel relatively long distances before transferring their energy. On the other hand, beams of heavy particles such as neutrons transfer their energy over short distances. **Linear energy transfer** (LET) is defined as the rate of energy transfer along the beam's track (de/dl). Linear energy transfer is proportional to Z^2/V^2 (Z = atomic number, V = velocity). Low LET radiation is sparsely ionizing. Electromagnetic radiation photons have a very low mass and high velocity and therefore low LET, while particles have a higher mass and lower velocity, and high LET. Beams of identical energy can have different LETs and therefore different tissue effects. The ability of tissues to repair radiation damage decreases with higher LET radiation.

The differences in beams can also be expressed according the their **relative biological effect** (RBE). Relative biological effect is the ratio of dosages of different LET beams required to reach the same biological endpoint. If twice the dose of a low LET beam is re-

quired to achieve the same kill rate as a high-LET beam, the relative biological effect of the high-LET beam is twice that of the low. With very high LET beams, the relative biological effect relationship is distorted because tumors begin to suffer more than one lethal hit per cell and the beam becomes less efficient.

CLINICALLY USEFUL BEAMS

Two forms of radiation therapy are commonly used. Brachytherapy involves placing a radiation source near the target (e.g., implant of I^{131} seeds), while teletherapy uses a distant radiation source (e.g., particle accelerators or x-rays). A variety of the beams mentioned earlier are used in both forms of delivery. One of the most relevant differences in beams is tissue penetration. Attempts to improve tissue penetration and reduce skin reaction has lead to the widespread use of supervoltage EM radiation beams. These are relatively easily produced in x-ray tubes by accelerating electrons between filaments. The electrons collide with the anode and give off energy as an x-ray photon. Typically, beams of 1–25 MeV are used. Advantages of supervoltage radiation include skin sparing, good penetration, and less scatter. Typical penetration curves for supervoltage radiation are compared to lower kilovoltage and gamma beams in Figure 24-2.

Particle beams are usually divided into electron beams and high-LET beams. Electron beams are advantageous because the depth of penetration can be controlled by varying electron energy. They are well suited for superficial tumors and for boosts following therapy with other beams. Calculating dose distributions is made relatively more difficult by the effect bone and air cavities have on electron beams. Bone absorbs electron beams well, while air cavities allow them to pass unattenuated.

A variety of linear accelerators have been developed, making high-LET beams practical. These utilize neutrons, protons, and α-particles, which have substantially greater mass than electrons. The primary advantages of high-LET beams are that they can be sharply focused at particular depths (the Bragg peak) and have a relatively great biological effect.

BIOLOGICAL EFFECTS

Beams can have their effects either directly or indirectly. Particle beams are of sufficient energy to break chemical bonds, and a small fraction of the damage caused by

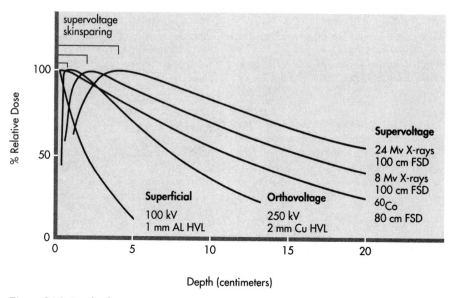

Figure 24-2 Depth of tissue penetration increases with increasing energy of the radiation beam. Supravoltage radiation therefore penetrates deeper into tissues before delivering its dose and is relatively skin-saving compared with superficial and other voltage radiation. (Reproduced from DeVita VT, Hellman S, Rosenberg SA. *Cancer—principles and practices of oncology.* Philadelphia: JB Lippincott, 1985:248.)

EM radiation is caused directly, primarily by supravoltage radiation. About 70% of the damage to chemical bonds is caused indirectly by **free radicals** and charged particles produced by the radiation. Since 70% of a cell's mass is water, many of the effects of radiation are mediated by free radicals formed by the excitation and ionization of water (Figure 24-3). All intermediary species are short-lived and must be in close proximity to biologically significant molecules to have an affect. The likelihood of causing damage to biological mole-

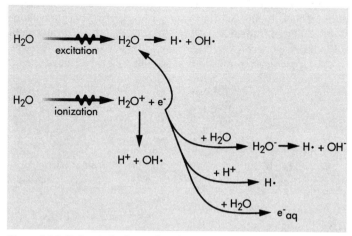

Figure 24-3 Pathways for free-radical formation. (Reproduced from Rubin P, ed. *Clinical oncology—a multidisciplinary approach.* East Syracuse, NY: American Cancer Society, 1983:42.)

cules can be enhanced by using agents that prolong the life of the reactive species.

Several classes of molecules can modify the efficacy of a dose of radiation. This is achieved by either prolonging or shortening the half-life of reactive species created by the radiation. **Radioprotective agents** include sulfhydryl compounds, which inactivate oxygen free radicals. **Radiosensitizers** include actinomycin D, adriamycin, halogenated pyrimidines, oxygen, and nitroimidazoles. Another agent commonly used to enhance the effect of radiation is hydroxyurea, which does not directly increase the sensitivity of cells to radiation but, rather, is more toxic to cells that have already been irradiated. Actinomycin D and adriamycin increase the efficiency of radiation by decreasing the cell's ability to repair radiation damage. Cells are more sensitive to radiation killing when halogenated pyrimidines, such as ido- or bromouracil-deoxyribose, have been incorporated into their DNA before irradiation. Postirradiation repair is also inhibited in these cells.

The single most studied radiosensitizer is oxygen. Oxygen prolongs the half-life of free radicals, improving the odds that a free radical will react with a biologically significant molecule. The most clinically significant radioprotectant is hypoxia. However, the partial pressure of oxygen must be very low to realize a protective effect, because radiosensitivity maximizes at the relatively low oxygen partial pressure of 20–30 mm Hg (Figure 24-4). **Hypoxic cells** require as much as 2.5–3.0 times the dose of radiation required by nonhypoxic cells to achieve a similar effect. Hypoxia is a problem in the center of a tumor mass. As a tumor grows, it outstrips its blood supply, leaving areas distant from capillaries hypoxic. There is a relative gradient of oxygen tension to a point approximately 150 nm from the capillary where the PO_2 approaches zero. The zone from 100 to 150 nm is relatively hypoxic. All tumors have hypoxic regions. However, after a dose of radiation kills oxygenated cells, usually those interposed between the blood supply and the hypoxic cells, the total number of tumor cells decreases for the given blood supply. This improves oxygenation to previously hypoxic cells, making them more susceptible to the next radiation dose (Figure 24-5). Some tumors may show a benefit from hyperbaric oxygen therapy with radiation, for example, tumors of the head and neck, and cervix. Generally, though the benefit of hyperbaric oxygen is greatest when the total dose of radiation is given in only a few fractions, the effect is minimal with normal fractionation schemes. It is generally believed that correcting an

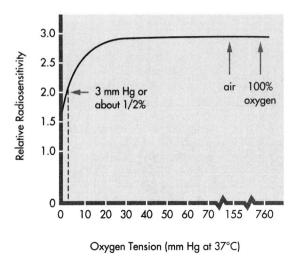

Figure 24-4 The oxygen effect. The oxygen effect is illustrated as the curve relating relative radiation sensitivity to oxygen tension in tissues. As the oxygen increases, the relative radiosensitivity of cells increases by a factor of 3 for the same radiation dose. (Reproduced from Rubin P, ed. *Clinical oncology—a multidisciplinary approach.* East Syracuse, NY: American Cancer Society, 1983:61.)

anemia before radiation therapy will improve oxygen delivery to a tumor, decrease its hypoxic component, and improve the cure rate. The protective effect of tumor hypoxia can further be overcome by using high-LET radiation, such as particle beams. These cause damage by directly ionizing biological molecules and are therefore less dependent on oxygen to stabilize the reactive agents produced by radiation. Other agents, like nitroimidazoles, have been developed to mimic the effect of oxygen. Some aims of current research are to find radiosensitizing agents that specifically concentrate in, or preferentially affect, tumor cells, and to find protectants that selectively protect normal tissue.

Several classes of molecules are damaged by radiation, including **nucleic acids, proteins,** and **lipids.** Nucleic acids suffer several types of damage that can potentially interfere with information storage and transfer. The DNA strands can be broken, or cross-linked, bases can be changed or lost, and the DNA can become bound to other associated molecules. Proteins suffer changes in their side chains that can affect their three-dimensional conformation. Lipids are converted to peroxides.

The exact cellular target responsible for cell killing remains to be definitively identified, but much evidence

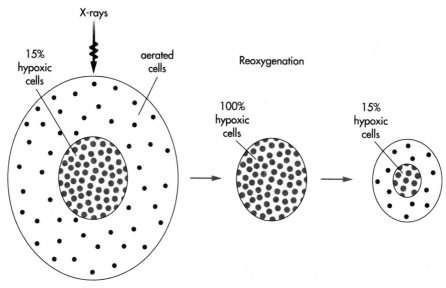

Figure 24-5 Reoxygenation of hypoxic cells with repeated dosing. (Reproduced from Moss WT, Cox JD, eds. *Radiation oncology—rationale, technique, results.* St. Louis: CV Mosby, 1989:30.)

points to the nucleus, and more specifically the DNA. This has been difficult to prove since the number of hits to DNA required for a biological effect is small and difficult to detect. Evidence includes microbeam studies focusing radiation on the nucleus, targeting radiation to the nucleus by incorporating radioactive species in nucleic acids, and transplanting irradiated nuclei into unirradiated cells and observing a transfer of the toxic effects. Indirect evidence includes the observation that radiosensitivity increases with increasing DNA content. It has also been described that cells lacking the ability to repair DNA damage are particularly sensitive. Other cellular targets important in cell killing are membranes. Cell survival is dependent on membrane integrity. Ionizing radiation can disrupt cell membrane components and destroy their integrity.

DNA REPAIR

DNA repair plays an important role in protecting a cell against the potentially lethal effect of radiation. This is demonstrated by the greater sensitivity of cells deficient in these repair mechanisms. Research suggests that the cells of some incurable tumors are better able to repair damage than normal cells. There are several forms of damage to DNA caused by irradiation. Irreparable damage includes strand cross-linking and formation of aber-

rant chromosomes as broken strands rejoin in abnormal combinations. This damage is not necessarily lethal, although it often is. Mechanisms exist in mammalian cells to repair other forms of damage, including strand breaks, deletions, formation of pyrimidine dimers, and base damage. Conditions that slow cell division allow more time to repair damaged DNA and have been shown to increase cell survival following a dose of radiation. Furthermore, dividing a given dose into two fractions separated by time will increase cell survival. Presumably this allows repair to occur between doses, avoiding a lethal number of hits in a cell at any one time. Similarly, a slow dosing rate can be significantly less effective, even if the total dose is large. Cell survival is most affected by changes in dose rate in the range of 1–100 rad/min. This is a clinically relevant issue in brachytherapy, where dose rates are generally slower.

CELL CYCLE AND GROWTH FRACTION

Irradiation affects the progression of the cell cycle. The cell cycle consists of five stages (see Figure 1-3). Irradiation will cause a growth delay by temporarily blocking cells in stage G_2. The duration of the block is related to the radiation dose, increasing until a plateau is reached. It may be due to damage to the proteins responsible for DNA replication, or due to a temporary change in the conformation of the DNA. This block causes cells to become synchronized in the cell cycle, accumulating in G_2. Theoretically it would be advantageous to time subsequent doses when the synchronized population has entered a sensitive stage. Unfortunately, the synchronization is incomplete and only temporary. Thus, currently it is of limited clinical significance. However, research is continuing on chemotherapeutic agents that may hold cells in a sensitive stage.

Radiosensitivity varies with the cell cycle. Although there are large differences between cell lines, sensitivity is generally greatest in the M and G_2 phases. There are peaks of relative resistance in early G_1 and late S. The cause of this variation is not clear.

In an idealized exponential model of tumor growth, all cells divide, doubling the number of tumor cells during the "doubling time." However, not all cells in a tumor are actively dividing. Growth fractions in human tumors can vary from 10% to 90%. As tumors grow large, the growth fraction decreases until the number of cell divisions approaches a stable plateau. The largest growth fraction occurs when the tumor is at about one third of its final size. Size is tumor specific and cannot be predicted prospectively. But as a rule the growth fraction is greater when tumors are small. This is a Gompertzian model of tumor growth. It helps explain why large tumors often appear less sensitive to cell-cycle-dependent therapy (more so with chemotherapy then radiotherapy) than small ones; their growth fraction, and therefore the fraction of sensitive cells, is smaller.

CELL DEATH

The ability of cells to continue dividing is critical in evaluating the effect of radiation. Cells suffering a lethal hit may either die an interphase or a reproductive death. **Interphase death** can occur in any stage of the cell cycle. **Reproductive death** occurs during mitosis. It may be the first mitosis after irradiation or several divisions later. Cells that survive the first mitosis rarely divide more than a few times. Reproductive death follows low to moderate radiation exposure, while interphase death requires large doses, typically greater than 5,000 rad.

Survival curves are the dose-effect curves of radiation therapy (Figure 24-6). They describe the radiation sensitivity of various cells as determined by in vitro experiments. A known number of cells are exposed to a dose of radiation and then cultured in appropriate medium. After an interval of time, growing colonies are counted, with each colony presumably arising from a single surviving cell. When assessing survival in bacteria, the fraction of surviving cells is a simple exponential function. The same fraction of cells, not total number, survive regardless of the starting number. If survival curves are plotted on a semilogarithmic graph (i.e., the ordinate, survival, is a logarithmic scale), the exponential dose-survival function is described by a straight line. Survival curves for mammallian cells are complicated by the cell's ability to repair small amounts of radiation damage. Therefore, mammallian cells are less sensitive to low doses of radiation. This adds a shoulder to the survival curve. At sufficient doses, mammalian survival curves also become exponential.

As noted in Figure 24-6, the slope of the survival curve relates to the sensitivity of the cells to radiation.

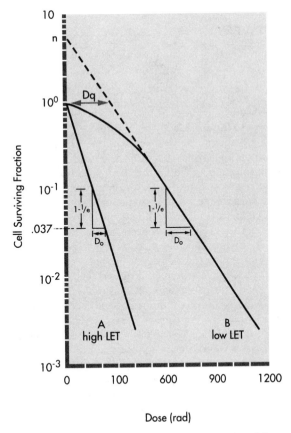

Figure 24-6 Dose-related cell survival. (Reproduced from Rubin P, ed. *Clinical oncology—a multidisciplinary approach.* East Syracuse, NY: American Cancer Society, 1983:59.)

D_0, **the mean lethal dose,** is the dose that will produce on average one lethal hit per cell. When such a dose is given, some cells receive more than one lethal hit and others none. Statistically the number of cells that receive no lethal hit is $1/e$. Thus, D_0 is the dose of radiation that kills $1 - 1/e$ (63%) and spares $1/e$ (37%) of the tumor cells. The dose required to achieve a log kill, killing all but 10% of the original number of cells, is 2.3 x D_0. The shoulder of a mammalian survival curve is described by D_q. It is the horizontal distance from the point of 100% survival on the y-axis to the straight line extrapolated from the exponential portion of the curve. Many factors affect the survival curve. Increased LET radiation decreases the ability of cells to repair damage, thus D_q is smaller. Since D_0 is smaller for high-LET radiation, the curve is steeper. Hypoxia and radioprotectors increase D_q, broadening the shoulder, and increase D_0, flattening the curve.

DELIVERY

Survival curves help describe the efficacy of different delivery protocols. A given dose of radiation can be administered many different ways with markedly different results. Doses must reach the exponential portion of the survival curve to be maximally effective. Early attempts to use radiation therapy employed single large doses. Although tumors were curable, the injury to surrounding normal tissues made this unacceptable. **Fractionation,** dividing the total dose into several smaller doses, spaced out over time, allowed similar cure rates with less damage to normal tissues. This approach, in particular, spares the acute effects on normal tissues, such as erythema of overlying skin, sloughing of gastrointestinal mucosa, and oral mucositis, while the long-term effects are largely unchanged. Long-term effects depend more on total dose and include fibrosis, CNS and bone effects, and carcinogenesis. Dividing the dose allows recovery of normal tissues between doses by repair of sublethal damage and repopulation through regrowth of cells. Normal tissues can even accelerate cell proliferation through a process called recruitment. Recruitment seems to be less significant in tumors than normal tissues. In addition, fractionation promotes the effect of radiation on tumor cells by permitting reoxygenation of central portions of the tumor.

Timing of fractional doses is critical to allow maximal recovery of normal cells while minimizing the recovery of tumor cells. If the interval between doses is too long, tumor cells may regrow to previous dimen-sions with no net benefit derived from radiation. In rapidly dividing tumors it may be necessary to adopt an accelerated fractionation protocol with more than one dose per day.

TISSUE EFFECTS

Much of the preceding material focused on cellular and subcellular effects of radiation. Ultimately clinical response and adverse side effects are observed at tissue, organ, and organism levels. The damage caused by radiation can occur directly within the target area or at a distant site. When a critical element of a tissue or an organ, in the target field, is damaged, it can lead to secondary damage at distant sites. This is called an **abscopal** effect. For example, endothelial cells are particularly sensitive to radiation. Damage to endothelial cells can cause occlusion of vessels supplying distal areas, resulting in necrosis of nonirradiated tissues. Similarly, many organs are dependent on other organs to maintain normal function. Damage to one organ may cause failure of a dependent organ. Tissues and organs are therefore usually as sensitive to radiation as their most sensitive cell type, and the maximum tolerated dose is determined by the most sensitive cells within the field.

Typically, the radiosensitivity of a tumor mimics the sensitivity of the normal tissue from which it is derived. Hematogenous tumors are very sensitive, sarcomas are highly resistant, with adenocarcinomas falling somewhere between. Well-differentiated cells are usually more radioresistant than rapidly dividing cells. This is related to the rate of cell division rather than intrinsic differences in the cells. Slowly dividing or dormant cells will often appear resistant initially but will demonstrate radiation damage when they attempt to divide. Cells can be categorized into four groups on the basis of these principles (Table 24-1).

Tumor curability is dependent on a number of factors including tumor volume and the radiosensitivity of the tumor cells. Radiation therapy is very effective at the periphery of a tumor but is less effective at its center. Central regions of a tumor are often hypoxic and relatively radioresistant. Furthermore, large target volumes increase the amount of normal tissue exposed and thus reduce the tolerated dose. For these reasons surgery is often indicated prior to radiation therapy to reduce the tumor volume. Excision of all gross tumor probably reduces the radiation dose required for a cure. Alternatively, when surgery is already planned, the extent of the resection can be reduced by preoperative radiation

TABLE 24-1. Categories of Mammalian Cell Sensitivity

Cell Type	Properties	Examples	Sensitivity[a]
Group I Vegetative intermitotic cells	Divide regularly; no differentiation	Erythroblasts Intestinal crypt cells Germinal cells of epidermis	High
Group II Differentiating intermitotic cells Connective tissue cells[b]	Divide regularly; some differentiation between divisions	Myelocytes	
Group III Reverting postmitotic cells	Do not divide regularly; variably differentiated	Liver	
Group IV Fixed postmitotic cells	Do not divide; highly differentiated	Nerve cells Muscle cells	Low

[a]Sensitivity decreases for each successive group.
[b]Intermediate in sensitivity between groups II and III.
Reproduced from Rubin, P. ed. *Clinical oncology—a multidisciplinary approach.* East Syracuse, NY: American Cancer Society, 1983:54.

therapy. This may allow preservation of critical structures that would otherwise need to be sacrificed. Furthermore, some tumors that are initially unresectable may be made resectable with preoperative radiation therapy. The radiocurability of a tumor depends on its intrinsic radiosensitivity. Doses for particular tumors are chosen based on the radiosensitivity of the

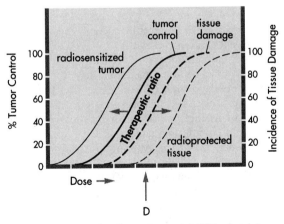

Figure 24-7 Dose-related tumor control (*solid lines*) and tissue damage (*dashed lines*) demonstrating the choice of dosage to maximize tumor killing and minimize tissue damage, and the effect of tumor sensitizing and tissue protectve interventions (see text). (Reproduced from Rubin P, ed. *Clinical oncology—a multidisciplinary approach.* East Syracuse, NY: American Cancer Society, 1983:70.)

tumor and normal surrounding tissues. Rates of both tumor control and normal tissue damage can be plotted as a function of total dose, yielding similar sigmoid curves (Figure 24-7). The distance between these curves is a measure of the **therapeutic ratio.** The therapeutic ratio can be increased, employing methods discussed earlier, such as surgical debulking; selecting beams to reduce scatter, increase penetration, and spare skin; minimizing the effect of hypoxia by using more densely ionizing particle beams; administering chemical modifiers such as radioprotectors and radiosensitizers; and using fractionation schedules.

When cure is not possible, there is still an important role for radiation therapy—palliation. The radiobiology of radiation used for palliation is the same as that for cure, only the endpoint is different. The goals are local shrinkage of tumor for relief of symptoms, usually caused by pressure or infiltration of sensitive structures.

Chemotherapy

Chemotherapy shares many basic principles with radiation therapy. Dose-response curves, cell death kinetics, and variation of sensitivity with the cell cycle are common to both modes of therapy. Additional important aspects of chemotherapy include pharmacologic properties of and interactions among chemotherapeutic agents. The key to successful chemotherapy is the use of

TABLE 24-2. Categories of Therapeutic Agents

Categories	Examples	Mechanism of Action
Alkylating agents	Cyclophosphamide Chlorambucil Busulfan	DNA crosslinking; base mismatches; reacts with sulfhydryl, phosphate, and amino groups
Antimetabolites	Methotrexate	Folic acid analog inhibiting dihydrofolate reductase
	5-Fluorouracil Cytosine arabinoside Mercaptopurine	Purine and pyrimidine analogs inhibiting nucleic acid synthesis
Alkaloids	Vincristine Vinblastine	Interfere with microtubule assembly in mitotic spindle formation, M-phase specific
Antibiotics	Doxorubicin Daunorubicin Bleomycin Dactinomycin	Intercalate in DNA, inhibit DNA and RNA synthesis, cause chromosomal breaks Binds DNA, causes strand breaks Binds DNA and inhibits translation of RNA
Enzymes	L-Asparaginase	Degrades asparagine, killing cells with no asparagine synthetase
Platinum complexes	Cisplatin	Cross links DNA
Substituted urea	Hydroxyurea	S-phase specific inhibition of DNA synthesis
Hormones	Estrogens Androgens Progestins Anti-estrogens Adrenocortocoids	Via cell surface receptors

agents that are cytoxic to tumor cells while sparing normal tissues. Most agents only approximate this ideal.

Some agents are only active against cells in a specific phase of the cell cycle, while other agents, such as the alkylating agents, kill cells in any phase. Many chemotherapeutic agents affect cell division and are therefore more effective against actively dividing cells.

DRUG RESISTANCE

Resistance can either be inherent in the tumor cells or acquired during growth or exposure to the drug. Tumors may have a heterogeneous population of cells with a certain fraction expressing drug resistance. This allows an initial clinical response to a course of chemotherapy followed by regrowth of a resistant tumor. The mechanisms of drug resistance include increased drug inactivation, decreased drug activation, more efficient repair mechanisms, switching to alternate enzymatic pathways to avoid blocked steps, alterations in the tar-

gets to decrease drug-target interaction, and amplification of genes for target enzymes.

Random mutations can impart drug resistance through any of these mechanisms. Under the selective pressure of exposure to the toxic agent resistant cells expand to replace sensitive ones. Resistance may be imparted by a single mutation or by the gradual accumulation of multiple mutations, each imparting an incremental resistance. Although drug resistance is often specific for single agents, there is a phenomenon of **multidrug resistance (MDR).** It has been demonstrated that some tumors that have gradually developed a drug resistance are then also resistant to many other drugs, often in unrelated classes. An *MDR* gene has been identified that is amplified in MDR tumor cells and is suspected to encode a transport pump. This pump may be responsible for removing many different cytotoxic agents from cells.

Techniques have been devised both to increase the therapeutic index of chemotherapeutic agents and to reduce the significance of drug resistance. Increasing the concentration of these drugs, specifically in the target tumor, will enhance their tumor-killing effect while reducing damage to normal cells. This can be done by delivering these agents directly to the tumors via catheters, for example, intrathecal and hepatic artery catheters. Research continues on linking cytotoxic agents to other ligands with a particular affinity for tumor cells, for example, tumor-specific antibodies. Multidrug regimens can minimize the effect of drug resistance by attacking tumor cells at several sites simultaneously. Different classes of drugs are usually used to increase the chances that a cell resistant to one drug will still be sensitive to another.

Chemotherapeutic agents fall into many categories summarized in a Table 24-2. Description of specific drug regimens is beyond the scope of this text.

TOXICITY

Although chemotherapeutic agents are often very effective in controlling tumors, they are associated with significant toxicities. Generally, the toxic effects of various chemotherapeutic agents are proportional to the concentration of drug times the length of exposure ($C \times T$). Most common are bone marrow suppression; immunosuppression; nausea; and gonadal, pulmonary, cardiac, liver, and neural toxicities. Chemotherapy is often used for palliation when cure is not possible. Whenever chemotherapy is being administered, but especially when palliation is the goal, close attention must be paid to these side effects and maximal effort made to insure good nutrition, adequate pain control, and psychological support.

Bibliography

DeVita VT, Hellman S, Rosenberg SA. *Cancer—principles and practice of oncology*. Philadelphia: JB Lippincott, 1985.

Moss WT, Cox JD, eds. *Radiation oncology—rationale, technique, results*. St. Louis: CV Mosby, 1989.

Rubin P, ed. *Clinical oncology—a multidisciplinary approach*. East Syracuse, NY: American Cancer Society, 1983.

Paul J. Turek and Edward B. Savage

25 KIDNEY AND URINARY TRACT PHYSIOLOGY

The anatomy and physiology of the kidney and urinary tract provide superb examples of structural-functional relationships within the body. Through its functional unit, the nephron, the kidney regulates body solute composition, blood pressure, acid-base balance, and extracellular fluid volume. The lower urinary tract, though not as complex, possesses unique physiologic processes concerning urine conduction, storage and micturition.

Anatomy

Situated in the retroperitoneal space, the kidneys are paired, solid organs. On gross sectioning, the kidney has a pale outer region, or **cortex**, and a darker inner region, the **medulla**. Histologically, the kidney is composed of functional units called **nephrons** (Figure 25-1). The filtering portion of the nephron, the **glomerulus**, consists of a capillary tuft with afferent and efferent arterioles situated within the urinary space (Figure 25-2). The human kidney contains $1-1.5 \times 10^6$ glomeruli. The **mesangium** consists of cells that form the stalk of the glomerulus as well as the matrix around it. At the vascular pole of the glomerulus, a specialized area of the ascending distal tubule, the **macula densa,** is in close proximity to the afferent and efferent arterioles. These three structures and a portion of the mesangium referred to as the extraglomerular mesangium constitute a specialized area called the **juxtaglomerular apparatus.** In 70% of cases, a single artery usually supplies each kidney, although accessory renal arteries are common. The renal artery divides into divisional and then segmental arteries. All segmental branches are true end arteries.

The ureter is formed as the renal pelvis tapers down into a muscular tube. The arterial supply of the ureter arises from the renal, aortic, gonadal, hypogastric, vesical, and uterine arteries. The ureter as a conduit is composed of three tissue layers cross-sectionally: **fibrous, muscular** and **mucosal.** The outer fibrous layer is contiguous with the renal capsule. A muscular layer consisting of roughly longitudinal and circular fibers is contained within the fibrous layer. A transitional epithelium continuous with that of the renal pelvis and bladder lines the inner muscular layer.

The bladder wall is similar in structure to the ureter and has three layers in cross section. The arterial supply to the bladder arises from the superior, middle, and inferior vesical arteries, branches of the hypogastric artery. Both autonomic nervous system divisions supply the bladder, the sympathetics arising from T11 to L2 and the parasympathetics from S2 to S4. Functionally, the bladder is divided into a **detrusor**, or body, and

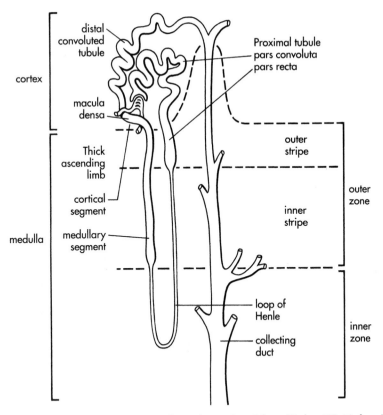

Figure 25-1 Diagram of a single nephron. (Reproduced from Tissher CC, Madsen KM. Anatomy of the kidney. In: Brenner BM, Rector FC, eds. *The kidney.* 3rd ed. Philadelphia: WB Saunders, 1986:9.)

trigone. The trigone is the area of the posterior bladder between the ureteral orifices and the bladder outlet. As the ureter enters the bladder, it is surrounded by 1–2 cm of an incomplete collar of detrusor muscle, referred to as **Waldeyer's sheath.** Connective tissue separates this sheath from ureteric muscle. This arrangement helps prevent ureteric reflux since the ureters are occluded as bladder pressure rises.

Cellular Physiology

KIDNEY

Epithelial Cells

Epithelial cells of the nephrons perform elaborate and necessary kidney functions. Their polarity and intercel-lular connections allow them to participate in the mass transport of substances. Through gap, intermediate, and tight junctions, cells can couple electrically or chemi-cally and form barriers of variable permeability. Renal epithelial cells also harbor specialized **pores** and pro-tein carriers for water and ion transport.

Juxtaglomerular Apparatus

The juxtaglomerular apparatus, with its constituent af-ferent and efferent arterioles, macula densa, and mesangium, is intimately involved with extracellular volume regulation. Large quantities of renin are stored within the juxtaglomerular cells (JG cells). Renin release appears to be mediated via several pathways, which in-clude the NaCl delivery mechanism, prostaglandins, sympathetic nerve activity, and the baroreceptor mech-anism. The macula densa senses NaCl concentration in

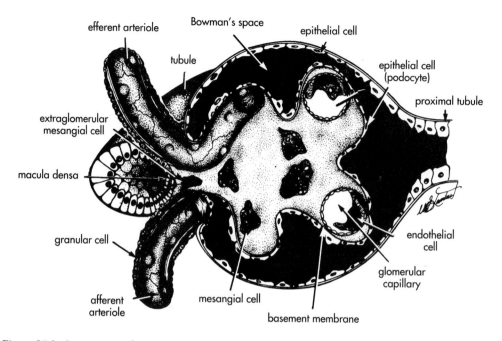

Figure 25-2 Cross section of the glomerulus. (Reproduced from West JB. *Best and Taylor's physiological basis of medical practice.* 11th ed. Baltimore: Williams & Wilkins, 1985:454.)

the distal tubule and responds to decreased NaCl delivery by stimulation of renin release from the JG cells. Renal nerve stimulation results in an increase in intrarenal renin release. Prostaglandin I_2 (PGI_2) and PGE_2 stimulate renin production from the JG cells, and this pathway may be important in the macula densa response. The JG cells, as modified smooth muscle cells, serve also as baroreceptors, secreting renin from granules in response to decreased stretch secondary to lower blood pressure. Through its activity on angiotensinogen to produce **angiotensin I**, and indirectly **angiotensin II** and **III**, renin regulates arterial blood pressure and volume (see below).

Nephron

Urine elaboration begins at the glomerulus with the formation of a protein-free ultrafiltrate of plasma. This ultrafiltrate then enters **Bowman's space** and consequently passes through the tubules, a process that involves the reabsorption and secretion of substances. For descriptive purposes, the rate of glomerular filtration is defined for a **single nephron (SNGFR)**, as micropunc-

ture studies first allowed quantitative measurements in solitary nephrons. Thus,

$$\text{SNGFR} = K_f[(P_G - P_T) - (\Pi_G - \Pi_T)]$$

In this equation, $(P_G - P_T)$, or glomerular capillary hydrostatic pressure minus tubular hydrostatic pressure, is a measure of the hydrostatic force that favors ultrafiltration. Alternatively, $(\Pi_G - \Pi_T)$, or the oncotic pressure within the glomerular capillary minus the oncotic pressure within the tubule, is a measure of the net colloid osmotic pressure or oncotic pressure that complements hydrostatic pressure. This oncotic pressure, or Π_G, reflects the contribution of plasma proteins in their various spaces to ultrafiltration: glomerular capillary plasma proteins create pressures that oppose transcapillary fluid movement, and tubular proteins create oncotic forces that favor fluid movement. Under normal conditions, no proteins are ultrafiltered and $\Pi_T = 0$.

The term K_f represents a combination of the permeability of the glomerular capillary and the total surface area of filtration, and is otherwise known as the **glomerular ultrafiltration coefficient**. The permeability of the "membrane" or glomerular capillary is a function of the combined permeabilities of its three components: the endothelium, basement membrane, and podocytes. The **pores** of the endothelium, with 50–100 nm fenestrae, serve as the initial barrier. The filtration slits between the podocyte foot processes, known as slit pores, with widths of 4–14 nm, contribute to size selectivity. In addition, negatively charged glycoproteins, sialic acid residues, and sulfate-rich proteoglycans on the basement membrane, endothelial, and epithelial surfaces act as a barrier by discriminating against molecules of differing electrical charge.

Once past the glomerulus, the ultrafiltrate of plasma then enters the proximal tubule. Like other tubule segments, the proximal tubule cells use energy to transport substances. The most important active transport mechanism is the Na,K-ATPase pump, which fuels the transport of sodium out of the cells and into the blood in exchange for potassium. Such ion movement creates a negative intracellular voltage, which secondarily drives the transport of other solutes like bicarbonate, sulfate, and phosphate. Glucose and amino acids are reabsorbed by carriers in a process powered by the sodium electrochemical gradient. Chloride transport is both active and passive and water is reabsorbed by osmosis.

In Henle's loop large amounts of solute are transported, but unlike the proximal tubule, very little if any active transport is involved. The thin descending loops are highly permeable to water, and as they descend into the highly osmolar medulla, the high osmotic pressure gradient drives water from the tubular lumen into the interstitium. Though the thin descending limb is freely permeable to NaCl and urea, the relatively greater efflux of water raises the intraluminal concentration of these substances. Thin ascending loop permeability differs from that of the descending loop in that it is highly permeable to salt and urea but not permeable to water. Salt permeability also exceeds that of urea. The result is passive NaCl reabsorption and urea secretion from the lumen, without the movement of water. This lowers the intraluminal concentration of solutes.

The fluid next enters the distal tubule. Distal tubule segments include the medullary and cortical thick ascending limbs and the convoluted tubules. The macula densa and associated renin release have been discussed earlier. In thick ascending limbs, NaCl is rapidly reabsorbed, primarily by Na,K-ATPase pumps. These tubules are impermeable to water; thus, the osmolality of tubular fluid decreases. Chloride concentration remains low as it diffuses out of cells down the estab-

lished voltage gradient. Chloride is also carried extracellularly by an active transport process. A third, complex active transport process in this tubule carries one sodium, one potassium, and two chlorides intracellularly, resulting in sodium, potassium, and chloride reabsorption. This pump is affected by loop diuretics (e.g., furosemide), which compete with chloride for the transporter, inhibiting its function. Thick ascending limbs are leaky and highly permeable to cations like K^+, Cl^+, Ca^{2+}, Mg^{2+}, and NH_4^+. These cations are passively reabsorbed, driven by the existing transepithelial voltage gradients.

As tubular fluid passes from the thick ascending limbs through the macula densa, it next reaches the distal convoluted tubule. Here, salt continues to be reabsorbed in the presence of Na,K-ATPase pumps. Water permeability is low, even when antidiuretic hormone (ADH) is present, and thus the tubular fluid becomes hypo-osmolar. Because of a negative transepithelial voltage, Cl reabsorption is mainly passive, but active pumps probably exist that contribute to its transport.

Once beyond the distal tubule, the luminal fluid, hypo-osmolar in character, enters the collecting duct. Through a Na,K-ATPase pump, cortical collecting duct cells reabsorb NaCl and secrete potassium. Collecting duct transport functions appear to be highly variable and strongly influenced by the hormonal milieu. Aldosterone acts on the distal tubule and collecting duct to promote sodium reabsorption. Water permeability of the collecting duct is routinely low unless ADH is present. When ADH is absent, duct pumps reabsorb the low amount of remaining NaCl in tubular fluid, decreasing its intraluminal concentration to around 15 mmol. With ADH present, water permeability increases and it is reabsorbed by osmosis. As a result, urine osmolarity increases.

URETER

Like other excitable tissues, the smooth muscle cells of the ureter exhibit resting and active membrane potentials (see Chapter 26). Excitatory stimuli causing membrane depolarization include those of an electrical, mechanical (stretch), or chemical nature. Located proximally within the collecting system, in the pelvicalyceal border, are specialized pacemaker smooth muscle cells. They are capable of spontaneously depolarizing. Contraction rhythms, generated by these cells, exist within the calyceal system and can be conducted down the ureter, promoting urine flow.

BLADDER

The transitional cell epithelial layer of the bladder is pleuristratified and underpinned by elastic fibers within a loose connective tissue. This permits considerable stretching of the mucosa, important in periods of bladder distention. The luminal surface of the mucosa secretes a layer of glycosaminoglycans, proteins that protect the bladder wall from infiltration by bacterial, carcinogenic, or cancerous agents.

There are several physical properties of the bladder wall that relate to its storage and emptying functions. The bladder is elastic and distensible because of **passive** and **active** elements found within its wall. Collagen, elastin, and certain smooth muscle elements account for the passive properties such that at normal intravesicular volumes, the pressure rise is small as volume increases. At the limits of bladder distensibility, however, increases in volume result in great increases in pressure. Bladder wall tension also varies with the rate of fill; at high rates rapid stretching occurs and higher tension is generated. However, the bladder accommodates with time to provide a low-pressure reservoir. The active properties of the wall are determined largely by the wall **tonus**. Tonus is maintained by contractile element activity within the muscle. The factors governing the degree of tonus include the intrinsic smooth muscle characteristics, local tissue factors or hormones, and tonic activity initiated by the autonomic nervous system. With these various inputs, bladder compliance during filling is determined and a low intravesical pressure maintained despite increasing bladder volumes.

The bladder is controlled by the autonomic nervous system. The bladder body and, more sparsely, the bladder base are innervated by the parasympathetic nervous system. The bladder neck and proximal urethra and, less so, the bladder body are innervated by the adrenergic or sympathetic nervous system. Of the two main kinds of adrenergic receptors, β-receptors are found predominantly in the bladder body and the α-receptors in the bladder neck and proximal urethra. The external, or striated, muscle sphincter of the proximal urethra is controlled by the somatic nervous system and is essential for bladder continence. During normal micturition, an orchestrated interplay of sympathetic, parasympathetic, and somatic nerve stimulation occurs, effecting bladder contraction and bladder outlet opening and sphincter release.

Organ Physiology

KIDNEY

Renal Blood Flow

Although they receive 20% of the cardiac output, the kidneys constitute only 0.5% of the total body mass. The renal circulation must accomplish bulk filtration, reabsorption, and selective regulation of normal urine constituents as well as deliver nutrition to the organ itself. These functions are accomplished through several microcirculations, including glomerular, peritubular, and medullary networks. To determine renal blood flow, the Fick principle is applied to the disappearance of an indicator substance from blood as it passes through the kidney and appears in urine. Ideally, the indicator should not be synthesized, stored, or metabolized and should also be totally secreted by the tubules. The most commonly used indicator for estimation of renal blood flow is para-aminohippuric acid. If the above conditions are met, then the appearance of indicator in the urine is equal to renal plasma flow (RPF) rate multiplied by the arteriovenous concentration difference, or

$$U_i Q_u = (A_i - V_i)RPF$$

where U_i = indicator concentration in urine; Q_u = urine flow rate; A_i = indicator concentration in arterial plasma; and V_i = indicator concentration in venous plasma. Since extraction is assumed to be complete, let $V_i = 0$. Incorporating this assumption

$$RPF = \frac{U_i Q_u}{A_i}$$

To convert RPF to renal blood flow (RBF),

$$RBF = \frac{RPF}{1 - HCT}$$

where HCT is hematocrit.

The renal circulation is regulated by resistance changes mediated by relaxation or contraction of vascular smooth muscle. Although humoral and intrarenal factors may exist, the evidence for neural input affecting blood flow is clear. Renal nerve stimulation causes smooth muscle contraction and simultaneous reduction in total renal blood flow. Sympathetic stimulation may result in a 50% decrease in renal blood flow. This effect can be abolished with α-adrenergic receptor blockade. Intrarenal β-adrenergic and dopaminergic receptors also exist, but their functions are less well delineated. Renal blood flow is maintained over a wide range of perfusion pressures by autoregulation. Within the blood pressure range of 80–180 mm Hg, glomerular filtration rate and renal blood flow change less than 10%.

Creatinine Clearance and Glomerular Filtration Rate

Urine elaboration begins at the glomerulus with the production of a plasma ultrafiltrate. As the filtrate progresses through the tubules of the nephron, substances are removed or reabsorbed and added or secreted. The term **clearance** is a quantitative description of the rate at which the kidney excretes a substance relative to its concentration in the plasma. It is expressed mathematically as the volume of blood or plasma that is completely cleared of a substance in a unit time. By measuring the amount of a substance removed by the kidney in a unit time and dividing this by the plasma concentration, a value for the clearance can be obtained. Thus,

$$C = \frac{UV}{P}$$

where P = plasma concentration of substance in mg/ml and V = volume of urine per unit time or ml/min. The clearance of a substance is equal to the **glomerular filtration rate** (GFR) if (a) it is freely filtered at the glomerulus (i.e., uncharged, inert, small) and (b) it is neither secreted nor reabsorbed by the tubules. Inulin is such a marker and has been employed for the precise measurement of GFR. However, inulin is impractical for common use, and urinary creatinine is used instead. Creatinine, derived from endogenous muscle catabolism, is produced at a relatively constant rate. It is not a perfect marker because it is secreted by the tubules, and at low GFRs and low flow rates, large calculation errors can result.

The various permeability factors affecting GFR have already been discussed and are functions of glomerular structure. Variations in arteriolar resistance with resultant changes in capillary hydraulic pressure are felt to contribute to regulation of the GFR. Several substances have been implicated in the control of arteriolar resistance changes. One involves a system of tubuloglomerular feedback. As described

earlier, the macula densa region of the distal tubule is closely juxtaposed with the afferent and efferent arterioles of that nephron. An intrarenal renin-angiotensin mechanism is the prime hormonal mediator of this feedback loop. Angiotensin II, a product of the renin cascade, probably acts locally on the arterioles and mesangium to reduce permeability and increase arteriolar resistance and thus decrease GFR. In addition, a wide variety of hormones and vasoactive substances are capable of modifying the GFR, including parathyroid hormone (PTH), ADH, serotonin, prostaglandins, (E series, I_2), histamine, adenosine, isoproterenol, dopamine, epinephrine, and papaverine. Finally, renal nerve stimulation of adrenergic terminals can produce dose-related, graded vasoconstriction as well.

The Countercurrent Mechanism

In the process of solute and water reabsorption, the vasa recta function as countercurrent exchangers and Henle's loop as a countercurrent multiplier (Figure 25-3). This allows the production of either dilute or concentrated urine. The concentrating mechanism revolves around the presence of an osmotic gradient within the medullary pyramids. As NaCl is reabsorbed in the relatively water impermeable ascending limb of Henle's loop, it is deposited in the interstitium, creating a horizontal osmotic gradient. This osmotic gradient results in water extraction from the relatively solute impermeable descending limb of Henle's loop. This gradient is protected by small nutrient exchanges between the limbs of the vasa recta, in which substances like O_2 and glucose are recirculated and thus unable to perturb the hypertonic medulla. Urea contributes to the osmotic gradient by circulating from the collecting duct through the interstitium to the ascending limb of Henle's loop. Because of active solute reabsorption in the distal tubule, the filtrate delivered to the collecting duct is hypo-osmolar. In the presence of ADH, collecting duct fluid equilibrates with a hypertonic medulla and urine osmolality rises. If ADH is absent, there is no equilibration of the hypo-osmolar fluid with the interstitium, and dilute urine results.

Mechanisms of Water and Solute Excretion

Sodium, Chloride, and Water
Sodium balance is maintained by several physiologic mechanisms. Glomerular filtration rate autoregulation

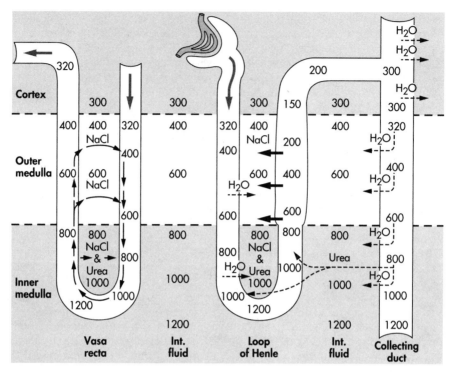

Figure 25-3 The countercurrent mechanism. (Reproduced from Guyton AC. *Textbook of medical physiology.* 7th ed. Philadelphia: WB Saunders, 1986:415.)

keeps the filtered sodium load constant despite changes in the blood pressure. The fraction of sodium absorbed in the proximal tubule can vary. Adrenergic nerve stimulation in the kidney can increase proximal tubule sodium reabsorption independently of changes in GFR or RPF. Reabsorption of sodium in the distal tubule is enhanced by the presence of aldosterone. Atrial natriuretic factor acts as a diuretic and natriuretic. Prostaglandins, made locally in the medulla, enhance sodium excretion by inhibiting sodium and urea transport and exchange, antagonizing the action of ADH and increasing renal blood flow.

Water excretion is linked to sodium excretion. Variations in sodium reabsorption can affect the generation of free water. **Free-water clearance,** used to quantify free-water balance, describes the excretion of the combined number of osmotically active particles relative to urine volume. Thus,

$$C_{osm} = \frac{U_{osm}V}{P_{osm}}$$

and

$$C_{H_2O} = V - C_{osm}$$

where C_{H_2O} = free-water clearance, C_{osm} = osmolar clearance, U_{osm} = urine osmolality, P_{osm} = plasma osmolality, and V = volume of urine/time. If urine and plasma osmolalities are equal, osmolar clearance will equal urine volume. In this case, water is neither retained nor secreted, and there is no net change in plasma osmolality. If the volume of urine increases but clearance remains stable, urine osmolality drops and water is lost in excess of solute.

The anatomic site of most free-water regulation is the distal nephron (distal tubule and collecting duct), and ADH is the principal regulating humoral factor. Water excretion is also dependent on solute load and can be altered by external influences on that osmotic load. Osmotic diuresis results from an osmotic load in the tubules that prevents water reabsorption. Osmotic diuretics include mannitol, urea, glucose, and NaCl. Thiazide and loop diuretic agents inhibit chloride reabsorption in the distal loop of Henle and distal tubule.

This prevents salt and water reabsorption and leads to their excretion.

Potassium

Ninety percent of plasma potassium is filtered at the glomerulus and only 10–20% is eventually excreted. It is reabsorbed mainly in the proximal tubule and Henle's loop. The final potassium content of urine results from tubular secretion in the late distal tubule and collecting duct. The rate of secretion is influenced by mineralocorticoids, urine flow rate, acid-base balance, and sodium load. Mineralocorticoids stimulate potassium secretion, possibly by enhancing Na,K-ATPase activity in the collecting duct. If urine flow rates are high, a steep potassium concentration gradient is maintained between tubular fluid and cells and secretion is promoted. Since potassium and hydrogen ion transport are linked, acidosis results in hydrogen ion secretion in lieu of potassium secretion. Alkalosis enhances potassium secretion, in an effort to conserve hydrogen ions. When increased amounts of sodium are presented to distal tubule reabsorptive sites, the sodium tends to move into the cells, and a large negative transmembrane potential is generated. This electrical gradient promotes the movement of potassium into the tubular lumen. Potassium depletion by thiazide and loop diuretics is related to the increased sodium load in the distal tubule.

Glucose

Freely filtered at the glomerulus, glucose is virtually completely reabsorbed early in the nephron in a transport mechanism linked to sodium reabsorption (as discussed above). Although urine is normally glucose free, at higher filtered loads, a tubular maximum glucose reabsorption rate (T_{MG}) is reached. Glucose loads in excess of the T_{MG} cause glucose to appear in the urine.

Calcium

Of total plasma calcium, 60% is filtered at the glomerulus. The remaining fraction is protein bound and therefore not filtered. Of the filtered load, 96–98% is reabsorbed. Calcium reabsorption occurs mainly in the proximal tubule and thick ascending limb of Henle's loop and is in part Na-dependent. Calcium reabsorption is dependent on phosphate, magnesium and PTH. Hypophosphatemia and hypermagnesmia decrease calcium reabsorption, the latter probably secondary to the saturation of a shared ion pump. Parathyroid hormone enhances calcium reabsorption and reduces phosphate reabsorption. As well, PTH stimulates the kidney to produce 1,25 dihydroxyvitamin D_3, which increases gut and bone calcium reabsorption.

Phosphates

Plasma inorganic phosphates are 80–90% ultrafiltered and eventually 85–90% reabsorbed in the nephron. Phosphate reabsorption occurs mainly in the proximal tubule, but further distal reabsorption is likely. Parathyroid hormone acts on the proximal tubule to inhibit phosphate reabsorption, resulting in increased phosphaturia.

Acid/Base Balance

Extracellular fluid pH is maintained by the renal regulation of plasma bicarbonate (HCO_3^-) concentration. Based on the pH, bicarbonate is either reabsorbed or generated anew as by-product of acid secretion. Of filtered bicarbonate, more than 99% is reclaimed, mostly within the proximal tubule. More specifically, bicarbonate is not reabsorbed as HCO_3^-, but in conjunction with the secretion of hydrogen ion (H^+) into the tubular fluid. Instrumental to bicarbonate reabsorption is the enzyme carbonic anhydrase, which catalyzes the hydration of CO_2 to form carbonic acid (H_2CO_3). Carbonic acid dissociates to form H^+ and HCO_3^-. This occurs in the proximal tubule cell. The hydrogen ion generated is secreted into the tubular lumen and the bicarbonate formed diffuses into peritubular capillaries. Bicarbonate in the tubular fluid combines with H^+ to form H_2CO_3. Adluminal carbonic anhydrase (not intracellular) then catalyzes the dehydration of H_2CO_3 to H_2O and CO_2, the latter of which is reabsorbed by the tubular cell. Carbonic anhydrase within the cell hydrates this CO_2 to H_2CO_3 and the process is renewed, causing a net reabsorption of bicarbonate and a net secretion of hydrogen ions. Factors that affect the bicarbonate reabsorption process include extracellular fluid volume, arterial P_{CO_2}, potassium stores, PTH, and phosphates. Decreased extracellular fluid increases and hypocapnia reduces bicarbonate reabsorption. Potassium depletion is a mild stimulant of bicarbonate reabsorption. Parathyroid hormone presence and phosphate depletion inhibit bicarbonate reabsorption.

Renal production of a hydrogen ion concentration gradient is limited; the kidney cannot generate urine with a pH less than 4.5. Thus, the ability of the kidney to excrete large amounts of acid depends on intraluminal buffering capacity. Intraluminal buffering mechanisms include the formation of CO_2 and H_2O discussed above, and the combination of hydrogen ions with inorganic phosphate and ammonia. Hydrogen ion reacts with dibasic phosphate (HPO_4^{2-}) to form monobasic phosphate ($H_2PO_4^-$) predominantly in the distal tubules and collecting ducts. Ammonia is secreted in the proximal and distal tubules and the collecting ducts. It is created principally by the deamination of glutamic acid and to a lesser extent other amino acids. After diffusing into the lumen, the ammonia (NH_3) combines with hydrogen ion to form ammonium ion (NH_4^+). This reaction also promotes ammonia excretion; ammonium ions are lipid insoluble and this reaction prevents back diffusion of secreted ammonia.

Urea

As the end product of protein catabolism, urea is freely filtered at the glomerulus. It is reabsorbed in the proximal tubule and medullary collecting ducts; reclamation at the latter location helps regenerate the hypertonicity of the medullary interstitium (as described above). Urea reabsorption is inversely proportional to tubular flow rate. Thus during water diuresis 60% to 70% of filtered urea is excreted; however, with low urine flow rates only 10–20% of filtered urea is excreted. A result of this is "prerenal azotemia." When urine flow is low there is a disproportionate increase in serum BUN relative to creatinine as a higher percentage of urea is reabsorbed.

Uric Acid

Uric acid, the final product of purine catabolism, is excreted predominantly by the kidney but also by the gut. It is freely filtered at the glomerulus and undergoes nearly complete tubular reabsorption. Of the amount reabsorbed, 50% is secreted back into tubular fluid. Postsecretory reabsorption then returns 80% of the secreted amount. The secretion mechanism involves organic anions and cations and various other substances which compete for these mechanisms, including penicillins, thiazides, cimetidine, and creatinine.

Amino Acids

Proximal tubular reabsorption reclaims mostly all of the circulating, freely filtered amino acids. Like glucose transport, the process is carrier mediated and related to Na transport. Complicated transport models have been proposed involving two or three pumps to describe the reabsorptive defects of cystine, arginine, lysine, and orinthine.

Endocrine Functions of the Kidney

Renin, Angiotensin, and Aldosterone

One of the major hormonal systems regulating blood pressure, sodium balance, and potassium balance is the renin-angiotensin-aldosterone system (Figure 25-4). It is a system that protects against sodium depletion but at the expense of vasoconstriction and decreased organ perfusion. Several angiotensin II receptor blockers have been elucidated and have confirmed several ideas about cascade functions. (1) Basal blood pressure maintenance does not depend on the cascade. This assumes, of course, true sodium balance in the individual. (2) Renin secretion is stimulated whenever cardiac output or blood volume are reduced in order to contract peripheral arteries and, through aldosterone, retain sodium. (3) Angiotensin (II or III) probably directly causes aldosterone secretion. Aldosterone, which binds cells predominantly in the distal tubule and collecting system, increases the rate at which sodium is reabsorbed from the tubule lumen. Aldosterone also enhances potassium secretion in a manner independent of sodium reabsorption.

Atrial Natriuretic Factor

Atrial natriuretic factor, a 28-amino-acid polypeptide derived from the atrium, inhibits aldosterone synthesis and release, acts as a diuretic and natriuretic factor, and also has vasorelaxant properties. Its release is stimulated by atrial stretch, volume expansion, increased sodium load or osmolality, and vasopressor agents.

Prostaglandins

The prostaglandin cascade, beginning with arachidonic acid as a precursor, is complex. Indeed, many of its putative roles in kidney function need validation. Two families of compounds or eicosanoids result from arachidonic acid metabolism: prostaglandins, prostacyclin, and thromboxanes from the cyclo-oxygenase pathway, and leukotrienes, from the lipoxygenase pathway. Prostaglandin synthesis occurs predominantly in the renal medulla. Data thus far show a role for prostaglandins in mediating renin release, acting as natriuretic factors, and opposing the action of ADH. More controversial is the importance of prostaglandins in the regulation of RBF. Renal vasculature behaves like other vascular beds and undergoes vasodilation with PGE_2, PGI_2, and PGD_2. Thromboxane A_2, however, is a potent vasoconstrictor of vascular beds. When administered exogenously, the effects of these compounds can be

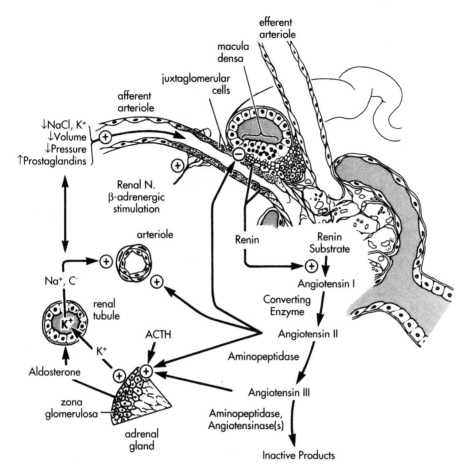

Figure 25-4 Diagram of the stimulatory and feedback mechanisms of the renin-angiotensin system. +, Stimulation; –, inhibition. (Reproduced from Biglieri EG, Baxter JD. In: Felig P, Baxter JD, Broadus AE, Frohman LA, eds. *Endocrinology and metabolism.* New York: McGraw-Hill, 1981:556.)

seen. Recently, it has been shown that RBF is prostaglandin-independent in situations of euvolemia and in steady, basal states. In these states, only low levels of endogenous prostaglandins are circulating and presumably their physiologic effect is minimal.

Kallikreins and Kinins

It is thought that two independent kallikrein-kinin systems exist: one in the general circulatory system that plays an important role in blood coagulation and blood pressure homeostasis, and the other confined to the kidney with a natriuretic role. Kallikreins are enzymes that release kinins from their precursor kininogens.

They are located predominantly in the renal cortex and specifically within the distal convoluted tubules. Renal kallikreins may serve to activate a precursor renin pool within the kidney and therefore influence the renin-angiotensin cascade. Bradykinin is known to be a renal vasodilator, the effects of which may be partially or completely mediated through the prostaglandins. The interaction of these compounds with many discussed above is shown in Figure 25-5.

Glucocorticoids

Glucocorticoid effects on kidney function are uncertain but they may change GFR and distal nephron perme-

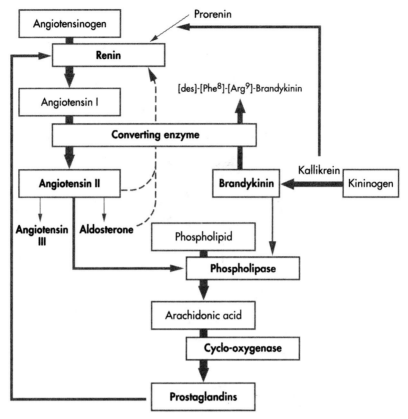

Figure 25-5 Interactions of renal hormones. *Solid arrows,* activators; *dashed arrows,* inhibitors. (Reproduced from Leslie BR, Vaugh ED. Normal renal physiology. In: Walsh PC, Gittes RF, Perlmutter AD, Stamey TA, eds. *Campbell's urology.* 5th ed. Philadelphia: WB Saunders, 1986:89.)

ability to water. In states of glucocorticoid depletion, GFR falls and water loads cannot be excreted because distal tubule water permeability is raised. These effects can be reversed by glucocorticoid administration.

Parathyroid Hormone and Calcitonin
Parathyroid hormone and calcitonin are important in the regulation of both calcium and phosphate homeostasis. Parathyroid hormone inhibits NaCl reabsorption in the proximal tubule and therefore inhibits reabsorption of all substances linked to sodium transport, including calcium and phosphate. Overall, sodium and calcium reabsorption remain unchanged because of compensatory reabsorption from elsewhere in the tubule and stimulated by PTH. Phosphate, however, is only reabsorbed in the proximal tubule and thus PTH causes phosphaturia. The effect of calcitonin on the distal tubule and collecting duct experimentally resembles PTH but its function is unknown.

Erythropoietin
Erythropoietin, a hormone responsible for increasing red cell mass, is produced within the kidney. The stimulus for production of erythropoietin appears to be decreased tissue oxygen tension. Erythropoietin induces primitive marrow cells to differentiate into erythrocytes.

URETER
The ureter functions as a muscular conduit for urine. It has a syncytial smooth muscle cell arrangement with pacemaker cells located in the pelvocalyceal border. At normal rates of urine production, the renal pelvis fills and pelvic pressure rises. Urine is then extruded into

the collapsed upper ureter, which expands to receive the pelvic urine. Peristaltic waves, originating high in the ureter, push the urine toward the bladder, effectively making a "bolus" of the urine volume. The ureterovesical junction (UVJ) assures one-way transport of urine propelled through it. The peristaltic contraction dissipates at the UVJ. When ureteral transport of urine fails, urine stasis and ureteral dilatation occur. As flow rates increase, the ureter initially increases peristaltic frequency to a maximum rate. After this, urine is transported by increases in bolus volume until dilatation occurs, at which time the ureter becomes a simple, wide-caliber conduit.

BLADDER

Functionally speaking, micturition can be described in two phases: bladder filling and storage and bladder emptying. The nervous system activity and physiology differ for each phase. Micturition is basically a function of the peripheral nervous system; however, ultimate control resides within the central nervous system.

The bladder and its associated sphincters are innervated by cholinergic, adrenergic, and somatic nerve fibers. During bladder filling, bladder pressure rises slowly despite large volume changes. This is ascribed to the passive and active properties of the bladder wall, with only a low level of neural efferent input present. At a certain intravesicular pressure, a spinal sympathetic reflex is activated. The efferent arm of the reflex results in increased outlet resistance by smooth muscle sphincter stimulation, a decrease in bladder contractility, and an inhibition of excitatory cholinergic innervation of the detrusor muscle. Outlet resistance is enhanced by α-adrenergic stimulation of the sphincter. Bladder relaxation is mediated directly via β-adrenergic sympathetic stimulation of the detrusor muscle and indirectly via sympathetic inhibition of parasympathetic stimulation of the bladder. To contain the urine at even higher pressures, the striated muscle sphincter is activated through somatic nerves. Thus, the combined effect of these maneuvers is to inhibit coordinated bladder activity and increase outlet resistance.

Bladder emptying involves many factors, but intravesical pressure, by producing a sensation of distension, is the primary stimulus for a voluntary bladder contraction. A coordination of several events follows: (1) efferent outflow, through the pelvic nerves, is stimulated and excitation of cholinergic detrusor nerve terminals in the bladder promotes bladder contraction; (2) somatic

neural discharge to the external sphincter is inhibited, allowing relaxation; and (3) the spinal sympathetic reflex is inhibited. What results is a coordinated contraction of the bulk of the bladder musculature with funnelling of the relaxed bladder outlet and proximal urethra.

The neuroanatomic details of micturition are still subject to debate. However, for normal filling to occur (1) bladder sensation must be intact; (2) the bladder must be able to accommodate increasing urine volume at low pressure; (3) the bladder outlet should be closed at all times during filling, even when sudden increases in intra-abdominal pressure occur; and (4) the bladder should not exhibit involuntary contractions. For normal emptying, a coordinated, adequate bladder contraction must occur with simultaneous lowering of the flow resistance in the smooth muscle and striated muscle sphincters. Finally, there must be no anatomic obstruction in the bladder, bladder outlet or urethra.

Pathophysiology

KIDNEY

Acute Renal Failure

Acute renal failure (ARF) is a common yet challenging clinical condition. It is defined as deterioration of kidney function that occurs over hours to days and results in nitrogenous waste buildup and disorders of fluid, acid-base, and electrolyte balance. It is generally agreed that a rise in serum creatinine of 0.5 mg/dL/day and a rise in BUN of 10 mg/dL/day over several days is a useful working definition of ARF. The causes of ARF can be divided into prerenal, renal, and postrenal (obstructive). Prerenal causes include hypovolemia, hepatorenal syndrome, and renal artery stenosis (bilateral). Among renal causes, there exist acute tubular necrosis, acute glomerulonephritis, interstitial nephritis, and vascular causes. Postrenal causes of ARF include lower urinary tract obstruction, or intrarenal obstruction. Obviously, many other possible causes for ARF exist.

Although there are many causes of ARF, the pathophysiologic changes that result in renal shutdown are limited to four: (1) changes in renovascular dynamics, (2) alterations in the permeability barrier for glomerular filtration, (3) back leak of filtered tubular fluid secondary to injured epithelium, and (4) tubular obstruction from debris. Changes in renal hemodynamics occur in nearly all forms of ARF, manifested as a decrease in total RBF. Two theories have been proposed to explain how vascular factors can maintain acute renal failure. In one, afferent arteriolar constriction occurs and GFR and RBF are reduced. Arteriolar constriction may be secondary to increased renin-angiotensin activity or to metabolic disturbances from injury, resulting in endothelial cell swelling and capillary lumen narrowing. The second theory involves the dilatation of efferent arterioles as a vascular factor maintaining ARF. If efferent arteriole resistance is reduced, then glomerular hydrostatic pressure falls and may reach a point at which glomerular filtration is not possible. If surface area for filtration is reduced or the ultrafiltration coefficient altered, GFR can be decreased in a manner independent of changes in RBF or capillary pressures. The tubular back-leak theory proposes that although GFR may be normal, filtered fluid leaks from the tubular system into the peritubular vasculature as the epithelial barrier integrity is lost. Theories of tubular obstruction by debris are based on the presence of tubular casts found within the kidney and urine in patients with ARF. Such tubular casts were thought to account for clinically observed oliguria in ARF. However, animal models of ARF only variably show increases in tubular intraluminal pressures with casts, a necessary condition for obstruction. Recent evidence suggests that filtration may be depressed as a result of tubular obstruction by debris. All of these processes probably contribute to ARF and the relative contribution of these effects is unknown.

Chronic Renal Failure

Defined as a progressive and irreversible impairment of renal function, chronic renal failure (CRF) differs from ARF in that ARF is often reversible but CRF is not. Since CRF is often a slowly progressive process, the kidney invokes many adaptive mechanisms for the maintenance of homeostasis until function is severely limited. Uremic symptoms occur with CRF when functions necessary for protein excretion, electrolyte, and acid-base balance fail. A plethora of disorders can cause CRF and can be classified anatomically as vascular, tubulointerstitial, and obstructive-infective in nature. Regardless of etiology, all forms of CRF have a major common denominator: the progressive destruction of nephrons.

In damaged kidneys, some nephrons atrophy, but surviving nephrons hypertrophy and become individu-

ally more active. It follows, therefore, that if normal renal function is to be maintained, each of the surviving nephrons must assume a greater portion of the total renal function, and hence process and excrete more solute than usual. This has been termed the "intact nephron hypothesis" and it serves to describe how altered whole kidney function must be reflected in, and depend on, similar alterations in single nephron function. There are four postulated mechanisms that, when integrated, allow remaining nephron units to increase their functional capacity: (1) RBF increases, (2) single nephron GFR increases, (3) undamaged nephrons increase in size, and (4) individual segments of nephrons adapt to the increased load.

As a result of perturbations in the composition of body fluids in CRF, endocrine and cardiovascular mechanisms are activated and contribute to an increase in RBF. There is evidence implicating prostaglandins in this process, through vasodilation of arterioles supplying remaining glomeruli. Demonstrated reductions in afferent and efferent arteriolar resistances exist in states of CRF, contributing to increases in capillary hydraulic pressures and therefore ultrafiltration. It is unclear whether the surface area for ultrafiltration or capillary wall permeability (both contributing factors to the ultrafiltration coefficient, K_f) in functioning nephrons change during CRF.

As RBF and GFR increase in CRF, so too does remnant kidney mass. This mass augmentation appears to be secondary to increases in length and diameter of the different nephron segments. Proximal tubules exhibit the most marked growth and with it increases in ultrafiltrate reabsorption, thus maintaining glomerulotubular balance. The phenomenon of remnant nephron hypertrophy is referred to as compensatory renal hypertrophy. The stimuli for tubule hypertrophy remain unclear.

Obstructive Nephropathy

Obstructive nephropathy describes renal abnormalities secondary to obstruction of the urinary tract. These can range from phimosis to uteropelvic junction or intrarenal blockage. Depending on whether the obstruction is partial or total, unilateral or bilateral, acute or chronic, changes in nephron function can differ. Proximal to the site of obstruction, dilatation of the ureters and calyces occurs; this is referred to as **hydronephrosis.** Causes of obstruction are divided into intrinsic and extrinsic categories. Intrinsic causes are those derived from the urinary tract. They can be intraluminal, intramural, functional, or anatomic in nature. Extrinsic causes are those involving adjacent organ systems, like the reproductive system, and include GI and retroperitoneal abnormalities. Common causes of urinary tract obstruction in men include prostatic hypertrophy and urinary calculi; pregnancy and pelvic malignancies are frequent causes in women.

The renal effects of obstruction vary with the type and degree of blockage. Renal blood flow, GFR, and tubular functions are altered to some degree in all forms of obstruction. With ureteral blockage, ureteric pressure rises and with time exceeds proximal tubular pressure. At this point, GFR will decrease, but it does not stop completely. The maintenance of filtration at about 2% of normal is allowed by the dilatory capacity of the collecting system, and by alterations in renal blood flow. Eventually, as the duration of obstruction becomes chronic, a progressive reduction in the number of functioning nephrons is seen. With three months of blockage, irreversible renal damage is assured and minimal recovery is often obtained upon release of obstruction. Removal of the blockage before three months usually results in graded increases in GFR, depending on the degree of obstruction and the condition of the contralateral kidney.

Tubule function is exquisitely sensitive to obstruction, as demonstrated by the increased osmolality of urine from an obstructed kidney. Partial obstruction can also be associated with a decreased ability to achieve a maximal urinary concentration, as the medullary osmolar gradient becomes disrupted. Once the blockage is released, especially in situations of bilateral ureteral obstruction, tubular cell damage is reflected by a postobstructive diuresis and natriuresis. Volume status and the plasma urea content also affect the degree to which a diuresis will ensue. In addition, a prolonged inability to concentrate urine in a manner unresponsive to ADH occurs after release of obstruction. Again, the disruption of medullary hypertonicity most likely plays a role in this pathologic process.

The hemodynamic response to ureteral obstruction can be separated into two phases; hyperemic and vasoconstrictive. During the first 1–2 hours of obstruction, especially unilateral, RBF increases secondary to decreased resistance at the glomerular afferent arteriole. This hyperemic reaction to blockage is most likely an autoregulatory response to maintain GFR and may be mediated through altered glomerulotubular feedback or vasodilatory prostaglandins. After 2–5 hours of blockage, the RBF declines. Two systems have been impli-

cated in this blood flow reduction: the renin-angiotensin cascade and renal prostaglandins, like thromboxane A_2. The common pathway is an increased afferent arteriolar resistance and subsequent decline in GFR. Renal blood flow then continues to decline as the obstruction becomes chronic, falling to 30% of normal after one month of blockage.

Vascular Renal Disease

Compromised renal function secondary to occlusion of the renal vasculature is a common clinical problem. Thrombosis of renal, branch, or segmental arteries can occur with trauma, inflammatory conditions, and various forms of embolization. The effects can range from undetected to renal infarction to overt, oliguric renal failure. In the case of thromboembolization, renal damage is ischemic in nature with nephron loss based on the degree and distribution of thromboemboli. Glomeruli become hyalinized and the renal tubules and parenchyma undergo atrophy. Renal vein thrombosis is caused by conditions of impaired blood flow or hypercoagulability. It is postulated that small venules of the kidney are initially affected by clots, with larger arcuate and interlobular veins sequentially becoming involved. Glomerular capillary permeability is altered because of elevated venous pressure and because of the presumed deposition of immune complexes on the glomerular capillary membrane. Tubular dysfunction is also associated with renal vein thrombosis, as hyperchloremic acidosis and glucosuria are often observed clinically. The mechanism for this is unknown.

Since the kidneys are critically involved in the regulation of systemic blood pressure, it is not unusual for diseases of the renal vasculature or parenchyma to lead to hypertension. Renovascular hypertension is the elevation of systemic blood pressure secondary to partial occlusion of the main or branch renal arteries. Multiple causes include atherosclerosis (60%) and various forms of fibromuscular dysplasia (35%). Trauma, inflammation, congenital abnormalities, and mass lesions may also be infrequent causes of hypertension. There is evidence that the renin-angiotensin system may play a significant role in human renovascular hypertension. As renal arterial pressure is reduced by occlusive disease, baroreceptor-mediated mechanisms result in plasma renin release, in an effort to increase the affected kidney's perfusion pressure. The cascade is initiated, and angiotensin II and aldosterone are produced. These factors are thought to be critical in the acute phase of renovascular hypertension. However, the exact mechanism by which the hypertension is sustained chronically is less clear. Volume-related factors secondary to long-term reduction in sodium and water excretion by the unaffected contralateral kidney are more likely involved in the chronic phase of this disease.

URETER

Several pathologic conditions can alter normal ureteral physiology. These include obstruction, reflux, infection, calculi, pregnancy, and anatomic abnormalities of ureterovesical and ureteropelvic junctions. Following obstruction of a ureter, there is a backup of urine proximal to the blockage and a resultant increase in resting intraluminal ureteral pressure and dimensions. A transient increase in amplitude and frequency of peristaltic waves occurs followed by a decrease as urine volume increases and the ureter dilates. At some point, the contractions become too weak and the ureteral walls are unable to coapt; urine transport through the ureter now depends on the kidney-generated hydrostatic forces. Within a few hours of obstruction, intraluminal pressures peak and then fall as adaptive changes occur in intrarenal hemodynamics and fluid is reabsorbed via the venous and lymph systems. Even though pressures are low, ureteral length and diameter continue to increase in a process referred to as creep. The ureteral muscular wall, after two weeks of obstruction, hypertrophies and exhibits increased contractility. The organization of ureteropelvic pacemakers is disrupted, producing uncoordinated pelvic contractions and further upper tract dilatation.

Functional blockage of the UPJ can occur solely from abnormal peristalsis. Propagation of an abnormal peristaltic wave may produce an adynamic segment that is unobstructed anatomically but physiologically blocked. Alterations in muscle bundle arrangement at the UPJ are thought to be the cause of this obstruction.

Vesicoureteral reflux is a pathologic state in which urine flow is reversed, with flow from the bladder back into the ureter. Many factors have been identified in the development of this condition, including UVJ anatomic abnormalities, high bladder pressures, and impaired ureteral peristalsis. As the length and caliber of the intramural ureter is critical in maintaining the one-way flow of urine, any destruction of the tunnel results in reflux. By sheer pressure effects, high intravesicular pressures (e.g., from prostatic obstruction of the bladder neck) can render the UVJ incompetent.

Infection in the urinary tract is known to impair ureteral transport by inhibiting peristalsis or producing irregular, decreased contractions. The toxins of several bacteria, like *Escherichia coli* and *Staphylococcus* species, have been implicated in this process. The passage of ureteral calculi makes important demands on the ureter. In order to transport a stone, the hydrostatic pressure behind the stone must be raised and the ureteral segment around the stone must be fully relaxed. Infection, inflammation, and edema of the ureter can inhibit ureteral efforts at stone passage. The hydronephrosis of pregnancy, common in the second trimester of gestation, is another common cause of impaired ureteral transport. The gravid uterus and hormonal effects on the ureter have been suggested as causes.

BLADDER

Bladder pathophysiology can be viewed as the failure to store urine and the failure to empty. Problems with urine storage can be related to bladder or bladder outlet dysfunction or both. Inappropriate bladder muscle contractions with or without decreased outlet resistance, or the reverse, constitute the main processes by which proper urine storage is not maintained. Among other causes, decreased bladder compliance is associated with bladder hyperactivity in interstitial cystitis, increased bladder muscle activity after pelvic surgery, and bladder instability with stroke, dementia, and spinal disease. Outlet resistance can be reduced secondary to structural or nerve damage to either the striated or smooth muscle sphincters, neurologic disease, or aging.

Failure to empty the bladder also implies pathology of the bladder or outlet. Painful stimuli such as an operation involving the pelvic or perineal areas often result in a central inhibition of micturition. Other bladder-specific pathologies include those of smooth muscle functional impairment from overdistension of the contractile elements, infection, and muscle replacement with fibrosis. Commonly, a failure to empty has its source in an anatomic obstruction of the outlet. Prostatic hypertrophy, bladder neck contractures, and urethral strictures or valves are frequent causes. Since the bladder is controlled by the central nervous system, processes within this system can go awry. Three interesting situations of bladder dysfunction involve the central nervous system and spinal cord. Lesions within the brainstem or spinal cord present with abnormal, but fairly typical, voiding patterns. Spinal cord transection results in uninhibited bladder contractions as brainstem inhibition is lost. The guarding reflex, whereby an individual increases external sphincter activity to prevent leakage as the bladder fills, is also lost with spinal cord injury. Autonomic dysreflexia is a massive sympathetic discharge in response to bladder filling in patients with spinal injuries at or above the T6 level. Here too, supraspinal moderating influences controlling sympathetic activity are lost as a result of the injury. Lastly, patients with multiple sclerosis can exhibit complicated voiding pathophysiology that may include failure to store and empty through hyperreflexia, smooth, and striated sphincter dyssynergia, and a sensory neuropathy.

Diagnostic Evaluation

KIDNEY

Several diagnostic studies are commonly used and underpin basic renal physiologic concepts. These include the intravenous urogram (IVU) and the battery of radionuclide studies currently available. For the IVU, a contrast material is chosen that is completely filtered at the glomerulus but not reabsorbed or secreted. Thus, 1 minute after injection, a nephrogram phase is obtained and radiograph made. The kidneys can be evaluated at this point for size, shape, and contour. The nephrogram can be delayed—signifying obstruction—or prolonged —signifying hypotension or low flow. At 3–5 minutes, during the pyelogram phase, calyceal distortion, irregularity or filling defects may be observed. From 5 minutes on, the lower urinary tract is imaged.

The selective use of certain radiopharmaceutical agents allows the assessment of many parameters of renal function. Unlike intravenous urography, structural detail is not an attribute of these studies, and for this reason, radiologic and radionuclide techniques complement each other. There is a wide variety of functional information obtainable using different radionuclides. Renal scans are divided into dynamic and static types. Dynamic scans are used to measure differential blood flow and renal function and to assess quantitatively outflow tract transit time. Agents chosen for these studies usually assess unique aspects of kidney physiology: Tc-DTPA is filtered similar to inulin and can be used to measure GFR; iodohippurate is filtered and secreted by tubules and closely approximates renal

plasma flow. Static renal scans involve agents that are taken up by the kidney and fixed within the kidney for prolonged time periods. In this way the functional renal tissue can be evaluated for defects, masses, and differential function.

Dynamic Tc-DTPA scans can differentiate vascular from intrarenal causes of ARF. A unilateral decrease or delay in kidney visualization implies a vascular etiology, whereas a bilateral delay or hypoperfusion may indicate acute tubular necrosis. Renal artery stenosis and emboli can be assessed with this technique. Decreased kidney perfusion, reduced concentration, and prolonged transit time are fairly diagnostic of these conditions. Iodohippurate is commonly used to assess renal function after transplantation. It is filtered in one pass through the glomerulus but is also secreted into tubular fluid after extraction from blood by proximal tubule cells. Thus it can generate both flow GFR and functional (tubule-cell processing) data. In cases of posttransplant oliguria or anuria, renal scans that show a total absence of flow and function along with a photopenic kidney image suggest renal artery stenosis, renal vein thrombosis, hyperacute rejection, or severe urinary obstruction. Decreased early iodohippurate uptake with increasing activity later, along with poor excretion, suggests tubular necrosis, acute rejection, or urinary obstruction. This pattern results from adequate blood flow but decreased tubular cell function. In acute tubular necrosis, iodohippurate is freely filtered but tubular function is blocked secondary to necrosis and thus function is impaired. Unlike rejection, blood flow is usually preserved in acute tubular necrosis. In addition, leaks in the urine-collecting system can be visualized as activity is observed outside the urinary tract. Photopenic areas around the kidney itself in static views may represent lymphoceles or hematomas.

Obstruction of urine flow is better visualized by ultrasound than renal scan. Renal ultrasound can demonstrate ureteral dilitation and hydronephrosis. Ultrasound can also be used to assess kidney size in the assessment of CRF or renal artery stenosis and to evaluate renal masses.

URETER

The assessment of ureteral patency is best accomplished with intravenous urography and retrograde contrast studies. At approximately 10 minutes after IVU dye injection, the full length of the ureters should be visualized. Delayed ureteral filling may result from hydronephrosis, and later films, up to 24 hours, are essential to help localize an obstruction. Through cystoscopy, dye can be injected in a retrograde fashion from bladder to renal pelvis. Although less physiologic than an IVU in evaluating hydronephrosis, retrograde urography assists in the assessment of ureteral transit time with drainage radiographs. Specialized radionuclide imaging of the ureters is best accomplished with Tc-DTPA and can help differentiate obstructing from nonobstructing forms of hydronephrosis. By using parenteral diuretics, radionuclide imaging of the ureters provides information concerning the ability of the dilated ureter to "wash out" urine. Ureteral dilatation with adequate washout suggests a nonobstructive hydronephrosis. Radionuclides are also an excellent method by which to evaluate vesicoureteral reflux in that nuclide activity in the ureters during voiding can be quantified and graded.

BLADDER

Bladder assessment with urodynamics is a basic, commonly employed diagnostic study that can identify and measure physiologic variables in the evaluation of storage or emptying disorders. As the bladder responds to a variety of pathologic processes by producing similar symptoms, this type of testing is essential. Four modalities constitute urodynamic testing: (1) cystometry, (2) uroflowmetry, (3) urethral pressure profilometry, and (4) combined studies. Not all studies are indicated for all patients. During cystometry, changes in bladder pressure are measured with increasing bladder volumes. This evaluates bladder storage function with respect to compliance, contractility, and capacity. Uroflowmetry measures urine flow rates or the volume of urine expelled per urethra per unit time. A flow pattern, and peak and average flow rates are obtained and give valuable data on the integrated function of bladder and outlet. In urethral pressure profilometry, urethral pressures are measured along its length, providing informa-

tion on functional outlet resistance at rest and during micturition. Combined studies tailor the urodynamic tests to fit the patient's symptom complex. Videourodynamics utilize urodynamic studies simultaneously with cystourethrography in the evaluation of complex lower urinary tract problems. By combining tests of bladder pressure, flowmetry, and sphincter-EMG activity with visualization of bladder and urethra appearance during filling and emptying, complicated forms of outlet obstruction can be identified and localized.

Bibliography

Brenner BM, Rector FC Jr, eds. *The kidney.* 3rd ed. Philadelphia: WB Saunders, 1986.

Chisholm GD, Fair WR, eds. *Scientific foundations of urology.* 3rd ed. Chicago: Year Book Medical Publishers, 1990.

Dixon J, Gosling J. Structure and innervation in the human. In: Torrens M, Morrison JF, eds. *The physiology of the lower urinary tract.* New York: Springer-Verlag, 1990:3.

First MR, ed. *Chronic renal failure.* Philadelphia: Medical Examination Publishing Co, 1982.

Ganong WF. *Review of medical physiology.* Los Altos: Lange Medical Publications, 1981.

Gillenwater JY, Grayhack JT, Howards SS, Ducket JW Jr, eds. *Adult and pediatric urology.* Chicago: Year Book Medical Publishers, 1987, vol 1.

Grainger RG, Allison DJ, eds. *Diagnostic radiology.* New York: Churchill Livingstone, 1986, vol 2.

Hamburger J Crosnier J, Grunfeld J, eds. *Nephrology.* New York: Wiley-Flammarion/John Wiley & Sons, 1979.

Humes HD, ed. *Pathophysiology of electrolyte and renal disorders.* New York: Churchill Livingstone, 1986.

Massry SG, Glassock RJ, eds. *Textbook of nephrology.* 2nd ed. Baltimore: Williams & Wilkins, 1989.

Schrier RW, Gottschalk CW, eds. *Diseases of the kidney.* 4th ed. Boston: Little, Brown & Co, 1988, vol 1.

Walsh PC, Gittes RF, Perlmutter AD, Stamey TA, eds. *Campbell's urology.* 5th ed. Philadelphia: WB Saunders, 1986, vol 1.

Donald J. Moyer

26 NEURAL PHYSIOLOGY

Man's activities are carried out through the actions of the nervous system. The neuron is the principal unit of the nervous system. It is composed of a cell body, or soma, and processes that lead from it. The axon is the process responsible for transmission of an impulse away from the soma, while dendrites conduct impulses toward it.

The central nervous system consists of the brain and spinal cord. It is composed of a complex network of interconnecting neurons forming a central processing unit for receiving and storing information and acting upon it in various ways. The peripheral nervous system consists of a network of nerves leading to and from the central nervous system. These nerves carry both afferent information from sensory receptors to the CNS and efferent impulses from the CNS to muscles, glands, and visceral organs.

Neurons are specialized cells designed for rapid transmission of impulses. They exist in an electrically polarized state at rest, the inside of the cell being negatively charged with respect to the extracellular space. Stimulation of the neuron results in an influx of positively charged ions, leading to depolarization and generation of an action potential or nerve impulse. The impulse is transmitted throughout the cell, but the net result is propagation of the action potential down the axon.

Throughout the nervous system are specialized areas

of near-neuronal contact called synapses. Once the action potential has reached the end of the axon, chemical substances called neurotransmitters are released and bind to receptors on the next neuron. This in turn results in depolarization of the cell membrane and subsequent generation of an action potential. It is in this manner that neurons communicate with one another. The seemingly endless number of neuronal connections account for functions as diverse as the patellar reflex, memory, and learning.

The nervous system differs greatly from other organ systems in its response to injury and disease. This occurs for many reasons, including the unique bony confines of the CNS, the inability of neurons to replicate or regenerate, the tendency of certain brain tumors to invade normal tissue insidiously, the inaccessibility of certain tumors or other mass lesions, and the exquisite sensitivity of neurons to hypoxia and ischemia. The goals of this chapter are to review the gross and microscopic anatomy of the nervous system, discuss the mechanisms of nerve impulse transmission, review the manner in which functional neuronal networks are grouped, and examine the ways the nervous system influences other organ systems. Finally, several general pathophysiologic states will be discussed, and some of the more commonly used diagnostic tests will be mentioned.

Microscopic Anatomy

NEURON

The neuron is the principal functional and anatomical unit of the nervous system (Figure 26-1). Each neuron consists of a cell body, or perikaryon, and several protoplasmic processes leading from it. Dendrites are typically short, branching processes that receive stimuli and conduct impulses toward the cell body. Neurons typically have one axon that conducts impulses away from the cell body. Axons vary greatly in length from neuron to neuron.

Many nerve fibers are covered with a myelin sheath. This sheath consists of a wrapping of many layers of cell membranes from a Schwann cell in the peripheral nervous system, and from an oligodendrocyte in the central nervous system. One Schwann cell covers one axon, while one oligodendrocyte contributes myelin to several axons.

NEUROGLIA

The nonneural supporting cells of the CNS are called glial cells. These are more numerous than neurons and, unlike neurons, are capable of undergoing cell division. They are of three types: astrocytes, oligodendrocytes, and microglia. The functions of astrocytes are poorly understood. Certain astrocytes have processes that are applied to blood vessels, forming part of what is known as the blood-brain barrier. Other astrocytic functions are thought to include: (1) the uptake of excessive amounts of extracellular potassium during periods of increased neuronal activity, (2) the regulation of the extracellular concentration of neurotransmitters, and (3) the transfer of metabolites from capillaries to neurons. Astrocytes are also the cells that form the "scar" that results from destruction of neuronal elements.

Oligodendrocytes, as previously mentioned, are responsible for forming the myelin sheaths of axons in the CNS, while microglia are phagocytic cells that form the nervous system's defense against injury and disease.

BLOOD-BRAIN BARRIER

The blood-brain barrier is a unique feature of the CNS. It is not a single, comprehensive barrier, but rather a functional system that exerts strict control over the movements of substances from the bloodstream to the brain and vice versa. The blood-brain barrier provides mechanisms for exclusion or transport of any solute, depending on the functional characteristics of the brain capillaries and the biochemical composition of the solute. The barrier is located primarily at the level of the capillary. Its existence is dependent on (1) tight junctions between capillary endothelial cells, (2) astrocytic foot processes encasing the capillaries, and (3) a large number of mitochondria in the endothelial cells, providing an energy source for active transport of substances across the barrier.

Gross Anatomy

SPINAL CORD

The spinal cord is a slender, cylindrical structure that resides within the bony confines of the vertebral column. It is divided into five regions: cervical, thoracic, lumbar, sacral, and coccygeal, which span its entire

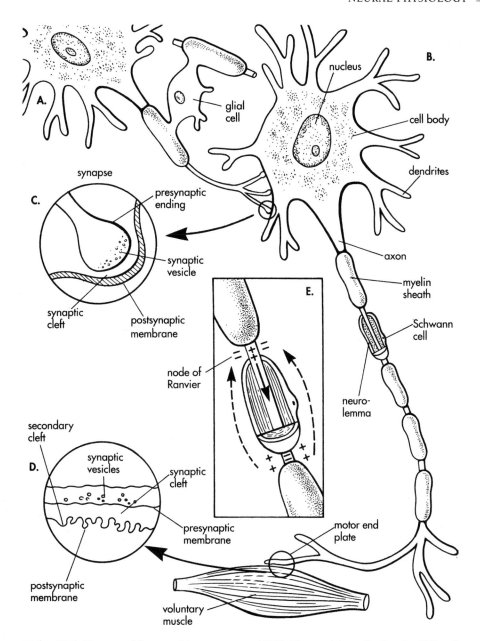

Figure 26-1 Neurons of the central nervous system (CNS). Neuron **A** is confined to the CNS and terminates on neuron **B** at a typical chemical synapse (**C**). Neuron B is a ventral horn cell; its axon extends to a peripheral nerve and innervates a striated (voluntary) muscle at the myoneural junction (motor end plate, **D**). In **E** the action potential is moving in the direction of the solid arrow inside the axon; the dashed arrows indicate the direction of flow of the action current. (Reproduced from Gilman S, Newman SW. *Manter and Gatz's essentials of clinical neuroanatomy and neurophysiology*. 7th ed. Philadelphia: FA Davis, 1987.)

length, from its connection to the medulla oblongata of the brainstem to its caudal termination. The lower cervical and lumbosacral regions of the spinal cord are enlarged, reflecting the increased number of neurons necessary to supply the upper and lower extremities, respectively.

Exiting segmentally from the spinal cord are the paired spinal nerves. There are 8 cervical, 12 thoracic, 5 lumbar, 5 sacral, and 1 coccygeal pairs in all. Each nerve consists of the union of a dorsal and ventral root. The dorsal root axons carry sensory impulses, while the ventral root axons transmit efferent impulses. Cell bodies of the axons of the dorsal root reside in the dorsal root ganglia, which lie alongside the vertebral column adjacent to the intervertebral foramina. The cell bodies for the axons of the ventral root lie inside the spinal cord.

The spinal cord does not continue to the end of the vertebral column distally but ends at the lower border of the first lumbar vertebra. This results from differential growth of the vertebral column and spinal cord during late fetal and early postnatal life. Thus, the spinal nerves of the rostral spinal cord exit through their appropriate foramina approximately horizontally, while those of the lumbar and sacral cord have very long roots that must travel caudally to leave the vertebral column. The collection of nerve roots below the termination of the spinal cord is known as the **cauda equina.**

Sectioning of the spinal cord perpendicularly to its long axis reveals an H-shaped area of gray matter surrounded by white matter. The white matter is primarily made up of longitudinally oriented nerve fibers, while the gray matter contains neuronal cell bodies. The cell bodies for the efferent fibers reside in the gray matter, and those of the afferent fibers are located in the dorsal root ganglia as previously mentioned.

BRAINSTEM AND CEREBELLUM

The brainstem is that part of the brain that remains after removal of the cerebral hemispheres and cerebellum. It consists of four subdivisions: the **diencephalon, mesencephalon, metencephalon, and myelencephalon** (Figure 26-2).

The **diencephalon** lies between the cerebrum and midbrain and envelops the third ventricle. It is made up of several structures, the largest of which is the thalamus. The **thalamus** is a large gray ovoid mass located on either side of the third ventricle. It is the major relay station interposed between many subcortical structures and the cerebral cortex.

Another important part of the diencephalon is the **hypothalamus.** This structure is located below the thalamus and forms the floor and ventral half of the lateral walls of the third ventricle. The hypothalamus is responsible for control and integration of the autonomic nervous system, and also for regulation of body temperature, appetite, endocrine functions, and some behavioral responses. The pituitary gland and its connection to the hypothalamus, the infundibular stalk, lie beneath the hypothalamus in a bony pit at the base of the skull called the **sella turcica.**

The mesencephalon, or midbrain, is located between the diencephalon and the pons. Its ventral surface is dominated by the cerebral peduncles, which contain nerve fibers of the main motor pathways—the **corticospinal** and **corticopontine** tracts. The dorsal surface is primarily occupied by the superior and inferior colliculi.

Exiting from the midbrain are the IIIrd and IVth cranial nerves. There are 12 cranial nerves in all, and like their counterparts in the spine, they are paired structures. They also transmit afferent and efferent impulses to and from the CNS. The cell bodies of the afferent fibers are in peripherally located ganglia, while those of the efferent fibers reside within the central nervous system. The Ist and IInd cranial nerves, the olfactory and optic nerves, respectively, are located higher in the neuraxis and will be discussed later.

The IIIrd (**oculomotor**) nerve exits ventrally between the cerebral peduncles. The IVth (**trochlear**) nerve exits dorsally below the inferior colliculus, then curves around the brainstem. These nerves send fibers to ocular muscles to produce movements of the eyes.

The **metencephalon** consists of the **pons** and **cerebellum.** The pons is located between the midbrain rostrally and the medulla caudally. The dorsal pons is concealed by the cerebellum, while the ventral portion bulges out in front of the rest of the brainstem.

Four cranial nerves exit from the ventral surface of the pons. The Vth (**trigeminal**) nerve is located on its lateral aspect. The VIth (**abducens**), VIIth (**facial**), and VIIIth (**vestibulo-cochlear**) nerves are located in a sulcus marking the inferior boundary of the pons. Nerves V and VII are composed of two roots, one sensory and one motor. The Vth nerve receives sensory input from the face and also innervates the muscles of mastication. Nerve VII primarily provides efferent innervation to the facial muscles but also receives afferent input from the taste buds. The VIth nerve provides purely motor innervation to the abducens muscle of the eye, while nerve

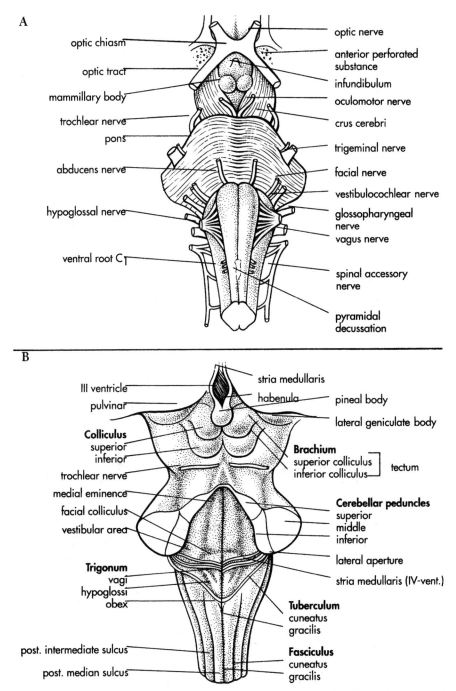

A

optic chiasm

optic tract

mammillary body

trochlear nerve

pons

abducens nerve

hypoglossal nerve

ventral root C₁

optic nerve

anterior perforated substance

infundibulum

oculomotor nerve

crus cerebri

trigeminal nerve

facial nerve

vestibulocochlear nerve

glossopharyngeal nerve

vagus nerve

spinal accessory nerve

pyramidal decussation

B

III ventricle

pulvinar

Colliculus
superior
inferior

trochlear nerve

medial eminence

facial colliculus

vestibular area

Trigonum
vagi
hypoglossi
obex

post. intermediate sulcus

post. median sulcus

stria medullaris

habenula

pineal body

lateral geniculate body

Brachium
superior colliculus
inferior colliculus — tectum

Cerebellar peduncles
superior
middle
inferior

lateral aperture

stria medullaris (IV-vent.)

Tuberculum
cuneatus
gracilis

Fasciculus
cuneatus
gracilis

Figure 26-2 A, Drawing of the anterior aspect of the medulla, pons, and midbrain. **B,** Drawing of the posterior aspect of the brainstem with the cerebellum removed. (Reproduced from Carpenter MB. *Core text of human anatomy.* 2nd ed. Baltimore: Williams & Wilkins, 1978.)

VIII carries auditory and vestibular input from the ear.

The cerebellum occupies most of the posterior cranial fossa, and attaches to the midbrain, pons, and medulla by three pairs of thick fiber bundles known as the superior, middle, and inferior cerebellar peduncles, respectively. The cerebellum is composed of two large lateral hemispheres and a midline portion called the vermis. It is primarily responsible for coordinating the actions of muscle groups throughout the body.

The **myelencephalon,** or **medulla oblongata,** is the most caudal part of the brainstem. The ventral surface is composed primarily of the pyramids, which contain the **corticospinal** motor fibers, and the more laterally placed **olives.** The fasciculus gracilis and cuneatis, two structures carrying sensory information from the spinal cord, make up the major part of the lateral surface of the medulla. The remaining cranial nerves, IX (**glossopharyngeal**), X (**vagus**), XI (**spinal accessory**), and XII (**hypoglossal**), exit from its ventral surface. The IXth and Xth nerves are complex and contain fibers carrying sensory impulses from the viscera, taste buds, carotid body and skin around the ear, and motor impulses to the branchial musculature (IX) and viscera (X). The XIth nerve supplies motor fibers to the sternomastoid and trapezius muscles, while nerve XII innervates the tongue.

CEREBRUM

The right and left cerebral hemispheres are the most conspicuous parts of the brain. They are composed of many eminences, called gyri, and furrows known as sulci, and are incompletely separated by a medial longitudinal fissure. The cortex is a layer of gray matter that covers the hemispheric surface (Figure 26-3).

Several sulci stand out owing to their size, location, or both. The **central (Rolandic) sulcus** runs from the dorsal brain surface obliquely downward and forward until it meets another major sulcus, the **lateral (Sylvian) fissure.**

The lateral brain surface is traditionally divided into four lobes. The frontal lobe is that portion anterior to the central sulcus, above the Sylvian fissure. The occipital lobe lies behind an imaginary line drawn from the

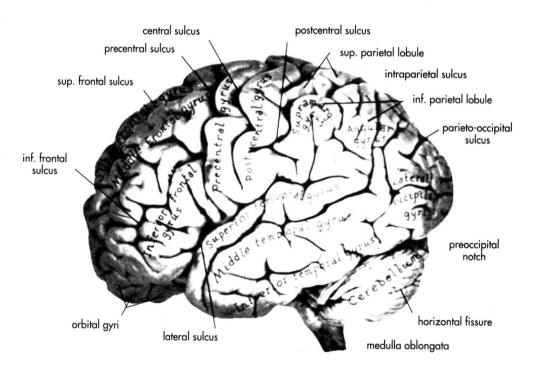

Figure 26-3 Illustration of the lateral surface of the brain. (Reproduced from Carpenter MB. *Core text of human anatomy.* 2nd ed. Baltimore: Williams & Wilkins, 1978.)

parieto-occipital fissure to the pre-occipital notch. The parietal lobe lies between the central sulcus and the parieto-occipital fissure and is separated from the temporal lobe below by an imaginary line drawn from the horizontal portion of the Sylvian fissure to the midpoint of the line demarcating the occipital lobe.

VENTRICULAR SYSTEM

The ventricular system is a series of four communicating cavities within the brain that are filled with cerebrospinal fluid produced by specialized tissue called the choroid plexus. The two rostral-most ventricles, known as the lateral ventricles, are contained within the cerebral hemispheres and communicate with the third ventricle below through the **interventricular foramina of Monro.** The third ventricle is a thin vertical chamber located in the midline between the lateral ventricles. The fourth ventricle is a rhomboid-shaped cavity overlying the pons and medulla. It is continuous with the **cerebral aquaduct (of Sylvius)** of the midbrain above, which connects it to the third ventricle. The fourth ventricle communicates with the subarachnoid space via three foramina—the two lateral foramina of **Luschka** and the medial foramen of **Magendie.** Once in the subarachnoid space, the CSF is able to flow over the surface of the brain and spinal cord before being absorbed over the superior surface of the hemispheres.

MENINGES

The meninges consist of three layers of nonneural connective tissue that enclose the brain and spinal cord. The **dura mater** is the outermost meningeal layer. It is composed of two layers around the brain and one around the spinal cord. The outer layer of dura, or periosteal layer, is actually the connective tissue membrane (periosteum) of the skull. The inner layer, or meningeal layer, folds into a double-layered partition in several areas of the skull. The **falx cerebri** is that double dural fold between the cerebral hemispheres in the midline. The falx cerebelli is similarly positioned between the cerebellar hemispheres. The **tentorium cerebelli** is horizontally oriented and lies between the occipital and medial temporal lobes above and the cerebellum and midbrain below. It contains an opening called the tentorial hiatus through which the brainstem passes. The diaphragma sellae is the dura that forms the roof of the sella turcica.

The **arachnoid** is the thin, delicate, middle meningeal layer and tends to follow the dura. The **pia mater** is the inner meningeal layer and is intimately applied to the brain and spinal cord.

The subarachnoid space exists between the arachnoid and pia mater. It is filled with CSF and contains the larger branches of the arteries of the circle of Willis (see below). The arachnoid separates from the base of the brain in several areas, forming large CSF-filled spaces known as **cisterns.**

BLOOD SUPPLY

The arterial supply of the intracranial contents is derived from branches of the two internal carotid and two vertebral arteries. The internal carotid arteries terminate in the anterior and middle cerebral arteries, which supply primarily the midline and lateral hemispheric surfaces, respectively. The vertebral arteries join posteriorly to form the basilar artery, which gives off branches to the brainstem and cerebellum and terminates in the posterior cerebral arteries, which supply mainly the posterior and posterior-basal portions of the cerebrum.

These arteries communicate with one another through the **circle of Willis.** This structure lies at the base of the brain and is formed by the anterior and posterior communicating arteries and the proximal portions of the anterior, middle, and posterior cerebral arteries. The function of the circle of Willis is to provide adequate blood supply should one of the parent arteries become occluded (Figure 26-4).

Cerebral autoregulation is an important intrinsic property of the arterioles of the brain. Adequate cerebral blood flow is ensured over a wide range of systemic blood pressures by constriction or dilation of these vessels. If severe hypotension or hypertension occurs, however, these vessels are unable to compensate, and cerebral blood flow will decrease or increase as blood pressure continues to fall or rise.

The veins of the brain all drain into the dural venous sinuses, which are epithelially lined spaces between the two layers of dura. The sinuses, in turn, drain chiefly into the internal jugular veins.

The largest unpaired sinus, the superior sagittal sinus, is also the site of CSF absorption from the subarachnoid space. This occurs via outpouchings of the arachnoid, called arachnoid granulations, which are located within the sinus.

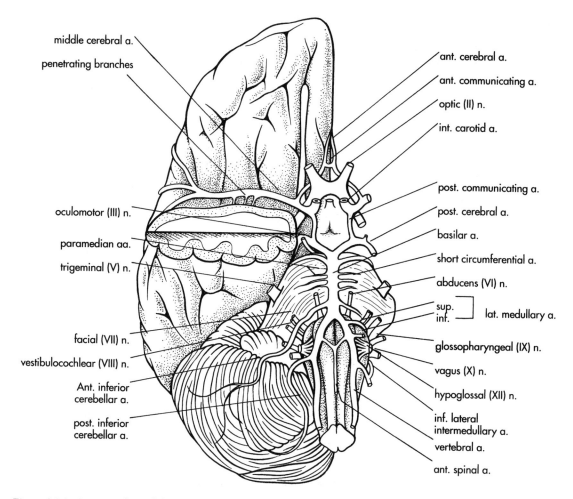

Figure 26-4. Arteries at base of the brain. (Reproduced from Pansky B, Allen DJ. *Review of neuroscience.* New York: Macmillan, 1980:119.)

Mechanisms of Nerve Impulse Transmission

MEMBRANE POTENTIAL

All cells of the body are bathed in extracellular fluid containing electrolytes. Unequal distribution of electrolytes results in the presence of electrical potentials across nearly all cell membranes. Nerve and muscle cells, in addition to having these potentials, are also "excitable." This means that they are capable of generating electrochemical impulses, and in some instances of transmitting these signals along their membranes.

The membrane potential of the resting neuron is determined by several factors that influence the distribution of ions across the membrane. The membrane potential is measured from the inside relative to the outside. The most significant contributors to the membrane potential are (1) the Na,K-ATPase pump in the cell membrane, (2) the tendency of ions to diffuse down their concentration gradients, (3) the difference in membrane permeability to sodium and potassium, and (4) the higher concentration of nonpermeable, negatively charged molecules such as organic phosphates, sulfates, and proteins inside the cell.

The Na,K-ATPase pump transports three sodium ions out of the cell for every two potassium ions pumped in.

Diffusion of sodium and potassium ions down their concentration gradients through a selectively permeable membrane also contributes to the maintenance of the membrane potential. Because of the large sodium concentration gradient from outside to inside, sodium ions diffuse inward, carrying a positive charge with them. Although the interior of the cell is electrically negative, this flow of sodium ions creates a relative electropositivity at the cell membrane. This electropositivity balances the tendency of ions to flow down their concentration gradient. The membrane potential at which these forces balance for each ion can be expressed by the Nernst equation. In the case of sodium,

$$EMF = -61.5 \log \frac{\left[Na^+ \right]_i}{\left[Na^+ \right]_o} \text{ at } 37°C$$

where EMF is electromagnetic force in mV, and $[Na]_i$ and $[Na]_o$ are the concentrations inside and outside the cell, respectively. An opposing situation exists for potassium ions that are highly concentrated inside the cell. Diffusion of the potassium ions to the outside causes a relative electronegativity at the cell membrane that counters the egress of potassium ions. The above-described relationships coexist in the cell. If the membrane were only permeable to sodium, based on the Nernst equation, the membrane potential would be +61 mV. Conversely, if the membrane were only permeable to potassium, the membrane potential would be -94 mV. Since the resting nerve cell is 50–100 times more permeable to potassium than to sodium, potassium is the major determinant of the cell's resting membrane potential.

The resting nerve membrane potential, then, comes about in the following manner. First, sodium is pumped outside the cell while potassium is pumped in. This occurs in a 3:2 ratio as previously mentioned. Since most of the negatively charged ions inside the cell are not diffusible, the inside of the nerve fiber becomes electronegative while the outside becomes electropositive. Sodium ions, in turn, will tend to diffuse back into the cell owing to the negative charge there. Eventually, the inward diffusion equals the outward pumping by the Na,K-ATPase pump, at which time the pump has reached its maximum capacity for transferring sodium ions to the outside. This occurs when the membrane potential is about -90 mV, which is the resting potential of the nerve fiber (Figure 26-5).

Potassium, on the other hand, is so readily diffusible that it tends to leave the cell as rapidly as the pump can pump it in. The main reason potassium exists in high concentrations intracellularly is the negative charge that exists there.

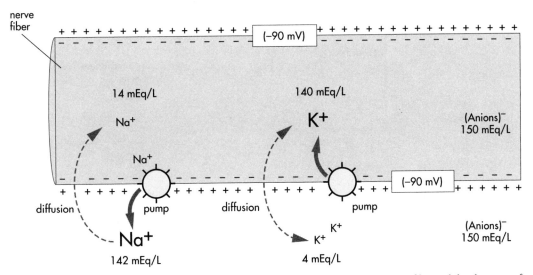

Figure 26-5 Establishment of a membrane potential of -90 mV in the normal resting nerve fiber and development of concentration differences of sodium and potassium ions between the two sides of the membrane. The *dashed arrows* represent diffusion and the *solid arrows* represent active transport (pumps). (Reproduced from Guyton AC. *Basic human neurophysiology.* 3rd ed. Philadelphia: WB Saunders, 1981.)

ACTION POTENTIAL

Most cells of the body generate a membrane potential of some degree, but nerve cells are capable of conducting changes in potential along their cell membranes. Impulse transmission results from a change in the membrane potential and a flow of electrical current across the membrane. This change in potential, which gives rise to the nerve impulse, is called the action potential (Figure 26-6). The action potential is characterized by an initial depolarization of the cell membrane (decrease of negativity of the cell interior relative to the extracellular space). A reversal of polarity then occurs, whereby the cell interior actually becomes positive relative to the cell exterior. This is followed by a slower process of repolarization back to the resting potential.

The action potential is initiated by a stimulus (such as a neurotransmitter) that transiently increases membrane permeability to sodium. This results in a rapid influx of sodium, causing a reversal of polarity across the cell membrane. The increase in sodium conductance is promoted by the opening of sodium-specific channels in the cell membrane. Immediately following the sodium influx is a corresponding increase in membrane permeability to potassium, allowing an efflux of potassium ions from interior to exterior. This eventually restores the original membrane potential, as the interior once again becomes negatively charged relative to the extracellular space. Membrane permeability to both cations then returns to baseline and concentration gradients are maintained by active extrusion of sodium by the Na,K-ATPase pump. This process is called repolarization. The action potential can be propagated for very long distances at constant velocity and is independent of the type of stimulus that initiates it.

A stimulus is any event that causes the generation of an action potential. The minimal stimulus intensity required to generate a nerve impulse is called the threshold stimulus. A stimulus below threshold is called a subthreshold stimulus, while one greater than threshold is called a suprathreshold stimulus. Once threshold has been reached, an action potential of the same magnitude, traveling at the same velocity, will be generated, regardless of how much greater than threshold the stim-

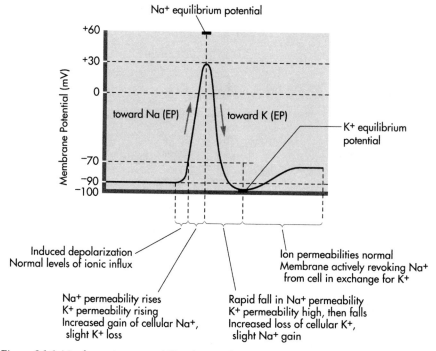

Figure 26-6 Membrane ion permeability changes during an action potential. (Reproduced from Pansky B, Allen DF. *Review of neuroscience*. New York: Macmillan, 1980:139.)

ulus is. Conversely, if the stimulus is below threshold, no impulse will be generated. The action potential is therefore an all-or-none event.

REFRACTORY PERIOD

Neurons possess a property called **refractoriness.** A stimulus that occurs during the early phase of the action potential will have no effect, no matter how great its magnitude. The time interval during which this holds true is called the absolute refractory period. Once the cell begins to repolarize, only suprathreshold stimuli will generate another impulse. As the membrane potential nears its resting value, stimuli of lesser and lesser magnitude are required for action-potential generation. This period following the absolute refractory period is called the relative refractory period. This is determined by a time- and voltage-dependent restoration of sodium channel function.

SALTATORY CONDUCTION

The action potential will propagate down the entire length of an unmyelinated fiber at a constant velocity, with a constant waveform. Myelinated fibers, however, are effectively insulated over large distances by their myelin sheaths. This sheath is periodically interrupted at points called nodes of Ranvier. It is only at the nodes of Ranvier (see Figure 26-1) that current flows. The myelin sheath allows changes in membrane potential to be quickly transmitted from node to node in a process known as saltatory conduction. This is a much faster and more efficient method of conduction than that which occurs in unmyelinated fibers.

SYNAPSES

Communication between neurons occurs at the synapse. This is typically a point of near contact between terminal axon branches of one neuron and the dendrites, soma, or axons of another. There are two types of synapses—**electrical and chemical.** Electrical synapses are most commonly found in invertebrate and lower vertebrate species. They are areas of very low resistance between membranes of two neurons, and they allow for the direct conduction of action potentials from one neuron to another. Chemical synapses involve substances called **neurotransmitters.** They are released from the presynaptic neuron, diffuse across the extracellular space, then bind to receptors on the postsynap-

tic neuron, resulting in a change of the membrane potential. The neurotransmitters are stored in vesicles in the terminal axons of the presynaptic neuron and released when the cell membrane is depolarized. This process is mediated by an inward calcium current that occurs in concert with, but less rapidly than, the sodium current.

The neurotransmitters are either excitatory or inhibitory. Excitatory neurotransmitters cause the generation of **excitatory postsynaptic potentials (EPSPs),** and inhibitory neurotransmitters cause **inhibitory postsynaptic potentials (IPSPs).** EPSPs are small depolarizations that occur in the postsynaptic cell, while IPSPs are small hyperpolarizations. Each EPSP or IPSP results from the deposition of one vesicle's worth, or quanta, of neurotransmitter on the postsynaptic neuronal receptors. Neither a single EPSP or IPSP is sufficient to produce any significant change in the membrane potential, but many summated EPSPs can reach the threshold potential, or summated IPSPs can cause significant hyperpolarization. Summation may be either temporal, as when two subthreshold stimuli occur in close succession, or spatial, as when two subthreshold stimuli occur simultaneously but at different loci on the neuron.

Many substances have been identified as probable neurotransmitters, including acetylcholine, γ-aminobutyric acid, glutamate, dopamine, norepinephrine, seratonin, and enkephalin, to name a few.

Functional Organization of the Nervous System

SOMATIC SENSORY SYSTEMS

The receptors mediating pain sensation are felt to be naked nerve fiber endings. Impulses generated by these receptors are conveyed into the CNS by small unmyelinated or slightly myelinated fibers. The cell bodies of these fibers, and all fibers that convey sensations from receptors below the head, are located in the dorsal root ganglia. The pain fibers synapse with secondary neurons within the gray matter of the spinal cord, which in turn give rise to axons that cross to the contralateral side of the cord and form a collection of fibers called the **spinothalamic tracts.** These fibers then supply input to a diffuse complex of nuclei (groupings of neuronal cell bodies) in the brainstem called the **reticular formation,** and also synapse with neurons in the thalamus. Pain fibers from the face are carried in the trigeminal nerve to the trigeminal ganglion and into the brainstem, where similar connections are made. Thalamocortical fibers relay impulses from the thalamus to the sensory cortex of the parietal lobe. The cortical input is not necessary to perceive the presence of pain but is important in the localization and characterization of it.

Visceral pain sensation is transmitted to the CNS via splanchnic autonomic and body wall somatic nerves. Intraperitoneal visceral pain can arise from ischemia, distension of a hollow viscus, or traction on the mesentery. Pain of visceral origin is often poorly localized. It is sometimes felt in a surface of the body far removed from its true source. This phenomenon is known as referred pain. An example of this is when pain resulting from irritation of the peritoneum covering the diaphragm is felt over the shoulder. Referred pain is thought to result from visceral sensory fibers entering the spinal cord at the same level as fibers from the skin. The brain has a better representation of the body surface than of the viscera and misinterprets the pain as arising from the skin covering the body surface supplied by nerve fibers of that particular spinal cord level. In contradistinction, anatomically localized abdominal pain is usually the result of irritation of the adjacent parietal peritoneum innervated by body wall somatic nerves.

The receptors in the skin for the sensations of cold and warmth consist of naked nerve fiber endings also, and, as in the case of pain receptors, their impulses are conveyed to the spinal cord via small unmyelinated or slightly myelinated fibers. The pain and temperature systems are, in fact, closely associated in the CNS and are difficult to distinguish from each other.

Information regarding limb position and movement, muscle action, body position, vibration, and tactile discrimination travels in two different sets of sensory pathways. The **spinocerebellar tracts** project to the cerebellum, where sensory information is used for the coordination of movement. The **lemniscal system** projects to the thalamus, then to the cortex where the proprioceptive (position sense), kinesthetic (sense of motion), and tactile information is consciously perceived and interpreted. The receptors mediating these sensations include **muscle spindles** and **Golgi tendon organs** (activated by muscle stretch and contraction, respectively) and encapsulated receptors such as **Pacinian corpuscles** in muscles, tendons, ligaments, joints, and skin.

The fibers that project to the cerebellum are large and myelinated and enter the spinal cord via the dorsal root. They then synapse within the gray matter and ascend to the cerebellum. Fibers of the lemniscal system are also large and myelinated and ascend in the fasciculus gracilis and fasciculus cuneatus, which carry fibers from the leg and arm, respectively. These fiber tracts occupy most of the posterior white matter of the spinal cord. The fibers then terminate in the lower medulla, synapse with secondary neurons whose fibers cross to the other side, and terminate in the thalamus. Thalamocortical fibers then project to the somatosensory cortex of the parietal lobe, where conscious recognition takes place.

MOTOR FUNCTIONS

Reflex Actions

The most basic motor activities are those involving reflex actions. The simplest reflex is called a **monosynaptic reflex** response and involves two neurons, one afferent and one efferent. The muscle stretch reflex is an example of a monosynaptic reflex (Figure 26-7). Special receptor organs called muscle spindles sense muscle stretch and send impulses via large, myelinated, afferent fibers that then synapse with motoneurons in the ventral gray matter of the spinal cord. These neurons then send impulses to their respective muscle groups, causing muscle contraction. At the same time, motoneurons to antagonistic muscle groups are inhibited. A reflex response mediated by more than two neurons is called a polysynaptic reflex. These reflexes result in more complex actions, such as that which occurs when a hand is rapidly withdrawn after contacting a hot object.

Muscle Tone

Muscle tone is the resting tension that exists in a muscle and results in a resistance to movement when a limb is passively moved. Two abnormalities of muscle tone exist—hypopotonia and hypertonia. Hypotonia results immediately if either the ventral or dorsal roots containing the fibers innervating a particular muscle are severed. Muscle tone, then, is regulated by the nervous system and is not an intrinsic property of the muscle itself.

Hypertonia usually results from loss of descending input to the lower motor neurons (see below) and is manifested as either spasticity or rigidity. **Spasticity** is

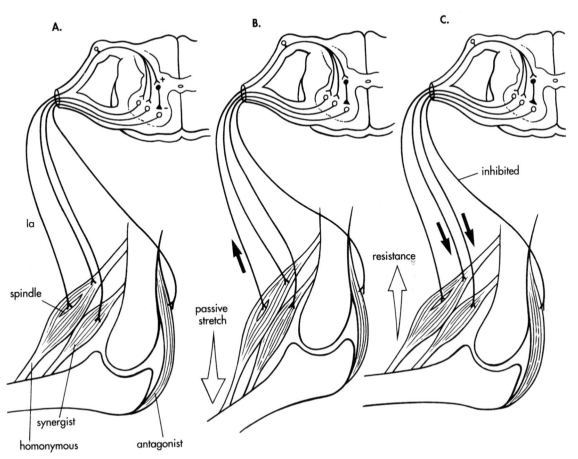

Figure 26-7 The role of Ia afferent fibers in the stretch reflex is exemplified by this reflex of flexor muscles. **A,** The connections of the Ia afferents excite the homonymous and synergist muscles and inhibit the antagonist muscles. **B,** Passive stretch of the limb (*open arrow*) gives rise to an increased Ia fiber discharge (*solid arrow*). **C,** The Ia fiber discharge causes homonymous and synergist α-motor neurons to fire (*solid arrows*), producing resistance to the stretch (*open arrow*). (Reproduced from Kandel ER, Schwartz JH. *Principles of neural science.* 2nd ed. New York: Elsevier, 1985:296.)

a state of increased tone that is usually accompanied by an increase in the deep tendon reflexes. It involves a "clasp knife" type of resistance to passive movement, where an initial increased resistance disappears as the limb is moved further. **Rigidity** involves a plastic or "cogwheel" type of resistance to movement and is not accompanied by changes in the deep tendon reflexes.

Descending Motor Pathways

The motoneurons of the spinal cord receive input from higher centers by way of descending motor pathways. The neurons of the brainstem and spinal cord that

directly stimulate muscle through myoneural junctions are called lower motoneurons. The descending pathways that act upon the lower motoneurons are termed upper motoneurons. Damage to lower motoneurons usually results in a flaccid weakness with accompanying atrophy of the involved muscle groups, while upper motoneuron disruption generally causes a spastic weakness without muscle atrophy.

The **corticospinal** tracts are concerned primarily with skilled movements of the distal muscles of the limbs. They are a collection of fibers that originate in the motor cortex, then travel through the internal capsule to the cerebral peduncles of the midbrain. The tracts then descend to the medulla, where their fibers form the pyramids. Most of the fibers cross in the lower medulla and descend in the spinal cord as the lateral corticospinal tracts. These neurons then terminate on the lower motoneurons of the spinal cord that supply primarily muscles of the distal extremities.

The **corticobulbar tracts** are anatomically similar to the corticospinal tracts, except that their fibers terminate on lower motoneurons of the cranial nerves. With the exception of the portion of the facial nucleus that is responsible for innervating the lower facial musculature, the cranial nerve motor nuclei receive bilateral innervation, while the motor nuclei of the spinal cord receive input mainly from crossed fibers.

THE VISUAL SYSTEM

Vision occurs when light reflected from an object reaches the eye, is refracted by the cornea and lens, and forms an image on the retina. Objects in the right visual field reflect light that strikes the temporal, or outer, side of the left retina, and the nasal, or inner, side of the right retina. The opposite is true for objects in the left visual field. The light stimulates receptor cells called rods and cones that then transmit impulses via other retinal cells to the optic nerves. **Optic nerve** fibers then pass directly to the **optic chiasm,** where crossing of fibers from the nasal half of each retina takes place. The fibers then continue as the optic tracts that terminate in the **lateral geniculate bodies** of the thalamus. From the thalamus, visual information is relayed to the visual receptive area of the occipital lobe via fiber tracts called the optic radiations. The visual pathways are organized such that images in the right visual field are represented in the left cortical visual area and vice versa. The right and left optic nerves carry impulses originating in the right and left eyes, while, posterior to the optic chiasm, the right and left optic pathways carry impulses from the left and right visual fields respectively (Figure 26-8).

Some fibers of the visual pathways project to the brainstem. The **Edinger-Westphal nucleus** of the midbrain receives impulses from the optic tracts, then gives rise to neurons that mediate pupillary constriction. This sequence of events is known as the pupillary light reflex.

The **superior colliculus** also receives input from the optic tracts and some projections from the visual cortex. Fibers coursing from the superior colliculus to the cerebellum (tectopontine tracts) convey visual information to the cerebellum while the fibers from the superior colliculus to the motoneurons of the spinal cord (**tec-**

tospinal tracts) mediate the reflex control of head and neck movements in response to visual stimuli.

THE AUDITORY SYSTEM

Sound waves enter the ear and strike the tympanic membrane, which causes movement of three tiny bones (malleus, incus, and stapes) in the middle ear. This results in a pressure wave of the fluid (perilymph) in the cochlea. Hair cells in the cochlea then generate impulses that travel by way of the eighth cranial nerve to the brainstem. The eighth nerve has two divisions, cochlear and vestibular, but only the cochlear division conveys impulses related to hearing. Once in the brainstem, the fibers synapse and ascend to the **inferior colliculus.** The fibers then project to the **medial geniculate body** of the thalamus and from there terminate in the **gyrus of Heschl** located in the temporal lobe. The ears are bilaterally represented in each temporal lobe.

CEREBRAL CORTICAL FUNCTIONS

The cerebral cortex is the site of man's advanced intellectual functions. It is involved in memory and learning, language execution and comprehension, and is responsible for perceiving and consciously understanding all sensations, and integrating one sensory modality with others. It is also involved in the planning and execution of complex motor acts, particularly those involving fine digital and hand movements.

The primary motor region is located in the **precentral gyrus** of the frontal lobe and contains a representation of the muscles of the body arranged in order. Neurons in this region give rise to the corticospinal tracts, which influence mainly fine movements of the distal extremities.

A supplementary motor area exists just anterior to the primary motor cortex and is felt to be responsible for the advanced planning of movements. The remaining part of the frontal lobe anterior to the motor areas is called the prefrontal region. Lesions in this area cause deficiencies in abstract thinking, foresight, judgment, and initiative.

There are three primary cortical sensory receptive areas that receive projections from sensory thalamic nuclei. These have all been mentioned previously and include the visual receptive area of the occipital lobe, the auditory cortex of the temporal lobe, and the primary somesthetic area contained in the postcentral gyrus of the parietal lobe. This area, like the primary

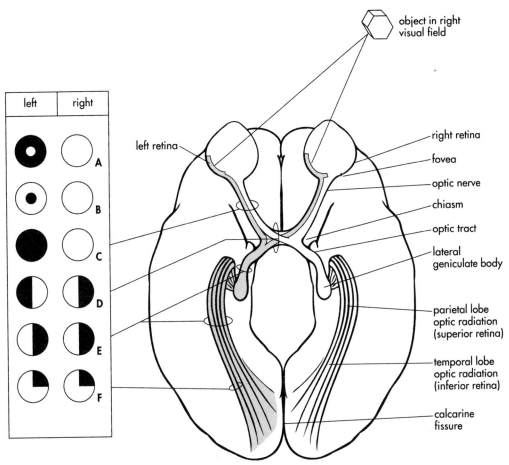

Figure 26-8 The visual pathways as seen from above the brain. **A–F** refer to visual field defects following lesions in the corresponding brain areas. Circles indicate what the left and right eyes see (the left and right visual fields). Black areas represent visual field defects. **A,** Constricted field left eye (e.g., end-stage glaucoma). When constricted fields are bilateral, it sometimes signifies hysteria. **B,** Central scotoma (e.g., optic neuritis in multiple sclerosis). **C,** Total blindness of the left eye. **D,** Bitemporal hemianopia (e.g., pituitary gland tumor). **E,** Right homonymous hemianopia (e.g., stroke). **F,** Right superior quadrantopia. (Reproduced from Goldberg S. *Clinical neuroanatomy made ridiculously simple.* Miami: Med Master, 1983.)

motor cortex, contains a topographic representation of body parts called a homunculus. In both the precentral and postcentral gyri, the face is represented ventrolaterally and the leg dorsomedially.

Secondary sensory areas are located near each primary receptive area and receive input from the thalamus and from their respective primary sensory cortices. These secondary sensory areas serve to elaborate and analyze sensory information.

One hemisphere is almost always "trained" early in life in the process of language function. The left hemisphere usually assumes this role, and the person becomes right-handed. Approximately 90% of people in the United States are right-handed, and nearly all have left-hemisphere dominance. About 10% are left-handed, but half of these have left-brain dominance as well. The remainder are right-brain dominant or have mixed right and left dominance.

Three regions of the dominant cerebral hemisphere are important for the production of language: **Broca's area, Wernicke's area,** and the **arcuate fasciculus** that connects them. Broca's area is located on the motor cortex just anterior to the motor representation of the face. Wernicke's area occupies the posterior part of the superior temporal gyrus and is responsible for recognizing speech patterns, then relaying this information to Broca's area via the arcuate fasciculus. Broca's area formulates the planned speech pattern and sends this information to the adjacent representation of the speech musculature for the production of meaningful speech.

AUTONOMIC NERVOUS SYSTEM

Smooth muscle, cardiac muscle, and glands are innervated by an important subdivision of the CNS called the autonomic nervous system (ANS). The ANS operates at the subconscious level and influences the activities of its effector organs. It is not, however, necessary for the basic functioning of these organs. Peristalsis of the intestinal tract or beating of the heart can both occur without autonomic input. The ANS comes into play when rapid changes in the activities of smooth muscle, cardiac muscle, or glands are necessary. The ANS also contains sensory neurons that convey impulses related to visceral sensation and whose cell bodies are located in the dorsal root ganglia.

There are two subdivisions of the autonomic nervous system: the sympathetic and parasympathetic nervous systems. The sympathetic nervous system mediates responses that prepare the body for a stressful situation. Its activation increases heart rate, cardiac output, and blood pressure; suspends functions of the gastrointestinal tract; decreases splanchnic blood flow; dilates bronchioles; and causes release of red blood cells from the spleen. This collection of events has been described as the "fight-or–flight" response.

Effector organs innervated by the autonomic nervous system receive impulses by way of a two-neuron chain. The first visceral motor fiber, called a preganglionic fiber, leaves the spinal cord, then synapses with a second neuron, known as a postganglionic fiber, which travels to the effector organ. Preganglionic sympathetic nervous system fibers leave the spinal cord at the thoracolumbar level, then synapse either in the chain ganglia of the sympathetic trunk (located on either side of the vertebral column) or travel as part of a thoracic or lumbar splanchnic nerve, terminating in one of the prevertebral ganglia of the abdomen and pelvis. This group of ganglia includes the celiac, superior mesenteric, aorticorenal, inferior mesenteric, and hypogastric ganglia, located at the root of the arteries for which they are named.

The neurotransmitter released by the preganglionic sympathetic neuron is acetylcholine, while that released by the postganglionic neuron is norepinephrine. The only exceptions to this are the postganglionic fibers that innervate the sweat glands, which secrete acetylcholine.

The adrenal medulla may be thought of as a large sympathetic ganglion. Its cells are functionally similar to sympathetic neurons, and stimulation by preganglionic fibers causes them to release epinephrine into the bloodstream. This adds to the effect of norepinephrine in producing the fight-or-flight response mentioned previously.

Activation of the parasympathetic nervous system causes more discrete, localized effects, while stimulation of the sympathetic nervous system mediates generalized physiological responses. Preganglionic neurons of the parasympathetic system emerge from the CNS at the brainstem and sacral levels, then travel to ganglia located either within or close to their effector organs. The postganglionic fibers are thus very short.

The preganglionic parasympathetic fibers emerging from the brainstem travel with cranial nerves III, VII, IX, and X, while those of the sacral division form the pelvic splanchnic nerves. Stimulation of fibers accompanying cranial nerve III causes pupillary constriction and changes the thickness of the lens of the eye. Those fibers of nerve VII and IX mediate lacrimation and salivation, while parasympathetic neurons of nerve X supply the heart, lungs, and abdominal viscera. Generally, the effects of the parasympathetic nervous system on the heart, lungs, and abdominal organs are "opposite" of the effects of the sympathetic nervous system. Activation of the vagus nerve slows the heart rate, constricts bronchioles, and stimulates intestinal peristalsis.

The pelvic splanchnic nerves supply fibers to ganglia located in the walls of the urinary and reproductive tracts, the colon and rectum. This division of the parasympathetic nervous system is principally concerned with mechanisms for emptying the bladder and rectum. The nerve terminals of both the preganglionic and postganglionic fibers of the parasympathetic system secrete acetylcholine.

▨▨▨▨▨▨▨▨▨▨

Pathophysiology

TRAUMA

Primary head injuries may be classified as either skull fractures, focal injuries, or diffuse brain injuries. Skull fractures themselves do not result in neurological injury, but accompanying brain injury may be present owing to stresses generated by the impacting force. Such neurological injury may be caused either directly by the impact or indirectly as a result of bleeding or swelling, causing mass effect.

There are two types of focal injuries—**contusions** and **hematomas.** **Coup** contusions occur beneath the impact site, while **contra-coup** contusions are found at sites remote from the point of contact. Coup injuries occur when local bending of the skull from contact forces causes local tissue strains that result in cortical brain and vascular injury. Contra-coup injuries occur when brain motion toward the impact site causes tensile strains at an area opposite the point of impact, resulting in contusion if the tissue strain exceeds the vascular tolerance. Unlike coup injuries, acceleration rather than impact is the critical mechanism for generation of a contra-coup contusion.

Hematomas may be epidural, subdural, or intracerebral. Epidural hematomas occur when a skull fracture or skull deformation results in disruption of dural or skull vessels. Blood then collects in the epidural space and, if the volume is large enough, can cause significant neurological impairment and death.

Subdural hematomas are of two general types. Acute subdural hematomas are often associated with contusion and laceration of the brain and result from the same contact and acceleration effects that cause the primary lesion. Chronic subdural hematomas usually occur when surface vessels, primarily veins carrying blood from the brain surface to the sagittal sinus, are torn.

Large traumatic intracerebral hematomas are uncommon and are often associated with extensive cortical contusion.

Diffuse insults include cerebral concussion and diffuse axonal injury. Concussion is a condition in which rotational acceleration of the head produces functional neuronal derangement without accompanying structural damage. Diffuse axonal injury, like concussion, is produced by inertial, not contact forces. Rotational acceleration of the head is again the responsible mechanism, but in the case of diffuse axonal injury the forces are severe enough to result in structural neuronal damage.

Head injuries cause neuronal dysfunction either because of direct neuronal injury, or because they are accompanied by an increase in intracranial pressure (ICP). The brain is enclosed by the bony confines of the skull. Consequently, only small increases in intracranial volume can occur before pressure begins to increase significantly. Hematomas and contusions, as well as the edema that may accompany them, act as space-occupying lesions and can result in significant elevations of ICP. Impaired cerebral blood flow will result if the intracranial pressure rises to a high enough level, causing abnormal neurological function. Cerebral blood volume increases in severe head injury owing to impairment of autoregulation and can itself contribute to elevations of ICP.

Shifts of the intracranial contents may also occur, resulting in herniation of the brain under the falx cerebri, over the tentorium cerebelli, or through the foramen magnum. Herniation of the medial temporal lobe (uncus) through the tentorial hiatus results in compression of the midbrain and causes the clinical syndrome of ipsilateral pupillary dilation (compression of the parasympathetic fibers of the IIIrd nerve) and contralateral hemiparesis (compression of the cerebral peduncle).

Therapeutic intervention in the head-injured patient involves operative treatment, medical management, or both. Linear fractures rarely require surgery, but compound fractures may if they are associated with an overlying scalp laceration or are significantly depressed and pushing on the brain surface. Lesions causing significant mass effect, such as hematomas, should be removed.

Many serious head injuries involve no surgical lesions but result in significant brain swelling either from edema or increased cerebral blood volume. Intracranial pressure monitors provide accurate ICP readings and may be placed in the subdural or subarachnoid space, or within the ventricle. Once elevated ICP is detected, several measures may be instituted to reduce it, if possible, to below 20 mm Hg. Elevation and straight positioning of the head and neck provide optimal venous drainage, while sedation and blood pressure control help to reduce ICP by limiting excessive cerebral blood flow. Osmotic diuretics such as mannitol reduce cerebral edema and ICP by decreasing brain water content. Hyperventilation lowers P_{O_2}, thus elevating the interstitial pH of the brain. This causes cerebral vasoconstriction, decreasing the cerebral blood volume and intracranial pressure. Drainage of CSF through a ventriculostomy may also be employed to lower ICP by decreasing the intracranial volume. High-dose barbiturate therapy is reserved for cases of intracranial pressure that are not controlled by these measures. These drugs probably lower ICP through a reduction in cerebral blood flow and blood volume, coupled to a fall in cerebral metabolism.

ISCHEMIA

Neurons are exquisitely sensitive to ischemia and hypoxemia. Within 10–20 seconds of the onset of ischemia, electrical activity stops. The Na,K-pump fails and glucose levels fall rapidly within 30 seconds. Sodium then enters the cell as a result of pump failure, and is accompanied by water, resulting in intracellular edema within 3 minutes of the ischemic onset. Intracellular glucose is depleted, and lactate levels rise fivefold by 10 minutes. These changes are all reversible if flow is restored at this point.

INTRACRANIAL VASCULAR ACCIDENTS

Most intracranial hemorrhages are classified by location. Epidural and subdural hematomas exert their effects by acting as space-occupying lesions, raising intracranial pressure, and possibly resulting in herniation of the brain.

Subarachnoid hemorrhages occur when blood leaks into the subarachnoid space. This may result primarily from rupture of vascular lesions such as aneurysms occurring on arteries of the circle of Willis, or secondarily when a hemorrhage into the brain parenchyma ruptures through to the subarachnoid space. These hemorrhages are not usually associated with significant mass effect but cause neurological dysfunction either early in the course of the illness as a result of meningeal or cortical inflammation, or late owing to delayed effects, such as cerebral vasospasm or hydrocephalus.

Intraparenchymal hemorrhages involve bleeding into the brain substance itself. The majority of these hemorrhages result from the rupture of end-arterioles weakened by the effects of chronic hypertension. The vessels most commonly involved are found in the basal ganglia (gray matter structures lying deep within the brain) and thalamus.

Other causes of intraparenchymal hemorrhages are large arterovenous malformations, blood dyscrasias, aneurysms, and trauma, to name a few. Occasionally, a hemorrhage of this type ruptures into a ventricle. The clot that forms may obstruct CSF flow, resulting in hydrocephalus.

HYDROCEPHALUS

Hydrocephalus is a condition that results from excessive amounts of cerebrospinal fluid within the ventricular system or subarachnoid space. If the CSF flow is impaired between its site of origin in the choroid plexus and its egress into the subarachnoid space at the foramina of Luschka and Magendie of the fourth ventricle, it is called obstructive hydrocephalus. If the flow is normal, but absorption of CSF over the cerebral hemispheres is hindered, communicating hydrocephalus occurs. When the volume increase caused by the excessive CSF accompanying either type of hydrocephalus becomes great enough, elevation of ICP results.

Obstructive hydrocephalus is most commonly treated by shunting CSF from the lateral ventricles to the pleural or peritoneal spaces, and sometimes to the right atrium. **Communicating hydrocephalus** may be similarly managed but also may be treated by diverting CSF from the lumbar subarachnoid space to the peritoneum.

DEMYELINATING DISEASE

Myelin is critical for the normal functioning of many neurons by ensuring rapid impulse transmission. Certain disease states such as multiple sclerosis cause injury and destruction of the myelin sheath through the actions of either exogenous or endogenous agents, or a combination of both.

Presently, two major theories, which are not necessarily mutually exclusive, exist regarding the etiology of multiple sclerosis. One rests upon the concept of an infection (presumably viral) with a long incubation period. The other cites an autoimmune mechanism as being responsible for the destruction of the myelin sheath. No clear etiology or definitive treatment is known at this time.

DEGENERATIVE DISEASE

There are a wide variety of diseases of the central nervous system of unknown cause, many of which have a hereditary or familial occurrence. They begin insidiously, after a long period of normal nervous system function, and gradually progress over many years. Alzheimer's disease is one of the most common of these disorders. It results in diffuse atrophy of the brain, especially of the frontal and temporal lobes, and eventually causes dementia and death. In addition to the cerebrum, other parts of the nervous system, including the basal ganglia, brainstem, cerebellum, motor neurons, peripheral nerves, and muscle, may be affected by neurodegenerative disease.

EPILEPSY

Epilepsy is an intermittent disorder of the nervous system caused by the sudden, excessive, and disorderly discharge of cerebral neurons. This discharge results in an almost immediate disturbance of sensation, loss of consciousness, convulsive movement, or some combination of the three. Seizures are often due to structural lesions, such as brain tumors, but may also occur secondarily as a result of fever, metabolic disturbance, or other effects of systemic illness. Seizures for which no pathologic entity or other cause can be found are called primary, or essential, and include certain types of grand mal and petite mal seizures.

TUMORS

Brain tumors cause neurologic dysfunction and death because of both tissue compression intracranially and breakdown of neurological architecture from local invasion. Primary brain tumors, in contrast to most other solid tumors, are a regional disease without capacity for systemic spread. These confined tumors often cannot be curatively resected owing to their tendency to invade normal brain tissue and their often inaccessible location. They are also notoriously chemoresistant and radioresistant, making many of the more malignant varieties universally lethal. Radiation therapy is often hampered by the radiosensitivity of normal brain, while the blood-brain barrier and systemic toxicity limit the effectiveness of most currently available chemotherapeutic agents.

INFECTION

The parenchyma, coverings, and blood vessels of the nervous system may be invaded by practically any pathogen. Pyogenic infections of the intracranial contents originate either by hematogenous spread or by direct extension from cranial structures. Infection of the pia mater and arachnoid and of the CSF they enclose is known as meningitis. Infection of the brain parenchyma is known as encephalitis.

Brain abscesses occur when areas of encephalitis become "walled off" by the formation of a capsule around the infected site. They are almost always secondary to a suppurative focus elsewhere in the body. Infection of the paranasal sinuses, middle ear, and mastoid air cells accounts for 40% of all brain abscesses. Treatment of all infections involves appropriate antibi-

otic therapy, but surgery may be required in cases of brain abscesses that cause persistent or progressive elevated intracranial pressure or that are simply not responding to antibiotic therapy.

Viral infections of the nervous system are invariably complications of generalized viral infections, with the possible exception of rabies. Many of the common viruses (herpes simplex, measles, varicella) cause only insignificant systemic illness but can have a devastating effect on the nervous system. Fortunately, when considering the large number of systemic viral illnesses, the proportion of cases of nervous system involvement is very low.

Diagnostic Studies

COMPUTED TOMOGRAPHY

Computerized axial tomography (CAT) scanning utilizes an accurately collimated x-ray beam that passes through the patient and strikes a series of detectors. The x-ray tube and detectors then rotate, and the degree of attenuation is determined by a computer that then generates an image. Dense objects, such as hematomas, highly cellular tumors, and bone, appear bright, while hypodense lesions, such as edema or infarcts, appear dark, owing to high and low attenuation, respectively, of the x-ray beam. Lesions with high blood flow and blood-brain barrier breakdown may be more readily demonstrated with the injection of an intravenous contrast agent. The contrast will "leak" through the disrupted blood-brain barrier and appear as an area of high attenuation (brightness) on the CAT scan image.

MAGNETIC RESONANCE IMAGING

Magnetic resonance imaging (MRI) is a recent, rapidly developing technology that utilizes a strong magnetic field to orient the protons of the body in a particular direction. A radiofrequency current is then passed through the area of interest and disturbs the proton alignment. Once the current stops, the protons realign with the magnetic field, emitting signals that are then detected. The result is an image of extraordinary anatomical detail.

While CAT scanning utilizes differences in density to demonstrate contrast between normal and abnormal tissues, MRI depends on the signal intensities of tissues to create images. The signal intensity is influenced by many factors, including proton density, flow and motion, paramagnetic effects, and others too detailed to mention here. An example of the difference between MRI and CAT is intracranial blood, which initially appears bright on CAT scans, then becomes progressively darker as the clot dissolves. The MRI appearance, however, is determined by the state of breakdown of the hemoglobin in the clot, and may appear bright or dark depending upon the imaging parameters and the time elapsed from the initial bleeding episode.

CEREBRAL ANGIOGRAPHY

Cerebral angiography is a procedure in which the arteries of the brain are studied by x-ray following injection of either the carotid or vertebral arteries with contrast material. It is useful for locating aneurysms, arterovenous malformations, or any other vascular anomalies of the larger branches of the arteries of the circle of Willis. Small terminal arteries generally are not visualized. Cerebral hemorrhage, infarction, tumors, and vasospasm also may be localized via changes in the arterial pattern. Injection of the internal carotid artery outlines the anterior and middle cerebral arteries, while the major branches of the basilar artery are outlined following injection of the vertebral artery.

MYELOGRAPHY

Plain x-rays of the spine are useful for evaluating bony changes of the spinal column, while myelography allows for visualization of the spinal cord and nerve roots as well. Radiopaque contrast material is introduced into the spinal fluid, usually by way of a lumbar puncture. The fluid can be made to move up or down the spinal canal by tilting the table on which the patient lies. X-rays and CAT scans are then taken that reveal the outline of the spinal cord and nerve roots.

ELECTROENCEPHALOGRAPHY

The brain's neuronal activity can be indirectly studied by recording the electrical activity from the scalp surface (electroencephalography) or from the brain surface at surgery (electrocorticography). Changes in potential within neurons cause current to flow in the extracellular fluid, which produces the potentials recorded at the electrode site. Action potentials, the largest signals generated by neurons, actually contribute little to the elec-

troencephalography potentials. Most of the activity recorded consists of extracellular current flow from summated postsynaptic potentials of cortical neurons. Electroencephalography is important in the diagnosis and treatment of epilepsy, head injury, stroke, and coma. The absence of electrical activity is required to meet most accepted criteria for the establishment of brain death.

EVOKED POTENTIALS

Evoked potentials are recorded from the scalp and result from a change in the ongoing neuronal electrical activity in response to stimulation of a sensory organ or pathway. The evoked potentials used clinically are the visual evoked potentials, brainstem auditory evoked potentials, and somatosensory evoked potentials. They are useful diagnostically, as when lesions of the visual pathways from multiple sclerosis cause delay in the cortical response after visual stimulation. They can also be a valuable surgical monitoring modality. Brainstem auditory evoked potentials provide a measure of the amount of brainstem manipulation occurring during certain posterior fossa operations. A decrease in amplitude or an increase in latency (delay) of the responses indicates excessive retraction and ischemia of the auditory pathways of the brainstem.

ELECTROMYOGRAPHY

Electromyography measures the activity of motor units (the total number of muscle fibers innervated by one motoneuron) in muscle both at rest and during contraction. Normal resting muscle shows no activity, but during increasing muscular contraction more and more motor units are recruited. The appearance of muscular activity at rest is usually secondary to denervation, and includes fibrillations and fasciculations. Fibrillations represent contractions of individual muscle fibers, and fasciculations represent contractions of individual motor units. When electrical silence is present at rest, and small motor unit potentials are recorded during voluntary contraction, a primary muscle disease is likely to be present.

NERVE CONDUCTION VELOCITY

The conduction velocity of peripheral nerves can also be recorded after electrical stimulation. Demyelinating neuropathies slow conduction, while axonal neuropathies have no effect on impulse velocity.

Bibliography

Adams RD, Victor M. *Principles of neurology.* 3rd ed. New York: McGraw-Hill, 1985.

Carpenter MB. *Core text of human anatomy.* 2nd ed. Baltimore: Williams & Wilkins, 1978.

Guyton AC. *Basic human neurophysiology.* 3rd ed. Philadelphia: WB Saunders, 1981.

Kandel ER, Schwartz JH. *Principles of neural science.* 2nd ed. New York: Elsevier, 1985.

Gilman S, Newman SW. *Manter and Gatz's Essentials of clinical neuroanatomy and neurophysiology.* 7th ed. Philadelphia: FA Davis, 1987.

Pansky B, Allen DJ. *Review of neuroscience.* New York: Macmillan, 1980.

Rowland LP, ed. *Merritt's textbook of neurology.* 6th ed. London: Lea & Febiger, Henry Kimpton Publishers, 1989.

Youmans JR. *Neurological surgery.* 3rd ed. Philadelphia: WB Saunders, 1990.

David H. Deaton

27 ENDOCRINE PHYSIOLOGY

The endocrine system is responsible for communication and regulation of spatially and functionally disparate cells and organs. Its existence is the consequence of ever-increasing cellular specialization and differentiation in the evolution of multicellular organisms. The "endocrine system" is unlike other body "systems" in that, while it is true that some cells and organs have more prominent, and even primary, endocrine functions, almost all cells are imbued with at least some endocrine role. This chapter is primarily concerned with the "classic" endocrine organ systems (e.g., thyroid, pituitary, etc.). Their structure, function, and regulatory pathways, as well as some more recent information on cell-surface-receptor interactions, intracellular mediators, and second signals, will be discussed. More recently discovered hormones and endocrine functions such as atrial natriuretic factor will also be covered. Endocrine function of the gastrointestinal tract is discussed in Chapter 18.

General Considerations

HORMONE CLASSIFICATION, SYNTHESIS, AND MECHANISMS OF ACTION

A hormone is defined as "a chemical substance that is released into the blood in small amounts and that, after delivery by the circulation, elicits a typical physical response in other cells." When this process occurs as a result of transport by simple diffusion in the extracellular fluid to other cells in the local microenvironment, it is termed **paracrine**. Substances affecting the same cell from which they were secreted are said to have **autocrine** function. Hormones secreted into the blood must be produced synchronously by a sufficiently large group of cells specialized to synthesize that hormone in

order to achieve effective concentrations in the blood. These groups of cells are what are classically referred to as the **endocrine** organs. Paracrine and autocrine mediators are secreted by individual cells, often dispersed throughout the body.

Most hormones fall into three general chemical categories: (1) derivatives of the amino acid tyrosine, (2) steroids (i.e., cholesterol derivatives), and (3) peptides and proteins. Table 27-1 gives examples of each of these.

Postsynthetic processing of hormones is common, and defects in these mechanisms can be responsible for endocrine disease states. Peptide and protein hormones undergo many of the posttranslational events common in other proteins (i.e., cleavage, folding, glycosylation, etc.). Proteins destined for secretion all appear to include a hydrophobic sequence at the amino-terminus that allows endoplasmic reticulum and Golgi uptake that results in their "packaging" for exocytosis. Some hormones undergo transformation outside their cell of origin (e.g., thyroxine→triiodothyronine) and in some cases within the target tissue (e.g., testosterone→dihydrotestosterone→estrogen).

Many hormones (e.g., epinephrine, insulin) are stored intracellularly in membrane-bound vesicles that

TABLE 27-1. Types of Hormones

Tyrosine Derivatives	Steroids	Peptides (<20 Amino Acids)	Proteins (>20 Amino Aacids)
Epinephrine	Testosterone	Oxytocin	Insulin
Norepinephrine	Estradiol	Vasopressin	Glucagon
Dopamine	Progesterone	Angiotensin	Adrenocorticotropic hormone
Tri-iodothyronine	Cortisol	Melanocyte-stimulating hormone	Thyroid-stimulating hormone
Thyroxine	Aldosterone	Somatostatin	Follicle-stimulating hormone
	Vitamin D	Thyrotropin-releasing hormone	Luteinizing hormone
		Gonadotropin-releasing hormone	Growth hormone
			Prolactin
			Corticotropin-releasing hormone
			Growth hormone-releasing hormone
			Parathyroid hormone
			Calcitonin
			Chorionic gonadotropin
			Chorionic somatomammotropin

Reproduced from Goodman HM. *Basic medical endocrinology*. New York: Raven Press, 1988:4.

are released into the blood by the process of exocytosis. The initiation of this process requires calcium influx and also involves cyclic adenosine monophosphate (cAMP) and protein kinase production and activation. Conversely, there is little storage of steroid hormones and it is unclear whether regulation of their secretion takes place at the synthetic or cellular release phase. Other hormones (e.g., thyroxine) have unique storage and secretion characteristics. Once secreted into the bloodstream, hormones may have varying fractions of free (i.e., unbound) and protein-bound hormone. Only unbound hormone can leave the intravascular space for delivery to the target tissue. The equilibrium between bound and unbound fractions thus buffers the delivery of many hormones. Protein binding also affects hormone half-life, which can vary from seconds (e.g., epinephrine) to days (e.g., thyroxine). Hormone degradation prior to excretion occurs by enzymatic cleavage in the bloodstream, extracellular fluid, or the target tissue. Some degradation pathways yield distinct and recognizable by-products that can be measured in the urine, while others are broken down to common precursors precluding assay.

Target tissues respond specifically and uniquely to hormones directed at their regulation, based on the possession of receptors specific for that hormone. Specificity of response is determined at this level of activation (i.e., hormone-receptor). Secondary intracellular activation steps (i.e., second messengers) are shared by cells with disparate end function.

Hormone-receptor interactions fall into two general categories, **hydrophilic** and **hydrophobic.** The hydrophilic hormones (e.g., proteins and catecholamines) bind to cell-surface membrane receptors that, when activated by hormone binding, initiate a cascade of intracellular reactions (i.e., "second messengers") that finally mediate the cellular response to hormone stimulus (Figure 27-1). Hydrophobic hormones (e.g.,

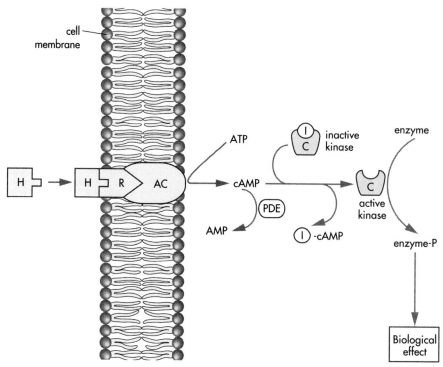

Figure 27-1 Mechanism of hydrophilic hormone binding and intracellular regulation. The hormone (H) binds a specific receptor (R) on the cell surface, which activates a series of intracellular regulation events common to many disparate cell types. Phosphodiesterase (PDE) I and C represent inhibitory and catalytic subunits of the kinase. AC, Adenylate cyclase. (Reproduced from Hedge GA, Colby HD, Goodman RL. *Clinical endocrine physiology.* Philadelphia: WB Saunders, 1987:20.)

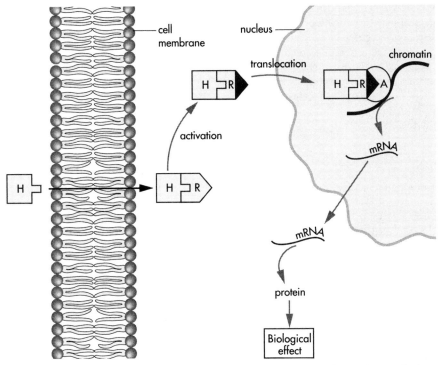

Figure 27-2 Mechanism of hydrophobic hormone binding and intracellular regulation. The hormone (H) binds an intracellular receptor (R). Binding of the H-R complex to chromatin effects mRNA synthesis and increased gene product expression. (Reproduced from Hedge GA, Colby HD, Goodman RL. *Clinical endocrine physiology.* Philadelphia: WB Saunders, 1987:18.)

steroids and thyroid hormone) are able to enter cells and, in most cases, are bound to intranuclear receptors that result directly in gene regulation, thus obviating the need for second messengers (Figure 27-2). The mechanisms by which second messengers (i.e., intracellular activation and regulatory signals) function to mediate the effects of hormonal stimulation are not completely elucidated. The mediators that are most understood, and are considered most important, are (1) **cAMP,** (2) **calcium,** (3) **phospholipase C,** and (4) **cyclic guanosine monophosphate (cGMP).** The postbinding intracellular activation events are not known for all hormones (e.g., insulin and prolactin).

Cyclic AMP is formed by **adenylate cyclase** on the inner membrane surface. Adenylate cyclase is one of three subunits of the hormone receptor complex. This complex consists of (a) a recognition component (i.e., the hormone-specific binding molecule), (b) a regulatory component, and (c) adenylate cyclase. The regulatory component binds guanine nucleotides, **guanosine**

diphosphate (GDP), and **guanosine triphosphate (GTP).** Guanosine diphosphate activates adenylate cyclase, while GTP inhibits it. Guanosine triphosphate also diminishes affinity of the recognition component for its hormone. Cyclic AMP activates **protein kinase A,** which catalyzes phosphorylation of serine hydroxyl groups of various enzymes, increasing or decreasing their activity.

Calcium in concert with **calmodulin** perform a variety of functions related to cellular activation. Calcium concentrations increase up to 1000-fold during hormonal stimulation. Calmodulin binds calcium and activates other catalytic proteins.

Phospholipase C is an enzyme that, when activated by hormonal stimulation, acts to split membrane phospholipid into **diacylglyceride** and **1,4,5-triphosphate.** Both of these compounds can act as second messengers. **Cyclic GMP** is also thought to play a role as a second messenger, but its catalytic pathways are not well understood.

Hydrophobic hormones pass directly through the cell membrane and into the nucleus. There they are bound by a closely related group of molecules that have a hormone-specific sequence on one end and a chromatin specific sequence on the other. Hormone binding stimulates activation of gene transcription. In this way hormone stimulation is realized by increasing enzyme concentration rather than by increasing the activity of enzymes already present.

REGULATION

The essential components of endocrine regulatory systems are

1. Detector of actual or threatened homeostatic imbalance
2. Coupling mechanism to activate the secretory apparatus
3. Secretory apparatus
4. Hormone
5. End-organ capable of responding
6. Detector that can recognize hormonal response and signal cessation of hormone requirement
7. Mechanism to clear and metabolize secreted hormone
8. Synthetic apparatus for hormone replenishment.

The most common form of hormonal regulation is **negative feedback.** In this regulatory loop, the elicited hormone or some elicited response inhibits further release of the hormone. This aspect of hormonal regulation is important in the pathogenesis of many endocrine disease states (e.g., the regulatory feedback has been interrupted in some way) and in their diagnosis (e.g., assay for excess or deficiency of specific hormones with appropriate stimulus). A single negative-feedback loop can regulate deviation in only one direction. For this reason many homeostatic functions are regulated by opposing negative-feedback loops that, together, effect a tight control of the concerned variable within a narrow range (e.g., blood sugar by insulin and glucagon).

Positive feedback is a less common regulatory pathway. By definition it results in ever-increasing hormone secretion until some threshold is reached that ablates the primary stimulus. A good example of this occurs with oxytocin and cervical dilatation. Oxytocin is stimulated by cervical dilatation, thus increasing uterine contractions, which increase cervical dilatation, etc., until delivery, which ablates the stimulus.

HORMONE MEASUREMENT

Early measurements of serum hormone levels were done by means of the **bioassay.** This technique capitalizes on the cross-reactivity between many human hormones and their counterparts in other species. Hormone levels are determined by administering serial dilutions of an unknown sample in a well-characterized animal model to determine the greatest dilution that will elicit the desired response. More recently, **radioimmunoassay** has become the method of choice. In this assay an unknown amount (i.e., the sample being tested) is mixed with a known amount of hormone-specific antibody and a known amount of radiolabeled hormone. The labeled and unlabeled hormone (i.e. sample) are thus in competition for antibody binding. The bound fraction is separated, and the level of radioactivity in the bound sample allows calculation of the amount of unlabeled hormone in the sample being tested. This method can be misleading in the evaluation of circulating bioreactive hormone in that it assays the immunoreactive site of the molecule rather than the biologically active site. Prohormone and certain nonbiologically active degradation products, possessing the immunoreactive but not the bioreactive site, may thus be included in these assays. Some of these compounds have half-lives far longer than the bioreactive hormone and are present in the serum in quantities many times greater than the bioreactive form. This artifact can be misleading, as in the case of parathyroid hormone, which has its biologic activity in the amino-terminal portion of the molecule and its immunoreactive portion in the carboxy-terminal portion. Renal-failure patients in particular will have very high circulating levels of the carboxy-terminal of parathyroid hormone, as a result of their inability to clear this compound effectively, the assay of which would be misleading in the evaluation of their parathyroid function. Despite this artifact, radioimmunoassay is generally quite useful in providing an accurate index of serum hormone concentrations if not the actual concentration of bioreactive substance. **Radioreceptor assays** utilize specific binding of water-soluble hormones to cellular membranes and thus *are* able to assay these hormones in their biologically active state. This is a relatively complex assay however, and does not offer enough advantages to warrant its use in most situations.

Blood levels of the various hormones are useful only in a well-defined clinical state and often only in relation to other physiologic variables that have been controlled (e.g., suppression of various hormone responses by exogenous administration of synthetic compounds, etc.). In addition, many hormones are secreted in pulsatile patterns or according to a defined circadian rhythm. In this circumstance the relative serial values of a given mediator yield more information than a solitary absolute value. Indeed, information can be transmitted through the rhythm or pattern of secretion as well as through the direct response elicited by hormone-receptor interaction.

Parathyroid Glands and Calcium Metabolism

Calcium homeostasis is influenced by several factors, most importantly parathyroid hormone. The parathyroid glands themselves are small yellow-tan ellipsoids of tissue positioned superiorly and inferiorly on the posterior surface of the thyroid gland. While most humans have four of these glands, as few as two and as many as eight have been reported. Their location in the neck is somewhat variable and glands outside the neck are not uncommon, the most common ectopic site being the mediastinum. The inferior glands originate from the third branchial pouch and the superior glands, which are most likely to be ectopic, originate from the fourth branchial pouch. The composite mass of the parathyroids is less than 150 mg. Each gland is composed primarily of **chief cells,** the cells responsible for the production of **parathyroid hormone (PTH),** arranged in cords and clusters. Other cells, known as **oxyphil cells,** appear singly or in small groups and have no known function. Oxyphil cells increase in number throughout life. The blood supply to the parathyroids is derived largely from the inferior thyroid arteries.

PARATHYROID HORMONE

Parathyroid hormone is a chain of 84 amino acids with no disulfide bonds. While up to 50 carboxy-terminal amino acids may be removed without a diminution in biologic activity, the removal of only a single serine at the amino-terminus renders the compound biologically inactive. The regulation of PTH secretion is somewhat unusual in that it takes place at the degradation stage rather than at production. Up to 90% of PTH is broken down within the chief cell that synthesized it, prior to secretion, in response to circulating calcium concentra-tions. The plasma half-life of secreted, biologically active hormone is only a few minutes. It is metabolized outside the parathyroids in the renal tubules. The degradation products have longer half-lives (i.e., hours) and can cause misleading results when measurements directed at the carboxy-terminus (i.e., the nonbiologically active terminus) of the molecule are used to assay serum PTH.

Parathyroid hormone is the hormone responsible for regulation of calcium concentration in the extracellular fluid. It regulates calcium through a variety of effects on bone (mobilization of calcium), kidney (excretion of calcium and phosphorous), and intestine (absorption of calcium). The acute response to PTH in the bone compartment is known as osteocytic osteolysis. Within several hours of PTH secretion, osteocytes begin reabsorbing calcium from the surrounding bone fluid compartment and subsequently secreting it into the extracellular space. Osteoclasts secrete acids that lower the pH and favor bone solubilization. Osteoblasts are inhibited. The second phase of PTH-induced activity begins after about 12 hours of exposure to increased PTH levels. In this phase osteoclastic activity predominates as bone is actively resorbed and new osteoclasts are recruited from monocytic precursors in reticuloendothelial organs.

The response to PTH within the kidney is divided into three distinct effects. Within the distal nephron, calcium reabsorption is enhanced. Only 10% of the filtered calcium is not reabsorbed in the distal tubule, making this mechanism of calcium regulation useful for small, rapid adjustments in serum calcium. It is this mechanism that provides the "fine tuning" to serum calcium concentration. In the proximal tubule, the primary site of phosphorous reabsorption, PTH exerts a powerful inhibitory effect on the reabsorption of phosphate. PTH also affects total body calcium balance through its activating effect on the renal enzyme responsible for the hydroxylation, and thus activation, of vitamin D, crucial in the intestinal absorption of dietary calcium.

Regulation of PTH secretion occurs within the chief cells and is inversely proportional to serum *ionized* calcium concentration. While PTH can affect serum phosphorous through its effects on the kidney, there is no evidence that serum phosphorous affects PTH secretion. The cellular mechanisms of PTH secretion are not well understood. While calcium is the primary intracellular mediator of extracellular secretion in most secretory cells, just the opposite is true in the chief cell. The reasons and mechanisms underlying this phenomenon are unclear.

CALCITONIN

Calcitonin (thyrocalcitonin) is secreted by the **parafollicular, or C cells,** of the thyroid. These cells are seen singly or in clusters interdigitated at the junctions of the thyroid follicles. They have a neuroectodermal origin and arise from the fourth branchial pouch. Parafollicular cells are the cell of origin of medullary carcinoma of the thyroid.

Calcitonin is a 32-amino-acid protein with a bioreactive serum half-life of approximately 10 minutes. It is cleared from the bloodstream primarily by the kidney. The function of calcitonin as a homeostatic hormone does not seem to be in acute regulation of serum calcium but, rather, in chronic calcium homeostasis and maintenance of bone. Calcitonin's primary activity is mediated through inhibition of osteoclastic activity in the bone. It, therefore, has very little effect outside periods when osteoclastic activity is high. There is some evidence that high concentrations of calcitonin can increase urinary excretion of calcium and phosphorous. This effect is minimal and in cases of prolonged exposure to increased calcitonin levels (i.e., tumor production of calcitonin), the kidney becomes refractory to its influence. The secretion of calcitonin is primarily controlled by serum calcium, with increasing concentrations seen when serum calcium rises above 9 mg/dL. Calcitonin secretion is also elicited by **gastrin** and to a lesser degree by a variety of other gastrointestinal hormones. This is the basis of the provocative test using gastrin in the diagnosis of medullary carcinoma of the thyroid.

VITAMIN D

"Vitamin D" is a derivative of vitamin D_3, whose proper name is 1,25-dihydroxycholecalciferol, or $1,25(OH)_2D_3$. This compound is vital for maintaining extracellular fluid concentration of calcium and in the mineralization of bone. Vitamin D deficiency is known as **osteomalacia,** and in children is often called **rickets.** In mammals, vitamin D is also known as **cholecalciferol.** Its synthesis begins with the unmodified vitamin D_3. This compound is chemically altered (i.e., photolysis of the bond between carbons 9 and 10 in 7-dihydrocholesterol, opening the B-ring in this steroid) in the skin when exposed to near-ultraviolet radiation (i.e.,

sunlight). While still biologically inert, it gains an strong affinity for vitamin D-binding protein, present in the serum, that its parent molecule lacked. The compound is next altered in the liver where it is oxidized at the carbon 25 position to yield **25-hydroxycholecalciferol (25-OH-D_3).** In the kidney a second hydroxylation takes place in the carbon 1 position, yielding the bioreactive compound, **$1,25(OH)_2D_3$.** This compound is approximately 1100 times more biologically active than its precursor (25-OH-D_3) and accounts for all the physiologic activity of "vitamin D". It has less affinity for vitamin D-binding protein than does its precursor and a consequently shorter half-life, about 15 hours compared to 15 days for 25-OH-D_3.

The primary physiologic action of $1,25(OH)_2D_3$ is to increase calcium and phosphate concentration in extracellular fluid. This action is realized through the compound's effects on intestine and bone, and to a limited degree, kidney. 1,25-Dihydroxycholecalciferol acts on the intestinal epithelium to increase the absorption of both calcium and phosphorous. While the exact mechanisms by which this increased absorption is achieved are unknown, $1,25(OH)_2D_3$ acts in a manner similar to steroid hormones in that it binds an intracellular receptor that induces the production of a variety of enzymes, presumably those responsible for calcium and phosphate absorption. The effects of $1,25(OH)_2D_3$ on bone are primarily indirect. Osteoid mineralization occurs spontaneously when the appropriate concentrations of calcium phosphate are present, which depends on adequate intake of calcium and phosphorous from the environment made possible by adequate $1,25(OH)_2D_3$. Vitamin D also increases both the number and activity of osteoclasts and is very similar to PTH in this regard. Indeed the actions of PTH and $1,25(OH)_2D_3$ on bone osteoclasts and osteoblasts are similar and synergistic when both are present, suggesting a common final pathway for their effects. $1,25(OH)_2D_3$ can increase both calcium and phosphorous absorption in the kidney when given to $1,25(OH)_2D_3$-deficient subjects. There is some evidence for a direct action by this compound on renal absorption of calcium, while the effect on phosphorous absorption is probably an indirect phenomenon and related to the reactive decrease in PTH secretion to $1,25(OH)_2D_3$ replenishment.

The regulation of $1,25(OH)_2D_3$ production is controlled primarily at the step of 1-carbon hydroxylation in the kidney. The enzyme responsible for this reaction, **1α-hydroxylase,** is induced and activated by PTH and falls to very low levels quickly when PTH levels are low. 1,25-Dihydroxycholecalciferol itself provides negative feedback at both the hepatic and renal stages of hydroxylation.

OTHER HORMONES AFFECTING CALCIUM HOMEOSTASIS

A variety of other hormones have less prominent roles in calcium homeostasis. The effects of these hormones are realized over relatively longer periods of time (i.e., months and years) and have little to do with acute calcium regulation. Some of the more important hormones include **growth hormone**, the **somatomedins, thyroid hormone,** and the **gonadal hormones.** The latter influence overall bone mass, and their diminution in the elderly often leads to osteoporosis. Hyperthyroidism has been correlated with decreased bone mass as well, the mechanism of which is poorly understood. Glucocorticoids can lead to loss of skeletal mass, an effect thought to be primarily mediated through these compounds' antagonistic effects on $1,25(OH)_2D_3$.

DISORDERS AFFECTING CALCIUM HOMEOSTASIS

Hypercalcemia can occur whenever there is excess calcium input, via bone resorption or intestinal absorption, that exceeds the capacity of the kidneys to excrete it. **Primary hyperparathyroidism** results when there is excess and unregulated secretion of parathyroid hormone from adenomatous or hyperplastic parathyroid tissue. The classic symptoms of this disease include osteitis fibrosa cystica (osteoporosis), nephrolithiasis, and peptic ulcer disease. Central nervous system depression, mental aberrations, fatigability, weakness, constipation, and anorexia can all be a result of hypercalcemia. **Secondary hyperparathyroidism** is the normal response to hypocalcemia and is therefore easily distinguishable based on high PTH levels and normal or low serum calcium levels. **Tertiary hyperparathyroidism** results after prolonged secondary hyperparathyroidism renders the parathyroids insensitive to regulatory input. In this condition the parathyroid glands secrete autonomously, resulting in elevated PTH and calcium levels and the symptoms of classic hyperparathyroidism.

Hypoparathyroidism can be either primary or secondary in nature. The secondary form is the response to pathologic hypercalcemia. Primary hypoparathyroidism is either iatrogenic (e.g., a complication of thyroid surgery) or idiopathic. Treatment consists of dietary calcium and vitamin D supplements.

Vitamin D deficiency results in decreased intestinal calcium absorption, disrupting calcium/phosphorous homeostasis. It results in bone demineralization and is called **rickets** in children and **osteomalacia** in adults.

Pituitary

ANATOMY

The pituitary lies within the **sella turcica,** a small, bony depression in the sphenoid bone. Its substance is derived from two quite different embryological origins. The **posterior lobe,** or **neurohypophysis,** is derived from the brainstem while the **anterior lobe,** or **adenohypophysis,** is derived from the foregut. The anterior lobe has large polygonal cells surrounded by a sinusoidal capillary network. The secretory cells within this lobe can be identified with respect to which hormone they secrete using various stains, but there does not appear to be any significance to their location within the anterior lobe. The posterior lobe is composed of the infundibular stalk and the infundibular process, or neural lobe. The posterior lobe is a collection of large nonmyelinated nerve fibers with secretory granules. These fibers originate within the hypothalamus. They are also surrounded by a fenestrated capillary network that potentiates their secretory capacity.

The blood supply to the anterior lobe plays a vital role in the regulation of its activity. The blood supplying the anterior lobe is that which drains from the hypothalamus. Thus, hypothalamic secretory products in high concentrations ($\approx$1000-fold higher than systemic) serve to regulate the activity of many anterior pituitary functions. The posterior lobe, on the other hand, receives a standard arterial supply from the inferior hypophyseal arteries.

ANTERIOR PITUITARY PHYSIOLOGY

There are six major hormones that originate in the anterior pituitary, all known as **-tropic** or **-trophic** hormones for their influence and regulation of other organs. The end-organ targets of these hormones are the *thyroid, adrenal, mammary glands, gonads,* and general *body stature.* All of these hormones are polypeptide hormones produced by specific cells within the anterior pituitary. These compounds are stored within secretory granules in amounts large enough to satisfy physiologic demands for several days. These hormones and their actions are listed in Table 27-2.

Glycoprotein Hormones

Three of the six anterior pituitary hormones are glyco-proteins: (a) **thyroid-stimulating hormone (TSH),** whose only known function is to stimulate thyroid hormone secretion, and (b) two gonadotropins, **follicle-stimulating hormone (FSH)** and **luteinizing hormone (LH),** both of which are vital to proper gonadal function in both men and women. Follicle-stimulating hormone promotes ovarian follicle growth in women and spermatogenesis by testicular germinal epithelium in men. Luteinizing hormone induces ovulation and formation of the corpus luteum and also stimulates synthesis and secretion of estrogen and progesterone in women. Luteinizing hormone is equally important in male gonadal physiology because it stimulates the secretion of testosterone by gonadal interstitial cells.

Growth Hormone and Prolactin

Growth hormone is a necessary hormone for the attainment of normal adult stature. It has a variety of metabolic effects that may not be directly related to its growth-potentiating activity. Some of these actions include mobilization of free fatty acids from adipose tissue and inhibition of glucose metabolism in muscle and adipose tissue. Growth hormone is the most abundant of the anterior pituitary hormones and represents up to 10% of the dry weight of the gland. **Prolactin** is structurally related to growth hormone and is necessary for the postpartum production of milk in women. The function of prolactin in nonlactating women and men is unknown.

Adrenocorticotropins

Portions of the adrenal cortex are controlled by the anterior pituitary hormone **ACTH,** also known as **corticotropin** or **adrenocorticotropin.** There are several other anterior pituitary hormones closely related, genetically and structurally, to ACTH: (a) β- and γ-**lipo-**

TABLE 27-2. Anterior Pituitary Hormones

Hormone	Target	Major Actions in Humans
Glycoprotein family		
Thyroid-stimulating hormone (TSH), also called thyrotropin	Thyroid gland	Stimulates synthesis and secretion of thyroid hormones
Follicle-stimulating hormone (FSH)	Ovary	Stimulates growth of follicles and estrogen secretion
	Testis	Acts on Sertoli cells to promote maturation of sperm
Luteinizing hormone (LH), also called interstitial cell-stimulating hormone (ICSH)	Ovary	Stimulates ovulation of ripe follicle and formation of corpus luteum; stimulates estrogen and progesterone synthesis by corpus luteum
	Testis	Stimulates interstitial cells of Leydig to synthesize and secrete testosterone
Growth hormone/prolactin family		
Growth hormone (GH), also called somatotrophic hormone (STH)	Most tissues	Promotes growth in stature and mass; stimulates protein synthesis; usually inhibits glucose utilization and promotes fat utilization
Prolactin	Mammary glands	Promotes milk secretion
Proopiomelanocortin family (POMC)		
Adrenocorticotropic hormone (ACTH), also known as adrenocorticotropin or corticotropin	Adrenal cortex	Promotes synthesis and secretion of adrenal cortical hormones
β-Lipotropin, β-Endorphin	?	Physiological role not established

Reproduced from Goodman HM. *Basic medical endocrinology.* New York: Raven Press, 1988:31.

tropin, (b) α- and β-melanocyte-stimulating hormones, and (c) β-endorphin. Of these hormones, only ACTH has a clearly delineated role in humans.

REGULATION OF ANTERIOR PITUITARY FUNCTION

The secretion of anterior pituitary hormones is determined primarily by stimulation from the CNS (i.e., hypothalamic input) and secondarily by hormones produced in peripheral target tissues. When CNS input is interrupted, secretion of all anterior pituitary hormones, except prolactin, ceases. Prolactin appears to be secreted at a continuous basal rate and is predominantly *inhibited* by CNS input.

Communication between the CNS and the anterior pituitary takes place as a result of **hypophysiotropic hormones** that are delivered to the anterior pituitary via the hypothalamo-hypophyseal portal vascular system. These hormones are present in vanishingly scarce amounts (i.e., 0.1% of the scarcest anterior pituitary hormones). The first of these hormones isolated was **thyrotropin-releasing hormone,** the hormone responsible for TSH secretion. The names and actions of these hypophysiotropic hormones are listed in Table 27-3.

Follicle-stimulating hormone and LH are under the control of a single hypothalmic decapeptide, **gonadotropin-releasing hormone (GnRH),** also called **luteinizing hormone-releasing hormone,** in reference to its ability to promote LH release. Other factors that affect FSH and LH secretion account for their differential regulation, as GnRH stimulates both.

Growth hormone is stimulated by a releasing hormone, **growth hormone-releasing hormone,** and a release-inhibiting hormone, **somatostatin** or **somatotropin release-inhibiting factor.** These and several other CNS hormones whose actions are unclear are closely related to gastrointestinal hormones. Somatostatin analogues are used clinically to control pancreatic secretions in patients with enterocutaneous fistulas.

The regulatory effect of hormones secreted in response to pituitary hormone stimulation (e.g., thyroid hormone on TSH) is largely one of negative feedback. In the absence of end-organ hormone feedback, anterior pituitary secretion gradually increases under the stimulatory input from the CNS. Thus, end-organ feedback, in the form of hormone secretion, provides the down-regulation necessary for physiological control of anterior pituitary function. Little is known about the mechanism of the various negative-feedback loops. This negative effect could be realized through decreased sensitivity of the anterior pituitary to hypothalmic releasing factors, to direct inhibition of the hypothalmus, or to direct inhibition of anterior pituitary function.

In summary, the anterior pituitary is stimulated by CNS centers through the delivery of various releasing factors via the local portal circulation, and inhibited by the end-products (i.e., peripheral organ hormones) of its hormones (i.e., pituitary stimulating hormones) (Figure 27-3).

TABLE 27-3. Hypophysiotropic Hormones

Hormone	Amino Acids	Physiological Actions on the Pituitary
Corticotropin-releasing hormone (CRH)	41	Stimulates secretion of ACTH, β-LPH, and β-endorphin
Gonadotropin-releasing hormone (GnRH), originally called luteinizing hormone-releasing hormone (LHRH)	10	Stimulates secretion of FSH and LH
Growth hormone-releasing hormone (GHRH), somatocrinin	40 or 44	Stimulates GH secretion
Somatotropin release-inhibiting factor (SRIF); somatostatin	14 or 28	Inhibits secretion of GH
Prolactin-stimulating factor (?)	?	Stimulates prolactin secretion
Prolactin inhibiting factor (PIF)	Dopamine	Inhibits prolactin secretion
Thyrotropin-releasing hormone (TRH)	3	Stimulates secretion of TSH and prolactin

β-LPH, β-lipotropin.
Reproduced from Goodman HM. *Basic medical endocrinology.* New York: Raven Press, 1988:37.

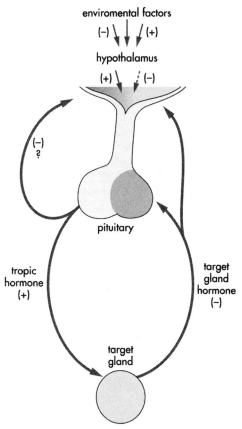

Figure 27-3 Environmental factors influence hypophysiotropic hormone secretion which, in turn, influences pituitary function. Negative feedback occurs through inhibition of pituitary or hypothalamic secretion by products of the end organ. (Reproduced from Goodman HM. *Basic medical endocrinology.* New York: Raven Press, 1988:40.)

POSTERIOR PITUITARY PHYSIOLOGY

The posterior pituitary secretes two products: **oxytocin** and **vasopressin** or **antidiuretic hormone (ADH)**. Both are nonapeptides whose structures differ by only two amino acids and probably originate from a single ancestral molecule. These hormones are stored in secretory granules in nerve terminals in the posterior pituitary gland bound to larger protein molecules called **neurophysins**. The neurophysins have no known physiological role. These hormones are synthesized within cell bodies located in the **paraventricular** and **supraoptic nuclei** of the hypothalamus and then transported down the axon to the nerve terminals in the posterior pituitary, where they are eventually secreted.

Oxytocin stimulates uterine contraction and mammary myoepithelial contraction. Oxytocin is released in response to sensory nerve input (e.g., cervical dilatation or infant suckling) and can be secreted as part of a conditioned response (e.g., secretion in a lactating mother in response to hearing a child's cry prior to suckling).

Vasopressin affects both the contraction of vascular smooth muscle to increase blood pressure and permeability of the renal tubule to promote water reabsorption in the face of hyperosmolality. Vasopressin is released as a result of increased osmolality sensed through cells located in the paraventricular and supraoptic nuclei, and through ill-defined intrathoracic volume receptors that relay their information via the CNS.

PITUITARY DISORDERS

Hypersecretion or hyposecretion of pituitary hormones may result from (a) developmental anomalies, (b) autoimmune disorders, (c) trauma, or (d) pituitary adenomas. Abnormal pituitary function can also be caused secondarily in the presence of end-organ or hypothalamic dysfunction. **Hypopituitarism** results in pituitary dwarfism when present in children and produces weakness, fatigability, headaches, and the signs and symptoms of decreased gonadotropin secretion (e.g., loss of menstrual cycles in women, loss of muscle mass and libido in men) in adults. **Acromegaly** or **gigantism** results from excessive growth hormone, usually from an adenoma. If it occurs before epiphyseal closure, a true giant results, whereas later in life it presents with thickened bone, skin, and overgrowth of visceral organs. **Hyperprolactinemia** is the most common form of excessive pituitary function and is the result of either multiple microadenomas or prolonged therapy with dopamine receptor blockers (e.g., often used in psychiatric disorders). Its primary symptoms relate to the disruption of gonadotropin function caused by excessive prolactin. In women it results in amenorrhea and galactorrhea, and in men, loss of libido and impotence.

Thyroid

The functions of the thyroid gland and its secreted hormones, **thyroxine (T_4)** and **triiodothyronine (T_3)**, are difficult to define specifically. Rather, these hormones are important *permissive* elements in the maturation and function of a number of body systems, most importantly, the musculoskeletal and nervous systems. Their function is best interpolated from the pathological manifestations seen in states of thyroid excess or deficiency.

ANATOMY

The thyroid gland lies below the strap muscles of the neck, inferior to the cricoid cartilage, adherent to the trachea at that level. It is composed of two lobes, right and left, connected by the isthmus. A variably present pyramidal lobe is found extending superiorly from the isthmus and is thought to represent an embryologic remnant of the thyroglossal duct. The thyroid normally weighs from 15 to 20 g but can hypertrophy to many times its original weight in pathologic conditions.

The blood supply to the gland is one of the richest in the body on basis of weight. Arterial supply is via paired superior and inferior thyroid arteries that arise from the external carotid artery and thyrocervical trunk, respectively. Paired superior, middle, and inferior thyroid veins drain into the jugular and innominate veins. The thyroid is also invested with rich lymphatic drainage and abundant autonomic innervation.

The gland itself is composed of follicles lined by cuboidal or columnar epithelium; the height is determined by the current state of epithelial stimulation. These epithelial cells are derived from pharyngeal endoderm. The follicles are filled with the glycoprotein **thyroglobulin**. Follicles are grouped into thyroid lobules that are supplied by a single artery. **Parafollicular, or C cells,** occupy positions between follicles and secrete calcitonin (see parathyroid section).

THYROID HORMONES

The thyroid hormones, T_4 and T_3, are both -amino acid derivatives of tyrosine. Both molecules are rich in iodine (i.e., T_3 has three iodine atoms; T_4 has four), which represents over half their molecular weight. T_4 was discovered first and is present in greatest quantity in the serum. T_3, discovered in 1953, is the more biologically potent of the two compounds.

The biosynthesis of the thyroid hormones has several unique and interesting aspects:

1. Concentration of a rare dietary constituent, iodine, is made possible by an iodide pump in follicular cells.
2. Partial synthesis occurs extracellularly at the luminal surface prior to deposition in follicles.
3. Previously synthesized thyroglobulin is taken up from the follicle for breakdown to T_3 and T_4, which

are then secreted into blood from the basal portion of the cell.
4. Extrathyroidal transformation of some T_4 to T_3 occurs.

The first step in this pathway is known as **iodine trapping.** Follicular cells can concentrate iodine up to 250 times serum levels. This is an active, energy-requiring process that can be competitively inhibited by other anions (e.g., pertechnetate, thiocyanate). **Thyroglobulin** is synthesized as a high-molecular-weight glycoprotein within the follicular cell and secreted into the lumen of the follicle via exocytosis. Iodination requires oxidation of iodine by a peroxidase on the apical border of the cells. It is on the apical surface of the cell at the time of, or shortly after, thyroglobulin exocytosis that iodination of this compound occurs. The tyrosine molecules of thyroglobulin ($\approx$20% of the amino acids) are either singly or doubly iodinated, through the action of the aforementioned peroxidase, to form monoiodotyrosine or diiodotyrosine. The next step, known as **coupling,** involves the joining of two diiodotyrosine molecules to form thyroglobulin-bound T_4. This occurs to about 20% of the iodinated tyrosine residues, the rest remaining as either monoiodotyrosine or diiodotyrosine or coupled as T_3, which is present in only very minute quantities. Once again, thyroid peroxidase plays an important role in this reaction, the exact mechanism of which is unclear. This precursor of the final T_4 remains incorporated in the much larger thyroglobulin molecule until the thyroid is stimulated by **TSH.** Under this influence, thyroglobulin is endocytosed by follicular cells into lysosomes where thyroglobulin is metabolized to its constituent amino acids, T_4, T_3, monoiodotyrosine, and diiodotyrosine. Thyroxine and T_3 (ratio 20:1) are then secreted via the basal membrane of the cell by simple diffusion down a concentration gradient. Monoiodotyrosine and di-iodotyrosine cannot be reutilized and are specifically deiodinated by a deiodinase allowing iodine recycling, which accounts for approximately twice the amount of iodine provided by the iodine pump. Follicular cells are thus able to participate in a simultaneous process of exocytosis and endocytosis of thyroglobulin in response to TSH and need for thyroid hormone (Figure 27-4).

REGULATION OF THYROID FUNCTION

Thyroid hormone secretion takes place autonomously but only in quantities insufficient to meet basal needs.

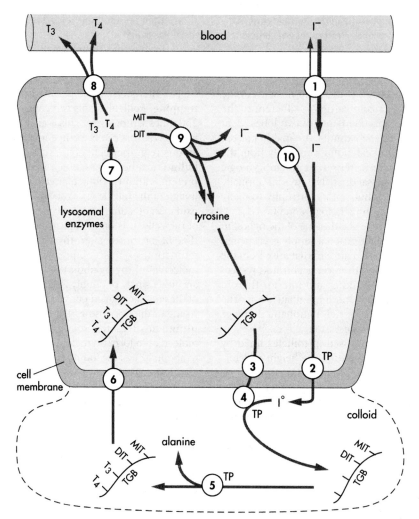

Figure 27-4 Follicular cell showing steps in synthesis and release of T_3 and T_4. TP, Thyroperoxidase; TGB; thyroglobulin. The numbers identify the major steps: **1**, trapping of iodide; **2**, oxidation of iodide; **3**, exocytosis of TGB; **4**, iodination of TGB; **5**, coupling of iodotyrosines; **6**, endocytosis of TGB; **7**, hydrolysis of TGB; **8**, release of T_3 and T_4; **9**, deiodination of monoiodotyrosine (MIT) and di-iodotyrosine (DIT); **10**, recycling of iodide. (Reproduced from Hedge GA, Colby HD, Goodman RL. *Clinical endocrine physiology.* Philadelphia: WB Saunders, 1987:105.)

The primary regulator of thyroid hormone secretion is **TSH,** a peptide secreted by the anterior pituitary. Under the influence of TSH, both thyroid blood flow and hormone secretion are elevated. Prolonged stimulation leads to thyroid hypertrophy and hyperplasia. Thyroid-stimulating hormone binds to specific receptors on the basal surface of follicular cells, stimulating intracellular cAMP production, which mediates an up-regulation of a variety of intracellular metabolic pathways. Phospholipid metabolism within the thyroid cell is also profoundly affected by TSH binding and may play a role in the activation of protein kinase C, another second messenger important in intracellular metabolic regulation.

Dietary iodine impedes hormone production when iodine is in short supply. Paradoxically, it temporarily also impedes production when present in excess. The gland eventually adapts and begins to increase production of thyroid hormone in the presence of excess iodine.

THYROID HORMONES IN BLOOD

Greater than 99% of thyroid hormone is bound to plasma proteins and is therefore biologically unavailable and not filtered by the glomerulus. Three proteins account for the vast majority of the binding: (1) **thyroxine-binding globulin,** which binds about 80% of both T_4 and T_3, (2) **thyroxine-binding prealbumin,** which binds about 15% of T_4 and 5% of T_3, and (3) **albumin,** which accounts for the rest. The remaining unbound hormone is responsible for all biologic activity and is in equilibrium with the bound hormone. Triiodothyronine is much less tightly bound by these proteins than is T_4.

THYROID HORMONE METABOLISM

The half-lives of T_4 and T_3 are 6.2 and 1.0 days, respectively. These values are increased in hypothyroid states and decreased in the milieu of hyperthyroidism. The first step in metabolism is the deiodination, usually in the liver or the kidney, of either the inner or outer rings of T_4 to form either reverse T_3 (rT_3, biologically inactive) or T_3, respectively. Considerable evidence suggests that the primary source of T_3 is the extrathyroidal metabolism of T_4. Thyroid hormones are also conjugated with glucuronic acid and secreted in the bile, from which they can be reabsorbed. Thyroxine is one of the few hormones sufficiently resistant to enteral digestion to permit effective oral therapy with the compound.

PHYSIOLOGICAL EFFECTS OF THYROID HORMONES

Thyroid hormone seems to play a role in the regulation of almost all cells, which is generally reflected as an increase or decrease in a given cell's primary function. An effect on gene regulation mediated by thyroid hormone has been postulated as a mechanism for this nonspecific effect.

Skeletal System

Thyroid hormone has profound effects on skeletal development. While independent of thyroid hormone in infancy, the skeleton is dependent on thyroid hormone for final maturation. Growth retardation and facial bone malformation may result in its absence (i.e., **cretinism**). It seems to be necessary for and synergistic with the secretion of growth hormone and several other hormones important to musculoskeletal growth.

Central Nervous System

The presence of thyroid hormone is vital to the proper development of the the brain and to the myelination of peripheral nerves during the fetal and infant stages of development. Excess or deficiency of the hormone leads to either hyperexcitability and restlessness or lethargy and apathy, respectively, in adult subjects.

Autonomic Nervous System

Many of the physical findings associated with hyperthyroidism (e.g., tachycardia, increased cardiac output) and hypothyroidism are a result of the pronounced effects of thyroid hormone on the sympathetic branch of the autonomic nervous system.

Metabolism

Thyroid hormone has profound effects on oxidative metabolism. The basal metabolic rate is quite sensitive to thyroid hormone. Heat sensitivity in patients with hyperthyroidism is thought to be a result of the excess energy released by oxidative metabolism within the mitochondria.

Carbohydrate and Lipid Metabolism

Numerous aspects of carbohydrate (e.g., glucose absorption from the gut, glycogenolysis, gluconeogenesis) and lipid metabolism (e.g., lipolysis) are all stimulated by excess T_3 and T_4. No specific mechanisms have been identified to explain this observation.

Nitrogen Metabolism

Degradative effects predominate in thyroid excess leading to severe muscle catabolism. In deficiency states there is a characteristic extracellular accumulation of mucuslike materials (e.g., hyaluronic acid and chondroitin) that lead to osmotic retention of water and the characteristic physical findings of **myxedema.**

Temperature Maintenance

Temperature maintenance is largely dependent on shivering and nonshivering (i.e., metabolic) thermogenesis. While the exact role of thyroid hormone is not well understood, it is felt that potentiation of the sympathetic nervous system by thyroid hormone is important in maintenance of the nonshivering component of thermogenesis.

MECHANISM OF THYROID HORMONE ACTION

Most evidence favors a role for thyroid hormone at the intranuclear level, where it binds to the genome and assists in regulating in gene transcription. Cytosolic and mitochondrial effects, while theorized, are even less well understood. Both T_3 and T_4 pass freely into the cell as a result of their hydrophobicity.

REGULATION OF SECRETION

Thyroid-stimulating hormone is responsible for the primary regulation of the thyroid gland and, in turn, is stimulated by **thyrotropin-releasing hormone** secreted by the anterior pituitary. Thyrotropin-releasing hormone appears to be secreted in a rather constant fashion. Regulation is therefore achieved via the negative feedback of T_3 and T_4 on the sensitivity of TSH secretion to thyrotropin-releasing hormone stimulation. It is for this reason that the evaluation of serum TSH is critical to the evaluation of thyroid dysfunction.

THYROID DISORDERS

Hyperthyroidism presents classically with symptoms of elevated basal metabolic rate, heat intolerance, warm skin, and excessive perspiration. Muscle wasting and weight loss often occur in the face of increased caloric intake. Hyperthyroidism has several etiologies, resulting from an abnormality in either the gland itself or in its regulation. **Grave's disease** is a form of hyperthyroidism in which patients have very low serum levels of TSH despite the fact that a factor present in their serum can be shown to directly stimulate the gland. This factor, often referred to as **long-acting thyroid stimulators (LATS)**, is an immunoglobulin (i.e., IgG) with specificity for the TSH receptor. It can thus simulate TSH in binding to the cell.

Hypothyroidism results in symptoms opposite those of hyperthyroidism—reduced basal metabolic rate; cold intolerance; cool, dry skin; coarse hair; and a coarse voice. Infiltration of the skin with mucopolysaccharides results in **myxedema.** CNS effects include slow mentation, slow speech, poor memory, and occasional personality disorders. Congenital hypothyroidism, **cretinism,** results in dwarfism, mental retardation, and a puffy face with a protruding tongue.

Male Gonadal System

The principal hormone of the male reproductive system is **testosterone.** This hormone is responsible for both promotion of spermatogenesis as well as physical and behavioral sexual differentiation necessary for effective procreative function.

ANATOMY

The testes are paired ovoid organs in the scrotal sac. Intratesticular temperature within the scrotal sac is approximately 2°C lower than the core body temperature and is essential for normal spermatogenesis. The two primary functions of the testis are sperm production and steroid hormone production. These functions are carried out in two morphologically different compartments. The sperm are generated within the seminiferous tubules, which constitute the bulk of testicular mass, while testosterone is produced by the interstitial cells, or **Leydig cells** dispersed between the seminiferous tubules. Blood supply is via paired spermatic arteries. Blood is cooled initially through heat exchange with venous blood in the pampiniform plexus, where both vessels intermingle in a tortuous fashion. The seminiferous tubules are composed of (a) **spermatogonia** (i.e., stem cells), (b) **spermatocytes** (i.e., immature sperm), and (c) **Sertoli cells,** responsible for a variety of functions necessary to nurture and promote spermatogenesis. The Sertoli cells are responsible for the "**blood-testis barrier,**" the physiological significance of which is unclear. The blood-testis barrier refers to the fact that developing spermatids rely solely on Sertoli cells for their vitality and that only certain molecules are permeable from the blood to the intraluminal portion of the seminiferous tubules. The spermatogonia are on the blood side of the barrier, while the spermatocytes are on the luminal side of the blood-testis barrier.

TESTICULAR ENDOCRINE FUNCTION

Follicle-stimulating hormone (FSH) and **LH** are pituitary hormones and the primary stimuli for testicular growth and function. Follicle-stimulating hormone acts on germinal epithelium, while LH exerts its stimulatory effects on Leydig cells. The primary function of Leydig cells is the synthesis and secretion of testosterone in response to stimulation by LH. Binding of LH on the surface of Leydig cells initiates a series of intracellular events mediated by cAMP, protein kinase A, and elements of the phospholipid-calcium-calmodulin system. The rate-determining step in the steroid synthetic pathway of testosterone is the conversion of cholesterol to pregnenolone.

Testosterone is the primary secretory androgen product of the mature male testis. Approximately 7 mg is secreted each day, of which less than 5% is of adrenal origin. Testosterone is present in concentrations comparable to adult values in fetal life, then regresses to very low levels until puberty, when it gradually rises to achieve its physiologic adult concentration. While there is some decrease in testosterone production with age, it is present in considerable quantity throughout male maturity, and there is no sudden decrease in production comparable to the cessation of estrogen production in postmenopausal women.

Testosterone is present as free hormone in the blood in only minute amounts (approximately 2–3%) with most bound to either albumin (30%) or **sex hormone-binding globulin,** also called **testosterone-estradiol-binding globulin.** Only unbound hormone is physiologically active and diffuses out of capillaries into both target and nontarget tissues. Various tissues convert testosterone to other steroid products (e.g., estradiol and estrone), depending on their metabolic capabilities.

Testosterone realizes its end-organ effects through the regulation of genetic elements within its target tissues. It is bound to the genetic material in complex with various intracellular proteins that, together, promote the transcription and eventual translation of specific genes.

Testosterone primarily promotes the growth, differentiation, and function of those organs involved in sexual function. It has profound effects on the differentiation of the genital tract in embryonic life and is responsible for maintenance of the body habitus, seminal vesicle secretory epithelium, and behavioral aspects of sexual function in adult life. Urogenital development in the fetus proceeds toward the female phenotype unless actively suppressed by the presence of testosterone and its by-products. Müllerian duct (female urogenital precursor) differentiation is suppressed by a factor from the wolffian ducts (male urogenital precursor), the differentiation and maintenance of which is dependent on testosterone.

The exact role of testosterone in spermatogenesis is unclear. Testosterone is permeable across the blood-testis barrier and is found in concentrations 40–50-fold higher in seminiferous fluid than in plasma. While FSH is vital to the initiation of spermatogenesis, once initiated, it can be maintained with sufficient levels of testosterone or LH alone.

REGULATION OF TESTICULAR FUNCTION

Testicular stimulation and maintenance is dependent on pituitary secretion of FSH and LH, which are in turn dependent on GnRH delivered from the CNS via the hypothalamic-hypophyseal portal circulation. Negative feedback is supplied via signals related to testicular function: steroidogenesis and gametogenesis.

Gonadotropin-releasing hormone is released in discrete pulses that range from 1 to 3 hours apart. The duration of each pulse is only several minutes. The pulsatile nature of GnRH secretion is essential to its activity, and the pituitary is rendered unresponsive to GnRH when a high concentration is maintained.

Testosterone functions as a mediator of negative feedback for the secretion of LH from its pituitary origin without affecting FSH production from the same cell. Feedback inhibition of FSH secretion is thought to occur as a result of a compound released during gametogenesis, **inhibin.** This compound is likely secreted by Sertoli cells, as well as ovarian granulosa cells. In addition, there are numerous other regulatory pathways relating to gonadal function.

DISORDERS OF MALE GONADAL FUNCTION

Postpubertal infertility is usually nonendocrine in origin, while prepubertal infertility is usually endocrine in nature, resulting from the failure of sexual maturation based on an endocrine deficiency. Endocrine hypogonadism is further divided into primary (gonadal) or secondary (pituitary) forms. The former is called **hypergonadotropic hypogonadism** since LH and FSH levels are elevated in the face of decreased serum testosterone levels and insufficient negative feedback. The latter is called **hypogonadotropic hypogonadism**, since it is a result of deficient LH and/or FSH secretion. **Klinefelter's syndrome** is a genetic abnormality in which the sex chromosome complement is XXY. Occurring in 0.2% of the population, it results in almost total loss of gonadal function.

Hypergonadism (true precocious puberty) can be either neural or idiopathic in origin. Neural etiologies of hypergonadism result from brain tumors that cause the deregulation of GnRH secretion and must be treated as aggressive malignancies. **Pseudoprecocious puberty** results from increased circulating androgen levels owing to ectopic LH or androgen production. The most common etiology of this disorder is **congenital adrenal hyperplasia (adrenogenital syndrome)**, which is the result of an enzyme deficiency preventing or decreasing glucocorticoid production and shunting precursors into the androgen-synthetic pathways.

Female Gonadal System

The ovaries are analogous to the testicles in their dual role as producer of gametes and hormones but, unlike the male, produce only a single gamete at a time for potential fertilization. The primary ovarian hormones are **estradiol** and **progesterone**, both steroids.

Ovarian function is dependent on two pituitary hormones, **FSH and LH**, which stimulate ovarian steroid production, growth of the follicle, ovulation, and corpus luteum development. These hormones are released as a result of hypothalamic stimulation in the form of **GnRH** and complex inhibitory and stimulatory input from the ovarian steroids.

ANATOMY

The **ovaries** are paired, flattened, ellipsoid structures approximately 5 cm in their greatest dimension. They are located within the pelvis, attached to the broad ligaments that extend from either side of the uterus by peritoneal folds called the mesovaria. The cortex of each ovary consists of primordial follicles, developing follicles, stromal or interstitial cells, and the corpus luteum. The medulla consists primarily of vascular elements that arise from collaterals between the uterine and ovarian arteries. Unmyelinated nerve fibers also enter the ovarian medulla with the blood vessels.

The human female has approximately 2–4 million primordial follicles, each consisting of a primary oocyte surrounded by a single layer of **granulosa cells,** encased by a basement membrane. Only a small fraction of these oocytes are recruited with each menstrual cycle for possible fertilization and only one actually matures to ovulation. Reproductive capacity continues until the supply of primordial follicles is exhausted at menopause.

Follicular development is a complex process that begins with the primordial follicle. Initially the granulosa cells begin to proliferate, which in turn gives rise to the stimulation of surrounding stromal cells that coalesce around the follicle. These stromal cells are called **thecal cells.** They develop many of the characteristics of steroid-producing cells, with a rich endoplasmic reticulum. The **theca interna,** or internal layer of thecal cells, is richly vascularized and is responsible for the nutrition and sustenance of the enlarging mass of granulosa cells surrounding the oocyte. The granulosa cells and oocyte are dependent on this transmembrane diffusion of oxygen and nutrients across the basement membrane that isolates them from the systemic blood stream. Gradually, fluid accumulates within the follicle and it becomes an **antral** or **graafian follicle.** As the follicle enlarges from its original diameter of 15 μm to its final diameter of 10–20 mm (i.e., 1000-fold increase in diameter), it migrates to the ovarian surface and finally ruptures, extruding a single oocyte surrounded by a corona of granulosa cells.

Following ovulation, there is ingrowth and differentiation of the remaining granulosa cells, thecal cells, and stromal cells to form a new structure, the **corpus luteum.** Unless a pregnancy ensues, the corpus luteum remains for approximately two weeks, leaving a small scar on the surface of the ovary.

Only about 500 follicles ever ovulate in the reproductive lifetime of a woman. More than 90% of primordial follicles undergo partial development and atresia during the prepubertal period. Many of the remaining follicles undergo a similar fate in adulthood. The physiological reasons behind this apparent underutilization of available gametes is not understood.

The **fallopian tubes (oviducts)** and **uterus** are the route of ova delivery and site of embryo development, respectively. They are both derived from the müllerian ducts, as is the upper portion of the vagina.

The fallopian tubes are paired tubular structures whose open ends terminate in fingerlike projections called **fimbriae** near each ovary. Ciliated cells line the fallopian tubes and are responsible for oocyte nutrition and delivery of the oocyte to the uterus for fertilization. The nongravid uterus is a small, pear-shaped structure approximately 6–7 cm in its greatest diameter. Its outer portion consists of smooth muscle, and its inner portion and secretory layer of **endometrial cells.** The endometrial layer varies in thickness, depending on the hormonal environment, and is sloughed with each menstrual cycle. The uterus is capable of massive hypertrophy and distension during pregnancy.

OVARIAN HORMONES

The principal ovarian hormones are **estrogens (17β-estradiol** and **estrone)** and **progesterone.** Estrogens are generally responsible for sexual receptivity. They vary 20-fold in serum concentration in the course of a reproductive cycle. As with most steroid hormones, little is stored intracellularly. In the blood, estrogens are loosely bound to albumin and tightly bound to **testosterone-estradiol-binding globulin.** The liver is the principal site of metabolic destruction of estrogens.

Progesterone plays its most prominent role during pregnancy. Outside the pregnant state, progesterone production is largely confined to corpus luteum cells. In the blood, progesterone is loosely bound to a number of plasma proteins but has a high affinity for **corticosteroid-binding globulin.** As with estrogens, the liver is the primary site of progesterone catabolism.

The production of **estrogen** and **progesterone** are intimately tied to the stimulation of the ovary and development of the oocyte. These hormones are responsible for the extra-ovarian changes in the female reproductive tract and other organs necessary to support potential fertilization and pregnancy. Estradiol stimulates the growth of reproductive tract structures that are responsible for sperm reception, facilitation of fertilization, and providing an environment for embryo development. Estradiol also acts to stimulate granulosa cell proliferation, with the ovarian follicle thus enhancing its own production. Progesterone is produced by the corpus luteum, a structure that arises from the ovarian follicle once the ovum is released. It prepares the uterus for implantation and embryo growth and is absolutely required for successful maintenance of pregnancy. These hormones are important in subprimate species as an impetus for copulation, but androgens alone provide libido in both the male and female human.

Estrogens and progesterone usually act in concert, both to enhance and to antagonize each other's actions. Estrogen production is usually necessary to prime target tissues for sensitivity to progesterone through the induction of progesterone receptors. Progesterone induces the turnover of estrogen receptors, thus decreasing the response to estrogens and eventually progesterone. The effects of estrogen and progesterone on the female reproductive tract are outlined in Table 27-4.

Estrogen and progesterone have a variety of effects on the body not directly related to reproductive function. Effects on the breast are discussed in the following section. Estrogen contributes to the pubertal growth spurt; the closing of the epiphyseal plates; widening of the pelvis; increased synthesis of steroid- and thyroid-hormone binding proteins; and, to a lesser degree, behavioral patterns. Progesterone has a thermogenic effect, raising basal body temperature approximately 1°C. This effect is the basis for temperature monitoring of the female to detect the time of ovulation in those trying either to conceive or avoid conception. Progesterone also has effects on the central nervous system, with changes in mood and behavior seen when it is withdrawn. This action of progesterone is postulated to be the basis of postpartum psychic depression.

Relaxin is a peptide ovarian hormone, originally described on the basis of its ability to relax the pubic ligament of pregnant guinea pigs. In the human it also relaxes myometrium. Its precise physiologic role has not been determined.

TABLE 27-4. Effects of Estrogen and Progesterone on the Female Reproductive Tract

Organ	Estrogen	Progesterone
Oviducts		
Lining	↑ Cilia formation and activity	↑ Secretion
Muscular wall	↑ Contractility	↓ Contractility
Uterus		
Endometrium	↑ Proliferation	↑ Differentiation and secretion
Myometrium	↑ Growth and contractility	↓ Contractility
Cervical glands	Watery secretion	Dense, viscous secretion
Vagina	↑ Epithelial proliferation ↑ Glycogen deposition	↑ Differentiation ↓ Proliferation

Reproduced from Goodman HM. *Basic medical endocrinology.* New York: Raven Press, 1988:292.

CONTROL OF OVARIAN FUNCTION

Follicular development beyond the antral stage depends on the pituitary hormones **FSH** and **LH** as well as estrogens and androgens. FSH and LH are also important in a variety of other ovarian functions, including (a) ovulation, (b) corpus luteum steroid production, and (c) luteinization. The regulation and differentiation of the preantral follicle is poorly understood.

The **ovarian cycle**, averaging 28 days, consists of two phases: (1) the **follicular phase** (14 days) and (2) the **luteal phase** (14 days). The granulosa cell is the principal target of FSH and is the only cell in the female known to have FSH receptors. Granulosa cells secrete estrogens in response to FSH. Thecal cells, especially those of the theca interna, are the primary target of LH. Luteinizing hormone stimulates these cells to secrete steroid hormones, which are responsible for adjacent stromal hypertrophy. Follicular development depends on estradiol, which acts in an autocrine or paracrine manner. One of its primary effects is to increase the sensitivity of granulosa cells to FSH. An interdependence between the theca and granulosa cells exists in the production of estrogen. Theca cells effectively produce large quantities of androgens, and granulosa cells, large quantities of 21-carbon steroid precursors. The granulosa cells have the enzymes the theca cells lack to convert the androgens to estrogens, and the theca cells have the appropriate enzymes to convert the 21-carbon precursors to androgens, which can then be metabolized to estrogens by the granulosa cells. Follicular development and hormone secretion is thus dependent on both pituitary hormones.

Luteinizing hormone is the physiologic signal for ovulation, its concentration rising sharply in the blood approximately 16 hours prior to ovulation. The initiation of ovulation is a complex process that requires both LH and FSH. Progesterone and prostaglandins also appear to play critical roles. Tissue plasminogen activator and other hydrolytic enzymes appear to participate in the dissolution of the collagen framework necessary for rupture of the follicle.

Luteinizing hormone also initiates the luteinization process, probably just prior to ovulation. Occasionally, luteinization occurs in the absence of ovulation leading to luteinization of unruptured follicles and infertility in the affected female. Steroid production by the corpus luteum depends on continued stimulation by LH.

REGULATION OF THE REPRODUCTIVE CYCLE

The central event of each menstrual cycle is ovulation, triggered by a massive surge in the serum levels of LH. Following ovulation the ovum can be successfully fertilized for a period of approximately 24 hours. If this does not occur, the cycle must be renewed and a new oocyte recruited for ovulation and potential fertilization. These events require a complex network of intercommunication between the pituitary, the ovaries, and the female reproductive tract which is mediated by hormones (Figure 27-5).

Follicle-stimulating hormone and LH both demonstrate a sharp peak in concentration at the time of ovulation, which must be timed with maturation of an ovarian follicle. These two hormones are otherwise at a basal level throughout both follicular and luteal phases of the cycle except for some minor variations in FSH concentrations. Estradiol levels rise gradually in the follicular phase at an increasing rate reaching a maximum approximately 12 hours prior to the LH peak. Following this, the level falls again to basal levels, then rises to approximately 50% of its peak concentration for a period of about seven days during the midluteal period of the cycle. Progesterone is low during the follicular phase, then rises gradually during the luteal phase before descending at about the same rate as the luteal phase concludes.

The regulation of FSH and LH secretion during the reproductive cycle is the result of a complex set of positive- and negative-feedback loops involving estrogen, progesterone, GnRH, and hypothalamic mechanisms responsible for the pulsatile secretion of GnRH. Estrogen acts as both a negative and a positive feedback to LH secretion during a given cycle. The attainment of a critical estrogen concentration necessary to achieve positive rather than negative feedback on LH secretion is the central event in the reproductive cycle, signaling readiness of the follicle for ovulation. The timing of reproductive cycles is not a result of pulsatile GnRH secretion, as one might expect. Rather the developing follicle is responsible for the signal (i.e., thecal production of estrogen) that allows the surge in LH resulting in ovulation. A discussion of the complex regulation of FSH and LH secretion, hypothalamic control of GnRH secretion, and other complex pathways in the female reproductive cycle is beyond the scope of this text.

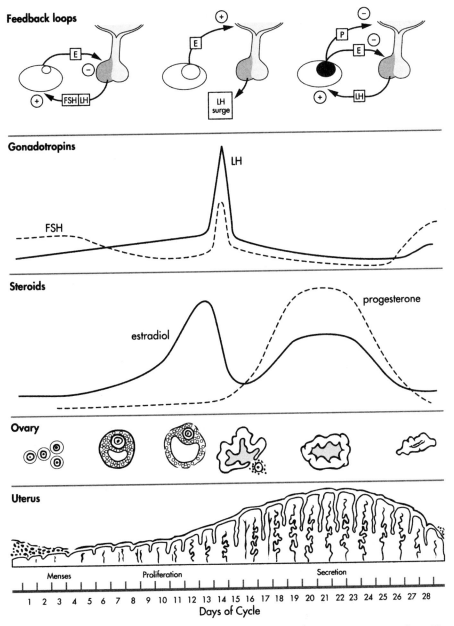

Figure 27-5 Events of the menstrual cycle. (Reproduced from Hedge GA, Colby HD, Goodman RL. *Clinical endocrine physiology*. Philadelphia: WB Saunders, 1987:211.)

FEMALE REPRODUCTIVE DISORDERS

Amenorrhea usually results from inadequate ovarian function. **Primary amenorrhea** is the absence of menses in women who have never menstruated, while **secondary amenorrhea** is the cessation of menses in menstruating women. While these two clinical presentations can represent identical pathologies, the incidence of etiologies is quite different in each. In patients with primary amenorrhea, developmental anomalies of the reproductive tract are common with **gonadal dysgenesis** being the most common. The most common cause of secondary amenorrhea is, of course, pregnancy. Hyperprolactinemia, extreme weight loss or gain, and psychological disorders can all be causes of pathologic secondary amenorrhea.

True precocious puberty and **pseudoprecocious puberty** can occur in females as in males. Pseudoprecocious puberty is especially important to recognize, as it can result from ovarian tumors, in contrast to the male situation, which is very rarely due to gonadal malignancy. Excessive ovarian hormone secretion results in symptoms similar to hypofunction—namely, oligomenorrhea and amenorrhea. The most common etiology of excessive ovarian function is **polycystic ovary syndrome,** the result of numerous atretic follicles in an ovary that secretes excess androgen but a paucity of estradiol.

Breast

ANATOMY

The breast is an exocrine gland derived from the skin of the chest wall. It is composed of 12–20 glandular lobes, or **acini,** each of which drains via a **lactiferous duct** to the surface of the breast at the **areola.** These lobes are composed of a network of **intralobar ducts,** which drain the **mammary alveoli.** The mammary alveoli are lined by milk-secreting epithelial cells and surrounded by a network of myoepithelial cells that effect milk secretion when they contract. The breast is innervated with sympathetic nervous fibers and has a rich sensory network to the nipple and areola. Extensive lymphatic drainage of the breast terminates in the (a) axillary, (b) interpectoral, and (c) internal mammary lymph node groups. Fibrous septa, known as **Cooper's ligaments,** interdigitate the glandular lobes of the breast and form a fibrous connection from the pectoral fascia to the skin.

GROWTH AND DEVELOPMENT

Growth and development of the human breast is sex-independent (i.e., identical in male and female) until the onset of puberty. **Estrogen** initiates growth and proliferation of the duct system. **Progesterone** in combination with estrogen influences lobuloalveolar growth. Both of these hormones can act only in the permissive environment of several other hormones: **prolactin, growth hormone,** and **cortisol.**

LACTATION

Lactation is dependent on (a) a well-developed secretory apparatus and (b) continued episodic stimulation with high concentrations of **prolactin.** Numerous other hormones are involved in a more peripheral manner (e.g., adrenal glucocorticoids, insulin, human chorionic somatomammotropin). Lactation is prevented during gestation by the interference of estrogen and progesterone, which are present in very high levels, on prolactin stimulation of the milk-secreting epithelium. At parturition this blockade is removed (as estrogen and progesterone levels fall precipitously) and prolactin receptors on the alveolar epithelium increase dramatically, allowing the high levels of prolactin to initiate lactation. Milk production is continued through the neuroendocrine reflex generated by suckling. Suckling initiates both prolactin secretion and **oxytocin** release. The prolactin release insures continued production of milk for future feedings. Oxytocin is a necessary stimulus for myoepithelial cell contraction that causes milk ejection, without which the milk would not be delivered to the feeding child.

PROLACTIN AND FERTILITY

Prolactin is secreted at low levels throughout life regardless of sex. Prolactin receptors are present in the gonads and reproductive tracts of both sexes. Physiological effects of prolactin, outside its role in lactation, are unknown. The high levels of prolactin seen in the nursing female correlate with the nursing mother's failure to resume normal ovarian cycles and thus her relative infertility. Prolactin-secreting tumors (i.e., pituitary microadenomas) cause infertility and amenorrhea. The mechanism by which prolactin suppresses ovarian function is unclear but has been correlated with suppression of gonadotropin release.

HORMONE RECEPTORS AND ENDOCRINE THERAPY IN BREAST MALIGNANCY

The intracellular receptors for the steroids, estrogen and progesterone, are routinely measured in breast-malignancy specimens to determine the patient's potential for response to hormonal therapy. **Estrogen receptor protein (ERP)** is the clinically most important and routinely measured. About 50% of all primary tumors are positive for this receptor, the most common being well-differentiated ductal and lobular carcinomas, of which approximately 90% are positive. Response to hormonal therapy correlates with the presence and quantity of ERP. Response to hormonal therapy (i.e., tamoxifen) in ERP-positive tumors is 50–60%; and in ERP-negative tumors, less than 10%.

Progesterone receptors are found in about 40% of all ERP-positive tumors. When both receptors are present the response to therapy is 77%. Tumors that are ERP positive and progesterone-receptor negative have a lower response rate, about 20–30%.

Tamoxifen, a nonsteroid amino-ether derivative of a polycyclic phenol, blocks the intracellular estrogen receptor and is the most widely used hormonal antitumor agent, largely because of its lack of toxicity and paucity of side effects. It is used with and without other chemotherapy as a prophylactic agent (i.e., patients with disease-free margins) and in advanced metastatic disease. It *can* effect a remission in advanced disease and increases the *disease-free survival* when used prophylactically, with or without other chemotherapy. Of note, it has *not affected overall survival* when used prophylactically, with or without other chemotherapy.

Other forms of hormonal therapy in breast cancer have included (a) castration, (b) hypophysectomy-adrenalectomy, (c) medical adrenalectomy (aminoglutethimide), and (d) additive hormonal therapy (i.e., supplemental estrogens, androgens, and progestational agents). Most of these therapies are directed at reducing circulating estrogens and androgens that are important to the hormonal maintenance of normal and, presumably, malignant breast tissue. Why the *addition* of these hormones occasionally induces regression is unclear but well documented. In general these forms of therapy are capable only of inducing a temporary regression in advanced metastatic disease, are fraught with multiple and serious side effects, and are not widely used.

Adrenal Glands

The adrenal glands are complex multifunctional organs that influence homeostatic mechanisms both acutely and chronically throughout the body. They are composed of a cortex responsible for steroid hormone synthesis and a medulla responsible for the production of a number of sympathomimetic compounds that are secreted in response to various forms of physiological stress. The steroid hormones are grouped into three general classes: (1) **mineralocorticoids,** whose actions defend the body content of sodium and potassium; (2) **glucocorticoids,** whose actions affect body fuel metabolism, responses to injury, and general cellular function; and (3) **androgens,** whose actions are similar to those of the hormone of the male gonad. Mineralocorticoid secretion is largely regulated by the kidney and the renin-angiotensin system, while glucocorticoid and androgen secretion is regulated by the anterior pituitary through the secretion of **ACTH.** The medulla functions in parallel fashion to the sympathetic nervous system and is best appreciated as a more central component of the sympathetic nervous response. In general, the cortical hormones are responsible for modulation of tissue sensitivity to medullary hormones and other hormones (i.e., chronic adjustments), while the medullary hormones are acute, fast-acting responses to physiologic stimuli (i.e., acute stress response).

ANATOMY

The adrenals are bilateral structures situated anatomically atop the superior pole of each kidney. The outer part, or **cortex,** of the gland accounts for approximately 75% of the total weight and is divided into three sections: (1) the **zona glomerulosa,** or outer zone, which produces the mineralocorticoid aldosterone; and (2) the **zona fasciculata,** a layer of radially aligned cells that shares responsibility for the production of cortisol and adrenal androgens with (3) the **zona reticularis,** an inner layer represented histologically as a tangled network of cells adjacent to the medulla. The cortex is derived from mesenchymal cells. The **medulla,** or central area of the adrenal, is a modified sympathetic ganglion responsible for the release of **epinephrine** and **norepinephrine** into the venous effluent of the adrenal in response to acute physiologic stress. The blood supply to the adrenals is rich and arises mostly from short arterial branches directly off the aorta or renal arteries, and venous return is via veins that empty directly into the vena cava or renal vein.

ADRENAL CORTEX

The adrenal cortex is a vital structure, the absence of which results in death within one to two weeks in all species. Surgical or pathologic destruction of the adrenal cortex results in profound dysfunction of almost every organ system, largely as a result of circulatory collapse initiated by severe hyponatremia (i.e., lack of mineralocorticoid) and hypoglycemia without active carbohydrate intake (i.e., lack of glucocorticoids). Indeed, the adrenal cortical hormones are divided into these two categories based on their ability to protect against these two causes of death.

Aldosterone is the most potent and physiologically significant mineralocorticoid produced by the adrenal cortex. **Cortisol** and, to a lesser extent, **corticosterone** are the physiologically important glucocorticoids responsible for maintaining carbohydrate reserves. Both mineralocorticoids and glucocorticoids may exhibit properties of the other class of hormones when present in high concentrations. Androgens are also synthesized in the adrenal cortex and are very similar to gonadal steroid products. In some abnormal conditions the adrenal may secrete any of the gonadal steroids.

All of the cortical hormones are steroids synthesized from a common precursor, cholesterol. The synthetic pathways and organic chemistry of these compounds is beyond the scope of this review. Cholesterol is taken up by the adrenal cell via receptor specific binding of **low-density lipoprotein**, a cholesterol-rich lipid transport molecule, and manufactured within the adrenal cell from carbohydrate and fatty acid precursors. The rate-limiting step of adrenal steroid synthesis is the series of reactions required to convert the 27-carbon cholesterol molecule to the 21-carbon **pregnenolone** molecule, the common precursor of all adrenal and gonadal hormones (Figure 27-6). By virtue of the fact that the zona glomerulosa cells lack a specific enzyme (17α-hydroxylase), they are capable only of producing corticosterone, aldosterone, and deoxycorticosterone. Steroid hormones can be generally grouped into three structural categories:

1. **21-Carbon atoms**
   Progesterone (see above)
   Deoxycorticosterone (potent mineralocorticoid but produced in small quantities)
   Corticosterone (glucocorticoid of minor importance in humans)
   Aldosterone (the primary human mineralocorticoid)
   Cortisol (the primary human glucocorticoid)
   Cortisone
2. **19-Carbon atoms**
   Generally have **androgenic** activity and serve as precursors for estrogens
   Testosterone (see above)
3. **18-Carbon atoms**
   Generally have **estrogenic** activity

As with all steroid hormones, there is no intracellular storage form of these lipid-soluble, membrane-permeable compounds. Increased demand is met by a direct increase in synthesis and the hormone is simply excreted down a concentration gradient across the cell membrane.

Adrenal cortical hormones are transported in blood bound to a specific plasma protein, **transcortin** or **corticosteroid-binding globulin,** as well as to albumin. **Corticosteroid-binding globulin** has a single steroid binding site with an affinity for glucocorticoids about five times higher than for aldosterone. Approximately 75% of glucocorticoids and 50% of aldosterone are protein-bound in the blood, which probably accounts for their relatively long half-lives (i.e., 90 and 30 minutes, respectively). Inactivation occurs through metabolic alteration of steroids in the liver. Breakdown products excreted in the urine include **17-hydroxycorticosteroids** from cortisol and **17-ketosteroids** from glucocorticoids and androgens.

MINERALOCORTICOIDS

Many of the adrenal cortical hormones have some mineralocorticoid activity, but aldosterone is the only physiologically significant mineralocorticoid. Absence of aldosterone causes a massive loss of sodium and consequently extracellular fluid. Secondary consequences of this primary insult include retention of water, which worsens the hyponatremia; impaired potassium excretion, leading to hyperkalemia; and diarrhea, which can aggravate the hypovolemia. Aldosterone is required for only 2% of the total sodium reabsorption from glomerular filtrate through its action on the cortical collecting duct. While seemingly small, this corresponds to the amount of sodium present in approximately 3.5 *liters* of extracellular fluid.

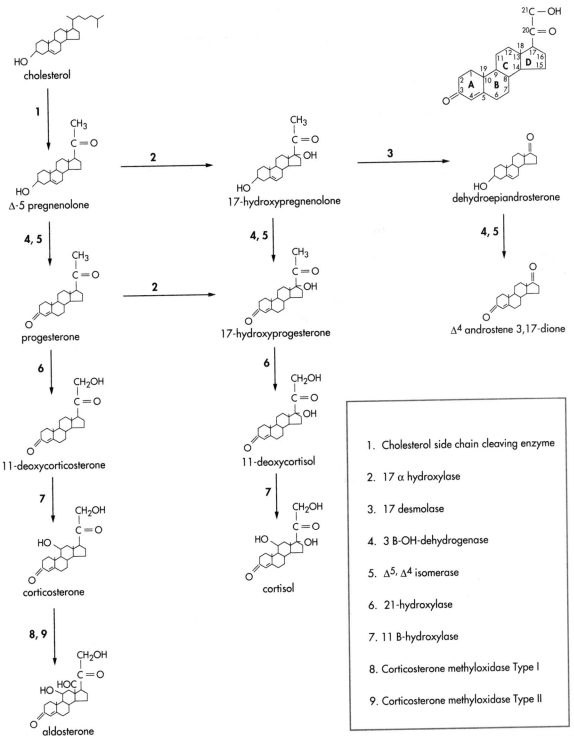

Figure 27-6 Steroid hormone biosynthetic pathways (Reproduced from Sabiston DC, ed. *Textbook of surgery: the biological basis of modern surgical practice.* 13th ed. Philadelphia: WB Saunders, 1986:660.)

The active site of aldosterone in the kidney is on epithelial cells of the cortical collecting duct, where it promotes the transport of sodium from the tubular fluid to the interstitium via an electrogenic sodium pump. The mechanism by which aldosterone induces increased potassium excretion by the kidney is unclear. Similarly, the increased excretion of hydrogen ion that results from aldosterone secretion is not well understood. Aldosterone has similar sodium retentive effects on sweat and salivary secretions that can be physiologically important in instances of excessive perspiration.

Angiotensin II is the single most important signal for aldosterone secretion (see Figure 25-5). Angiotensin II is an octapeptide product of the **angiotensinogen pathway**. The rate-limiting step in this pathway is the cleavage of angiotensinogen to angiotensin I by renin secreted by the juxtaglomerular apparatus of the kidney in response to hypovolemia and hyponatremia as well as to increased sympathetic stimulation. There are a multitude of other factors that influence aldosterone secretion. Small increases in serum potassium can result in a measured increase in aldosterone secretion independent of angiotensin. Although ACTH is much more crucial to maintaining secretory activity of the inner zones of the adrenal cortex, it can enhance aldosterone production.

GLUCOCORTICOIDS

Glucocorticoids play a critical role in the maintenance of carbohydrate reserves but also have a large variety of activities throughout the body (Table 27-5). In the absence of glucocorticoids, relatively short periods of fasting may result in catastrophic hypoglycemia accompanied by depletion of muscle and liver glycogen. This results from loss of the ability to produce sugar from nonsugar sources (i.e., gluconeogenesis) and decreased ability to rely on alternate fuel substrates (i.e., fatty acids and protein) for metabolism. Glucocorticoid effects favor proteolysis and lipolysis peripherally and increase the activity of gluconeogenic pathways within the liver.

Other than energy metabolism, the glucocorticoids' most profound effects are anti-inflammatory, at least when given in sufficient doses. As pharmaceutical preparations they have been important components of immunosuppressive regimens for a variety of disorders, including transplant rejection and autoimmune disease. While not completely understood, glucocorticoids have proven inhibitory effects on (a) prostaglandin synthesis, (b) lysosomal degranulation in inflamma-

TABLE 27-5. Glucocorticoid Effects

Tissue	Effects
Central nervous system	Taste, hearing and smell ↑ in acuity with adrenal cortical insufficiency and ↓ in Cushing's disease ↓ Corticotropin releasing hormone ↓ Antidiuretic hormone secretion
Cardiovascular system	Maintain sensitivity to epinephrine and norepinephrine ↑ Sensitivity to vasoconstrictor agents Maintain microcirculation
Gastrointestinal tract	↑ Gastric acid secretion ↓ Gastric mucosal cell proliferation
Liver	↑ Gluconeogenesis
Lungs	↑ Maturation and surfactant production during fetal development
Pituitary	↓ ACTH secretion (acute) and synthesis (chronic)
Kidney	↑ Glomerular filtraton rate Needed to excrete dilute urine
Bone	↑ Resorption ↓ Formation
Muscle	↓ Fatigue (probably secondary to cardiovascular actions) ↑ Protein catabolism ↓ Glucose oxidation ↓ Insulin sensitivity ↓ Protein synthesis
Immune system	↓ Mass of thymus and lymph nodes ↓ Blood concentrations of eosinophils, basophils, and lymphocytes ↓ Cellular immunity
Connective tissue	↓ Activity of fibroblasts ↓ Collagen synthesis

Reproduced from Goodman HM. *Basic medical endocrinology.* New York: Raven Press, 1988:90.

tory cells, (c) interleukin-1 and interleukin-2 secretion, (d) immunoglobulin synthesis, and (e) lymphocyte mitogenesis.

As with other steroid hormones, intracellular glucocorticoid binding leads to modulation of genomic translation. It is thought that glucocorticoids bind the same receptor in a wide variety of functionally disparate cells and that the cell's primary function ultimately determines the glucocorticoids' stimulatory or inhibitory effect.

Glucocorticoid secretion is regulated by ACTH from the anterior pituitary. Without ACTH, the two inner zones (i.e., the zona fasciculata and zona reticularis) of the adrenal cortex atrophy. Adrenocorticotropic hormone release is dependent on **corticotropin-releasing hormone (CRH)**, which is released by the paraventricular nucleus of the hypothalamus into the hypophyseal-portal capillaries. Adrenocorticotropic hormone release stimulates adrenal secretion of cortisol, which inhibits further ACTH release through negative effects on anterior pituitary corticotropes and neurons responsible for CRH release (Figure 27-7).

Adrenocorticotropic hormone has a stimulatory effect on the adrenal cortex through receptor-specific binding to cell surfaces that results in cAMP production

and a variety of secondary intracellular activation steps. The increased conversion of cholesterol to pregnenolone is the critical consequence of ACTH binding.

Adrenocorticotropic hormone is a primary regulator of both glucocorticoid- and androgen-hormone synthesis. The mechanisms by which androgens can be secreted in disproportionately larger amounts in certain circumstances (e.g., puberty) is unclear. Adrenocorticotropic hormone has secondary effects beyond its direct effect on steroid biosynthetic pathways, including (a) enhanced cholesterol storage, (b) increased esterase activity that liberates more intracellular cholesterol, (c) increased blood flow to the adrenal glands, and (d) hypertrophy of adrenal mass with continued stimulation.

The circadian rhythm seen in plasma ACTH and cortisol concentrations is thought to be a function of the sensitivity of CRH-releasing neurons to inhibitory feedback from cortisol. In the beginning of the awake or alert period these neurons become resistant to negative feedback, resulting in increased ACTH and cortisol levels. For the remainder of the 24-hour period, these neurons gradually become more responsive to negative feedback, resulting in a gradual decline in ACTH and cortisol until the next cycle begins. The mechanism of this central regulatory effect on the CRH-releasing neurons is unknown.

DISORDERS OF THE ADRENAL CORTEX

Excessive cortisol production is known as **Cushing's syndrome.** Patients with this syndrome present with hypertension, centripetal obesity, atrophied skin, and easy bruisability. If excessive pituitary secretion of ACTH is the cause of Cushing's syndrome, it is called **Cushing's disease.** Cushing's syndrome can also be caused by autonomously functioning adrenal tumors or ectopic ACTH-secreting tumors (e.g., commonly in the lung). In either case, adrenal hyperfunction causes abnormal nitrogen excretion and muscle wasting, resulting in the spindly extremities seen in the typical Cushing's body habitus.

Congenital adrenal hyperplasia, or the **adrenogenital syndrome,** encompasses a group of disorders resulting from an enzymatic deficiency in an adrenal steroidogenic pathway. Adrenocorticotropic hormone secretion is stimulated as the result of insufficient negative feedback from the hormones whose synthesis is blocked, which results in adrenal hyperplasia. The most common form of congenital adrenal hyperplasia is 21-

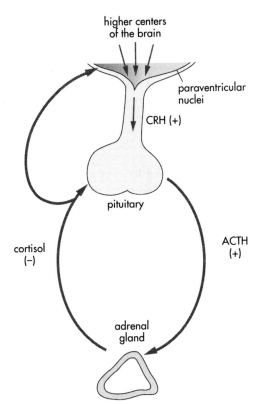

Figure 27-7 Feedback inhibition of glucocorticoid secretion. (Reproduced from Goodman HM. *Basic medical endocrinology.* New York: Raven Press, 1988:102.)

hydroxylase deficiency, which blocks the production of cortisol and aldosterone, shunting steroidogenesis down the androgen pathway, which results in virilization.

Hyperaldosteronism is the result of either a tumor, **primary hyperaldosteronism (Conn's syndrome),** or inappropriately high activity of the renin-angiotensin system, **secondary hyperaldosteronism.** The primary symptoms of either condition are hypertension, hypokalemia, and metabolic alkalosis.

Adrenocortical hypofunction can be caused by a defect within the adrenal cortex, preventing adequate steroid synthesis (**Addison's disease**), or from insufficient ACTH secretion (**secondary adrenocortical insufficiency**). Weakness, fatigability, weight loss, hyperpigmentation, hyponatremia, and hypokalemia are all frequent presenting features of adrenocortical insufficiency.

ADRENAL MEDULLA

The adrenal medulla accounts for approximately 10% of adrenal mass and is functionally, anatomically, and embryologically distinct from the adrenal cortex. Termed chromaffin cells for their affinity for chromium salts in histological preparations, the cells of the adrenal medulla are innervated by sympathetic nerves whose cell bodies lie within the thoracolumbar portion of the spinal cord. These cells are often referred to as "modified postganglionic neurons." Their principal secretory products are **epinephrine** and **norepinephrine,** which are present in a ratio of 5:1. Of interest is the fact that only norepinephrine is released by other synthetic synapses and the adrenal is the only source of epinephrine in the blood. While vital in the response to acute stress, the catecholamines (i.e., epinephrine and norepinephrine) of the adrenal medulla are redundant elements of the sympathetic nervous system and are not required for life so long as the rest of the sympathetic system is intact. Regulation of adrenal medullary hormone release generally parallels that of sympathetic tone and stimulation.

Epinephrine and norepinephrine are derivatives of the amino acid tyrosine. Hydroxylation of tyrosine results in **dihydroxyphenylalanine,** which is pumped into storage granules where norepinephrine is synthesized. Epinephrine synthesis requires exit of the norepinephrine from the granule back to the cytosol, where it is methylated and then pumped back into a storage granule. These two catecholamines are then secreted through degranulation and exocytosis.

Catecholamines are stored in secretory granules with ATP in a molar ratio of 4:1, along with a variety of opioid peptides including enkephalins, β-endorphin, and their precursors. The half-lives of these catecholamines is on the order of 10–15 seconds. As much as 90% of blood catecholamines are removed with a single passage through a capillary with a significant portion of the clearance performed by sympathetic neuronal reabsorption of theses compounds. **Monoamine oxidase (MAO)** is the principal enzyme within the neuronal cytosol responsible for degradation of excess absorbed catecholamine. It is for this reason that persons receiving monoamine oxidase inhibitors must avoid tyrosine-containing foods. **Catecholamine-O-methyltransferase** is the principal enzyme responsible for catecholamine degradation in non-neuronal tissue. The assay of urinary metabolites of catecholamines (i.e., **vanillylmandelic acid** and **3-methoxy-4-hydroxyphenylglycol**) is a valuable index of their aggregate secretion.

Tissues responsive to catecholamines make no distinction as to their source (i.e., adrenal or sympathetic neurons). The action of these compounds is of rapid onset with immediate (i.e., seconds) dissipation. While adrenal cortical hormones express their activity with a lag time on the order of 30 minutes or longer, medullary catecholamines provide an immediate response to "stress." Together they provide for immediate and continued homeostasis in the face of physiologic challenge.

Receptors for catecholamines are called adrenergic receptors and are subdivided into α1, α2, β1, and β2 subsets. These subsets were defined based on their capacity to be blocked by various pharmacological agents. The intracellular sequelae of catecholamine binding of these receptors serve to facilitate the affected cell's ability to contribute to the body's need to face a serious physical or mental challenge. Blood flow is diverted to the brain and working muscle mass, cellular metabolism is modulated to provide copious energy-rich substrates, bronchial muscles are relaxed to facilitate ventilation, and ocular effects increase visual acuity. Some typical responses to adrenal medullary stimulation (i.e., sympathetic response) are listed in Table 27-6.

DISORDERS OF THE ADRENAL MEDULLA

Adrenomedullary dysfunction is rare, the most common form being a catecholamine-secreting tumor, **pheochromocytoma.** The most common symptoms of pheochromocytoma are hypertension (paroxysmal), headache, excessive sweating, palpitations, gastroin-

TABLE 27-6. Responses Elicited by Adrenal Medulla Stimulation

Target	Responses	Receptor
Cardiovascular system		
Heart	↑ Frequency and rate of contraction	β
	↑ Conduction	β
	↑ Blood flow (dilation of coronary arterioles)	β
	↑ Glycogenolysis	β
Arterioles		
Skin	Constriction	α
Mucosae	Constriction	α
Skeletal muscle	Constriction	α
	Dilation	β
Metabolism		
Fat	↑ Lipolysis	β
	↑ Blood free fatty acid and glycerol	β
Liver	↑ Glycogenolysis and gluconeogenesis	β and $α_1$
	↑ Blood sugar	β and $α_1$
Muscle	↑ Glycogenolysis	β
	↑ Lactate and pyruvate release	β
Bronchial Muscle	Relaxation	β
Stomach and Intestines	↑ Motility	β
	↑ Sphincter contraction	α
Urinary bladder	↑ Sphincter contraction	α
Skin	↑ Sweating	α
Eyes	Contraction of radial muscle of the iris	α
Salivary gland	↑ Amylase secretion	α
	↑ Watery secretion	α
Kidney	↑ Renin secretion	β
Skeletal muscle	↑ Tension generation	β
	↑ Neuromuscular transmission (defatiguing effect)	β

Reproduced from Goodman HM. *Basic medical endocrinology*. New York: Raven Press, 1988:111.

testinal disturbances, and hyperglycemia. If left untreated, pheochromocytoma is almost invariably fatal.

Atrial Natriuretic Peptide

Atrial natriuretic peptide (ANP) is the most recently discovered hormone involved in the maintenance of sodium and water homeostasis. It is found primarily within myocytes of the right atrium and secreted via exocytosis of ANP-containing granules. Secretion is stimulated by volume expansion and sodium chloride intake. It is found in the blood initially as a 28-amino-acid peptide, the cleavage product of a 128-amino-acid precursor, which is then cleaved to a 20-amino-acid peptide, **atriopeptin II**, perhaps the most potent form of the hormone. Atrial natriuretic peptide has a serum half-life of approximately 3 minutes.

Atrial natriuretic peptide exerts its physiological effect in the kidney, where it increases the glomerular filtration rate without increasing renal blood flow and decreases reabsorption of water and salt in the proximal tubule by an as yet little understood mechanism. Atrial natriuretic peptide also has vasodilatory effects on peripheral arterioles, effecting a decrease in systemic blood pressure. Atrial natriuretic peptide directly and indirectly inhibits renin secretion, thus preventing significant aldosterone secretion. Receptors for ANP are found on juxtaglomerular, adrenal glomerulosa, and antidiuretic hormone-secreting cells. It is unclear what direct regulatory functions ANP has on these cells.

Multiple Endocrine Neoplasia (MEN)

TYPE I—WERMER'S SYNDROME

Wermer described the familial occurrence of tumors involving the pituitary gland, parathyroids, and pancreatic islets in 1945. **Hyperparathyroidism** occurs in approximately 90% of all cases and represents the most common endocrine abnormality in this syndrome. **Gastrinomas** are the most common islet lesion, followed by **insulinoma.** Pituitary tumors, usually **chromophobe adenomas,** occur in 60–70% of patients. Chromophobe adenomas are nonsecreting tumors that compress adjacent pituitary cells, diminishing their secretion. They usually manifest as secondary amenorrhea in women and hypogonadism in men. Other, less common lesions include (a) adrenal tumors, 40%; and (b) thyroid disorders of a mixed variety, 10–15%.

TYPE II—SIPPLE'S SYNDROME

This classification was originally introduced to describe a group of patients that presented with **medullary thyroid carcinoma (MTC), pheochromocytomas,** and **parathyroid hyperplasia.** More recently a subclassification to MEN-IIa and MEN-IIb has been made, the latter being a more rare condition characterized by **MTC, pheochromocytomas, multiple mucosal neuromas, ganglioneuromatosis,** and a **characteristic physical appearance.** Both of these diseases are inherited as autosomal dominant traits and are diagnostic considerations in any patient diagnosed with either MTC or pheochromocytoma. While the incidence of the various tumors is variable, MTC is present in almost 100% of patients presenting with MEN-IIa or MEN-IIb.

Bibliography

DeVita VT, Hellman S, Rosenberg SA. *Cancer—principles and practice of oncology.* Philadelphia: JB Lippincott, 1989.

Goodman HM. *Basic medical endocrinology.* New York: Raven Press, 1988.

Griffin JE, Ojeda SR. *Textbook of endocrine physiology.* New York: Oxford University Press, 1988.

Hedge GA, Colby HD, Goodman RL. *Clinical endocrine physiology.* Philadelphia: WB Saunders, 1987.

Sabiston DC, ed. *Textbook of surgery: the biological basis of modern surgical practice.* Philadelphia: WB Saunders, 1986.

Steven R. Buchman

28 PHYSIOLOGY OF WOUND HEALING

General Concepts

Perhaps nothing is as central to the science of surgery as wound healing. Wound repair is a complex and dynamic process that incorporates physiologic, biochemical, biomechanical, and immunologic forces into a network of coordinated interactions. These interactions work to restore the injured tissue toward its healthy, functional, and structurally sound preinjured state.

The healing process is initiated by an array of mechanisms triggered at the moment of injury (Figure 28-1). These mechanisms cascade into a series of reactions that activate and mediate wound repair. The detailed feedback network regulating this process is tempered by the unique characteristics of each wound. Perturbations in the environment of the injured tissue may disrupt the delicate balance directing repair and inhibit wound restoration.

The wound-healing process is often described in terms of stages (Table 28-1). Description in terms of stages compartmentalizes wound healing; however, the reconstitution of violated tissue results from a continuum of interactions and overlapping phases that contribute to the healing process. Although the duration of each phase may be specified, it is in most cases variable. Owing to the lack of uniform and specific gradations in wound repair, continued reference to stages or sharp demarcations will be avoided, and a more descriptive approach will be employed.

Macroscopic Aspects of Wound Repair

At the time of injury, energy is transferred and the resultant force is dissipated into the tissue. The rate, duration, magnitude, and direction of force delivered, with respect to the surface area contacted, determines the extent of the injury.

At the time of injury, multiple events occur within the wound. Soft tissue structures are violated and blood vessels are ruptured. The blood supply is compromised and hematoma forms at the site of injury. This may cause pain and tenderness.

The nascent wound is a milieu of devitalized tissue, clot, and necrotic debris and may contain bacteria or foreign material. As the healing process commences, the nonviable elements are degraded and digested and the hematoma liquefies and resorbs. In full-thickness wounds, **epithelialization** is initiated from the edges of the wound, providing a barrier to desiccation and toxic foreign materials (especially bacteria), as well as a degree of thermoregulation.

After three to four days, the affected area is **revascularized**. This is manifested grossly as the formation of **granulation tissue**. Granulation tissue helps to bridge the gap of the wound, incorporating surface irregularities. **Inflammation**, as evidenced by swelling, warmth,

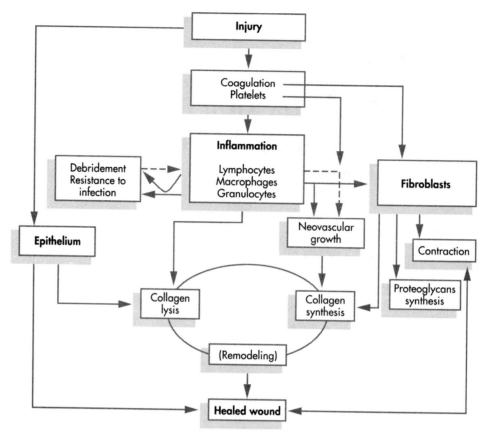

Figure 28-1 Schematic representation of key events in wound healing. (Reproduced from Hunt TK, Knighton DR, Thakral KK, et al. Cellular control of repair. In Hunt TK, Heppenstall RB, Pines E, et al, eds. *Soft and hard tissue repair.* New York: Praeger, 1984:5.)

and erythema, is a clinical sign associated with the revascularization process. If the wound edges are not approximated primarily, **contraction** during the first week of injury aids in closing the wound. Over the next month, collagen production fills the defect, forming a **scar.** The scar gradually increases in tensile strength and may take on an amorphous appearance without smooth contour.

The process of **remodeling** begins to replace the irregular scar. Slowly, old collagen is resorbed and new collagen is deposited in an attempt to change the shape and contour of the wound to its original form. This process may take years, but gradually the orientation of the components of the healed wound begins to reflect the stresses applied to it. In the case of a large, disfiguring wound, these processes can only approximate the nor-

mal structure and work primarily to restore the physical integrity and function of the injured tissue.

Histologic and Cellular Aspects of Wound Repair

Traumatic forces lead to fragmentation of soft-tissue elements and shearing and division of blood vessels and lymphatic channels. The disruption of the blood supply leads to tissue ischemia and cell death. The extent of wound necrosis correlates with the amount of ischemia caused by the injury.

The energy absorbed by the injured tissue results in demonstrable damage to protective barriers. Breach of

---

TABLE 28-1. Wound Healing

Stage	Time	Events	Cell(s)
Inflammation (0–4 days)			
Reaction lag	0–2 hours	Hemostasis	Platelets
			Erythrocytes
			Leukocytes
	0–4 days	Phagocytosis	Neutrophils
			Macrophages
Proliferation (2–22 days)			
Fibroblastic regeneration	1–4 days	Epithelialization	Keratinocytes
	2–7 days	Neovascularization	Endothelial
	2–22 days	Collagen synthesis	Fibroblasts
	2–20 days	Contraction	Myofibroblasts
Maturation (21 days to 2 years)			
Remodeling		Collagen remodeling	Fibroblasts

Reproduced from Wysocki AB. Surgical wound healing. A review for perioperative nurses. *AORN J* 49:508, 1989. Copyright © AORN Inc., 10170 East Mississippi Avenue, Denver, CO 80231.

---

these barriers is associated with leakage and egress of body fluids as well as possible ingress of foreign materials. Local cell death results in release of lysosomal enzymes that destroy collagenous and noncollagenous components of the organic matrix.

Extravasated blood forms hematoma in the wound. Mechanisms controlling hemorrhage include retraction of local blood vessels and spasm of perivascular smooth muscle, leading to reduction of luminal diameter and thrombosis. Blood-borne elements constituent to the hematoma provide the first population of reparative cells at the wound site. Erythrocyte adhesion can be seen histologically as **rouleaux formation.** Platelets are deposited and **platelet plugs** are formed. **Fibrin** incorporates these elements into a fibrous coagulum that bridges the defect. The fibrin is arranged as a scaffold that allows migration of new cells to the site of injury from the wound periphery. Local tissue reaction results in vasodilatation and an associated increase in vascular permeability. This creates tissue **edema** and allows the microcirculation adjacent to the wound to provide access for the early influx of inflammatory cells.

Neutrophils appear in the wound a few hours after injury and usually peak in number at 28–48 hours. These inflammatory cells serve to remove necrotic debris, engulf foreign material, and attack infiltrating bacteria—performing an initial wound debridement. Although neutrophils are active in the wound-healing

process, neutropenia does not itself interfere with healing. **Mast cells** are also seen early but play a regulatory role in the evolution of the repair.

Macrophages, derived from circulating monocytes, move into the wound and peak in number at approximately 72 hours post-injury. These cells resorb hematoma, digest necrotic debris and restore a level of immune competence to the sequestered wound. Macrophage secretory products play a vital role in directing the normal response to injury. Macrophages have been shown experimentally to be essential for wound healing and may be the most important cells in the process.

Lymphocytes appear early in the inflammatory response to an injury. Although the lymphocytes do not play an essential role in wound repair, recent experimental evidence has demonstrated a major modulating influence of these cells in the wound healing scenario.

Few structural cells are present at the time of injury and many more are needed for successful repair. Precursor **mesenchymal cells** and mature **fibroblasts** proliferate and migrate into the wound from adjacent tissue. These initiate the formation of collagen at the site of injury. The blood supply to the wound is initially derived from the periphery, but as the clot continues to organize, **endothelial cells and smooth muscle cells** migrate along the fibrin scaffold. The microcirculation is restored as endothelial cells coalesce with existing vascular channels and sprout new capillary buds. Granulation tissue is formed by the development of this new capillary system with its surrounding supportive framework consisting of fibrin and collagen. The neovascularization provides the pool needed for ongoing replacement of cells during wound repair. There is an influx of **pluripotent cells.** These precursors differentiate into the cells needed to manufacture the matrix and building blocks essential for wound repair. **Fibroblasts** synthesize **collagen, proteoglycans,** and **elastin. Osteoblasts** and **chondroblasts** produce bone and cartilage, respectively.

The growing collagenous matrix is initially random in organization and forms an amorphous mass without obvious structure. An immature scar is created that acts to bind the wound and provide tensile strength. Although the immature scar fills the defect, the architecture of the healing wound still does not resemble that of the original tissue. In addition, the tissue in the injured area is not as strong and stable as before injury. In an attempt to restore the wound to its original form and function the scar undergoes a process of **remodeling.** Remodeling refers to cell-mediated breakdown and replacement of the wound matrix. The immature scar is composed of cross-linked collagen that haphazardly follows the patterns of capillary ingrowth rather than lines of force. A more highly organized, mature collagen framework gradually replaces the irregular architecture of the immature scar along the lines of mechanical stress. The remodeled scar exhibits a restoration of the delicate weaves of normal collagen fibers and an increase in strength and efficiency. The maturation of the scar completes the sequence of events in wound healing.

Epithelialization and Contraction

While the reparative processes progress in the depths of the wound, there is also a rapid mobilization of cellular reserves to restore integrity at the wound's surface. The processes of epithelialization and contraction aid to close the gap created by a traumatic injury. Epithelial replication occurs within hours of injury. Cells migrate from the wound edges and spread across the defect, employing a collagenase to cleave a plane between viable tissue and superficial necrotic debris. In the case of a partial-thickness skin wound, epithelial cells are derived from both the wound edges and the adnexa

within the wound bed. In most cases epithelial cells have bridged the gap by 48 hours after injury. After the migrating cells have merged to form a solid sheet, they become columnar in shape, commence mitosis, and migrate upward to fill the defect. The epithelium seals the wound and acts as a barrier to contamination and desiccation, and may provide an element of thermoregulation to the injured tissue. An open wound may remain in an inflammatory phase with little effective collagen synthesis until epithelial coverage is complete.

Contraction is an additional force at work to close the wound. Through the interaction of cells with the collagenous matrix at the edges of the injured tissue, the wound is drawn together, resulting in a decrease in the size of the defect. The main cell responsible for wound contraction is a specialized actin-myosin complex containing unit called a **myofibroblast.** Myofibroblasts are modified fibroblasts able to exert a contractile force; they resemble smooth muscle cells in function and morphology.

Contraction begins approximately one week after wounding. In the case of skin injury, full-thickness wounds contract more than partial thickness wounds and in direct proportion to depth. The contraction process is a key element in the body's ability to heal large wounds and may be responsible for up to a 40% decrease in the size of a defect. On the other hand, severe contraction can lead to functional disability as well as cosmetic deformity and may be inhibited by the use of full-thickness skin grafts or flaps.

Peptide Growth Factors and Mediators of Wound Healing

Growth factors influence cellular activity through cell-surface binding to specific receptors, leading to biochemical activation and response at the level of the gene. The cellular response to an injury may translate into activities that are mitogenic, oncogenic, chemotactic, or hemostatic. Certain mediators of wound repair recruit mesenchymal pluripotent cells into the wound. Others may activate cells at the site of injury. Many different growth factors and regulatory protein complexes have been isolated and found to influence various portions of the wound healing cascade (Table 28-2). The timing, release, and differential effect of specific growth factors on isolated cell lines illustrates the complex interactions involved in the normal sequence of wound healing.

TABLE 28-2. Growth Factors

Factor	Source	Target
TGF-β (Transforming growth factor β)	Platelets Macrophage Lymphocyte Bone Most tissues	All cells
PDGF (Platelet-derived growth factor)	Platelets Macrophage Endothelial cell Smooth muscle cell	Fibroblast Smooth muscle cell Glial cells
aFGF and bFGF/HBGF (Acidic fibroblast, basic fibroblast/heparin-binding growth factors)	Macrophage Cartilage (CDGF) Brain (ECGF)	Endothelial cell Fibroblast Chondrocyte Glial, etc.
EGF (Epidermal growth factor)	Saliva Urine	Epithelial cell Fibroblast
TGF-α (Transforming growth factor α)	Platelets Keratinocyte Macrophage	Epithelial cell Fibroblast Endothelial cell
AGF (Angiogenesis growth factor)	Macrophage	Endothelial cell
EDF (Epidermal cell-derived growth factor)	Epithelial cell	Epithelial cell Fibroblast
MAF (Macrophage activating factor)	T lymphocyte	Macrophage
MDGF (Monocyte/macrophage-derived growth factor)	Macrophage	Fibroblast Smooth muscle cell
FGF (Fibroblast growth factor)	Macrophage	Fibroblast
IGF-I/Sm-C (Insulinlike growth factor/somatomedin C)	Plasma Liver Fibroblast	Fibroblast Endothelial cell Fetal tissues
TNF (Tumor necrosis factor)	Macrophage	Fibroblast
IL-1 (Interleukin-1)	Macrophage	Fibroblast Synovial cell
IL-2 (Interleukin-2)	T lymphocyte	?
MIF (Macrophage migration inhibition factor)	T lymphocyte	Macrophage
FAF (Fibroblast activating factor)	T lymphocyte	Fibroblast

CDGF, Cartilage-derived growth factor; ECGF, endothelial cell growth factor.
Modified from Miller SH, Rudolph R. Healing in the irradiated wound. *Clin Plast Surg* 1990; 17:503–508.

Mediators are delivered to target cells in three ways: (1) autocrine, interacting with the cell which produced it; (2) paracrine, interacting with a nearby effector cell; and (3) endocrine, traveling via the bloodstream to influence distant cellular activity.

As soon as a tissue is injured, a local network of fac-tor interactions is initiated. In fact, much of the failure of wound repair may be due to perturbations in the activation of local factors. Cellular injury leads to release of **phospholipase A,** which converts membrane phos-pholipids to arachidonic acid. Resultant metabolism of arachidonic acid to prostaglandins and leukotrienes initiates the humoral response to injury. **Prostaglandins** and **leukotrienes** influence microvascular permeability and chemotaxis of white blood cells and fibroblasts. They may serve as the final mediators of acute inflammation by fine tuning regulatory feedback mechanisms.

As blood and blood-borne elements pool in the wound, the clotting cascade is activated and platelets are deposited. Platelets adhere to exposed collagen and are activated by thrombin to aggregate and degranulate. **ADP, thromboxane** A_2, and **serotonin** are released and foster further platelet aggregation. In addition, platelets release proteolytic enzymes capable of initiating complement activation. **Complement** promotes unidirectional migration and demargination of inflammatory cells. The **C3a** and **C5a** elements of the complement system are specifically chemotactic for neutrophils and monocytes. Additional properties of complement that influence the wound-healing process include capillary vasodilatation and the promotion of specific and nonspecific opsonization.

Aside from stimulating the complement system, platelets also release a variety of factors that mediate wound repair. **Platelet-derived growth factor,** which is also synthesized by macrophages, endothelial cells, and smooth muscle cells, is released from the α-granules of platelets. Platelet-derived growth factor promotes the migration and proliferation of fibroblasts and in so doing stimulates collagen synthesis. Platelet-derived growth factor is also chemotactic for smooth muscle cells, neutrophils, and mononuclear cells.

Transforming growth factor-β, first isolated from transformed neoplastic cells, is a regulatory peptide. Transforming growth factor-β is released from platelets during aggregation and induces fibrosis and angiogenesis as well as collagen and proteoglycan synthesis. It fosters increased tensile strength, promotes granulation tissue formation, and may work in concert with other growth factors to stimulate or inhibit cell growth. Platelets also release **transforming growth factor-α**, which stimulates the proliferation of epithelial cells, fibroblasts, and endothelial cells. Transforming growth factor-α also acts as a chemoattractant by recruiting macrophages and lymphocytes into the wound. Transforming growth factor-β and platelet-derived growth factor may work together to induce cell transformation.

Fibronectin, a glycoprotein synthesized by regional fibroblasts and endothelial cells, is also produced in the wound. It helps to mediate macrophage promoted angiogenesis and also serves as a nonspecific opsonin for macrophage phagocytosis. One of the earliest events in wound healing is the combination of fibronectin with fibrin to form a matrix. This matrix provides structural support for cell migration. The fibronectin moiety assists in fibroblast adherence to collagen. **Fibrin,** in addition to its interplay with fibronectin, is active in attracting macrophages and fibroblasts into the wound.

Mast cells and neutrophils also appear early in the wound and provide a number of mediators of wound repair. They release **histamine,** which promotes vasodilatation and increased vascular permeability. Granulocytes release **kallikrein,** an enzyme that initiates the release of **kinins** and **kallidin** from α$_2$-globulin in plasma. Kinins may work in concert with complement to stimulate and sustain local inflammatory vascular responses. Activation of the kinin system may result in alterations in local blood supply, increased vascular permeability, and egress of circulating proteins and cells into the wound.

Lymphokines and **monokines** derived from blood-borne elements in the hematoma can act as mitogens, recruiting and directing cell lines to move into the wound and expand. Macrophages synthesize and release **interleukin-1,** a monokine that increases fibroblast stimulation and is thought to influence angiogenesis. Interleukin-1 also fosters lymphocyte proliferation and induces helper T cells to secrete **interleukin-2.**

T lymphocytes enter the wound after macrophage infiltration and produce lymphokines such as interleukin-2 and **fibroblast activating factor,** which work actively and directly to stimulate fibroblast growth. Other important lymphokines include **macrophage migration inhibition factor** and **macrophage activating factor,** which stimulate and direct macrophage function.

An array of macrophage secretory products have been shown to act as chemotactic agents, cell-stimulating agents, and agents leading to cell migration. These diverse functions establish the macrophage as one of the most important cells in wound healing. **Angiogenesis growth factor,** a macrophage derived mediator of wound repair, promotes the formation of endothelial buds and microvascular ingrowth. Macrophages also produce **fibroblast growth factor,** a mitogen for endothelial cells and another potent factor contributing to angiogenesis. Other inductive agents released by macrophages include **tumor necrosis factor** and **monocyte/ macrophage-derived growth factor,** which stimulate fibroblasts and influence collagen synthesis. Clearly, T lymphocytes and macrophages have an important modulating effect on the sequence of successful wound healing. Therefore, impaired immune function secondary to disease or therapeutic regimens could be expected to impair the normal wound-healing process.

Fibroblasts are another source of soluble mediators, such as **insulinlike growth factor-1** and **somatomedin C**, which affect wound repair. These factors stimulate target receptors on endothelial cells and may act as autocrine regulators by maintaining homeostatic feedback mechanisms.

Another inductive agent impacting on healing at the wound site is **epidermal growth factor**. Although its tissue source is unclear, epidermal growth factor has been studied extensively and shown to mediate a multitude of actions which enhance wound healing. Epidermal growth factor stimulates mitosis and glycosaminoglycan synthesis in cell culture, increases granulation tissue formation, and may enhance epidermal repair. Epidermal growth factor has also been shown to promote glycolysis and nutrient transport into cells as well as increased synthesis of fibronectin, DNA, and RNA. There is little doubt that many more chemoattractants and regulatory factors play a role, yet to be completely elucidated, in the complex process of wound repair.

Oxygen Tension

Oxygen tension plays a role at the site of injury and must be considered an integral part of any unified theory of wound repair. Tissue destruction at the site of injury leads to ablation of blood supply and curtails oxygen delivery. Local oxygen tension falls and glycolytic metabolism ensues, resulting in an increase in the concentration of lactate and a concomitant decrease in pH. Centrally, the wound exhibits critical levels of hypoxia, hypercarbia, and acidosis. As neutrophils and macrophages marginate from the adjacent blood pool into the wound, there is a simultaneous increase in the energy requirement (10–20 times normal) as active phagocytosis depletes the oxygen supply. Systemic circulatory compromise, if present, further contributes to wound hypoxia by reducing tissue oxygen delivery.

A gradient of oxygen tension extends from the perfused wound periphery to the hypoxic microenvironment at the center of the wound. This gradient may not be deleterious to normal wound healing. In fact, the energy gradient spanning across the normal and injured tissue may actually drive wound repair. The low partial pressure of oxygen in a fresh wound may signal the release of growth factors, promoters, and metabolites, thus providing stimulus for induction of wound healing. For example, the local changes in oxygen and lactate concentration and pH stimulate macrophages to secrete angiogenic growth factors, spurring vascular ingrowth. In a similar fashion the conditions prevailing at the wound center stimulate fibroblast synthesis.

The temporal changes in oxygen supply are important in controlling the various phases of wound repair. While oxygen gradients may be critical in the initial phases of wound healing, a persistent state of hypoxia will leave the injured tissue vulnerable and interfere with normal repair of the wound. The reparative capability of the cellular response may be compromised by hypoxia. The killing capacity of phagocytozing leukocytes is proportional to local oxygen concentration because the creation of high-energy free radicals necessary to destroy bacteria is oxygen dependent. Thus, there is an increased probability of infection in hypoxic wounds.

Oxygen is a necessary fuel for protein synthesis and cell replication. Oxygen is required for the hydroxylation of proline and lysine residues of collagen. Hydroxylization is required for the release of collagen from cells, for helix and subsequent fibril formation, and the formation of molecular cross-links.

Cellular Adhesion

Many of the cells involved in the healing process can reversibly adhere to tissue components. For example, after an injury, epithelial cells become migratory in an effort to re-epithelialize the wound. This ability is based on a locally regulated and reversible anchoring process. Cellular adherence may be expressed via matrix receptors that allow distinct and selective adhesion. The theoretical rationale for cellular adherence led to the discovery of cell-surface adhesion receptors called **integrins**. Integrins provide a bond between a cell and its surrounding extracellular matrix. Different structural permutations of a receptor translate into differing specificities for individual proteins. For example, an altered amino acid sequence at a receptor site would determine the affinity for a desired molecule such as fibronectin, fibrinogen, or collagen. The exact role of selective cellular attachment in the initiation and promulgation of wound repair remains to be elucidated.

Scar Formation

With the exception of certain tissues such as bone and liver, which have regenerative capabilities, wounds heal by the process of scar formation. Fibroblasts play an essential role in the formation of a scar. These cells must proliferate, synthesize **proteoglycans, collagen,** and **elastin,** and then incorporate these building blocks into a matrix with some semblance to the pre-injured state.

Glycosaminoglycans are large, repeating disaccharide units that are attached to proteins to create **proteoglycans.** Proteoglycans are the main component of **ground substance** and help to organize and direct collagen deposition and synthesis. Proteoglycans may be sulfated as **chondroitin sulfate, heparan sulfate,** and **kerato sulfate,** or remain nonsulfated as **hyaluronic acid, chondroitin,** and **fibronectin.** The sulfated varieties are more pronounced during the initial phases of wound healing, while the nonsulfated components dominate later in the process.

Collagen is composed of three similar or identical polypeptide chains. These polypeptides are unique because every third amino acid is glycine, and the other principal amino acids include hydroxyproline and hydroxylysine. Three of these polypeptide chains are wound together into a right-handed helix. Cross-links are formed within collagen molecules and between collagen fibers by bonds between two hydroxylysine molecules. In addition to the oxygen dependence of hydroxylation, there are a number of other cofactors crucial to the successful synthesis of collagen, including vitamin C (ascorbic acid, necessary to hydroxylate proline to hydroxyproline), iron, α-ketoglutarate, copper, and pyridoxine.

At least five distinct types of collagen have been identified. Each type is tissue specific and may change in concentration in different phases of wound repair. Type I collagen is associated with mature adult dermal and tendinous connective tissue; type II collagen is a major component of cartilage matrix; type III collagen is found in aorta, lung and skin and in embryonic and immature tissue; and type IV collagen is a constituent of basement membranes. Types I, II, and III are the principal components of the healing wound. Type III collagen is the first to be deposited in wound repair. As the scar matures, this is replaced by the more stable type I collagen. A mature scar will contain approximately 85% type I collagen and only 15% type III.

Eventually the cellularity and vascularity of the scar is decreased as it matures. The tensile strength of a scar increases at different rates depending on the tissue injured. Most tissues regain 50% of their original strength by six weeks after wounding. In any case, the strength of the repair approaches but never reaches that of uninjured tissue.

Miscellaneous Factors Affecting Wound Healing

The time from the initiation of wound repair to the restoration of structural integrity is dependent on the site of injury, the type and size of the wound, and the characteristics of the tissue injured. Healing time is related to the logarithm of the area of the wound. Wounds inflicted by destructive techniques such as laser surgery or cautery heal more slowly than wounds created by a scalpel. There is a vast array of systemic and local factors that have also been implicated in the promotion and impedence of wound healing (Table 28-3). Efficacy of wound healing can be modified by almost any endogenous or exogenous factor that influ-

---

TABLE 28-3. Factors Affecting Wound Healing

Systemic	*Local*
Age	Surgical technique
Smoking	Blood supply
Obesity	Mechanical stress
Stress	Suture materials
Anemia	Suture technique
Uremia	Radiation
Malnutrition	Infection
Corticosteroids	Oxygen tension
Chemotherapeutic agents	Antiseptics
Length of preoperative stay	Presence of drain
Vitamin deficiency (C, A, B, K)	Preparation of operative
Trauma	site
Hypovolemia	
Hypoxia	
Mineral deficiency (zinc,	
copper, magnesium)	
Underlying pathology	
(diabetes, cancer)	
Surgery (more than 3 h)	

ences the metabolism of the effector cells. Despite experimental evidence for factors that retard the healing process, in clinical practice healing tends to proceed with a degree of predictability and is modified by relatively few influences.

Bibliography

Wound Healing. *Nurs Clin North Am* 1990;25:163-277.

Barbul A, Pines E, Caldwell M, et al., eds. *Growth factors and other aspects of wound healing: Biological and clinical implications.* New York: Alan R. Liss, 1988.

Brighton CT. Principles of fracture healing. In: Murray JA, ed. *Instructional course lectures.* St. Louis: CV Mosby, 1984: 60–82, vol 33.

Eckersley JR, Dudley HA. Wounds and wound healing. *Br Med Bull* 1988;44:423–436.

Falanga V, Zitelli JA, Eaglstein WH. Wound healing. *J Am Acad Derm* 1988;19:559–563.

McCarthy JG. *Plastic surgery.* Philadelphia: WB Saunders, 1990.

Miller SH, Rudolph R. Healing in the irradiated wound. *Clin Plast Surg* 1990;17:503–8.

Peacock EE. *Wound repair.* Philadelphia: WB Saunders, 1984.

Wysocki AB. Surgical wound healing. A review for perioperative nurses. *AORN J* 1989;49:502, 504–506, 508 passim.

M. Pia DeGirolamo and
Patrick J. Brennan

29 PRINCIPLES OF SURGICAL INFECTIOUS DISEASE

Infectious diseases remain an important cause of morbidity and mortality among surgical patients a century after the development of aseptic technique in surgery. Infectious morbidity may ensue from the surgical procedure itself but is the result of the mechanism of injury that requires surgical intervention. Factors such as the cellular immunity of the host, virulence of the organism, and the use of antibiotics as well as other characteristics of the host and nosocomial environment interact to predispose to infection. An understanding of the mechanisms of normal immunity and the pathogenesis of infection is essential to surgical practice in order to prevent and treat the infections that threaten this vulnerable population.

In this chapter we shall provide an overview of normal and impaired host defense mechanisms in surgical patients, and the pathogenesis of the major classes of infectious diseases. Additionally, we shall review the principles underlying the use of the infectious diseases armamentarium: the laboratory and antimicrobial agents and vaccines.

Host Defense Mechanisms

BARRIER AND MECHANICAL DEFENSES

The skin and mucous membranes are the first line of defense against infection. The intact integument and mucosae act as mechanical barriers to microbes. The integrity of their cell structure serves to keep microorganisms from penetrating into deeper tissues. The relative dryness of the skin itself is inhibitory to the growth of micro-organisms. When the skin is breached and becomes inflamed, it tends to become more water permeable, and in turn, more susceptible to infection. The acid pH of certain barriers such as the skin, the stomach, and the vagina is antimicrobial. When the pH is altered, these organs can become infected or serve as portals for infection. For example, after gastrectomy, in the presence of antacid medications, or in the achlorhydric state, the incidence of infection by mycobacteria and salmonella rises. Mucosal surfaces produce enzymes such as lysozyme, found in all mucosal secretions, that break down linkages in bacterial cell walls and destroy them. Mucosal secretions also contain immunoglobulins, particularly IgG and IgA, that bind to organisms and block their attachment to host cells.

Whole organ systems function in an integrated mechanical way to expel foreign substances, including micro-organisms. Upper airway turbulence in the respiratory tract, ciliary action in the lower respiratory tract, and the coughing mechanism are able to clear 90% of deposited material within an hour. Alteration of these defenses, as occurs with endotracheal intubation, postsurgical atelectasis, and pollutants, tips the balance in favor of colonization and subsequent infection of the respiratory tract. The propulsive action of peristalsis in the gut appears to be necessary for limiting infection; when peristalsis is slowed by anticholinergic drugs, infectious diarrheas are prolonged. The repetitive flushing of the urinary tract mechanically washes out micro-organisms that flourish in the presence of obstruction. Table 29-1 provides a summary of host defenses.

CELLULAR DEFENSES

Once the host's barrier or mechanical defenses are overcome, its second line of defense is the inflammatory response, a concerted operation that involves the cells of the immune system. Drawn to the site of injury or infection by chemotactic factors, granulocytes arrive to begin the process of phagocytosis and destruction of micro-organisms. Chemoattractants include microorganism components, products of the clotting system, tissue factors, collagen fragments, and complement (particularly C3 and C5a). The granulocyte moves along a gradient of these chemotactic factors toward the source of inflammation. The invading micro-organisms are usually coated with opsonins, substances that facilitate phagocytosis, the most important being IgG, C3, and C5. Phagocytosis is initiated by contact with the microorganism, which activates the contractile proteins forming the cytoskeleton of the granulocyte. Cytoskeletal assembly alters the conformation of the cell membrane so that it may engulf the invader and trap it in a vacuole. Granules containing lytic enzymes such as acid hydrolases, lysozyme, and myeloproxidase fuse with the vacuole, releasing their contents into it. Oxygen radicals are generated that combine with the enzyme myeloperoxidase to kill the organisms. In defending against the infection, the granulocyte expends itself completely and ultimately dies in the attempt.

The monocyte-macrophage system, formerly called the reticuloendothelial system, is composed of phagocytic cells that act as scavengers of dead cells, microorganisms, and foreign substances but also is very important in the defense against intracellular pathogens, including *Salmonella, Legionella, Listeria, Brucella,* and mycobacteria. The mechanism of killing is thought to involve both oxidative and nonoxidative processes similar to those in granulocytes.

Intracellular pathogens, viruses, and fungi are not easily disposed of by means of phagocytosis by granulocytes and the monocyte-macrophage system or by complement lysis. The host draws on the defenses of cell-mediated immunity in this situation. Cell-mediated immunity refers to the action of antigen-sensitized T lymphocytes. Two major mechanisms of cell-mediated immunity are direct cytotoxicity and natural killer cell activity. Direct cytotoxicity involves killing of human leukocyte antigen compatible targets, requires cell-to-

TABLE 29-1. Host Defenses

Barrier and Mechanical	Cellular	Humoral
Skin/mucosal integrity	Phagocytosis	Opsonization
Acid pH	Degranulation	Lysis
Bile/digestive enzymes	Oxidative burst	Adherence inhibition
Mucosal enzymes/immunoglobulins	NK cells	Virus neutralization
Airway turbulence	Direct cytotoxicity	Toxin neutralization
Ciliary action	ADCC	ADCC
Peristalsis		Complement activation
Urinary flow		

ADCC, Antibody-dependent cell-mediated cytotoxicity.

cell contact, and is antibody independent. Natural killer cells are large lymphocytes with the ability to destroy human leukocyte antigen incompatible targets. T lymphocytes ultimately control the immune response, modulating it via the action of T-helper and T-suppressor cells and their cell products.

HUMORAL DEFENSES

The host also generates a humoral response to infecting micro-organisms. B lymphocytes recognize unique structural components of a microorganism and elaborate specific immunoglobulins against them. IgG antibodies serve as opsonins, inhibit bacterial adherence to cell walls, and participate in a process called antibody-dependent cellular cytotoxicity. With antibody-dependent cellular cytotoxicity, granulocytes, macrophages, and certain T lymphocytes make contact with their targets via an immunoglobulin molecule and kill them without phagocytosis. IgA inhibits bacterial adherence and neutralizes viruses, and also acts as a weak opsonin for alveolar macrophages. The roles of IgD and IgE in host defense are less clear.

The complement system is a nonspecific humoral defense system activated by a number of substances, among them antigen-antibody complexes, tissue proteins, and bacterial lipopolysaccharides. Activation results in cleavage of complement into components that have a variety of functions. Complement components act as opsonins and as chemoattractants for granulocytes. They also combine to form a membrane attack complex that is able to destroy some gram-negative bacteria. They stimulate histamine release and increase vascular permeability and vasodilation.

Impaired Host Defenses in Surgical Patients

CELLULAR IMMUNODEFICIENCIES

The risk of postoperative infection in the surgical patient increases when host defenses are impaired. The defects in host defenses encountered in surgical patients are largely those acquired through injury, underlying disease, or iatrogenic factors.

Disorders of granulocyte function are grouped into three general categories—disorders of migration, intracellular killing, and opsonization. Impaired leukocyte migration most commonly results in prolonged and recurrent infections of the skin and soft tissues. Pulmonary, hepatic, and renal infections also occur to a lesser extent. The most common offending agents are *Staphylococcus aureus, S. epidermidis,* fungi, and gram-negative enteric bacilli. Acquired defects in motility are observed in patients with diabetes mellitus, malnutrition, trauma, and burns. Recently, an acquired disorder of macrophage immunoglobulin Fc receptor function has been described in uremic patients. This defect was associated with an increased incidence of infection among those patients most severely impaired.

Chronic granulomatous disease is marked by an absence of oxidative activity in granulocytes that leaves the patient susceptible to pathogens that require intracellular killing, such as *S. aureus, Escherichia coli, Pseudomonas, Serratia, Salmonella,* and fungi. Impaired phagocytosis can be seen in patients with diabetic ketoacidosis.

Disorders of opsonization typically result in severe infections such as meningitis and septicemia with highly virulent encapsulated organisms. Patients with sickle cell disease exhibit opsonization defects that leave them vulnerable to infection by encapsulated organisms, such as pneumococcus, *Haemophilus influenzae,* and meningococcus. Though it appears that burn victims and patients with overwhelming infection acquire diminished opsonic capability, it is unclear whether this is of clinical significance.

Impairment of cell-mediated immunity leaves the host vulnerable to infection by intracellular pathogens such as *Listeria* and *Salmonella,* fungi, mycobacteria, viruses, and parasites. Cell-mediated immunity is diminished in the neonate and in the aged, and is significantly impaired in congenital disorders, including DiGeorge syndrome (thymic aplasia) and severe combined immunodeficiency disease. Viral infection (e.g., Epstein-Barr virus, cytomegalovirus), malignancy, steroids, chemotherapeutic agents, and radiation can all cause acquired disorders of cell-mediated immunity.

HUMORAL DEFICIENCIES

Immunoglobulin defects predispose to infection with encapsulated bacteria; toxin-producing bacteria (e.g., tetanus, diptheria); and viruses such as polio, hepatitis, and rubella. Bruton's agammaglobulinemia is an autosomal recessive disease in which immunoglobulins are produced in extremely low levels. Chronic lymphocytic leukemia is an acquired disorder marked by antibody defects. Regular administration of immunoglobulin appears to be somewhat protective in both congenital and acquired immunoglobulin deficiency states.

NOSOCOMIAL FACTORS, INCLUDING SURGERY AND ANESTHESIA

Surgical procedures necessarily involve the breach of cellular integrity and the disruption of mechanical processes that clear infection. Previously sterile regions of the host are brought into contact with nonsterile ones, increasing the risk of infection. Spillage of gastrointestinal contents into the peritoneum, entrance into the genitourinary tract or biliary tree in the presence of infected urine or bile, and surgery in the oropharynx all allow micro-organisms to enter spaces they normally do not inhabit and that often do not have adequate means of defense.

Depression of immune function following surgical procedures performed under general anesthesia has been demonstrated. In the postoperative period, lymphocytes are less responsive to various antigens including purified protein derivative of tuberculosis (PPD), and appear to have reduced capability to lyse antibody-coated target cells. Anergy in the postsurgical patient correlates with increased rates of sepsis and death. Anergic serum appears to inhibit neutrophil chemotaxis via as yet unidentified serum mediators. Depressed neutrophil chemotaxis also correlates with sepsis and death.

Other factors adversely affect the immune function of the surgical patient. Malnutrition causes a wide range of defects in cellular and humoral immunity that may be corrected with aggressive enteral and parenteral nutrition. In 1932, Studley demonstrated that preoperative weight loss of 20% correlated to a tenfold increase in postoperative mortality. Infection was the cause of death in the majority of these patients. Age, shock, hemorrhage, metabolic derangements such as uremia, infections, trauma, burns, and immunomodulating drugs all contribute to acquired deficits in immune function.

TRAUMA AND BURNS

Trauma and burn victims represent a unique subset of patients who have undergone drastic alteration in their host defense mechanisms. Burns alter the protective integument, creating oozing, moist surfaces vulnerable to intense bacterial colonization. Diminished neutrophil chemotactic activity, decreased lysosomal enzymes, lowered serum immunoglobulins, and a reduction in the absolute number of T lymphocytes and the T helper/suppressor cell ratio results in a profoundly immunocompromised state.

The breach of skin and mucous membrane barriers provides an important portal of entry for infection in trauma victims. Areas of impaired blood supply, hemothorax, and hematoma become excellent growth media for bacterial pathogens. In severe trauma, anergy develops as a function of the patient's age and severity of the injury. Neutrophil chemotaxis is also reduced.

PHARMACOLOGIC IMMUNOSUPPRESSION AND TRANSPLANTATION

The transplant patient is pharmacologically immunosuppressed in order to prevent the rejection of donor organs. The price paid for graft survival is an increased risk of infection. Steroids, cyclosporine A, azathioprine, antilymphocyte globulins, and monoclonal antibodies are used in various combinations in organ transplant recipients. Each impairs host defenses against infection. Steroids can cause atrophy of the skin and mucosa, which can lead to breaks in the skin and poor healing. They affect humoral defenses to some degree, but their major impact is on cellular immunity. There is a decreased accumulation of granulocytes at sites of inflammation probably as a result of decreased adherence and diminished chemotaxis. At very high doses, steroids impair phagocytosis and intracellular killing, but this is not thought to be clinically significant. Monocytes and lymphocytes appear to be decreased in number. Monocytes also have diminished chemotactic ability.

Cyclosporine A affects T cells preferentially. It diminishes the cytotoxic and proliferative capabilities of T-helper cells, probably by decreasing the production of interleukin-2 and its lymphocyte receptors. It may also block early B-cell activation. Antithymocyte globulin and monoclonal antibodies employed as immunosuppressive agents are directed against lymphocytes, suppressing cell-mediated immunity. Azathioprine causes lymphocytopenia and produces a moderate suppression of both humoral and cellular immune responses.

Infections occurring in the first month following transplant surgery are related to processes antedating the surgery or are related to the surgery itself. Postoperative wound infection, nosocomial pneumonia, urinary tract infection, or intravenous catheter-related bacteremia and fungemia are complications that stem from the surgery itself. Opportunistic infections during this time are unusual and often signal a nosocomial epidemic. The recipient may harbor infections such as tuberculosis and hepatitis B that may become fulminant following transplant. A variety of pathogens, including bacteria, viruses, and fungi, may be transmitted with the donor organ to the recipient. After four to six weeks, infections relating to the iatrogenic depression of cellular immunity are seen. Viruses, especially of the herpes group (in particular cytomegalovirus), intracellular bacteria such as *Listeria* and *Salmonella,* fungi, and the protozoa *Pneumocystis carinii* cause disease during this period.

ASPLENIA

The loss of an important immunologic organ, the spleen, leaves patients vulnerable to life-threatening infection with encapsulated bacteria. Patients undergoing splenectomy are at greatest risk for overwhelming postsplenectomy sepsis in the first two years following surgery but continue to have an overall lifetime risk of about 5%. In general, the risk of overwhelming sepsis in splenectomized patients is 60 times that of nonsplenectomized individuals. Patients who present with sepsis are usually otherwise healthy and typically develop a syndrome that begins with a mild upper respiratory tract infection and fever and progresses within hours to include nausea, vomiting, headache, confusion, shock, coma, and death. Though the mechanism of overwhelming postsplenectomy sepsis is not entirely clear, it appears to result from the loss of the valuable immune functions of the spleen. The microcirculation of the spleen strains micro-organisms from the blood, which are then engulfed by splenic macrophages. Tuftsin and properdin, factors crucial in the activation of the alternative complement pathway, are produced in the spleen, and this organ is the site of primary humoral response. At least 50% of the mass of the spleen is necessary to protect against encapsulated bacteria.

HUMAN IMMUNODEFICIENCY VIRUS INFECTION

One final aspect of host defense that has become a new challenge in the practice of surgery is the pandemic of human immunodeficiency virus (HIV), which was recognized in 1981.

The virus is a member of the lentivirus family of retroviruses. The spectrum of infection with HIV ranges from an acute mononucleosis-like illness to a protracted period of asymptomatic infection, terminating in a profound immunodeficiency state marked by the development of opportunistic infections, tumors, neurologic diseases, and a wasting syndrome. The singular characteristic of the disease is the inexorable loss of CD4 lymphocytes—the target cell of HIV infection. The CD4 or T-helper cell plays a central regulatory role in the cellular immune system. The CD4 antigen is the receptor on the surface of T-helper lymphocytes that binds the viral envelope glycoprotein and facilitates the entry of the virus into the host cell cytoplasm. Most individuals infected with the virus will begin to mount a detectable antibody response within six to twelve weeks. Prior to the development of a humoral response free virus circulates in very high titers. As humoral immunity develops, free viral titers drop significantly and the host enters a latent period of infection that may last from months to more than ten years. During this period of latency patients remain remarkably asymptomatic. Later in the course of infection CD4 cell counts fall dramatically and viral titers rise again. The amount of circulating virus may have some bearing on infectivity.

With the onset of the HIV epidemic, a heightened awareness has developed of the danger of occupationally acquired disease in health-care workers. A recent report from San Francisco indicates that accidental exposure to patient blood occurred during 6.4% of surgical procedures. Risk factors for blood exposure included procedures lasting longer than 3 hours, blood loss greater than 300 cc, and vascular or intraabdominal gynecologic procedures. Since patients with HIV can remain asymptomatic with the disease for years while still remaining infectious, it is difficult to identify those patients for whom special precautions are needed. A report from the emergency room at one institution identified victims of violent crime and drug overdose as the highest-risk patients in terms of HIV carriage. The Centers for Disease Control recommends that all patients be treated as if they were infected with HIV or other blood-borne organisms. To minimize risk of transmission, it recommends that health-care workers protect themselves with gloves, gowns, masks, and protective eyewear as is appropriate to the clinical setting when exposure to the blood and body fluids of any patient is likely.

Pathogenesis of Infectious Disease

BACTERIAL PATHOGENESIS

Colonization Versus Infection

Microorganisms are successful in causing disease when a combination of host and microbial factors exists. The host must be susceptible and the microbe abundant and virulent enough to produce infection. The skin and mucous membranes are colonized with microflora that coexist with the host. Hospitalization leads to colonization with nosocomial flora, the gram-negatives, and resistant staphylococcal species that are not normally part of the host's resident flora. However, the presence of bacteria cannot be of itself equated with infection. Critical inoculum size coupled with a breach or impairment in barrier defenses or a defective immune system allow invasion to occur.

Virulence Factors and Invasion

In addition to inoculum size, there are specific characteristics of each type of microorganism that contributes to its virulence. These factors include adherence, ability to escape phagocytosis or intracellular killing, elaboration of exotoxins, and extracellular enzymes, and presence of endotoxins. Cells often have receptors for bacterial and viral components that allow the organisms to stick to their surfaces. For example, influenza viral hemagglutinin attaches to muramic acid receptors on cells. Other micro-organisms have special structural components that enable them to adhere to mucosal surfaces, such as the pili of *Neisseria gonorrheae*. Micro-organisms have evolved ways of evading or neutralizing the immune system. The encapsulated organisms, such as pneumococcus, *H. influenzae, E. coli, Salmonella typhi, Klebsiella,* and fungi are better able to resist phagocytosis. Others have proteins that interfere with effective phagocytosis, such as the M protein of *Streptococcus pyogenes* and protein A in *S. aureus,* which block IgG-Fc on the opsonized organism and prevent it from binding to the Fc receptor of granulocytes. S. aureus makes the enzyme catalase that degrades H_2O_2 and impairs oxidative intracellular killing. *Mycobacterium tuberculosis, Toxoplasma, Aspergillus, Chlamydia* and staphylococci inhibit the fusion of lysosomes and phagosomes, also compromising intracellular killing. Table 29-2 lists a number of virulence factors.

TABLE 29-2. Virulence Factors

Factor	Effect
Hemagglutinins	Adherence
Pili	Adherence
Capsule	Resist phagocytosis
Surface proteins	Resist phagocytosis
Enzymes	Impair intracellular killing
Inhibition of lysosome-phagosome fusion	Impair intracellular killing
Toxins/enzymes	Cellular injury

Exotoxins

Numerous bacteria manufacture exotoxins and enzymes that destroy host tissue or cause disruption of normal organ functions. Table 29-3 lists a number of these organisms and their toxic products and harmful effects.

Endotoxins

Endotoxin is a lipopolysaccharide derived from the outer layer of the cell wall of gram-negative bacteria. Released upon the death of the bacteria, endotoxin causes fever directly by acting on the hypothalamus and indirectly by releasing the endogenous pyrogens interleukin-1, interferon, and tumor necrosis factor from phagocytic cells. Endotoxin also activates a cascade of events resulting in septic shock, including disseminated intravascular coagulation, complement activation, release of vasoactive substances such as serotonin, release of macrophage products such as collagenase and prostaglandin, and transient neutropenia followed by leukocytosis.

Host Factors

Variation in local host defenses influences infection. Lower extremity lesions may be more likely to become infected than upper extremity lesions, possibly related to differences in blood flow. Areas of venous insufficiency and lymphedema are more prone to infection because of reduced clearance of micro-organisms through impaired vascular channels. Embedded foreign bodies are a constant irritant and nidus for microorganisms that cannot be reached by the cells of the immune system. The diabetic foot is an excellent example of the alteration in local host factors that create conditions for infection. Diabetic peripheral neuropathy diminishes proprioception and sensation and exposes the extremity to traumatic injuries, which often go

TABLE 29-3. Representative Bacterial Toxins and Enzymes

Organism	Toxin/Enzyme	Effect
Staphylococcus aureus	Hyaluronidase	Hydrolyzes hyaluronidase component of connective tissue
	Catalase	Destroys H_2O_2
	Coagulase	Clots plasma
	Exfoliation	Desquamation of skin
	TSST-1	Toxic shock
	Enterotoxins	Food poisoning
Streptococcus pyogenes	DNAases	Degrade DNA
	Streptolysins	Hemolysis
	Pyrogenic toxin	Scarlet fever rash
	Streptokinase	Dissolves clot
Clostridium tetani	Tetanus toxin	Decreases neurotransmitter release from inhibitory neurons; spastic paralysis
Clostridium botulinum	Botulinum toxin	Decrease presynaptic acetylcholine release; flaccid paralysis
Clostridium perfringens	Alpha toxin	Hemolysis; necrosis
Corynebacterium diphtheria	Diphtheria toxin	Inhibits protein synthesis
Pseudomonas aeruginosa	Exotoxin A	Inhibits protein synthesis
Shigella dysenteriae	Shiga toxin	Inhibits protein synthesis
Escherichia coli	Heat labile enterotoxin	Activates adenylate cyclase; secretory diarrhea
Vibrio cholerae	Cholera toxin	Activates adenylate cyclase; secretory diarrhea

Adapted from Mandell G, Douglas RG, Bennett JE, eds. *Principles and practice of infectious diseases.* 3rd ed. New York: Churchill Livingstone, 1990:3; and from Howard RJ, Simmons RL, eds. *Surgical infectious diseases.* 2nd ed. Norwalk, CT: Appleton & Lange, 1988:9.

unnoticed. Arterial insufficiency in diabetics leads to ischemia of distal extremities that when injured become fertile territory for bacteria. Ischemia also delays wound healing and impedes the transport of antibiotic medications to infected wounds.

FUNGAL PATHOGENESIS

Special risk factors predispose to infection with fungi. The normal host is usually not subject to serious fungal infection beyond relatively minor skin diseases and vaginal infections during antibiotic administration. Risk factors for the development of serious fungal infection include intravenous cannulas, prolonged antibiotic use, hyperalimentation, pharmacologic immunosuppression, burns, trauma, and malnutrition. The use of broad-spectrum antibiotics alters normal flora and allows competing fungi to proliferate on skin and mucosa where they can then enter through breaks in

the surface. Steroids, chemotherapeutic agents, and other immunosuppressive factors depress the cellular arm of the immune system in particular, which weakens host defense against fungal invasion. Antineoplastic agents not only compromise the immune system but frequently cause a mucositis throughout the gastrointestinal tract. Autopsies of patients who die after prolonged postsurgical illness often reveal mucosal necrosis in areas throughout the gastrointestinal tract. In these circumstances, colonizing fungi cross the boundaries of the gastrointestinal tract to create local infections such as peritonitis and abscesses, or to disseminate via the bloodstream. In addition, when the density of fungal micro-organisms in the gut reaches about 10^9/mL, they can migrate through intact intestinal mucosa.

It is often difficult to make a definitive diagnosis of fungal infection. Positive blood or tissue cultures, biopsies, or ophthalmologic examination demonstrating fungal retinitis may provide a definitive diagnosis, but these are often absent. Blood cultures may be negative in over half the cases of widely disseminated disease. Candidal retinitis is only identified in about 25% of cases of disseminated candidiasis. There are currently no serologic tests available with adequate sensitivity and specificity to be clinically useful in the diagnosis of disseminated candidal infection. Serologic tests for other fungal diseases such as cryptococcosis and coccidioidomycosis are sensitive and clinically useful. The clinician is frequently left to make a judgment regarding the need to initiate antifungal therapy based on the number of sites colonized and the presence of risk factors, as previously mentioned.

VIRAL PATHOGENESIS

Viral infections can be grouped into three main categories—acute, latent, and slow. In acute infection, virus can remain localized to its portal of entry, spreading from cell to cell, or it can undergo replication at the entry site and then disseminate throughout the body through the blood and lymphatic system and attack a distant organ. Latent infection establishes the virus as a permanent resident in the host. Evading the host's immune system by replicating within host cells, certain viruses can also intercalate their genomes into host DNA and use the machinery of the host cell to reproduce themselves. Slow viral infections result in disease that develops over a prolonged period of time, usually several years. Warts and the common cold are examples of localized acute infections. Hepatitis and influenza are acute infections that disseminate. Viruses of the herpes family—herpes simplex, varicella-zoster, and cytomegalovirus—are responsible for latent infection that lies dormant until reactivated by various stimuli.

The members of the herpes family of viruses figure prominently in diseases arising in immunosuppressed transplant patients. Cytomegalovirus is the most common opportunistic pathogen found in transplant patients. It can cause asymptomatic infection; a variety of symptomatic syndromes, including a flulike illness and pneumonia; predispose to fungal and bacterial infections; and may precipitate graft rejection. Cytomegalovirus may be acquired via infected blood products or from the donor organ itself and cause acute disease. More commonly, the recipient already harbors the virus, and suppression of the cellular immune system reactivates viral replication. Varicella-zoster virus reactivates with increased frequency in transplant patients. The vesicular eruption is usually confined to a dermatomal distribution, but the disease can disseminate and cause severe systemic illness. Herpes simplex viruses reactivate in the oral and genital regions but can cause more extensive local disease, such as herpes esophagitis, and on occasion may disseminate as well. Epstein-Barr virus is latent in B lymphocytes and in transplant patients may cause a lymphoproliferative syndrome characterized by the development of a malignant B-cell clone. The lymphoproliferative syndrome can sometimes be aborted by the reduction or cessation of immunosuppression and the removal of the transplanted organ.

SEPTIC SHOCK

Pathogenesis

Severe uncontrolled infection can produce systemic responses that are life-threatening to the host. Septic shock represents the condition in which severe infection leads to hypotension and metabolic abnormalities. Studies of gram-negative bacteremia have elucidated some mechanisms for shock that appear to be applicable to other organisms as well. Endotoxin from the cell walls of gram-negative bacteria trigger a chain of reactions involving the complement, clotting, fibrinolytic, and kinin pathways that leads to hemodynamic instability, increased vascular permeability, metabolic derangements, and disorders of hemostasis. Upon exposure to endotoxin, macrophages release cytokines, including interleukin-1, γ-interferon, and tumor necrosis factor, which are among the mediators of septic shock. Tumor necrosis factor is a very important mediator of gram-negative sepsis. It is not specific to gram-negative infections but can be associated with other types of infection as well. Endotoxin-mediated activation of complement releases neutrophil chemoattractant factors, particularly C5a, which in turn leads to release of anaphylatoxins that increase vascular permeability. Clotting and fibrinolytic systems are turned on and lead alternatively to bleeding and thrombosis, often with resultant tissue ischemia and organ failure. Endotoxin activates Hageman factor in the clotting cascade, which also activates the kinin system. The end product of the kinin pathway is bradykinin, a vasoactive peptide that causes vasodilation and increased vascular permeability and leads to hypotension and third-space losses of fluid into the tissues.

Septic Physiology

In septic shock, the heart, peripheral vasculature, and the tissues are all affected, each to a different degree. Septic shock can present with one of two hemodynamic patterns. The first is a high flow state in which the patient appears flushed, warm, and has bounding pulses. Central hemodynamic monitoring reveals that the patient's cardiac output is high, the peripheral vascular resistance low. The second is a low-flow state in which the patient is cool, with mottled, cyanotic limbs. The cardiac output is diminished and the peripheral vascular resistance is elevated. Which pattern will ensue is unpredictable, although some preexisting factors may influence the hemodynamic state. Hypovolemia caused by third-space losses can lead to peripheral vasoconstriction, and preexisting cardiac disease in the face of the stress of infection can lead to impaired cardiac output, both of which can be seen in the low-flow state of septic shock.

When abnormalities develop in cardiac performance, they do so late in the course. The stress on the heart caused by a hyperdynamic state may cause ischemia and ultimately failure. The arteriovenous O_2 difference ($A-VO_2$) across the coronaries may be narrowed, decreasing oxygen release to tissues and causing ischemia. There is strong evidence that one or more myocardial depressant substances are produced that suppress myocardial contractility. It appears unlikely that gram-negative bacterial endotoxin itself depresses myocardial function.

In the hyperdynamic state, the vasodilatory response may well be a maladaptive one mediated by circulating factors. In the low-flow state, the vasoconstrictive response initially preserves blood flow to the brain and heart, but as it is maintained it leads to ischemia in the underperfused liver, kidney, and gut. Renal and hepatic failure and gastrointestinal hemorrhage often are the result.

Peripheral tissues are underperfused in septic shock, but they also do not appear to be able to utilize oxygen efficiently. The $A-VO_2$ difference decreases in the face of increasing metabolic needs, and the hyperdynamic state is not able to compensate. A highly catabolic state ensues in which the metabolism switches from aerobic to anaerobic glycolysis and fat and muscle are broken down into triglycerides, ketones, and amino acids. A refractory hyperglycemia develops that is resistant to insulin administration, and lactic acid and pyruvate levels increase.

Abnormalities in the clotting system result in disseminated intravascular coagulation, with either hemorrhage or thrombosis produced by the excessive consumption or coagulation of clotting factors. Microthrombi and hemorrhages damage the tissues and lead to organ failure.

In the lung, thrombosis and hemorrhage, and increased vascular permeability result in adult respiratory distress syndrome, and lead to respiratory failure. Gas exchange across damaged, fluid-filled membranes is severely impaired and mechanical ventilation with increased amounts of inspired oxygen and positive end-expiratory pressure are required to maintain an adequate PO_2.

PATHOGENESIS OF NOSOCOMIAL INFECTIONS

Up to 4% of hospitalized patients may acquire a nosocomial infection. The hospital environment exposes patients to a plethora of resistant organisms. The use of antibiotics selects for resistant bacteria that can be spread from patient to patient via intermediaries in the hospital environment. Potential sources of contagion include supplies, instruments, and hospital staff. Intravascular catheter infections, pneumonias, urinary tract, wound, and transfusion-related infections are common in the hospitalized patient. Infection control measures such as hand-washing and isolation and avoidance whenever possible of the impairment of host defenses are important in preventing nosocomial disease.

Intravascular Catheter Infections

Intravenous catheters are associated with a range of infectious complications, including cellulitis around the catheter entry site, septic thrombophlebitis, abscess, bacteremia, and endocarditis. Organisms can gain access to the bloodstream at any point in the intravenous system from the infusate to the skin insertion site, though the latter is thought to be the most common portal of entry. A number of risk factors are associated with development of infection. Stiff catheters appear to be more thrombogenic and are associated with a higher risk of infection than more flexible ones. Microorganisms adhere more easily to certain catheter materials; staphylococci and *Candida* species adhere better to polyvinyl chloride than to Teflon. Increased number and size of lumens in central venous catheters and repeated manipulation of these devices by frequent blood drawing or central pressure monitoring promotes infection. Bacterial and fungal overgrowth at the skin insertion site, contaminated ointments applied to the site, and poor aseptic technique by hospital staff providing catheter care also increase the incidence of infection. Placement of the catheter in the lower extremities, especially in the femoral area, is associated with a higher infection rate. Catheters left in place for greater than 72 hours are more likely to become infected. Prolonged central venous catheterization poses a significant risk in debilitated patients requiring total parenteral nutrition. The composition of the infusate itself supports the growth of organisms, especially fungi and coagulase-negative staphylococci. The hypertonic infusate promotes thrombus formation and subsequent infection. The catheter can also be seeded by hematogenous spread from a distant source.

The most common pathogens associated with intravascular catheter infections are the staphylococcal species, primarily *S. epidermidis,* followed in incidence by *S. aureus. Staphylococcus epidermidis* produces a polysaccharide biofilm that may contribute to its ability to adhere to plastic catheters and shield it from antibiotics and host defenses. The staphylococci are followed in order of frequency by the gram-negative enteric bacilli, including *Enterobacter, Klebsiella,* and *Serratia,* and then by *Candida* species, *Pseudomonas, Citrobacter,* and *Corynebacteria,* particularly the JK species.

The diagnosis of catheter-related infection is not always clear-cut. Other sources of infection must be eliminated. Factors that help differentiate catheter-related bacteremias from other infectious processes are listed in Table 29-4.

Pneumonia

Pneumonia is the most common fatal nosocomial infection. Fifteen percent of all hospital deaths are ascribed to this complication. The major route of acquisition of nosocomial pneumonia is via aspiration of oral flora. Mouth flora rapidly becomes colonized with nosocomial gram-negative rods in about half of all intensive care unit patients. Colonized patients are more likely to develop pneumonia than noncolonized patients.

Endotracheal intubation, even for brief periods, is associated with increased risk of aspiration pneumonia. Aspiration may occur when the endotracheal tube is removed. Long-term intubation and placement of a tracheostomy tube disturb the normal barrier defense mechanisms of the respiratory tract and prevent clear-

TABLE 29-4. Factors Differentiating Device-Associated Bacteremia from Other Septic Syndromes

- Local phlebitis/inflammation at catheter insertion site
- No other source for bacteremia
- Sepsis in patient not at high risk for bacteremia
- Septic emboli distal to arterial cannula
- *Candida* endophthalmitis in patient receiving total parenteral nutrition
- Greater than 15 colonies of bacteria on catheter tip culture
- Sepsis refractory to appropriate antimicrobial therapy
- Defervescence after device removal
- Typical (staphylococci) or unusual (gram-negatives) microbiology

Adapted from Mandell G, Douglas RG, Bennett JE, eds. *Principles and practice of infectious diseases.* 3rd ed. New York: Churchill Livingstone, 1990:2191.

ance of organisms by the filtering system of the nose, airway turbulence, and cough. Irritation and inflammation of the respiratory epithelium may promote colonization of the injured surfaces. The postsurgical patient is also deprived of the normal clearance mechanisms when coughing is limited by incisional pain and splinting. Antibiotic use selects more resistant pathogens. Advanced age, sedation, and head trauma are additional predisposing factors for aspiration pneumonia. Some additional risk factors are listed in Table 29-5.

Gram-negative bacilli are by far the most common pathogens in the etiology of nosocomial pneumonia,

TABLE 29-5. Predisposing Factors for Hospital-Acquired Pneumonia

- Intubation
- Intensive care unit
- Antibiotics
- Surgery
- Chronic lung disease
- Advanced age
- Immunosuppression
- Sedation
- Head trauma

Adapted from Mandell G, Douglas RG, Bennett JE, eds. *Principles and practice of infectious diseases.* 3rd ed. New York: Churchill Livingstone, 1990:2200.

causing more than 60% of these infections. *Pseudomonas* and *Enterobacter* species are frequently seen in most institutions, followed in frequency by *S. aureus* and other gram-negatives.

Urinary Tract Infection

Urinary tract infections are the most common infections occurring in hospitals and nursing homes. Eighty percent of nosocomial urinary tract infections are associated with bladder catherization.

The bladder catheter system leads to infection in several different ways. Both the inner and outer surfaces of the catheter act as a pathway for ascending bacterial infection. The mechanical trauma of the catheter against urethral epithelium inflames the mucosal surface, damaging its normal protective mechanisms and facilitating colonization by micro-organisms. Within 24 hours of catheterization, gram-negative rods and enterococci colonize the periurethral area, conditions that predispose to bacteriuria in up to two thirds of patients. The invading bacteria are able to adhere to mucosal surfaces as well as to the catheter material itself via their fingerlike fimbriae, and by producing glycocalyx, a biofilm that anchors the bacteria to surfaces and protects them from the flow of urine, host defenses, and antibiotics.

The enteric gram-negative rods as a group are responsible for the majority of urinary tract infections. *Escherichia coli, Pseudomonas, Klebsiella, Proteus mirabalis* and enterococci are most frequently isolated. More unusual organisms such as *Providentia stuartii* and other *Proteus* species become prevalent with catheterizations of longer than a month's duration. Mixed populations of bacteria with high colony counts are also more common after long-term catheterization.

The main complication of bacteriuria is progression to symptomatic infection. Ascending bacterial infection can progress to pyelonephritis and bacteremia, though cystitis may also on occasion lead to bacteremia.

Bacteriuria can also lead to obstruction of the bladder catheter from a conglomeration of bacteria, glycocalyx, and Tamm-Horsfall protein. Bacteriuria and infection with *Proteus mirabilis,* which hydrolyzes urea, alkalinizes the urine and causes crystallization of struvite and apatite into obstructing stones in the catheter or in the rest of the urinary tract.

Other complications of bladder catheterization include infection of structures in proximity to the urinary tract, resulting in prostatitis, prostatic abscess, epididimytis, and scrotal abscess.

Wound Infections

Bacterial colonization and virulence are major determinants of surgical wound infection. Increased numbers and virulence of the colonizing bacteria are correlated with increased risk of infections. Aseptic surgical techniques and the institution of appropriate preoperative antibiotic prophylaxis have decreased the incidence of surgical wound infections to approximately 1% for clean-contaminated cases.

Despite the advances in prevention, surgical wound infections have not been totally eliminated. The physical removal of organisms from the skin with antiseptic soaps and solutions succeeds in removing only the transient, surface-dwelling organisms on the skin at the operative site, but not the resident flora living deep in the sebaceous glands and follicles. These deeply buried organisms serve as a reservoir that recolonizes the skin and can infect wounds.

Contaminated instruments, supplies, and the hands of staff members can act as vehicles for the introduction of bacteria into wounds.

Devitalized tissues damaged by trauma, burns, or ischemia; the presence of a hematoma; and the placement of foreign material into the wound all provide fertile ground for the development of wound infection. Out of the reach of the cellular and humoral arms of the immune system, organisms grow unchecked. Debridement, drainage, and removal of foreign bodies are necessary for cure.

Methicillin-resistant *S. aureus, S. epidermidis,* fungi, and resistant gram-negative rods, including *Acinetobacter calcoaceticus* and *Pseudomonas* species are the cause of surgical wound infections with increasing frequency.

Hematogenous seeding is the least likely mechanism of postoperative wound infection and is thought to be the cause of some later postoperative infections. However, hematogenous spread is difficult to prove. In some postoperative wound infections, such as those seen in prosthetic valves and total hip replacements, organisms are more likely introduced at the time of surgery and lie dormant for years before causing infection.

Transfusion-Related Infections

Transfusion of blood and blood products may be associated with the transmission of disease from donor to recipient. Viruses such as hepatitis B, hepatitis C, cytomegalovirus, and HIV-1 are transmitted via transfusion, and there are reports of hepatitis A and Epstein-Barr virus as well as spirochetes and protozoa, including *Treponema pallidum*, malaria, and babesia being transmitted through this route. Screening for hepatitis B surface antigen started in 1972 and greatly decreased the incidence of posttransfusion hepatitis caused by this agent. Screening for the surrogate markers of hepatitis, such as elevated alanine aminotransferase, has lowered the incidence of posttransfusion hepatitis secondary to non-A, non-B types of hepatitis. A screening test is now available for hepatitis C, which will eliminate many cases of non-A, non-B hepatitis. Screening measures have not succeeded in completely eliminating posttransfusion hepatitis. Patients who receive numerous transfusions are at particularly high risk. Non-A, non-B posttransfusion hepatitis accounts for 90–95% of cases, and figures on attack rates of non-A, non-B hepatitis range from 1% to 11.5% per unit of blood. Blood-processing techniques using heat and chemicals inactivate viruses but do not totally eliminate the risk of infection.

Risk of transmission of cytomegalovirus (CMV) is estimated at 2–3% per unit of whole blood. Granulocyte transfusions in bone marrow transplant patients are also associated with a high rate of CMV infection. Patients receiving granulocyte transfusions develop CMV infection twice as often as patients who do not receive the transfusions. Transfusion-associated CMV infection is usually asymptomatic but can produce a febrile systemic illness with the characteristics of mononucleosis.

Testing for HIV-1 antibody in blood and blood products and heat treatment of clotting factors begun in 1985 greatly diminished the number of transfusion-related HIV-1 infections. In determining a patient's HIV risk, it is important to elicit a transfusion history, noting in particular if the transfusion took place prior to the start of routine screening. The blood supply is very safe at this time; however, a small number of HIV-infected individuals who have not developed antibody can be expected to slip through the screening net. When time permits, autologous blood donation should be encouraged.

The Use of the Laboratory

OBTAINING CULTURES

Definitive diagnosis of infectious disease is made in the microbiology laboratory, where pathogens are cultured and then identified by morphological characteristics and chemical tests. Blood, body fluids, and secretions can be cultured for bacteria, viruses, and fungi, and stained for protozoa, spirochetes, and parasites. As with any laboratory method of diagnosis, results must be interpreted in light of the individual patient's clinical situation. The positive culture may alternatively reflect true infection, colonization, or contamination. The clinician must make the final judgment regarding the significance of an isolate based on a number of factors, including the organisms, site of infection, and the clinical status of the patient.

Blood Cultures

Infections of the vascular structures, the heart and blood vessels, are accompanied by the release of microorganisms into the bloodstream that can be sampled for culture. Infections in the deeper tissues and organs can also make their way into the bloodstream. Bacteria are the organisms that are most commonly and easily cultured from the blood, though fungi and viruses can be cultured as well. Bacteremias originating from deep-seated infections are characteristically intermittent and low grade. Cultures of blood, therefore, must be temporally spaced and of sufficient volume to capture bacteria. On the other hand, bacteremias in the setting of endocarditis or endovascular infection are continuous, but multiple temporally spaced blood cultures are still necessary, as repetitively positive cultures will be diagnostic of this type of infection.

Sterile technique must be used to obtain the cultures to avoid contamination with skin flora. Three separate sets of blood cultures should be drawn within a 24-hour period. At least 15 minutes should elapse between cultures. A set of blood cultures includes one aerobic vial that is vented when it reaches the microbiology laboratory to permit the growth of aerobic organisms, and one anaerobic vial that remains unvented. Both aerobic and anaerobic organisms may grow in the unvented vial. A volume of 20 mL of blood per set is recommended for adults; 1–3 mL per set for infants and children. In the setting of endocarditis, the sensitivity of a single blood culture is approximately 80–90%; the sensitivity is greater than 95% if two to three sets are drawn within 24 hours. Volume of blood and number of cultures are independent variables, so obtaining a larger volume of blood at one time in order to avoid taking multiple blood cultures later will not have the same yield as the recommended protocol.

Large studies have been done that classify positive blood cultures as representing true infection versus contamination, and as a result of these studies guidelines can be provided for the interpretation of positive cultures. The presence of a particular type of organism in the blood and the number of positive cultures are important in determining true infection and also helpful in deciding whether the bacteremia arises from an endovascular infection or another source. The isolation of gram-negative organisms and fungi rarely represents contamination and is thus always significant. The presence of *S. aureus* in one study represented true infection 75% of the time, while *S. epidermidis,* a common skin isolate, was usually a contaminant. *S. pneumoniae* and the group B streptococci always represented infection. The viridans streptococci were judged to represent infection only about half the time. Gram-positive bacilli were almost always contaminants, except for *Listeria monocytogenes,* which was always a true pathogen. Anaerobic gram-positive bacteria were variously associated with infection or contamination, depending on the clinical situation, but gram-negative anaerobes all were indicative of true infection. Most fungal isolates were judged to be truly infective.

The patterns of positive blood cultures predict whether a bacteremia is representative of a true infection or of contamination. Illustrative of contamination is the pattern that initial positive cultures are usually not followed by subsequent positive cultures. At the other extreme, when one blood culture turns positive in a patient with endocarditis or endovascular infection, the likelihood that the subsequent cultures will be positive is 95–100%. Bacteremias from other sources of infection resulted in positive blood cultures 75–80% of the time.

In summary, the clinical setting, the type of organism cultured, and the number of cultures positive should be evaluated together to determine whether the patient is infected.

Urine Cultures

For the diagnosis of urinary tract infection, clean catch midstream urine is recommended. The specimen must be processed in the lab within 2 hours or be refrigerated until processing can take place. The urine is plated onto general-purpose and gram-negative differential media, upon which colonies of bacteria arise. Quantitative colony counts are performed to determine whether infection is significant. Colony counts of greater than 10^5/mL usually represent significant infection, but even counts as low as 10^2 can be significant if the patient is symptomatic.

Urinalysis

Microscopic examination of the urine provides information that can be used to interpret the results of urine culture and should be performed concurrently to make the diagnosis of urinary tract infection. The presence or absence of white blood cells can be used to distinguish between true infection and asymptomatic bacteriuria. Five to ten white blood cells per high-power field are considered the upper limit of normal, and higher numbers are indicative of infection. However, pyuria may be found in patients without urinary tract infection. White cell casts of renal tubular epithelium may form in the presence of pyelonephritis. Red cells may be associated with infection but can also be representative of other processes such as urinary tract calculi or tumor. The presence of squamous epithelial cells usually indicates contamination from the perineal area or from the vagina in females and makes interpretation of the urinalysis difficult. It is recommended to repeat the specimen in this case, obtaining a catheterized specimen if necessary. A Gram's stain of the resuspended sediment is useful in distinguishing gram-positive from gram-negative bacteria. The presence of one bacterium per oil immersion field is correlated with greater than 10^4 colony-forming units/mL in a centrifuged specimen, and 10^5 colony-forming units/mL in an unspun sample.

In patients who are not able to provide properly collected midstream specimens, urine may be obtained by catheterization or suprapubic aspiration. Since these samples are less likely to be contaminated, lower colony counts may be significant and indicative of true bacteriuria. The patient with a chronic indwelling foley catheter is frequently colonized with gram-negative bacteria. Treatment is not indicated unless pyuria is present or the patient is febrile without another source.

Sputum Cultures

The microbiologic diagnosis of pneumonia is fraught with uncertainty. Sputum may become contaminated with oral flora during the collection process. Diagnostic sputum samples must come from the deeper portions of the respiratory tree. A Gram's stain of a heat-fixed sputum smear is scanned under low power for squamous epithelial cells. Generally, 25 epithelial cells/low-power field are used as the cutoff point in determining the suitability of the specimen for culture. The presence of greater than 25 cells indicates an unacceptable specimen that is made up primarily of saliva and will therefore grow mouth flora. Samples with fewer than 25 cells are processed for culture. The Gram-stained smear is then examined under high power to identify pathogens and guide antimicrobial therapy. Though more than one type of organism may be seen on the smear, the predominant organism is felt to be the primary pathogen. If an abundant variety of organisms are equally represented on the slide, then a diagnosis of aspiration pneumonia should be considered if the clinical situation is appropriate, as the organisms may represent aspirated mouth flora. An abundance of granulocytes with a paucity of bacteria in the appropriate clinical setting should suggest the possibility of an atypical or viral pneumonia.

Viral Diagnostics

All body fluids, tissues, and secretions may be cultured for viruses. To increase the sensitivity of the cultures, samples should be taken as early as possible in the course of the illness, brought to the laboratory promptly, and transported in special media depending on the specimen type. Fluid specimens may be sent directly to the virology laboratory, while dry swabs or tissues should be placed in special fluid viral transport media.

The technique for growing viruses utilizes a battery of previously prepared cell cultures. A specimen is inoculated into the culture tubes, and virus from specimen infects the various cell monolayers that line the bottom of the tubes. The cells are incubated for 7–21 days and examined microscopically every day for the effects of viral replication. Rapid detection techniques are also available that considerably speed the identification process. Immunofluorescence, radioimmunoassay, and enzyme-linked immunosorbent assay are among the processes used to detect viral antigen within the incubating cell cultures.

Viral serologies can also be used to diagnose acute infection; however, convalescent serology is rarely available in time to impact upon patient management. Paired acute and convalescent sera, taken two to three weeks apart, are compared for a fourfold rise in IgG antibody to confirm recent infection. IgM antibody can be assayed in certain instances and provide a timely diagnosis of acute infection.

A new technique that is being used by some research laboratories to detect virus is the polymerase chain reaction. With the polymerase chain reaction, a single copy of viral DNA can be replicated over a million times, and the amplified DNA can easily be identified with specific gene probes or by restriction endonuclease analysis. Human immunodeficiency virus is one of the viruses that have been detected in this manner.

Fungal Diagnostics

Most of the common varieties of yeasts, such as the *Candida* species, are easily grown in conventional aerobic blood culture bottles, with preliminary results generally available within three to five days. Lysis centrifugation techniques are somewhat more sensitive and rapid and are useful for those fungal species which are harder to grow.

Surfaces can frequently be colonized with fungi in the absence of a true infection. While fungi are often visible on Gram's stain, they are also easily seen on KOH preparations, which eliminate cellular debris that might otherwise mask the fungal elements. It has been shown that the repeated culturing of *Candida* from three separate sites is associated with the presence of true infection. Histopathology is often necessary to distinguish between colonization and infection. For example, *Aspergillus* species, molds that may colonize the upper respiratory tract, require biopsy to diagnose invasive disease. Fungal elements seen in tissue sections treated with hematoxylin-eosin and methenamine silver stains are diagnostic.

The immune system's humoral response to fungal invasion may provide diagnostic evidence of infection. Serodiagnosis should be used as an adjunct to other methods of detection, such as culture and biopsy. As with other serologic tests, a single antibody titer is insufficient to diagnose current illness, and paired acute and convalescent sera must be drawn several weeks apart to document a fourfold rise in titer. Serologic detection of fungal antigen may be indicative of current active infection, particularly if the fungus is not a common colonizing organism. For example, a positive latex agglutination test for cryptococcal antigen in the serum or CSF is presumptive evidence of cryptococcosis. Currently, serologic detection of antibody to *Candida* species is not a useful clinical tool.

THE LABORATORY AS AID TO ANTIBIOTIC SELECTION AND MONITORING DRUG LEVELS

Susceptibility Testing

Resistance to antimicrobial agents requires that micro-organisms be tested against a panel of antibiotics to determine their susceptibility. Aerobic bacteria are almost always tested in this manner. Other micro-organisms, such as fungi, viruses, and anaerobic bacteria, are usually not tested against anti-infective agents. In vitro resistance patterns may not clearly correlate with in vivo observations, and only reference laboratories have the capability of testing the susceptibility of these pathogens.

Minimal Inhibitory Concentration

Automated systems currently in use for susceptibility testing utilize the dilution method. A fixed inoculum of bacteria is incubated with serial dilutions of a drug, and the minimal concentration needed to inhibit growth of the organism is determined. High minimal inhibitory concentrations (MIC) generally indicate resistance to a drug; low MICs, susceptibility. Previously determined cutoffs, or breakpoints, categorize the MICs as representing susceptibility, moderate susceptibility, intermediate susceptibility, or resistance to a specific drug. There are few instances when the clinician needs to know the actual MIC numerical value itself. The MIC is useful in a case such as Streptococcal endocarditis, where it has been shown that penicillin-sensitive organisms with higher MICs than usual require the addition of an aminoglycoside and the prolongation of therapy with penicillin to insure rapid and complete bactericidal activity.

The traditional method of determining antimicrobial susceptibility is the Bauer-Kirby disk diffusion technique. Antibiotic-impregnated paper discs are dropped onto a previously inoculated agar dish, and a zone of bacterial inhibition forms. The diameters of the zones of inhibition correspond with previously defined categories of susceptibility and resistance.

Pharmacokinetics

Plasma antibiotic levels are obtained for a limited number of commonly used drugs in order to insure that therapeutic levels are maintained and toxicity avoided.

The aminoglycosides and vancomycin are two of the drugs thus monitored.

Dosing intervals are determined by the half-life ($T_{1/2}$) of a drug, that is, the time it takes for the drug level to decrease by half as it is eliminated from the body. Given a fixed rate of elimination of drug from the body, drug peak and trough levels reach constant steady-state levels in about four half-lives. Once a drug reaches steady-state levels, plasma peak and trough concentrations can be measured with the knowledge that these levels will be constant, barring a change in the drug dose or a change in the rate of elimination, as may be the case with development of renal or hepatic failure. If a drug dose is increased or decreased it follows that steady state will again be reached after approximately four half-lives.

Therapeutic effectiveness and threshholds of toxicity have been correlated with ranges of plasma concentration of certain drugs. Following measurement of peak and trough levels, drug doses and dosing intervals can be adjusted to target specific ranges. Raising or lowering a peak concentration is usually accomplished by increasing or decreasing the drug dose, while raising or lowering the trough requires lengthening or shortening the interval between doses.

Use of Antimicrobial Agents

The therapeutic armamentarium against infectious diseases is extensive and includes an often bewildering array of anti-infective agents. Anti-infective drugs can be divided into three major categories, including antibacterials, antivirals, and antifungals. Drugs are categorized by chemical structure and spectrum of action. The use of anti-infective agents can be classified as empiric, therapeutic, or prophylactic. Passive and active immunization with immunoglobulins and vaccines are a major component of infectious disease prophylaxis. In the future, the clinician can expect to see the advent of biologic response modifiers that act to blunt the effects of the host immune response in such situations as gram-negative shock.

The choice of anti-infective agent encompasses knowledge of the drug's applicability to the clinical situation, activity, toxicity, and cost. General characteristics of the major classes of antimicrobials are discussed below and summarized in Table 29-6.

CLASSES OF ANTIMICROBIALS

Antibacterials

β-Lactam Agents

The β-lactam antibiotics are so named because of the four-sided β-lactam ring that forms the core of their chemical structure. This four-sided ring confers bactericidal activity that is lost if the ring is disrupted. Penicillins and cephalosporins as well as the newer monobactam and carbapenem drugs possess the β-lactam ring. The β-lactams are distinguished from one another by virtue of different side chains, which confer pharmacologic properties and spectrum of activity.

The drug binds to and impairs the function of the penicillin-binding proteins, enzymes located in the bacterial cell membrane responsible for synthesizing the peptidoglycan component of the cell wall. It is not clear how lysis is induced.

Bacteria have developed a number of different mechanisms of resistance to β-lactam antibiotics, the chief of which is disruption of the β-lactam ring. Inducible enzymes known as β-lactamases hydrolyze the amide bond of the β-lactam ring. Newer antibiotics have built into their chemical conformation structures that resist hydrolysis by β-lactamases.

The spectrum of action of the β-lactams is broad. Penicillin G is active against most streptococcal and *Neisseria* species. Semisynthetic penicillins, such as nafcillin, cover primarily penicillinase-producing *S. aureus* (except methicillin-resistant *S. aureus)*, and streptococci. The aminopenicillins such as ampicillin and amoxicillin retain gram-positive coverage but are also effective against common gram-negative bacilli, particularly urinary tract pathogens. The carboxypenicillins, which include ticarcillin and carbenicillin, and the ureidopenicillins, including mezlocillin and piperacillin, possess a wider spectrum of activity against gram-positive and gram-negative organisms, including *Pseudomonas.*

The cephalosporins are commonly described as first-, second-, or third-generation agents. First-generation agents such as cefazolin possess excellent activity against *S. aureus* and streptococci and a number of gram-negatives, particularly *E. coli, Proteus,* and *Klebsiella.* It should be noted that the oral-first generation agents possess higher MICs against most staphylococcal isolates than other antistaphylococcal drugs and may not be as effective against *S. aureus* for that reason. The gram-negative spectrum increases with succeeding generations, while the gram-positive activity is less than that of the first-generation agents. Cefoperazone and ceftazidime are third-generation drugs with significant antipseudomonal activity. Anaerobic sensitivity varies from one cephalosporin to another, but it should be remembered that none of these drugs are active against MRSA or enterococcal species.

β-Lactam related drugs of major importance include the carbapenems and monobactams represented by imipenem/cilastatin and aztreonam, respectively. Imipenem is resistant to many β-lactamases and has excellent activity against gram positive cocci, many enterococcal species, most of the gram-negative bacilli, including Citrobacter, Enterobacter, Acinetobacter, and Pseudomonas. It also covers most anaerobes very well. It is not active against MRSA. Aztreonam, a monocyclic β-lactam, has a narrow spectrum of coverage limited to gram-negative aerobic bacteria.

Compounds which combine a β-lactam with a β-lactamase inhibitior have recently been marketed. These include amoxicillin/clavulanate, ticarcillin/clavulanate and ampicillin/sulbactam. Clavulanate and sulbactam are weakly antibacterial agents in their own right which also possess a β-lactam based structure. Coupled to other antimicrobials, their function is to bind B-lactamases and prevent them from hydrolyzing the β-lactam ring of the more active agent. The β-lactamases of *S. aureus, Klebsiella, Haemophilus influenzae, Bacteroides* species and others are inhibited in this manner. Unfortunately, bacteria possess other mechanisms of resistance and in many cases the β-lactamase inhibitors provide little advantage over agents that do not possess the inhibitor.

Aminoglycosides

The aminoglycosides consist of two or more amino sugars coupled via glycoside bonds to 6-membered aminocyclitol ring. They inhibit bacterial protein synthesis by binding to ribosomes and interfering with transcription of mRNA. The general spectrum of activity includes gram-negative bacilli and *S. aureus,* although there are much more effective and less toxic drugs that are used for the latter. Individual aminoglycosides have different properties. Streptomycin has activity against Mycobacterium tuberculosis. Amikacin is active against many gram-negative rods otherwise resistant to β-lactams and other aminoglycosides.

Aminoglycosides can act synergistically in combination with β-lactams to combat serious enterococcal

TABLE 29-6. Characteristics of Major Antibiotic Classes

Class	Structure	Action	Excretion	Toxicity/Interaction
		ANTIBACTERIALS		
β-*Lactam Agents*	4-Membered lactam ring	Interfere with bacterial cell wall formation		
Penicillins			Renal	Rash, diarrhea, neutropenia, platelet dysfunction, interstitial nephritis
Cephalosporins			Renal, except cefoperazone and ceftriaxone	Similar to penicillin, coagulation disorders
Penicillins with β-lactamase inhibitors (amoxicillin clavulanate)			Renal, lung, fecal	Similar to penicillin
Carbapenem (imipenem-cilastatin)			Renal	Similar to penicillin, seizures in renal failure, without dose adjustment
Monobactam (aztreonam)			Renal	Rash, elevated transaminases
Aminoglycosides	Aminocyclitol	Binds ribosome	Renal	Nephro-, ototoxic; rare neuromuscular paralysis
Glycopeptides (*vancomycin*)	Carbohydrate and peptide	Inhibit bacterial cell wall synthesis	Renal	"Red man syndrome"— flushing of face and upper body with rapid I.V.admin; oto-, nephrotoxic
Macrolides (*erythromycin*)	Macrocyclic lactone ring	Binds to ribosome, inhibits protein synthesis	Renal, biliary	GI; hepato-, ototoxic; incr. levels of digoxin, warfarin, theophylline, cyclosporine, methylprednisolone, carbamazepine
Quinolones (*ciprofloxacin*)	Bicyclic 6-member ring	Attack DNA gyrase	Renal, biliary	GI, neurotoxic, Stevens-Johnson syndrome
Sulfonamides (*TMP-sulfa*)	Benzene ring with sulfonyl group	Inhibit folic acid synthesis	Renal	Rash, marrow suppression
Metronidazole	Nitroimidazole	Toxic metabolite interacts with bacterial DNA	Renal, fecal	Antabuse effect with ETOH, peripheral neurotoxicity

(Continued)

TABLE 29-6. *Continued*

Class	Structure	Action	Excretion	Toxicity/Interaction
		ANTIVIRALS		
Acyclovir	Guanosine analogue	Terminates viral DNA replication	Renal	Encephalopathy, renal dysfunction
Ganciclovir	Guanosine analogue	Stops DNA elongation	Renal	Leukopenia, cytopenia, CNS toxicity
		ANTIRETROVIRALS		
Zidovudine	Dideoxy-nucleosides	Inhibits viral reverse transcriptase	Renal	Bone marrow suppression, GI; acetaminophen increases zidovudine level
		ANTIFUNGALS		
Amphotericin B	Polyene	Binds to ergosterol in fungal cell membrane	3% Renal, rest unknown	Hypotension, GI, rigors, nephrotoxic, anemia
Azoles	Imidazole	Inhibit de-methylation of lanosterol to ergosterol	Fecal, renal	
Miconazole				GI, neuro-, cardioresp., hematologic toxicities; pruritis; increases warfarin, phenytoin levels
Ketoconazole				GI, hepatotoxic, gynecomastia, oligospermia, rare corticosteroid deficiency, increases cyclosporine levels, rifampin, and isoniazid increase ketoconazole levels
Fluconazole	Triazole		Renal	GI, transaminitis, increases warfarin, phenytoin, rarely cyclosporine levels; oral hypoglycemics, and rifampin decrease fluconazole levels

infections. The latter agents target bacterial cell walls and facilitate entry of the aminogylcoside which disrupts the internal mechanisms of protein synthesis. Similar combinations are frequently used in the treatment of gram-negative infections to assure that resistant nosocomial pathogens are treated and to prevent emergence of β-lactamase producing organisms during therapy.

Glycopeptides

Vancomycin is the major drug in the class of glycopeptides. It acts by inhibiting cell wall synthesis at a different step than the β-lactams. Vancomycin has a fairly narrow antimicrobial spectrum and is active against gram positive organisms exclusively. It is the drug of choice for methicillin-resistant *S. aureus* and coagulase-negative staphylococci.

Macrolides

Erythromycin belongs to the class of macrolides whose structure is based on a 14-membered macrocyclic lactone ring. Erythromycin binds to ribosomes and interferes with protein synthesis. It is the drug of choice against the *Legionella* species, *Mycoplasma pneumoniae, Ureaplasma urealyticum,* and *Bordetella pertussis.* It is also active against the *Chlamydia* species, *Treponema pallidum,* some *Rickettsia* species, sensitive *S. pneumoniae* and *S. pyogenes.*

Quinolones

Two six-membered rings form the bicyclic structure of these antimicrobials. Ciprofloxacin and norfloxacin are the two representatives of this class currently in active use. They are both oral drugs. Quinolones target DNA gyrases, the enzymes that supercoil DNA to fit into the bacterial cell.

Norfloxacin and ciprofloxacin have a similar spectrum of activity, with the latter having broader coverage and better tissue penetration. They are both very active against gram-negative enteric organisms, with ciprofloxacin having greater antipseudomonal activity.

Sulfonamides

The sulfonamides possess a benzene ring with a sulfonyl group attached. They are bacteriostatic and act by interfering with folic acid synthesis. Folic acid is required for the production of nucleotides for bacterial DNA.

Sulfamethoxazole is coupled to trimethoprim and the combination inhibits sequential steps in the folate pathway. Trimethoprim/sulfamethoxazole is active against a broad spectrum of gram-positive and gram-negative organisms. It is also the treatment of choice for *Pneumocystis carinii* pneumonia.

Metronidazole

Metronidazole is a nitroimidazole drug with a complex mechanism of action involving the reduction of the drug into a form that is rapidly bactericidal for anaerobes but not aerobes. It is effective against certain protozoa, including *Trichomonas vaginalis, Giardia lamblia,* and *Entamoeba histolytica.* Its major use is in the treatment of infections involving gram-positive and gram-negative anaerobes.

Antivirals

Acyclovir

Acyclovir is a guanosine analogue that is first monophosphorylated by viral thymidine kinase and then triphosphorylated by cellular enzymes. The triphosphorylated form inhibits viral DNA polymerase and also intercalates into the viral genome and terminates replication. It is active against members of the herpesvirus family, primarily herpes simplex types I and II, and varicella-zoster. It is the drug of choice for herpes simplex encephalitis and may arrest disease if given early in the course. Acyclovir decreases the duration and severity of mucocutaneous herpes simplex infection and reduces duration of viral shedding in immunocompromised hosts.

Ganciclovir

Like acyclovir, ganciclovir is a guanosine analogue that becomes incorporated into viral DNA and interrupts chain elongation. It has strong activity against the herpesviruses, in particular against CMV.

Antiretroviral Agents

Zidovudine (AZT) and the still investigational dideoxyinosine (DDI) and dideoxycytidine (DDC) are dideoxynucleosides used in the treatment of HIV-1. The dideoxynucleosides are phosphorylated by cellular kinases and in this form inhibit viral reverse transcriptase which is responsible for the production of proviral DNA from RNA.

Zidovudine has been shown to prolong survival and decrease the incidence of opportunistic infections in patients with AIDS and AIDS-related complex, and delay progression of disease in patients with mild symptoms or who are asymptomatic, with CD4 lymphocyte counts of less than 500 cells/mm^3.

Antifungals

Amphotericin B

Amphotericin B is an insoluble fungicidal antibiotic with a macrocyclic lactone ring. It is chelated to the bile salt deoxycholate to enhance its solubility. The bile salt is responsible for most of the immediate adverse reactions that occur during amphotericin administration. The drug binds to ergosterol, a sterol present in the plasma membrane of fungi, causing changes in membrane permeability and leakage of intracellular contents, resulting in cell lysis. Amphotericin is the treatment of choice for systemic and severe, deep-seated fungal infections, though promising new azole antifungals are currently being tested that appear to be efficacious and have fewer side effects.

The major acute side effects of amphotericin B include hypotension, nausea, vomiting, fever and rigors. Those stemming from more prolonged use include nephrotoxicity and normochromic normocytic anemia secondary to inhibition of erythropoietin production. Multiple mechanisms exist for the development of nephrotoxicity, the most important side effect, which to some degree affects all patients receiving the drug. Amphotericin appears to cause vasoconstriction, cortical ischemia, and a fall in the glomerular filtration rate. It also damages renal tubules, causing losses in potassium, magnesium, and bicarbonate, and can induce renal tubular acidosis in patients receiving total doses from 500 to 1000 mg or more. In most instances, renal failure and tubular defects are reversible. Because of the significant nephrotoxicity of this drug, patients on amphotericin should be kept well hydrated with all electrolytes in the normal range. As a general rule, the drug should be stopped if the creatinine rises significantly, and restarted after two to five days. Dialysis should be instituted and amphotericin B continued in the face of renal failure in the patient with severe fungal infection for which amphotericin is the only appropriate drug available.

Azoles

The azoles are a class of antifungal agents that function by inhibiting the demethylase enzyme responsible for ergosterol synthesis. Miconazole was the first available agent of this class. It is toxic, not widely used, and is now reserved only for amphotericin-resistant fungi. Clotrimazole, another azole, is used only in the management of superficial fungal infections, including cutaneous, oral, and vaginal candidiasis. Ketoconazole was the first oral antifungal agent but its use is limited because of variable absorption and poor tissue penetration. It is not useful for serious infections. Fluconazole, the most recently released azole, has better tissue penetration and achieves excellent levels in the CSF and urine. It currently carries indications for the treatment of oropharyngeal and esophageal candidiasis and for cryptococcal meningitis. Its effectiveness in systemic candidal infections has not been adequately evaluated.

FACTORS INFLUENCING THE EMPIRIC CHOICE OF AN ANTIMICROBIAL AGENT

Acquisition of infection in the hospital rather than in the community will influence the site and severity of infection and the pathogens involved. The patterns of susceptibility within an institution must be known in order to make empiric choices, since resistance to antimicrobials varies from one hospital to another. Toxicity of the drug must be weighed against the likely susceptibilities of the organism and the severity of illness. If equally efficacious drugs are available once the susceptibilities of the organism are known, then the least expensive agent should be chosen in most instances.

PREVENTION

Surgical Prophylaxis

Prevention of postoperative infections is achieved by reducing the number of micro-organisms at the wound site to levels below which they are likely to cause infection. This is accomplished by means of aseptic technique, avoidance of tissue necrosis, and preoperative antibiotic prophylaxis.

Timing and Choice of Preoperative Antibiotics

Effectiveness of prophylactic antibiotics is dependent on the type of drug used and on the timing of administration in relation to surgery. It is recommended that one dose of the appropriate antibiotic be given within a half-hour prior to surgery. Animal studies of antibiotic prophylaxis of wounds have shown that delaying antibiotic administration by several hours provides no protection against development of infection. There is some controversy regarding whether there is any added benefit to continuing the prophylactic antibiotic for several days after surgery.

Prophylactic antimicrobials are targeted toward the

organisms most likely to cause infection after surgery. Agents with a gram-positive spectrum are useful for cardiac, orthopedic, and vascular surgery where skin flora are the major problems postoperativeley. Agents with gram-negative and anaerobic spectra are used in bowel surgery. Cefazolin, a first-generation cephalosporin with good staphylococcal and gram-negative coverage and a long half-life, is the prophylactic drug of choice for cardiac, orthopedic, head and neck and vascular cases. Vancomycin is fast becoming a substitute for cefazolin as the incidence of infections with resistant staphylococci increases. Cefoxitin, a second-generation cephalosporin with a broader gram-negative and anaerobic spectrum than cefazolin, is often used in clean-contaminated and contaminated bowel surgery. The third-generation cephalosporins are currently not recommended for prophylaxis because of their inferior staphylococcal coverage, an unnecessarily broad spectrum, and increased cost.

In addition to parenteral preparations, oral antibiotics are given directly the day preceding elective bowel surgery to reduce the numbers of intestinal flora. Neomycin and erythromycin base are recommended for this purpose.

Traumatic Wound Prophylaxis
Cefazolin is effective against the skin flora that would be the primary cause of infection after traumatic skin wounds. Animal and human bite wounds, however, are contaminated with mouth anaerobes, requiring alternative prophylaxis. Penicillin is effective for human, dog, and cat bites.

Postsplenectomy Prophylaxis
The loss of the spleen creates an opsonic defect that leaves the host vulnerable to encapsulated organisms, particularly S. pneumoniae. These infections are usually overwhelming in the asplenic individual and may cause death within hours. Pneumococcal vaccine (discussed below) should be administered before splenectomy whenever possible to take advantage of the spleen's antibody production. Although the risk of infection is highest in the two years following splenectomy, there is a lifelong risk of serious infection. Penicillin prophylaxis in daily oral form or as intramuscular injections given at several-week intervals has been effective in preventing overwhelming infection. All forms of prophylaxis have been associated with failures, and for this reason asplenic patients should keep a supply of penicillin at home and begin to take it for any febrile illness.

Vaccines
Two methods of immunization exist. Active immunization stimulates the host's immune system to elaborate protective antibodies against an antigenic challenge. Passive immunization offers transient protection conferred by the administration of immunoglobulin preparations. Active immunization is accomplished either with vaccines consisting of live attenuated organisms, or of inactivated whole organisms or their component parts.

Pneumococcal
Pneumococcal vaccine is a polyvalent preparation composed of capsular polysaccharide from 23 types of pneumococci. Most of the bacteremias in the United States are caused by these strains. The vaccine appears to be protective in about 70% of immunocompetent patients over 55 years old. It should be given to patients over 65 and those who are at high risk from immunosuppression or chronic disease. It is most effective when it is administered prior to alteration of the immune system by splenectomy, chemotherapy, or transplantation. Patients who received the earlier 14-valent vaccine or received the 23-valent vaccine six or more years ago should be revaccinated if they are still at increased risk.

Influenza
Influenza vaccine is composed of inactivated virus. It decreases morbidity and mortality from the disease and should be administered yearly to persons over the age of 65 and those who have chronic illnesses or are immunosuppressed.

Tetanus
After the primary series of tetanus immunization in childhood, patients should receive a tetanus toxoid booster every ten years, and in the event a contaminated wound is sustained and it has been greater than five years since the last dose. It is generally given in a preparation including diphtheria toxoid. Tetanus immunoglobulin should be given to provide immediate protection to persons who have never received vaccination, or whose vaccination status is unknown and who have sustained a contaminated wound. It should be followed by immunization with the complete series of three injections of tetanus-diphtheria toxoid.

Rabies
Rabies vaccine is given pre-exposure to workers such as veterinarians who may have contact with rabid animals,

and to those bitten or licked on an open wound or mucosal surface by animals with known or suspected rabies. An inactivated-virus vaccine, it is produced in human diploid cell culture. Postexposure, five doses of the vaccine are given over the course of a month. Human rabies immunoglobulin is always given concomitantly, with half the dose infiltrated around the wound, the other half given intramuscularly.

Hepatitis B

Hepatitis B vaccine is recommended for individuals at high risk of exposure to blood and body fluids, including health-care workers. Composed of inactivated particles of surface antigen, initial vaccines were derived from pooled human plasma. The current vaccine is a product of recombinant DNA technology.

Bibliography

Abramowicz M, ed. Drugs for HIV infection. *Med Lett Drug Ther* 1990;31(811):11–13.

Abramowicz M, ed. Drugs for the treatment of fungal infections. *Med Lett Drug Ther* 1990;35:17–29SS.

Abramowicz M, ed. Fluconazole. *Med Lett Drug Ther* 1990; 32(818):50–52.

Abramowicz M, ed. Routine immunization for adults. *Med Lett Drug Ther* 1990;32(819):54–56.

Abramowicz M, ed. The choice of antimicrobial drugs. *Med Lett Drug Ther* 1990;32(817):41–48.

Abramowicz M, ed. Antimicrobial prophylaxis in surgery. *Med Lett Drug Ther* 1989;31(806):105–108.

Abramowicz M, ed. Recommendations for prevention of HIV transmission in health-care settings. *Morbidity and Mortality Weekly Report* 1987;36(2S):3–18SS.

Centers for Disease Control. CDC surveillance summaries. *Morbidity and Mortality Weekly Report* 1986;35:17–29SS.

Dinarello CA, Cannon JG, Wolff SM. New concepts in the pathogenesis of fever. *Rev Infect Dis* 1988;10(1):168–189.

Gerberding JL, Littell C, Tarkington A, Brown A, Schecter WP. Risk of exposure of surgical personnel to patient's blood during surgery at San Francisco general hospital. *N Engl J Med* 1990;322(25):1788–1793.

Howard RJ, Simmons RL, eds. *Surgical infectious diseases.* 2nd ed. Norwalk, CT: Appleton & Lange, 1988.

Kelen GB, Fritz S, Qaqish B, Brookmeyer R, Baker JL, Kline RL, Cuddy RM, Goessel TK, Floccare D, Williams KA, Sivertson KT, Altman S, Quinn TC. Unrecognized human immunodeficiency virus infection in emergency department patients. *N Engl J Med* 1988;318(25):1645–1650.

Kim JH, Perfect JR. Infection and cyclosporine. *Rev Infect Dis* 1989;11(5):677–690.

Kucers A, Bennett NM. *The use of antibiotics.* 4th ed. Philadelphia: JB Lippincott, 1987.

Mandell G, Douglas RG, Bennett JE, eds. *Principles and practice of infectious diseases.* 3rd ed. New York: Churchill Livingstone, 1990.

Meakins JL, Pietsch JB, Christou NV, Maclean LD. Predicting surgical infection before the operation. *World J Surg* 1980; 4:439–450.

Parrillo JE, Parker MM, Natanson C, Suffredini AF, Danner RL, Cunnion RE, Ognibene FP. Septic shock in human beings. Advances in the understanding of pathogenesis, cardiovascular dysfunction, and therapy. *Ann Intern Med* 1990; 113(3):227–242.

Rubin RH, Young LS, eds. *Clinical approach to infection in the compromised host.* 2nd ed. New York: Plenum, 1988.

Sabiston DC, ed. *Textbook of surgery. The biological basis of modern surgical practice.* 13th ed. Philadelphia: WB Saunders, 1986.

Shires GT, Dineen P. Sepsis following burns, trauma, and intraabdominal infections. *Arch Intern Med* 1982;142: 2012–2022.

Solomkin JS, Simmons RL. Candida infection in surgical patients. *World J Surg.* 1980;4:381–394.

Van Der Valk P, Herman CJ. Biology of disease. Leukocyte functions. *Lab Invest* 1987;57(2):127–137.

Weinstein MP, Reller LB, Murphy JR, Lichtenstein KA. The clinical significance of positive blood cultures: A comprehensive analysis of 500 episodes of bacteremia and fugemia in adults. A. Laboratory and epidemiologic observations. *Rev Infect Dis* 1983;5(1):35–50.

Russell F. Sassani

30 PRINCIPLES OF PHARMACOLOGY

Basic Pharmacokinetics

Pharmacokinetics is the study of the time course of a drug and its metabolites in the body following drug administration through the process of absorption, distribution, and eventual elimination. It involves following the rate of change of the concentration of the drug in the various body compartments, including the plasma.

Drugs are administered to achieve a therapeutic effect. In order for this to occur, an adequate concentration of drug must be achieved at the site of action. The attainment and maintenance of this adequate concentration is dependent on the pharmacokinetics of the drug, which considers how the body acts on the drug, rather than how the drug acts on the body.

BIOAVAILABILITY

Bioavailability is an absolute term that denotes both the total amount of drug and the true rate at which the drug reaches the systemic circulation from an administered dosage form. **Equivalence** is a relative term that compares one drug product with another or with a set of established standards. For example, bioequivalence indicates that a drug in two similar dosage forms reaches the systemic circulation at the same relative rate and to the same relative extent.

Once a drug is absorbed, it may combine with receptors to elicit a pharmacologic response. The **onset time** is the time interval from drug administration to pharmacologic response and reflects the time interval needed to achieve a **minimum effective concentration (MEC)** (Figure 30-1).

A pharmacologic response will be observed as long as the drug concentration remains above the MEC. This length of time over which a pharmacologic response is seen is called the **duration of action.**

Toxic effects may be seen if the drug concentration exceeds the **minimum toxic concentration (MTC).** The range of drug concentrations over which a normal therapeutic response will be seen is the **therapeutic window** and is depicted as the range between the MEC and the MTC.

The **peak time** of plasma drug concentration is related to the rate of drug absorption. The faster a drug is absorbed, the faster the peak time is reached. The **peak concentration** is the plasma drug concentration at the peak time and is related to the intensity of the pharmacologic response that is elicited. The total area under the curve (AUC) reflects the total amount of drug absorbed and has the units of concentration-time. The more drug that is absorbed, the greater the AUC.

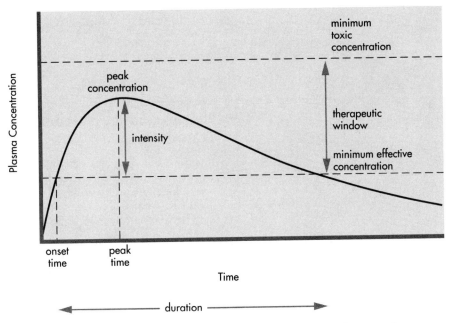

Plasma Concentration

minimum
toxic
concentration

peak
concentration

therapeutic
window

intensity

minimum effective
concentration

onset
time

peak
time

Time

duration

Figure 30-1 Typical plasma-level curve of a drug vs. time. Onset time, peak time, peak concentration, intensity, duration, MEC, MTC, and therapeutic window are defined. (Adapted from Disanto A. Bioavailability and bioequivalency testing. In: Osol A, ed. *Remington's pharmaceutical sciences.* 16th ed. Easton, PA: Mack Publishing Co, 1980: 1370.)

RATES AND ORDERS OF REACTIONS

The **rate of a reaction** is the speed with which it occurs. It is expressed as the change in concentration with respect to change in time (dC/dt).

The **order of a reaction** refers to the way in which the concentration of a drug influences the rate. In pharmacokinetics, only zero-order and first-order processes are important.

A **zero-order reaction** is one in which the rate of a reaction is independent of the concentration of the drug; thus the concentration of the drug changes with respect to time at a constant rate according to this straight-line equation:

$$C = -k_o t + C_o$$

where C is the drug concentration, k_o is the zero-order rate constant in units of concentration/time, t is time, and C_o is the initial concentration. When this relationship is plotted on a graph with C on the vertical axis and time on the horizontal axis, the slope of the line is $-k_o$, indicating that the slope is decreasing (Figure 30-2).

A **first-order reaction** is one in which the rate of a reaction depends on the concentration of a drug, such that the drug concentration changes with respect to time as the product of the rate constant and the concentration of drug remaining, according to this equation:

$$C = C_o\, e^{-kt}$$

or

$$\log C = (-kt/2.303) + \log C_o$$

where C is the drug concentration, C_o is the initial drug concentration, k is the first-order rate constant in units of reciprocal time, and t is time. This equation states that in a first-order reaction, drug concentration decreases exponentially with time. If this equation is plotted on a graph with $\log C$ on the vertical axis and time on the horizontal axis, a straight-line relationship is obtained with a slope of $-k/2.303$ (Figure 30-3).

The **half-life** of a reaction is the time required for the concentration of a drug to decrease by one half ($t_{1/2}$). For a first-order reaction, the half-life is a constant and

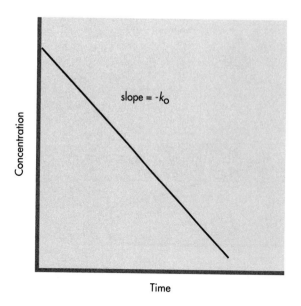

Figure 30-2 Linear plot of concentration (C) versus time (t) for a zero-order reaction. The slope of the line is equal to the zero-order rate constant, $-k_o$.

is related to the first-order rate constant by the following equation:

$$t_{1/2} = 0.693/k$$

Pharmacokinetic Models and Compartments

A **model** is a mathematical description of a biologic system that is used to express a quantitative relationship.

A **compartment** is a group of tissues with similar blood flows and drug affinities. It is not a real physiologic or anatomic region. Drug can distribute into "compartments," such as the plasma, cerebrospinal fluid, interstitial fluid, renal tubules, and individual cells. Fortunately, the rates of distribution among these various tissues are not markedly divergent, and drug kinetics are such that a drug behaves as though it were distributed to one, two, or at most a few compartments.

Drug distribution occurs rapidly to those tissues with high rates of blood flow and slowly to those tissues with low rates of blood flow. Drug permeability across capillary membranes varies from tissue to tissue. Drugs

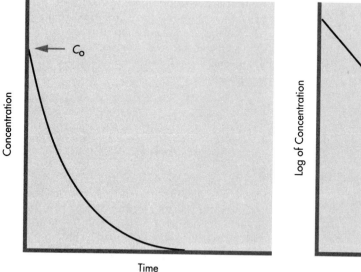

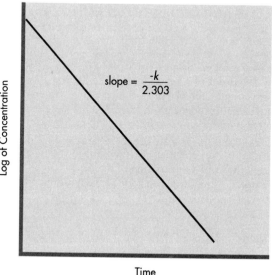

Figure 30-3 For a first-order process, a curvilinear relationship is obtained when concentration versus time is plotted on a graph. As can be seen, the concentration rapidly declines from an initial concentration of C_o, and at lower concentrations the rate of decline is slower (*graph at left*). When this relationship is plotted on a log scale (logarithm of concentration, log C, versus time), a linear plot with a slope equal to -k/2.303 is obtained for a first-order reaction (*graph at right*).

can cross membranes by passive diffusion and hydrostatic pressure, and cross readily through the glomerulus of the kidney and the sinusoids of the liver. In contrast, polar or ionic drugs pass very slowly across lipid membranes such as the blood-brain barrier. The physicochemical characteristics of a drug allow it to accumulate in certain tissues, as is the case with lipid-soluble drugs accumulating in fat tissue. Finally, protein binding can affect drug distribution, since protein bound drug cannot cross capillary or cellular membranes. Drugs must be displaced from protein binding sites in order to interact with drug receptors.

The **volume of distribution (V_d)** is a hypothetical volume of body fluid into which a drug is dissolved or distributed. Likewise, this is not a real physiologic or anatomic volume.

ONE-COMPARTMENT MODEL

In this model, the body is assumed to behave as if it were a single compartment. Thus it is assumed that there are no barriers to movement of drug within the body and the final distribution is achieved instantaneously. This model is depicted in Figure 30-4.

Formulas for time-related changes in concentration for the one-compartment model are given below. Different pharmacokinetic situations will be reviewed, including a single intravenous (IV) bolus injection, a single oral dose, IV infusion, and a multiple-dose regimen. For simplicity's sake, it is convenient to think of absorption and elimination occurring separately and then to add them algebraically to determine the overall pharmocokinetic effect.

IV Bolus Injection

When a drug is given via an IV bolus injection, the entire dose enters the body and the rate of absorption is ignored in calculations. The entire body acts as a single compartment, in that the drug quickly equilibrates in all body tissues. Drug elimination after an IV bolus injection is a first-order kinetic process according to this equation previously described and presented graphically in Figure 30-5.

$$\log C = (-kt/2.303) + \log C_o$$

The **first-order elimination rate constant (k)** in the above equation is the sum of all the elimination rate constants for drug removal from the body:

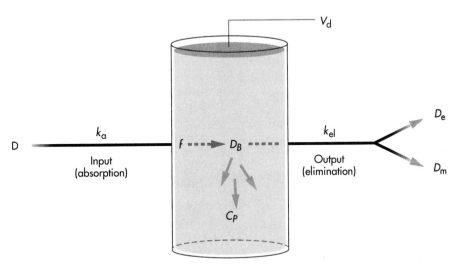

Figure 30-4 Diagram of the open one-compartment pharmacokinetic model. An amount of drug, D_B, is absorbed from the administered dose, D, with a rate constant of k_a into a compartment with volume V_d and is distributed instantaneously to reach a plasma concentration, C_p. V_d is obtained by dividing D_B by C_p. D_B = the dose D times f, the fraction absorbed. Drug is eliminated from the compartment with a rate constant k_{el}. D_e is the amount excreted into urine, feces, expired air, sweat, milk, etc.; D_m is the amount of drug metabolized. (Adapted from Harvey S. Basic pharmacokinetics. In: Osol A, ed. *Remington's pharmaceutical sciences.* 16th ed. Easton, PA: Mack Publishing Company, 1980:684.)

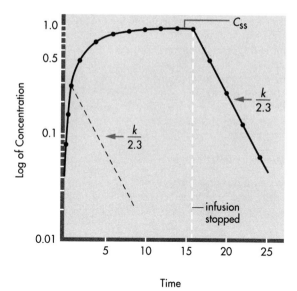

Figure 30-5 Pharmacokinetic plot for an IV infusion showing zero-order absorption and first-order elimination. C_{ss} is the steady-state concentration and k is the elimination rate constant. (Adapted from Gibaldi M, Perrier D. *Pharmacokinetics.* New York: Marcel Dekker, 1982:30.)

$$k + k_e + k_m$$

where k_e is the rate constant for excretion and k_m is the rate constant for metabolism. The elimination half-life ($t_{1/2}$) is determined by the previously described equation:

$$t_{1/2} = 0.693/k$$

The apparent volume of distribution (V_d) previously discussed is a hypothetical volume and is used to relate the amount of drug in the body to the concentration of drug in the plasma:

$$V_d \times C_p = D_b$$

where V_d is the volume of distribution, C_p is the plasma drug concentration, and D_b is the amount of drug in the body. This equation can be rearranged to calculate the volume of distribution after an IV bolus injection:

$$V_d = D_b^o/C_p^o$$

where D_b^o is the dose (D_o) of drug given IV and C_p^o is

the extrapolated drug concentration at time zero on the y-axis.

Single Oral Dose

When a drug is given in a single oral dose, it is rapidly absorbed by first-order kinetics, followed by elimination by first-order kinetics. The plasma drug concentration can be determined by the following pharmacokinetic equation:

$$C_p = \frac{FD_o k_A}{V_d(k_A + k)}\left(e^{-kt} - e^{-kt}A^t\right)$$

where k_A is the first-order absorption rate constant and F is the fraction of drug bioavailable. Changes in F, D_o, V_d, k_A, and k can all affect plasma drug concentration (C_p). The time to reach maximum concentration (T_{max}, or peak time) is given by the equation

$$T_{max} = \frac{2.3 \log\left(k_A / k\right)}{k_A - k}$$

From this equation, it can be seen that T_{max} depends only on k_A and k and not F, D_o, or V_d. The area under the curve (AUC), or total amount of drug absorbed, is given by the equation

$$AUC = \frac{FD_o}{V_d k}$$

From this equation, it can be seen that any changes in F, D_o, V_d, or k will affect the AUC.

IV Infusion

For drugs given by IV infusion, zero-order absorption and first-order elimination occur. The plasma drug concentration can then be determined at any time after the start of an IV infusion by the following formula:

$$C_p = \frac{R}{V_d k}\left(1 - e^{-kt}\right)$$

where R is the zero-order rate of infusion given in the units of drug amount per unit of time (e.g., mg/h or mg/min). Once the IV infusion stops, the plasma drug concentration decreases by a first-order process. The elimination half-life can be determined from the plasma drug concentration versus time curve (Figure 30-5).

As drug continues to be infused, the plasma drug concentration reaches a plateau or *steady-state concentration* (C_{ss}). At this point the amount of drug absorbed equals the amount of drug eliminated. The steady-state plasma concentration (C_{ss}) can be calculated from the following formula:

$$C_{ss} = R/V_d k$$

A **loading dose** (D_L) can be given at the initiation of an IV infusion so that C_{ss} can be reached more rapidly. A loading dose is the amount of drug that produces the desired steady-state concentration when dissolved in the apparent volume of distribution:

$$D_L = C_{ss} V_d$$

Intravenous infusions are often ideal because they produce relatively constant plasma drug concentrations that do not fall below the MEC or rise above the MTC.

Multiple-Dose Regimen

Many drugs are given at discrete intervals using a multiple-dose regimen. This allows for a sustained therapeutic effect. By using this regimen, the drug concentration will accumulate and rise to a steady-state level. Drug accumulates because a new dose is given before a prior dose can be eliminated completely. When steady state is achieved, plasma drug concentration will fluctuate between a maximum (C_{max}^{∞}) and a minimum (C_{min}^{∞}). In designing a multiple-dose regimen, the only variable that can be altered with any facility is the dosing rate. Dosing rate depends on the size of the dose (D_o) and the time interval between doses (τ):

$$\text{dosing rate} = D_o/\tau$$

As long as the dosing rate is the same, the average drug concentration at steady state (C_{av}^{∞}) will be the same. For example, a dose of a drug of 600 mg given every 12 hours gives the same C_{av}^{∞} as a dose of 300 mg given every 6 hours because the dosing rate is the same (50 mg/h) (Figure 30-6).

The maximum serum drug concentration at steady state (C_{max}^{∞}) is determined with the following equation:

$$C_{av}^{\infty} = \frac{D_o / V_d}{1 - e^{-k\tau}}$$

The minimum serum drug concentration at steady state (C_{min}^{∞}) is given by

$$C_{min}^{\infty} = C_{max}^{\infty} e^{-k\tau}$$

And the average drug concentration at steady-state (C_{av}^{∞}) is

$$C_{av}^{\infty} = \frac{FD_o}{kV_d\tau}$$

For IV injections and readily bioavailable drugs $F = 1$. For drugs administered by multiple oral doses, steady-state plasma concentrations can be approximated by using the above equations, provided the drug is readily absorbed and slowly eliminated (i.e., k_A is much greater than k). Another useful calculation is to determine the fraction of drug remaining in the body (f) after a dosing interval. This can be derived by using the equation below:

$$f = e^{-k\tau}$$

As with IV infusion, a loading dose (D_L), can be given in order to achieve a steady state more rapidly. For multiple oral doses, D_L can be determined by

$$D_L = D_M \frac{1}{1 - e^{-k\tau}}$$

where D_M is the maintenance dose. If a maintenance dose is given at a dosage interval equal to the drug's biologic half-life, then D_L will be twice the maintenance dose.

MULTICOMPARTMENT MODELS

Multicompartment pharmacokinetics describes drugs that distribute into different tissues at different rates. Tissues with high blood flow equilibrate with drug more quickly than tissues with low blood flow. In addition, the drug's physicochemical characteristics and the nature of the tissue determine tissue drug concentrations.

In the *two-compartment model*, a drug distributes rapidly into highly perfused tissues (central compart-

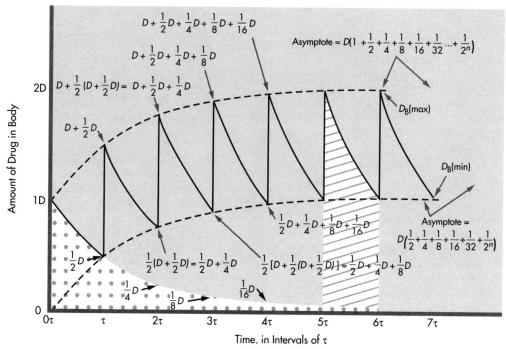

Figure 30-6 The accumulation of drug in the body during a regimen of multiple dosing. Dose, D, is administered intravenously at intervals (τ) equal to the half-life ($t_{1/2}$). Thus after each dose, the amount in the body, D_B, has decreased to half the previous peak amount at the time each does is administered. When the cumulated amount in the body after injection reaches $2D$, the body content will fluctuate from $2D$ to $1D$ during each dose interval thereafter. Approximately 5 half-lives are required before this leveling off (plateau) of the body content occurs. The *stippled area* is the area under the elimination curve after a single injection if no second dose had been given. The *cross-hatched area* is the area under the curve during a single dose interval. The two areas are equal. (Adapted from Harvey S. Basic pharmacokinetics. In: Osol A, ed. *Remington's pharmaceutical sciences.* 16th ed. Easton, PA: Mack Publishing Company, 1980: 691.)

ment) and more slowly into peripheral tissues (tissue compartment). The distribution phase is an initial rapid decline in the plasma drug concentration, followed by the elimination phase, which is a more gradual decline in drug concentration. In a *three-compartment model,* the drug slowly distributes into a deep-tissue space.

Nonlinear Pharmacokinetics

In nonlinear kinetics, first-order kinetics are not observed as the dose is increased. Additionally, the AUC is not proportional to the dose, the amount of drug excreted in the urine is not proportional to the dose, and the elimination half-life increases at higher doses. Saturation of an enzyme or a carrier-mediated system may account for these observations. **Michaelis-Menten kinetics,** which is used to describe the velocity

of enzyme reactions, is also used to describe nonlinear pharmacokinetics. Under Michaelis-Menten kinetics, drugs may exhibit first-order elimination at low drug concentrations, a mix of zero- and first-order elimination at intermediate concentrations, and zero-order elimination at very high drug concentrations.

Drug Action and Drug Effect

In order for a drug to act, it must first be absorbed and subsequently carried to the correct locus of action, where it can elicit its effect.

The **effect** of the drug is an alteration of function of the structure or process upon which the drug acts. The term **action** should not be confused with effect, since action precedes effect. Action is the alteration of condition that brings about the effect.

Most drugs elicit multiple effects, although these multiple effects may stem from a single mechanism of action. Despite these multiple effects, one effect is usually more readily elicited than others. **Selectivity** is the word used to describe this difference in responsiveness.

The **dose** of a drug is the amount administered. **Potency** of a drug is the reciprocal of the dose required to obtain a specific effect and has little use other than to provide a means of comparing the relative activities of different drugs.

Efficacy or **intrinsic activity** describes the ability of a drug to achieve its desired effect. Efficacy is one of the primary determinants in the choice of a drug.

DRUG RECEPTORS AND RECEPTOR THEORY

Receptors are cellular or extracellular constituents that combine or interact with drugs to trigger a series of events that lead to a pharmacologic effect. A receptor is a macromolecule such as an enzyme, protein, lipoprotein, or nucleic acid that may be membrane bound or intracellular. These receptors govern the spatial orientation of enzymes, compartmentalization of the cytoplasm, contractile properties of subcellular structures, or membrane properties such as permeability or electrical state.

Various physicochemical forces attract a drug to a receptor and bind the drug to the receptor, which eventually leads to the pharmacologic response. Ionic forces between oppositely charged atoms are often very important in the approximation of the drug to the receptor site. Subsequently, hydrogen bonding and van der Waals' forces are responsible for the proper alignment and stabilization of the drug-receptor complex. Covalent bonds between the drug and receptor yield stable, long-lasting complexes.

In contrast, certain drug actions are not mediated by drug-receptor interactions. For example, the chelation of heavy metals by drugs and the neutralization of hydronium ions by antacids are chemical reactions and are not mediated by a drug-receptor interaction. Likewise, local and general anesthetics do not interact with cellular or organelle membrane receptors. The mechanism involved here is mediated by the lipid solubility of the drug in the cellular lipid membrane. Drugs of this type are called structurally nonspecific, since their physical properties rather than their chemical structure are responsible for their mechanism of action. Structural nonspecificity implies that a drug-receptor interaction is not responsible for the mechanism of action.

Structurally specific drugs bind directly to a receptor, resulting in a pharmacologic effect. Drug-receptor interactions and receptor theory are concerned with the fraction of drug bound to the receptor. Only when the receptor is "occupied" by the drug can a response be elicited. In addition, the intensity of this response is directly related to the number of occupied receptors. This is called the **occupation theory.**

Another receptor-site theory is the **lock-and-key theory.** In this theory, the drug "fits" into an active or catalytic site of a receptor (such as an enzyme) and is responsible for its activation, leading to a biologic or pharmacologic effect.

An **agonist** is a drug that combines with a receptor to produce a pharmacologic response. The **affinity** of an agonist or drug is its ability to bind to a receptor.

A **partial agonist** is a drug that can elicit some effect but not a maximal effect. At low concentrations it can activate receptors, but at high concentrations it blocks the receptor binding of more efficacious agonists. Therefore, it has good affinity, but low intrinsic activity. For example, at low doses of dichloroisoproterenol, β-adrenergic effects similar to isoproterenol are produced, but at high concentrations it blocks β-adrenergic receptors, similar to propanolol.

Likewise, **antagonists** are drugs that have affinity but lack intrinsic activity. They may interact with a receptor but do not initiate a pharmacologic effect. A **competitive antagonist** competes with a drug for the same receptor sites. Thus, a larger dose of agonist will be needed to produce the desired pharmacologic effect. For example, naloxone is a competitive antagonist of morphine.

A **noncompetitive antagonist** does not necessarily prevent drug-receptor interactions, but it does prevent the interaction from initiating a pharmacologic response. For example, a noncompetitive antagonist may form a covalent bond to the receptor, which alters the receptor and prevents attachment or interaction of the agonist from eliciting a response.

Tolerance is a reduction in the responsiveness to a drug following repeated administration and implies the need to increase the size of subsequent doses to achieve the same previously obtained effect. Causes of tolerance include genetic, physiologic, and pathophysiologic factors as well as changes in the receptor, changes in postreceptor events or in other aspects of the cell. Rapidly developing tolerance to repeated doses of the same drug is called **tachyphylaxis.**

MECHANISMS OF DRUG ACTION

Drugs can act to alter many metabolic or physiologic functions. The mechanism by which the functions are altered, however, should not be confused with the site of action. In the strictest sense, mechanism of action refers to the first event that is the alteration of receptor function that subsequently leads to the desired pharmacologic effect. A drug may be excitatory or inhibitory, but these terms describe an effect and not the action of the drug on receptor function. Several types of drug mechanisms are discussed here.

The mechanism of action of many drugs involves enzymes because of their important role in cellular function. Drugs can activate or inhibit enzymes. **Enzyme activation** occurs when a drug induces a conformational change in the enzyme system and alters its affinity for substrate binding. For example, epinephrine, through binding with the β-adrenergic receptor modulates the activity of adenyl cyclase to increase the production of cAMP. Coenzymes such as vitamins and cofactors such as metallic ions (Mg^{2+}, Ca^{2+}, Z^{2+}, and Fe^{2+}) optimize enzyme activity by complexation and stereochemical interactions.

In contrast, drugs can also inhibit enzymes by destroying their protein configuration, reacting with their coenzymes or by binding with the enzyme, making it unable to bind substrate. In **competitive inhibition,** a drug or antimetabolite competes with an endogenous substrate for the active site of the enzyme. Inhibition can be overcome by increasing the concentration of the natural substrate, which will displace the drug from the binding site. These antimetabolites can react with enzymes to yield abnormal nonfunctional products. For example, sulfonamides compete with para-aminobenzoic acid and interfere with its incorporation into folic acid. Methotrexate competes with folic acid for folate reductase and interferes with formation of nucleotides and nucleic acids.

In **noncompetitive inhibition,** the drug combines with the enzyme at a site removed from the active site to prevent the binding of substrate. In contrast to competitive inhibition, an excess of substrate will not reverse this inhibition. For example, cyanide is a noncompetitive inhibitor.

Drugs can work through **nuclear or extranuclear genetic mechanisms** to inhibit nucleotide synthesis, DNA synthesis, or RNA synthesis. Antifolate drugs and purine and pyrimidine analogues inhibit nucleotide synthesis. Antifolate drugs, such as methotrexate, inhibit folate reductase, which leads to inhibition of purine and thymidylic acid synthesis. Purine analogues like 6-mercaptopurine and 6-thioguanine inhibit purine synthesis. Pyrimidine analogues, such as 5-fluorouracil, inhibit thymidine synthetase. Some antineoplastic agents inhibit DNA synthesis. Intercalating agents, such as adriamycin, alkylating agents, such as nitrogen mustards, and antimetabolites, such as methotrexate, all interfere with DNA replication. DNA polymerase inhibition occurs as a result of drugs such as novobiocin and cytarabine. Transcription is inhibited by drugs like cisplatin. Mitosis is inhibited by vinca alkaloids that affect microtubule assembly.

Drugs can work through the **inhibition of protein synthesis.** Tetracycline inhibits the binding of transfer RNA to the ribosome and blocks the release of a synthesized protein from the ribosome. Aminoglycosides bind to the ribosome, prohibiting amino acid incorporation into the peptide chain. They also cause misreading of the mRNA template. Chloramphenicol and erythromycin bind to ribosomes and inhibit peptidyltransferase, preventing translation.

Many drugs act through alterations in the physical and structural properties of membranes. There are several ways in which drugs can alter cellular membranes. The drug may be able to disperse itself throughout the lipid phase of the membrane to increase cellular permeability, as occurs with the antifungal agents amphotericin B and nystatin, and certain antibiotics such as colistin and polymyxin B. The drug may cause a change in the conformation of a membrane constituent so that pore size and permeability are affected. This is the case with acetylcholine, which increases membrane permeability to cations. Drugs are also known to affect ion movements through membranes by their action on enzymes. For example, digitalis glycosides inhibit the Na,K-ATPase pump. Ions are critical in maintaining the function of membranes and the excitability of cells. Drugs may disrupt these ionic movements. For example, local anesthetics block nerve cell conduction by interfering with membrane permeability to Na and K. Also, quinidine acts by affecting the membrane potential of the myocardial cell.

Chelation and complexation are important mechanisms of action in heavy-metal poisoning. Ethylene diamine tetraacetic acid is used to chelate lead and calcium; penicillamine chelates copper; and dimercaprol chelates mercury, gold, and arsenic.

Many drugs have simple mechanisms that do not involve an action at the cellular level and are said to have a **nonspecific mechanism** of action. Examples of these drugs include bulk and saline cathartics; osmotic diuretics; general anesthetics, such as nitrous oxide; skin emollients; and many antiseptics, such as alcohol.

Biotransformation (Metabolism) and Excretion

Biotransformation and excretion provide a mechanism for removal of drugs and their metabolites from the body.

BIOTRANSFORMATION

Biotransformation is the mechanism by which drugs are converted to metabolites by the action of enzymes or hydrolysis. Metabolism usually results in compounds that are more polar and less lipid soluble. This leads to their inactivation and rapid excretion from the body. This is the usual scenario by which drugs are biotransformed into inactive metabolites, detoxified, and eliminated from the body.

Some metabolites, however, may retain pharmacologic activity similar to their active parent compound. Examples of the conversion of active parent drugs to active metabolites includes the conversion of allopurinol to alloxanthine, codeine to morphine, digitoxin to digoxin, imipramine to desipramine, procainamide to N-acetyl procainamide, and propranolol to 4-hydroxypropranolol, to name just a few.

Likewise, a pharmacologically inactive compound, or prodrug, may be biotransformed into an active metabolite. Examples of biotransformation of an inactive prodrug to active metabolites include the conversion of acetylsalicylic acid to salicylic acid, prednisone to prednisolone, primidone to phenobarbital, and phenylbutazone to oxyphenbutazone.

The principal site of biotransformation is the smooth endoplasmic reticulum of the liver. Other sites of biotransformation include the kidney, skeletal muscle, plasma, and intestine.

The smooth endoplasmic reticulum (also called the microsomal drug-metabolizing system) contains a complex of many enzymes responsible for the biotransformation of drugs and endogenous substances. NADPH is a required cofactor in oxidation and reduction reactions of microsomal enzymes. A drug may bind to the oxidized form of cytochrome P450. This complex is then reduced by NADPH-cytochrome reductase. The reduced complex then combines with O_2. The oxidized metabolite is then liberated and the oxidized form of cytochrome P450 is regenerated.

TYPES OF BIOTRANSFORMATION

Biotransformation can be divided into two main categories. These categories are **nonsynthetic** (also called phase I reactions) and **synthetic** (also called phase II reactions).

Nonsynthetic, or phase I, reactions involve the processes of oxidation, reduction, or hydrolysis. Metabolites formed by one of these processes usually enter a second step of biotransformation in the form of a synthetic (or phase II reaction) before elimination from the body. The metabolites formed from nonsynthetic pathways may retain some pharmacologic activity, as previously discussed.

Oxidation is the most common type of biotransformation and occurs primarily in the liver microsomal system. This reaction is catalyzed by NADPH-dependent mixed-function oxidases of the cytochrome P450 system previously discussed. Microsomal oxidation reactions catalyzed in this way include aliphatic side-chain hydroxylation; aromatic hydroxylation; oxidative N-, O-, and S-dealkylation; oxidative deamination; sulfoxidation; dehydrohalogenation; and desulfuration. Nonmicrosomal oxidative processes can occur elsewhere and include the oxidation of alcohols by alcohol dehydrogenase, the oxidation of aldehydes by aldehyde dehydrogenase, and the oxidation of purines. Oxidized metabolites are more polar and thus more water soluble. This reduces their tubular reabsorption and enhances their urinary excretion. Oxidized metabolites also enter phase II reactions to be further biotransformed.

Reduction is relatively uncommon compared to oxidation. It occurs mainly in the liver microsomal system but may occur elsewhere. Reduction reactions include azoreduction and nitrosoreduction.

Hydrolysis is responsible for the enzymatic biotransformation of esters and amides. Esterases are enzymes that may be found microsomally and extramicrosomally in the plasma, erythrocytes, and nerve terminals. Esterases catalyze the hydrolysis of esters, such as procaine, into an alcohol and an acid that are more polar and water soluble. Amidases are primarily microsomal and catalyze the hydrolysis of amides, such as procainamide, into amines and acids.

Synthetic, or phase II, reactions involve the conjugation of a drug or its metabolite from a phase I reaction with a highly polar, water-soluble, naturally occurring endogenous substance. These polar, endogenous substances include glucuronic acid, glycine, glutamine, glutathione, and sulfate. These conjugation products are usually biologically inactive and very polar, resulting in their rapid excretion in the urine and bile. Phase II conjugations also include methylation or acetylation of a parent drug or its phase I metabolite with a methyl or acetyl fragment. These conjugations usually lead to products that are less polar than their parent compound and may retain some of their pharmacologic activity. Conjugation reactions require a high-energy molecule that consists of a coenzyme bound to the endogenous substance. Transferase enzymes catalyze the transfer of the endogenous substance to the parent drug or its phase I metabolite.

Glucuronidation is the most common synthetic reaction. It is the only phase II reaction to occur in the hepatic microsomal enzyme system. Other phase II reactions occur in the liver (extramicrosomal), the intestines, and other tissues. Glucuronic acid is an abundant product of glucose metabolism found in the liver. Glucuronyl transferase catalyzes the transfer of glucuronic acid from uridine diphosphate glucuronic acid to hydroxyl or carboxyl groups of a nonpolar drug. This results in a very polar metabolite that is water-soluble, poorly reabsorbed, and readily eliminated in the urine and secreted in the bile.

Amino acid conjugation, catalyzed by transacylase, involves the transfer of glycine or glutamine from S-acyl-coenzyme A to aliphatic or aromatic acids to form amides.

Glutathione conjugation, catalyzed by glutathione transferase, involves the transfer of glutathione to halides or nitrates to yield a mercapturic acid.

Sulfation, catalyzed by sulfokinase (or sulfotransferase), involves the transfer of sulfate from 3'-phosphoadenosine-5'-phosphosulfate to phenols and alcohols to yield an ethereal sulfate.

Acetylation, catalyzed by N-acetyltransferase, involves the transfer of an acetyl group from acetyl-coenzyme A to aromatic amines, aliphatic amines, or heterocyclic nitrogen compounds. In conjugations of this type, however, the metabolite is usually less water soluble than the parent drug. Sulfoamides are metabolized in this way, and for this reason may accumulate in tissues such as the kidney, resulting in kidney damage.

Methylation, catalyzed by methyltransferase, results from the transfer of a methyl group from S-adenosylmethionine to amines, phenols, and heterocyclic compounds, yielding N-, O-, and S-methylated metabolites. The methylated products are usually less polar and thus usually biologically active, sometimes more so than the parent compound.

Desulfuration involves the replacement of sulfur by oxygen in the liver. Thiopental is converted to pentobarbital in this way.

Dehalogenation of halogenated hydrocarbons and certain insecticides also occurs in the liver.

EXCRETION

Excretion is the mechanism by which drugs and their metabolites are eliminated from the body. Some drugs are excreted unchanged. Other drugs are biotransformed into more polar metabolites and then eliminated from the body. The kidney is the most important excretory organ, responsible for eliminating many water-soluble polar substances. Next in importance is the biliary system. Other routes of elimination include saliva, sweat, gastric and intestinal secretions, breast milk, and exhaled gases; but the overall contribution of these pathways is very small.

Renal excretion is the most important route of elimination for water-soluble compounds and drugs with low molecular weight. Overall excretion by the kidney is governed by glomerular filtration, tubular reabsorption, and active tubular secretion.

Glomerular filtration is the process by which plasma, along with small drug molecules, are passively filtered through glomerular pores. Drugs bound to plasma proteins are not filtered. Only unbound drug is present in the glomerular filtrate.

Tubular reabsorption is the process whereby drugs are passively reabsorbed by diffusion as they pass along the renal tubules. Polar, water-soluble substances and ions cannot diffuse through the tubular cells back into the circulation unless a transport mechanism exists for their reabsorption, such as for glucose, vitamin C, and vitamin B. Lipid-soluble drugs are readily reabsorbed. Reabsorption and excretion are also affected by pH. The nonionized forms of weak acids and weak bases are readily reabsorbed from the glomerular filtrate. If the urine is acidified, weak acids will become predominantly nonionized (and reabsorbed), whereas weak bases will become predominantly ionized (and eliminated). The opposite effect occurs when the urine is alkalinized. These effects are useful to enhance elimination of drugs when an overdosage has occurred. For example, alkalinization of the urine enhance the urinary excretion of the weak acids phenobarbital and aspirin.

Active tubular secretion is an energy-dependent process in the proximal tubule. It is an important process in the elimination of drugs such as penicillin. Anions and cations are handled by separate active transport mechanisms. The active secretory transport mechanism can become saturated at high concentrations. It is also susceptible to competitive effects, as evidenced by various anionic compounds that compete with one another for secretion. This mechanism is capitalized upon therapeutically by giving probenecid, which competes with penicillin for tubular secretion, resulting in higher plasma penicillin concentrations by decreasing penicillin excretion.

Hepatic clearance is the volume of plasma containing a drug cleared by the liver per unit time. Hepatic clearance is affected by hepatic blood flow, intrinsic clearance, and protein binding. Normal hepatic blood flow is about 1.5 L/min. Any process that enhances or diminishes hepatic blood flow, such as exercise, liver disease, food, or other drugs can affect drug delivery and thus drug elimination by the hepatic route. Intrinsic drug clearance is primarily a function of the biotransformation enzymes and their ability to metabolize drugs as they enter the liver. Protein binding decreases hepatic clearance because only free drug is available to cross the hepatocyte membrane to be cleared by metabolism and excretion.

Hepatic clearance is also dependent on biliary excretion of drugs. Biliary excretion is an active secretory process whereby drugs and their metabolites are transported across the biliary epithelium against a concentration gradient. Biliary elimination occurs for drugs of higher molecular weight (greater than 300–500 mol wt), for polar drugs, and for glucuronic acid conjugates. Drugs undergoing biliary excretion may be recycled by enterohepatic circulation. This is especially true for glucuronide conjugates, which are excreted into the bile and hydrolyzed in the GI tract by bacteria. The drug is then liberated and can be reabsorbed, thus completing an enterohepatic cycle.

Alveolar excretion accounts for the elimination of volatile liquids and gases. The large alveolar surface area and high blood flow make the lungs an ideal location for excretion of these substances. Gaseous and volatile anesthetics are essentially completely eliminated by this route.

Clinical Physiological and Pathological Factors Affecting Drug Metabolism and Excretion

In the presence of disease or pathological conditions, absorption, distribution, metabolism, or elimination can be altered. Clinical pharmacokinetics is the science that deals with the effect of physiologic, pathologic, and environmental factors on these different pharmacokinetic phases. Each of these factors is discussed below.

Body weight and body composition affect the plasma drug concentration achieved after a given dose. Intersexual, interracial, and interethnic differences exist in body weight. Lipophilic drugs will achieve a higher plasma drug concentration in a person with little fat tissue as compared to a person of the same weight with considerable fat tissue.

Blood flow rates affect absorption, volume of distribution, rate of metabolism, and excretion. Drugs absorbed by passive diffusion depend on a concentration gradient. When blood flow rates are high, the absorbed drug is carried away, maintaining the high concentration gradient necessary for absorption. Similarly, absorption is decreased if blood flow rates are decreased. Hepatic blood flow determines the rate of hepatic metabolism. Any disease that decreases hepatic blood flow will decrease metabolism and excretion.

Gastric emptying rate (GER) is the time it takes for a drug to leave the stomach. Thus, GER can affect the rate and extent of absorption. Fast GER is desired when the drug might be inactivated or decomposed by the acidic environment of the stomach, as occurs with certain penicillins. A rapid GER is also desired if the drug is irritating to the stomach mucosa (i.e., aspirin) or if the drug is required in the intestine in high concentration for effectiveness (i.e., anthelminthics or neomycin in intestinal antisepsis).

Body temperature changes can alter organ perfusion and thus alter absorption, metabolism, and excretion.

Protein binding of drugs to albumin can affect drug distribution, metabolism, and elimination. Diseases that alter albumin synthesis will change the fraction of bound to unbound drug. An increase in plasma albumin leads to an increase in bound drug fraction; thus, there is less free drug available to exert a pharmacologic response, less drug metabolized, and less drug excreted. The opposite scenario occurs when plasma albumin concentration decreases.

Age is known to affect the rate of drug metabolism. In neonates, liver function and drug-metabolizing capacity are immature. Drugs will thus have a more prolonged biologic half-life. Children have mature drug-metabolizing capacity, and drugs may be less active than in adults. This is so because in children the liver develops faster than the increase in general body weight and represents a greater fraction of total body weight. In the aged, the drug-metabolizing capacity declines, leading to a lower rate of drug elimination.

Gender appears to affect the metabolic rate of certain drugs such as erythromycin and phenytoin. The lower blood levels seen in women appear to be a result of lower blood flow rates, decreased gastric motility, increased metabolic rate, and possibly greater distribution into fat.

Circadian rhythm affects the pharmacokinetics of drugs as a result of the rhythmical changes in bodily functions occurring during the course of the day.

Exercise also influences absorption, metabolism, and excretion. Exercise augments cardiac output and increases blood flow to muscle and decreases blood flow to the kidneys and liver.

Environmental factors affect drug-metabolizing capacity by regulating enzyme activity. Many environmental pollutants and organic insecticides can promote enzyme induction and thus augment drug elimination. Other chemicals, such as halogenated hydrocarbons, cause liver and kidney damage and thus prolong the biologic half-lives of some agents.

Nutritional status affects the activity of the hepatic metabolic enzymes. Low-protein diets can lead to amino acid deficiencies (some of which are important in conjugation reactions) and a reduction in the activity of the cytochrome P450 mixed-function oxidase system. Malnutrition can also reduce the levels of other conjugating agents, such as sulfate, glutathione, and glucuronic acid. Dietary deficiencies of essential fatty acids and minerals such as Ca, Mg, and Zn can also decrease drug–metabolizing capacity.

Pregnancy and lactation affect the volume of distribution and elimination of some drugs. The increase in body fat, change in tissue composition, and the presence of the fetus itself may affect the volume of distribution. Decreased renal blood flow may decrease renal elimination. Drugs may be excreted into the breast milk by passive diffusion and active transport.

Genetics can affect many of the pharmacokinetic phases, particularly biotransformations. An example of this genetic variation in metabolic rate is the acetylation of drugs, such as isoniazid, sulfonamides, and hydralazine. The population is about evenly divided between fast and slow acetylators.

Obesity appears primarily to affect the volume of distribution and elimination. Drugs with high lipid solubility partition readily into fat; thus a higher dose is needed to achieve a therapeutic concentration.

Cardiovascular diseases, particularly congestive heart failure, decrease renal and hepatic blood flow, thereby decreasing renal elimination and hepatic metabolism. In addition, the rate of absorption of drugs from all sites is diminished in congestive heart failure.

Renal disease can lead to drug accumulation if a drug is primarily eliminated by renal clearance. Likewise, liver disease can cause impairment of elimination, since the liver is the primary organ of biotransformation.

Enzyme induction and **enzyme inhibition** are responsible for alterations in metabolic rate when several drugs are administered concurrently. Phenobarbital is a known enzyme inducer and leads to increased metabolism of other drugs. Enzyme inducers increase the synthesis or decrease the degradation of drug-metabolizing enzymes. On the other hand, some drugs can decrease the metabolism of other drugs by destroying or inactivating the enzymes, or inhibiting their synthesis. A well-known example of enzyme inhibition occurs when cimetidine is coadministered with theophylline. Cimetidine inhibits the enzyme for theophylline metabolism, thereby leading to an increase in plasma theophylline levels.

First-pass effect occurs when a significant proportion of administered drug is metabolized on its passage from the portal system to the systemic circulation. Thus much of the drug is metabolized before it is able to reach its site of action. Drugs that exhibit a significant first-pass effect include propranolol, isosorbide, and nitrogen.

Shock, burns, and trauma all can lead to circulatory stress. This leads to delayed absorption, decreased volume of distribution, decreased metabolism from diminished hepatic blood flow, and decreased renal elimination from diminished renal blood flow.

Bibliography

Berkow R, Fletcher A. *The Merck manual of diagnosis and therapy.* 15th ed. Rahway, NJ: Merck, Sharp and Dohme Research Laboratories, 1987.

Evans W, Schentag J, Jusko W, eds. *Applied pharmacokinetics—principles of therapeutic drug monitoring.* 2nd ed. Vancouver: Applied Therapeutics, 1986.

Gibaldi M, Perrier D. *Pharmacokinetics.* New York: Marcel Dekker, 1982.

Gilman A, Goodman L, Gilman A. *The pharmacologic basis of therapeutics.* 6th ed. New York: Macmillian, 1980.

Harvey S. Basic pharmacokinetics. In: Osol A, ed. *Remington's pharmaceutical sciences.* 16th ed. Easton, PA: Mack Publishing Company, 1980.

Irene D. Feurer

31 FUNDAMENTALS OF STATISTICS

This discussion is intended to review the basics of data classification, analysis, and reporting, and to assist the reader in interpreting published reports and selecting appropriate statistical designs and procedures. Statistical analyses may be considered either **descriptive** or **inferential**. Descriptive statistics characterize data. Inferential statistics draw conclusions about the population(s) represented by a sample or samples. Depending on the research design and purpose of the report, statistical analyses serve one of three basic functions: information summary; estimation of the significance of observed differences among treatment programs; or the determination of relationships among sets of data.

Scales of Measurement

Measurement scales refer to the "type" of data:

1. **Nominal** data are defined as mutually exclusive categories that do not have any hierarchical order, e.g., gender.
2. **Ordinal** data convey relative position along a con-

tinuum, but do not signify true distance between ordered points or categories. For example, a rank ordering of runners completing a race does not convey any information about precise finish time.
3. **Interval** data are expressed according to a scale having equal distances between units of measurement and an arbitrary zero point. Examples of interval scales are temperature and standardized test scores. An important characteristic of interval scales is that they can be manipulated mathematically without affecting relative distances among scores.
4. **Ratio** data extend the properties of interval scales to include an absolute zero point. Many physiologic variables are measured along ratio scales.

The scale by which data are measured defines to a large extent the type of statistical procedures that may be performed. In general, nominal and ordinal data are analyzed using **nonparametric** techniques; **parametric** procedures are typically applied to interval and ratio data. Interval and ratio data are more "rich" in the quantitative sense than data measured on nominal or ordinal scales. When there is the option, it is generally more meaningful to measure a variable by an interval or ratio scale as opposed to a nominal or ordinal scale. Conversion of interval or ratio data to a categorical scale (nominal or ordinal) generally reduces the level of empirical conclusions that can be drawn from a set of observations.

Descriptive Statistics

Descriptive statistics encompass measures of **central tendency** and measures of **variability**. Measures of central tendency express a collection of observations on a particular variable or attribute as one number:

1. The **mode** is the most frequent score in the distribution. As such, it is the measure of central tendency that is most subject to fluctuation when a few values change. It is the only measure of central tendency used to describe nominal data, but it can be applied to any other scale of measurement..
2. The **median** is based upon rank order and is the point on a distribution below which 50% of observations fall. It is the preferred measure of central tendency when ordinal data are described but can also be used with interval- and ratio-scaled data.
3. The **mean,** the most commonly used measure of central tendency, is the arithmetic average of all observations within a sample. It is most often used to describe interval- and ratio-scaled data. It is the most stable measure of central tendency because it takes each observation into account, but it can be influenced by extreme values or "outliers" when computed on small samples.

Measures of variability express the degree of deviation from the central tendency inherent in the data set. The smaller the variability, the more representative the measure of central tendency. Some common measures of variability are discussed below.

1. The **range** is simply the quantitative difference between the highest and lowest value of a given attribute and, as such, may fluctuate markedly if the highest or lowest observation changes. It is applied to data measured along interval or ratio scales.
2. The **semi-interquartile range** is used to describe the variability of ordinal-scaled data. It is half the distance between the first quartile (25th percentile) and third quartile (75th percentile).
3. **Variance** is defined as the sum of the squared arithmetic deviations from the mean of all observations in a sample divided by the number of cases minus one. The calculation of variance is fundamental to parametric inferential statistical procedures. Since it considers the entire sample, it and its direct arithmetic derivatives are the most stable measures of variability.
4. The **standard deviation (SD)** is simply the square root of the variance. Of note, the standard deviation is closely related to the normal or Gaussian distribution in that approximately two thirds of all observations fall within the mean ±1 SD; roughly 95% fall within ±2 SD of the mean; and the mean ±3 SD encompasses practically every observation in the normal distribution.
5. The **standard error of the mean (SEM)** is the standard deviation divided by the square root of the sample size. This statistic is naturally smaller than its corresponding standard deviation and will, at first glance, give the reader an impression of little variability. When the standard error of the mean is reported, it is often useful to calculate the standard deviation in order to gauge more clearly variability in relation to the normal distribution.
6. The **observed sample mean** is really an estimate of the actual population mean (which is assumed to be unknown). If the observed frequency distribution closely approximates a normal or Gaussian distribution, one may compute **confidence limits** or **intervals** that define the range of values within which the true mean will reside in a given percentage of instances (typically 95%). Confidence intervals are interpreted such that one could claim to be 95% confident that the true mean lies within the stated range.
7. The **coefficient of variation** is most commonly used to describe the reliability (or reproducibility) of a measurement. It is defined to be the standard deviation of repeated measurements expressed as a percentage of the mean. Since the units are percentage points, one can compare coefficients of variation of different attributes or those of one attribute as measured by several methods.

Frequency Distributions and Their Graphic Representation

A data set is often reported as a frequency distribution, a tabular presentation of values or ranges of values and the number of observations achieving each level. The **histogram** (bar plot) and **frequency polygon** (continuous curve) are graphical representations of interval or ratio data with frequencies depicted on the ordinate (y-axis) and data values on the abscissa (x-axis). As was suggested in the preceding description of the standard deviation, a frequency distribution having great importance in statistical inference is the normal, or Gaussian, distribution, with its characteristic "bell-shaped" curve. Because many attributes of large populations tend to be normally distributed, this distribution is at the center of probability theory inherent in many statistical tests. Normal distributions are exactly symmetrical, with the mean, median, mode, and 50th percentile lying at the center, or peak, of the frequency curve.

Most frequency distributions are to a certain extent asymmetrical or **skewed,** meaning that scores are more frequent or "pile up" at one end of the distribution. Negatively skewed distributions are those having a preponderance of high scores, while positively skewed distributions have a preponderance of scores at the lower end of the measurement scale. Empirical procedures such as the χ^2 goodness-of-fit and Komogorov-Smirnov tests can be used to evaluate whether an observed frequency distribution deviates significantly from normal. **Kurtosis** refers to the flatness or peakedness of a frequency distribution. **Leptokurtic** distributions are narrow with high peaks; **platykurtic** distributions are broad and flat. A rectangular distribution appears as its name suggests.

Test Accuracy in the Clinical Setting

The "accuracy" of clinical measurements can be discussed in a variety of manners. The **reliability** of a measurement, often reported in the biomedical literature as coefficient of variation, is the reproducibility of the measurement on repeated occasions, under "identical" circumstances. Imperfect reliability is the reason that laboratories provide data concerning the possible range of "true" test values. **Validity** refers to the degree to which a test is measuring the intended parameter. A measure must be reliable in order for it to be valid, but reliability does not mandate validity. Validity is typically assessed by comparing reliable measurements to some "gold standard" value for the parameter in question.

The **sensitivity** of a test (clinical positivity) refers to the probability of true positive test results when the test is applied to patients known to have the disease or condition. The **specificity** of a test is the probability of true negative test results among patients known to not have the disease or condition. **Prevalence** refers to the number of patients per 100,000 in the population known to have the disease at a particular point in time. The **incidence** of a disease is the number of persons per 100,000 of the population who develop the disease over a one-year period.

Test sensitivity and specificity are not related to the prevalence of a disease or condition. It is the test's **predictive value** which considers both test accuracy as well as the overall probability of the disease or condi-

tion occurring within the population. The predictive value of a positive test is the proportion of positive test results that are true positives in a sample including persons with and without the disease or condition. Similarly, the predictive value of a negative test is the proportion of negative results that are true negatives in a similarly diverse group.

Inferential Statistics

Hypothesis testing refers to the application of statistical techniques to draw conclusions about populations from sets of randomly selected observations known as samples. This is the general domain of **inferential statistics.** Hypothesis testing and statements of statistical conclusions generally follow a pattern of reverse logic. One begins by formulating a **null hypothesis** that states that the samples under consideration do not differ from each other with respect to a given variable or variables. The next step is to specify the level of significance or degree of improbability that will be deemed necessary to cast sufficient doubt upon the truth of the null hypothesis (typically <5%). This probability is known as the **α-level or Type I error rate**; it is the risk of being wrong when rejecting the null hypothesis and declaring "statistically significant" differences to exist. The obtained α-level is reported as the *p* value. A straightforward mathematical statement known as the rejection rule can then be formulated, which outlines the qualities of the data with respect to the mean and standard deviation necessary to reject the null hypothesis with a probability of erring at less than the accepted α-level or type I error rate (e.g., $p < .05$). Table 31-1 depicts the possible conditions encountered as a result of hypothesis testing.

The accepted convention is to consider an α-level (*p* value, Type I error rate) of <.05 to be sufficient evidence to reject the null hypothesis and declare a statistically significant effect, difference, or relationship to exist. While this is the usual case, a few circumstances would warrant setting a lower, more conservative, α-level, e.g.,<.01 (when the risks of being "wrong" carry extreme consequences) or a higher α-level, e.g., <0.10 (as with some behavioral data or occasional clinical pilot investigations when the measures have poor sensitivity). This decision is based on the investigator's knowledge of the field as well as the characteristics of the data in terms of measurement reliability.

TABLE 31-1. Possible Decisions and Outcomes of Hypothesis Testing

True State of the Universe	Your Decision	Condition/Probability
Null Hypothesis True No differences exist	Accept Null Hypothesis Declare no differences **(Correct Decision)**	$1 - \alpha$
Null Hypothesis True No differences exist	Reject Null Hypothesis Declare differences **(Incorrect Decision)**	Type I Error α
Null Hypothesis False Differences exist	Accept Null Hypothesis Declare no differences **(Incorrect Decision)**	Type II Error β
Null Hypothesis False Differences exist	Reject Null Hypothesis Declare differences **(Correct Decision)**	Power $1 - \beta$

Adapted from Young RK, Veldman DJ. *Introductory statistics for the behavioral sciences.* 3rd ed. New York: Holt, Rinehart and Winston, 1977:141.

Statistical power is the quantitative index of the sensitivity of the experiment, which should, in most circumstances, be .80 or greater. The importance of this concept is sometimes overlooked and can result in an erroneous impression of no effect or association among a set of variables when, in fact, the experimental design was simply not sufficiently sensitive to detect the effect. A related point is that failure to reject the null hypothesis does not mean that comparison groups are equivalent (e.g., treatments A and B are equally effective); it simply means that they were not shown to be significantly different given the conditions of the investigation with regard to sample size, required α-level, and measurement techniques. The **Type II error rate (β)**, which is inversely related to power, is simply the probability of failing to detect an existing difference or effect. Statistical power is a function of four aspects of the experiment:

1. **α-Level or Type I error rate.** A reduction in the type I error rate acceptable to the investigator increases the likelihood of making a Type II error, thereby reducing power.
2. **Sample size.** Power increases with sample size and the ratio between the number of subjects to variables in correlational analyses. Consequently, the question of sample size and its effect on power is crucial when planning an experiment or interpreting a report of "no effect." The inclusion of an excessive number of variables similarly reduces power in correlational research. The most straightforward solution to poor power is to increase the number of subjects or, while holding sample size constant, to reduce the number of variables studied.
3. **Effect size.** Effect size refers to the known effect of an experimental treatment or condition on the variable(s) being studied. Effect size can be expressed in SD units as the difference between groups means. Simply put, experiments involving treatments that result in small effects will have poor power unless the sample size is large.
4. **Error variance.** All things being equal, power (experimental sensitivity) is inversely related to the variability around group means, or within group error variance.

A balance between the accepted Type I error rate and experimental power must be struck. However, since Type I error rates of <.05 are the accepted standard in most instances, investigators are faced with finding ways to increase power other than adopting a more lenient (larger) Type I error rate. Straightforward steps to increase power while keeping the Type I error rate constant include (1) increasing sample size; (2) eliminating extraneous variables; (3) the use of one-tailed tests when a directional hypothesis is supported in the literature; and (4) reducing within group variability (error variance) by increasing the homogeneity of the subject sample, using "factorial" designs, covariates, blocking, or repeated measures designs.

Selecting an Experimental Design

The term *design* refers to the logical and statistical aspects of the investigation, including subject selection, Type I and II error rates, timing of observations, and control groups, all of which collectively dictate the statistical tests employed. The degree to which an investigation may be logically interpreted is dependent on the statistical control (over error variance and alternative explanations) implicit in the design. **Internal validity** refers to the degree to which one can logically interpret the outcome in the context of **the given experiment.** At a very minimum, an investigation must have reasonable internal validity. **External validity** refers to the generalizability of the experimental conclusions to the "real world" or outside situations. No investigation can be externally valid unless it is designed to have appropriate internal validity.

True experimental designs require **random** selection and assignment of subjects to the various experimental or control conditions. As such, true experiments are always considered to be **prospective.** Quasi-experiments lack various degrees of experimental control but are often useful when true experimentation is either impossible or impractical. Quasi-experiments employ logical design controls, such as repeated measures or random assignment procedures, but lack the element of random subject selection. Consequently, quasi-experiments may be either prospective or retrospective in nature. Examples of **retrospective** investigations are chart reviews or other analyses of existing databases.

Investigative control refers to those aspects of the design that reduce error variance and preclude alternative explanations that could be ascribed to events unrelated to the treatment conditions. Types of control include experimental manipulation, subject selection, and statistical control (mathematic "partialing"). A design is selected on the basis of the research question or null hypothesis and practical considerations such as data or subject availability, time required for completion, and cost.

The distinction between **independent** and **dependent** variables is a useful one. Independent, or predictor, variables are those that can be manipulated by the investigator. The outcomes, or dependent variables, are the effect parameters of interest. For example, if 300 men with hypertension evidenced by a diastolic pressure >90 mm Hg were selected at random to receive either a placebo or one of two antihypertensive medications for a period of three months (experimental conditions A, B, and P), the independent variable is "medication" (with its three possible "levels," groups, or conditions). The dependent variable is diastolic blood pressure after three months of study.

As stated previously, the choice of statistical tests or procedures is intimately related to the overall design of the investigation. The following brief summaries of commonly used statistical tests are intended to present the essentials of each.

Parametric Procedures

Parametric procedures are applied to interval or ratio scale data. In general, they assume that the data have normal frequency distributions and comparable or "homogeneous" variance among groups or variables. Their advantages include increased power and the fact that they are generally "robust" or relatively immune to minor violations of their inherent mathematic assumptions.

The familiar **Student's *t* test** is used to analyze the results of two-group studies or designs involving pairs of observations on each individual. A *t* test of group means would be appropriate in our antihypertensive medication study if we were evaluating the effect of one medication versus a placebo. If we were interested in evaluating the effect of one medication that all subjects received by measuring blood pressure before and after treatment, we could use a **paired *t* test.**

The two-tailed, or nondirectional, *t* test is most often appropriate and is the most "conservative." However, when prior research dictates a directional hypothesis, i.e., that a specific treatment effect is likely not only to result in a difference but in a clearly smaller or larger mean value, a one-tailed test may be employed. The advantages of a one-tailed test are that power is increased without increasing sample size and it is "easier" to demonstrate statistically significant effects. (If p equals .1 in a two-tailed test, it equals .05 in the one-tailed test). However, the investigator's rationale for using the one-tailed procedure must be well-substantiated in the literature.

The *t* test is nothing more than a special case of the "one-way" **analysis of variance (ANOVA).** Analysis of variance and its test statistic, the F test, evaluates whether differences exist among three or more treatment groups on one outcome measure. The three-group antihypertensive medication data (two medications plus placebo) could be analyzed by one-way ANOVA to test the null hypothesis that there was no between-group difference in posttreatment diastolic blood pressure. It is important to note that a statistically significant F test tells us only that the treatment regimens in all probability do not have the same effect on blood pressure. It does not tell us that medication A is has a statistically different effect from medication B, or that either are any more effective than the placebo (even though group means may suggest this interpretation). Some investigators mistakenly attempt to answer this question by using multiple t tests. This has the effect of markedly increasing the actual type I error rate with each successive t test. For instance, if t tests were applied to all possible pairs in the above example having three unique between-group comparisons, the actual type I error rate, the likelihood of finding a difference by chance, would be increased almost threefold, from a presumed .05 to .15. A correct method for evaluating which group pairs are significantly different following a significant overall F test is the use of "post hoc" comparisons. Examples, in decreasing order of statistical conservativeness (strictness) are the Tukey, Scheffe, and Dunn procedures.

As you might infer from the term "one-way" ANOVA, there exist "n-way" analyses of variance, also known as **factorial designs.** The value of these designs is that they allow the researcher to test for **interaction effects.** For example, if the subjects in the three-group antihypertensive drug study were simultaneously assigned at random to either a weight reduction diet or no dietary manipulation, we would have a two-factor design that could be analyzed by a two-way ANOVA. The two independent variables or factors are medication regimen (treatment groups A, B, and P) and dietary regimen (treatment groups diet and no diet), for a total of six unique experimental conditions. The dependent variable remains diastolic blood pressure after three months. The two-way ANOVA would test the statistical significance of the two possible **main effects** (of factors 1 and 2), via F tests no different from one-way ANOVAs. The new twist, evaluation of an interaction effect, would answer the question whether weight reduction in any way influenced the effect of the medications on blood pressure. These points are illustrated in Figure 31-1, which depicts mean values for the main effects and interaction analysis. Standard deviations have been omitted for the sake of this illustration; normally they would be reported and graphed.

Figure 31-1A depicts the overall means for the three medication treatment groups and a statistically significant main effect (overall F statistic) for factor 1. In this hypothetical example, patients receiving medication B had a slightly lower average posttreatment diastolic pressure than did patients receiving medication A, but this was not statistically significant. Via the Scheffe test, both medications A and B resulted in statistically lower posttreatment pressures when compared to the placebo group. Overall group means for factor 2, dietary regimen, were not significantly different (Figure 31-1B) so there was no main effect for this factor. The F test for an interaction effect (Figure 31-1C) was statistically significant because medication B was markedly more effective than medication A when coupled with weight loss but only equally effective as medication A in those patients who did not lose weight. This point is obscured when the data are "pooled" for the analyses of main effects.

Correlational designs investigate degrees of association between two variables or a set of independent variables and one dependent variable. This section will focus on **linear relationships** among variables, but tests of fit to functions other than a straight line can be performed. It is always important to remember that the presence of a correlation *does not* indicate a cause-and-effect relationship. Two variables, X and Y, may be correlated because X influences Y, Y influences X, or an unmeasured variable or group of variables impact both X and Y (making the X Y relationship **spurious**). An expansion of multiple regression known as **path analysis,** popular among social scientists, attempts to construct parsimonious models of causative relationships on the basis of theory and multiple regression statistics.

Associations between dichotomous (two-category) variables can be analyzed by **tetrachoric correlations** or **phi coefficients;** relationships between dichotomous and continuous variables by **biserial** or **point-biserial correlations.** However, this discussion will focus on correlations among interval or ratio data that are typically reported in the biomedical literature.

Correlational models evaluate the strength of the association (r), the proportion of variance in the dependent variable that can be accounted for in the independent variable(s) (r^2), the direction of the association (+ or −), and the degree to which the relationship may be due to chance (p). For example, in normal-weight women, there is a statistically significant ($p < .01$) correlation ($r = +.61$) between body weight and resting energy expenditure (REE). This may be interpreted as being a moderately strong relationship (r value between

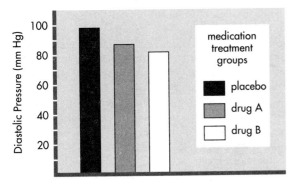

A. Main effect of factor 1 (medication)

medication
treatment
groups

■ placebo

▨ drug A

□ drug B

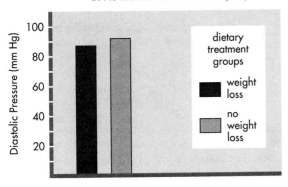

B. No main effect of factor 2 (diet)

dietary
treatment
groups

■ weight
loss

▨ no
weight
loss

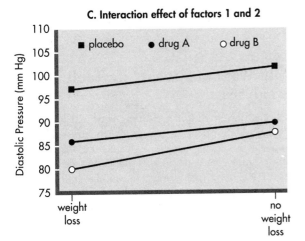

C. Interaction effect of factors 1 and 2

■ placebo   ● drug A   ○ drug B

Figure 31-1 Hypothetical data illustrating analyses of main and interaction effects in a factorial design having two independent variables.

.6 and .8), where 37% ($.61^2$) of the change in REE can be explained by change in body weight. The positive sign simply indicates that REE increases with increasing weight. Negative correlations exist when the value of one variable decreases with increasing values of the second variable.

Multiple regression models evaluate associations between two or more independent variables or predictors and a dependent variable. A variety of stepwise algorithms may be used (forward selection, backward elimination, etc.). These are usually referred to as "methods" in statistical software packages and define the mathematic rules for sequentially entering or dropping independent variables from the possible set to formulate the final regression equation. A good set of predictor variables is one where the predictors are only weakly correlated with each other, thereby eliminating redundant information, and each is well correlated with the dependent variable. An example of a multiple regression equation, developed by J. Harris and F. Benedict on a sample of 103 normal-weight women in the early 1900s, is REE (in kcal/day) = 655 + 9.6 x (weight in kg) + 1.8 x (height in cm) – 4.7 x (age in years). The multiple correlation coefficient (R) was approximately .73, which, given this sample size, was statistically significant ($p < .001$). We can assume that of all the independent variables measured by the investigators, height, weight, and age individually contributed significant new information to warrant their inclusion in the final formula. Any excluded variables were either highly correlated with a variable or variables already present in the equation, (e.g., body surface area) or did not correlate sufficiently well with REE. Also note that age carries a negative coefficient or "weight," indicating that REE declines with increasing age.

Two important points relating to correlational research are that the strength of relationships calculated on one sample of subjects are likely to "shrink" when recalculated on a similar set of subjects and that correlations characterize relationships among a collection of observations. Shrinkage is due to the manner in which multiple correlations are calculated; they are biased to obtain the maximum R value. For this reason it is not surprising that correlations decline or even disappear when regression equations are applied to groups unlike the original sample. Similarly, one can expect a reasonable level of inaccuracy when applying such formulae to individuals as opposed to groups.

Strong elements of control that reduce error variance can be introduced into quasi-experimental designs.

Blocking refers to the addition of a fixed classification variable that cannot be manipulated but serves to group like subjects. For instance, a heterogeneous sample could be blocked according to gender if there were some evidence that gender were related to the dependent variable of interest.

A similar technique, **analysis of covariance (ANOVA),** is a cross between regression and analysis of variance. It mathematically adjusts for differences existing between subjects at the start of an investigation. The covariate is a trait or stable characteristic that is not affected by the study, but is notably correlated with the dependent variable. For instance, it would make sense to use analysis of covariance in a study evaluating the relative efficacy of three weight-loss regimens through measurements of posttreatment weight loss. Starting weight, being correlated with the dependent variable (weight lost), would be a useful covariate.

Nonparametric Procedures

Although parametric procedures are generally more powerful, they are not always appropriate. **Nonparametric** tests, known as "distribution-free" techniques, do not assume the data to be normally distributed and are robust (their accuracy is retained), regardless of the shape of the frequency distribution. Nonparametric tests are typically used to test relationships among categorical variables (nominal or ordinal scales) or when the distribution of interval- or ratio-scaled data deviates significantly from normal. In the latter circumstance, one would first reduce the data to meaningful categories, e.g., convert age in years to categories such as 20–40, 41–65, >65. Brief discussions of a few nonparametric procedures follow.

The χ-**square** procedure may be used to test whether two frequency distributions are alike or whether a distribution deviates substantially from normal. Data are measured as frequencies. In the typical test for association between two categorical variables, data are cross-classified and the pattern of frequencies within cells evaluated in relation to some expected frequency pattern. For instance, if persons having symptomatic gallbladder disease were classified by gender and most pervasive type of stone (fully calcified versus not fully calcified) we could use the χ-square statistic to evaluate whether gender was in any way associated with

this gallstone characteristic. In this example there are four possible cross classified conditions, and the test would evaluate whether the obtained frequency pattern deviated substantially from random (equal number of individuals in each of four cells). **Fisher's exact test** is an alternative to the χ-square procedure that can be used with two dichotomous variables (2 x 2 cross-tabulations) when the sample size is small (≤ 20).

Log-linear and **logistic** models are useful with large samples of dichotomous data (categorical variables having two categories). Log-linear models can be thought of as extending the χ-square test to evaluate relationships among greater than two variables simultaneously. Logistic models extend this analysis and consider the variables to be either dependent or independent. Dregelid et al., in 1988, used these techniques to evaluate characteristics of 202 patients having surgery for suspected arterial embolism and noted an interaction between gender and several clinical characteristics.

The **Mann-Whitney** test (also called the **Wilcoxon** test) is used with ordinal-scale data to test whether two random, independent samples come from populations having the same distribution. This procedure is analogous to the more powerful two-sample t test for normally distributed interval or ratio-scale data. The **Kruskal-Wallis** test extends the Mann-Whitney procedure to three or more random samples and is analogous to the parametric one-way ANOVA. Interval- or ratio-scaled data can be converted to rank orders and the Mann-Whitney or Kruskal-Wallis tests computed if warranted when the data have distributions that are significantly different from normal.

Survival Functions, Life Table Analyses

Clinical investigations involving repeated follow-up measures lend themselves naturally to **survival** or **life table** analysis. This methodology examines the progress of the sample at regular intervals following the initiating event, e.g., long-term patency of vascular grafts. Not all patients will enter the study at the same point in time and not all will have experienced the predefined endpoint or termination event (not necessarily death) at the time of study termination, but all will have experienced the same initiating event and will have been followed in a standardized fashion. Close follow-up is critical.

Those cases that have not experienced the termination event at the time of data analysis are termed "censored." While their exact "life span" is not known, it is at least the amount of time since the initiation event. Censored observations also occur when patients die from unrelated causes or are simply lost to follow-up. Survival analysis makes use of both censored and uncensored observations when calculating survival times. Each survival score is then used to draw comparisons between treatment groups to determine whether differences in survival exist.

Meta-Analysis

Meta-analysis, a quantitative method for systematically combining data from many different sources, is being used with increased frequency in biomedical research. As noted by Thacker in 1988, traditional literature reviews may be fraught with problems: (1) sampling bias owing to reporting and publication policies; (2) the absence in published studies of specific desired data; (3) biased exclusion of studies by the investigator; (4) the uneven quality of the primary data; and (5) biased outcome interpretation. In general, meta-analyses pool data from a variety of sources after (1) defining the required experimental conditions of included studies; (2) comprehensive literature reviews; (3) coding study characteristics; (4) measuring study characteristics on a common scale; and (5) analyzing aggregate findings across included studies in light of study characteristics. The backbone of the meta-analytic technique is the set of study inclusion criteria. Its advantages include increased generalizability of conclusions resulting from the expanded "sample," as well as the elimination of potential subjectivity in literature review and interpretation.

Summary

The preceding discussion was intended to give the reader a sense for some key considerations to be mindful of when interpreting reports or planning an investigation and analyzing data. Statistical software packages make it simple to compute reams of tests. The challenge is to apply these procedures parsimoniously and appropriately, and to report data in a clear fashion so that they may be readily understood.

Bibliography

Campbell DT, Stanley JC. *Experimental and quasi-experimental designs for research.* Boston: Houghton Mifflin, 1963.

Colton T. *Statistics in medicine.* Boston: Little, Brown, 1974.

Dregelid EB, Strangeland LB, Eide GE, Trippestad A. Characteristics of patients operated on because of suspected arterial embolism: A multivariate analysis. *Surgery* 1988;104: 530–536.

Fienberg SE. *The analysis of cross-classified categorical data.* 2nd ed. Cambridge: The MIT Press, 1980.

Galen RS, Gambino SR. *Beyond normality: the predictive value and efficiency of medical diagnosis.* New York: Wiley, 1975.

Howell WH. Statistical analysis. In: Post-graduate course #10, getting started in clinical research. *Eleventh Clinical Congress of the American Society for Parenteral and Enteral Nutrition,* 1988.

Ingelfinger JA, Mosteller F, Thibodeau LA, Ware JA. *Biostatistics in clinical medicine.* 2nd ed. New York: Macmillan, 1987.

Keppel G. *Design and analysis: A researcher's handbook.* 2nd ed. Englewood Cliffs, NJ: Prentice-Hall, 1982.

Thacker SB. Meta-analysis: a quantitative approach to research integration. *JAMA* 1988;259(11):1685–1689.

Young RK, Veldman DJ. *Introductory statistics for the behavioral sciences.* 3rd ed. New York: Holt, Rinehart and Winston, 1977.

James D. Luketich, David Rigberg, and Eline Luning Prak

32 NUTRITION

Over the past decade, increasing emphasis has been placed on the study of nutrition and maintenance of optimal nutritional status in hospitalized patients. This is a consequence of a number of observations. First, we now have a better understanding of the natural history of starvation, beginning with subtle changes in muscle mass and visceral proteins, eventually leading to organ failure and death. Secondly, it was recognized that malnourished patients are frequently encountered in hospitalized populations and that these patients have an increased morbidity and mortality compared to normonourished groups. Finally, the advent of parenteral and enteral nutrition has allowed widespread nutritional intervention and has improved outcome in some patient populations.

The goals of this chapter are to discuss body composition; fuel reserves; response to simple starvation; nutritional requirements, including macronutrients and micronutrients; and review the essentials of nutritional assessment.

Body Composition

Body composition analysis quantitates the size of specific body compartments. A simple approach divides the body into two components; fat mass and nonfat mass (the lean body mass). Lean body mass can be subdivided into the extracellular mass and a cellular component, the **body cell mass.** The body cell mass has been described as the sum of all cellular components of the body including the oxygen-exchanging, glucose oxidizing, work-performing tissues of the body. The body cell mass composes 40% of the body weight of a normal adult. It is composed of 60% skeletal muscle mass and 20% visceral cell mass (liver, pancreas, kidney). The remaining 20% includes red blood cells, and the cellular makeup of cartilage, bone, tendons, and adipose tissue. Nutritional depletion always adversely affects the body cell mass.

There is no direct measure of the body cell mass, but it is possible to measure the lean body mass, which contains both extracellular fluid and the body cell mass. A number of methods exist to determine the size of the lean body mass, including isotopic measurement of water and potassium, densitometry and anthropometry, measurement of muscle metabolites, and electrical conductivity and impedance of tissues. Most of these techniques require an accurate assessment of total body water, which is usually performed by isotope dilution. In health this approach is satisfactory since water occupies a constant fraction (73.2%) of the lean body mass and is not present in stored triglyceride. This allows one to estimate lean body mass (LBM) from total body water (TBW):

$$LBM = TBW/0.73$$

In disease states and malnutrition, there is often a variable but significant increase in the extracellular fluid compartment. This increases the water content of the lean body mass compartment above the normal 73%, making the above formula unreliable. Newer methods of body composition analysis that utilize a four-compartment model (water, protein, bone mineral, and fat) overcome some of the limitations of the simple two-compartment model, but presently are limited to the research setting owing to prohibitive cost and complexity.

Fuel Reserves and Starvation

The fuel reserves of the body include carbohydrates, proteins, and fats. Carbohydrates and proteins reside in the aqueous environment of the lean body mass; fats in the water-free fat compartment. Carbohydrates are stored in the form of glycogen, primarily found in the liver and skeletal muscle. This fraction of the total energy reserve is small but essential, for example, in the production of high-energy phosphates during limited periods of anaerobic metabolism. The total caloric value of the glycogen stores in a 70-kg man is only about 1000 kcal. Since the metabolic requirement for a 70-kg man is approximately 2000 kcal/day, **glycogen stores are used rapidly** unless an alternate fuel source becomes available.

The caloric value of the total protein present in a 70-kg man is approximately 24,000 kcal. However, long before this amount of energy could be utilized, serious compromise in bodily function would occur, since each molecule of protein in the body has an enzymatic, structural, synthetic, or other function.

Fat represents the major fuel depot in the body. Its efficient storage in a nonaqueous environment makes available a much greater energy source without the additional volume of the aqueous storage form of carbohydrates. For example, 1 g of fat yields 9.4 kcal compared with approximately 4 kcal/g for carbohydrate and protein. In the 70-kg man there is about 15 kg of fat, mostly stored as triglycerides in adipose tissue, representing a potential of approximately 141,000 kcal. Assuming a metabolic rate of 2000 kcal per day, enough energy is present for a 70-day period of fasting.

During a fasting period the initial energy sources are glycogen and skeletal muscle protein. Since glycogen stores are limited and the use of protein for energy requires the breakdown of important structural and functional molecules, the key to survival during a prolonged fast is the **rapid adaptation to a fat-burning state.** Along with this adaptation other important mechanisms that facilitate survival during starvation include a **decrease in energy expenditure** and a shift from glucose to ketone bodies as a primary fuel source in the brain.

Initially, glucose requirements are high to fuel the brain, erythrocytes, leukocytes, bone marrow, and adrenal medulla. As the blood glucose level declines, insulin levels decrease and glucagon levels increase. The low insulin level favors peripheral lipolysis and proteolysis; the increased glucagon stimulates glycogen release and hepatic uptake of alanine, which is then used as a major substrate for gluconeogenesis by the liver. The increased level of glucagon plays an important role in the conversion to a ketone-producing state by inhibiting fatty acid synthesis and stimulating the uptake of acetyl-coenzyme A by mitochondria.

The **conversion to a fat-burning state** during starvation can be followed by measuring urinary losses of nitrogen. Since glycogen stores are rapidly burned, muscle breakdown supplies energy by releasing glucogenic amino acids for gluconeogenesis, the urinary excretion of nitrogen increases concurrently. In the fed state, urinary nitrogen losses average 4–6 g daily; this increases to 8–11 g/day during the first few days of simple starvation. If one considers the source of each gram of nitrogen as approximately 15 g of protein, in the aqueous state in the body this represents about 60 g of wet lean muscle. Therefore, during the first few days of starvation, when nitrogen losses are about 10 g/day, up to 600 g (1.3 lbs) of wet lean muscle mass can be lost per day.

If this rate of protein catabolism were to continue, death would ensue in a matter of weeks. However, as starvation continues, fatty acid mobilization, ketone body formation, and the brain along with some other tissues adapt to ketone body utilization to reduce glucose requirements and net protein losses. With this conversion, urinary nitrogen losses decrease to a nadir of 2–4 g/day, representing a daily loss of 80 g of wet lean muscle, much more compatible with survival during prolonged starvation.

Nutrient Requirements

CALORIES

Metabolic rate can be estimated based on age-, sex-, height-, and weight-matched controls (e.g., the Harris-Benedict equation) or it can be measured using an indirect calorimeter. Harris-Benedict predictions of resting energy expenditure are adequate for healthy populations where most predicted rates fall within 10% of actual measurement. However, in sick patients this formula is often inaccurate, and it may be helpful to measure energy expenditure using a bedside indirect calorimeter.

Resting energy expenditure is defined as the energy expenditure measured 2 hours postprandially with the patient at rest for at least 30 minutes in the supine position. This quantity is 10% higher than the **basal metabolic rate,** which is measured in the morning before activity commences and follows a 12-hour fast. In a normal but relatively sedentary individual the resting energy expenditure accounts for approximately 75–80% of the total daily energy expenditure. Activity-related energy expenditure makes up 20–25% of the total and the thermic response to food ingestion accounts for less than 5% of the total. In the bed-ridden hospitalized patient, resting energy expenditure may account for up to 90–100% of the total daily energy expenditure. It is significantly influenced by nutrient infusions, ambient room temperature, fever, disease states, and other factors.

After determination of energy expenditure, the caloric requirement can be administered as carbohydrate, in the form of dextrose solutions, or as fat in the form of lipid emulsions. The proportion administered as fat or carbohydrate can vary considerably. The maximum efficiency of glucose utilization occurs at a rate of 7 mg/kg/min. Delivery in excess of this amount leads to increased fat synthesis, hyperglycemia, and glycosuria. Maximal delivery of lipid should be less than 2.0–2.5 g/kg of bodyweight per day; infusions in excess of this amount may be associated with hypertriglyceridemia. To avoid essential fatty acid deficiency, it is recommended that at least 5% of required calories be administered as linoleic acid.

PROTEIN

Protein requirements have traditionally been estimated from nitrogen balance studies. Simply put, **nitrogen balance** equals nitrogen intake minus nitrogen output. If the balance is positive, the organism is presumed to be in an anabolic state with adequate protein intake and retention of nitrogen. The daily requirement in unstressed normals is approximately 1 g of protein per kilogram of body weight. If depletion of muscle stores is present, the requirement increases to 1.5 g/kg to facilitate repletion. In the stressed and depleted patient 2.0–2.5 g of protein per kilogram of bodyweight (ideal body or current body weight, whichever is lowest) should be administered.

ELECTROLYTES AND MINERALS

A number of other nutrients are required in the diet to maintain structure and optimal function. Sodium, potassium, calcium, magnesium, and phosphate are all required in amounts exceeding 200 mg/day. Optimal utilization of nitrogen requires a proper balance and intake of these micronutrients in addition to protein and calories. The requirement for electrolytes and minerals can vary significantly with the clinical course, and frequent measurements of the serum levels with appropriate replacement may be necessary. Some guidelines do exist for estimating the daily requirements in a healthy adult. For example, the retention of 1 g of nitrogen is associated with the retention of 0.08 g of phosphorus, 3.1 mEq potassium, 3.5 mEq sodium, and 2.7 mEq of chloride. Sodium chloride intake ranges from 100 to 300 mEq daily (2–3 mEq/kg/day) in a 70-kg healthy adult. The usual intake of potassium is somewhat less, averaging 50–150 mEq daily (1–2 mEq/kg/day).

Phosphorus and calcium are required in the diet to maintain structure and function of muscle, nervous system, and red blood cell function. Phosphorus is also necessary for the synthesis of high-energy phosphate bonds. The recommended daily allowance for both of these minerals is 800 mg if ingested orally; parenteral requirements are much less. Estimates of daily parenteral requirements of phosphorus range from 15 to 25 mEq, and 0.25 mEq/kg/day for calcium. Magnesium is an important component of many enzyme systems and is required for protein synthesis and neuromuscular transmission. The recommended daily allowance in health is 300–350 mg; parenteral requirements are estimated at 2 mEq per gram of administered nitrogen.

TRACE ELEMENTS

Essential trace elements include iron, iodine, cobalt, zinc, copper, chromium, and manganese. Clinical deficiency states have been identified when these substances are lacking from the diet; these can be reversed with replacement. Table 32-1 lists the important trace elements, their recommended daily allowance, function, and common deficiency syndromes.

VITAMINS

Vitamins are defined as organic molecules required in small amounts (less than 50 mg/day) for metabolism, which cannot be synthesized in adequate amounts. The water-soluble vitamins include all the B vitamins (thiamine-B1, folate, biotin, B12, etc.) and vitamin C; they function as coenzymes (Table 32-2). The fat-soluble vitamins include A, D, E, and K (Table 32-3).

Nutritional Assessment

BODY WEIGHT

Body weight is often the first variable considered in the assessment of nutritional status. Current body weight is compared with ideal body weight and to usual body weight. Current body weight is the patient's weight at the time of the nutritional assessment. Ideal body weight is determined by comparison to age-, height-, and sex-matched, healthy controls. Usual body weight is the patient's estimate of his or her "normal" body weight (i.e., when the patient was well.).

Weight loss may indicate a loss of fat mass or lean body mass consistent with malnutrition, or may simply be due to water compartmental shifts. Significant depletion of lean body mass may be present in the face of little or no change in body weight. Body weight may even increase in the presence of significant malnutrition, for example, in the cirrhotic patient with ascites. Similarly, significant loss of fat weight can occur with relative maintenance of the body cell mass, for example, the obese individual who has been on a sensible weight-reduction program. The rate of weight loss is also important; chronic loss of weight is often less detrimental than a loss of equal or lesser magnitude that occurred more acutely.

ANTHROPOMETRY

Anthropometric measurement is an inexpensive, noninvasive method to **assess fat and muscle stores** by measuring skinfold thickness and muscle circumfer-

---

TABLE 32-1. Trace Elements

Name	Function	Deficiency
Zinc	Enzyme component, growth	Dermatitis, diarrhea alopecia, psychosis, growth arrest, immunodeficiency, impaired wound healing
Copper	Erythropoesis, growth, enzyme constituent	Anemia, bone demineralization, ataxia, neutropenia
Chromium	Potentiates insulin reaction with tissue receptors	Hyperglycemia, neuropathy
Selenium	Antioxidant, enzyme systems	Uncertain
Manganese	Enzyme systems	Dermatitis, coagulopathy
Iodine	Thyroid hormone	Goiter, hypothyroidism
Iron	Heme synthesis	Glossitis, stomatitis, anemia
Molybdenum	Enzyme cofactor	Headache, irritability, lethargy, coma, night blindness
Fluoride	Teeth, bone	Caries, possible osteoporosis

TABLE 32-2. Water Soluble Vitamins

Name	Function	Deficiency
Bl (thiamine)	Part of coenzyme (TPP); used in decarboxylation reactions	Glossitis, beriberi, Wernicke's encephalopathy
B2 (riboflavin)	Electron carrier (FAD, FMN)	Glossitis, angular stomatitis
B3 (coenzyme A, pantothenic acid)	Transfers acyl groups	Rare
B5 (niacin)	Coenzyme in redox reactions	Pellagra
B6 (pyridoxal phosphate)	Used in transamination reactions	Glossitis, hypochromic anemia, peripheral neuropathy, convulsions
B7 (biotin)	Carboxylation	Rare
B9 (folate, THFA, contains pteridine, PABA and glutamic acid)	Carrier of l-carbon compound important for purine biosynthesis	Macrocytic megaloblastic anemia
B12 (cyanocobalamin)	Carrier of l-carbon compounds; needed for DNA synthesis	Similar to folate; can also have decreased myelin formation
C (ascorbic acid)	Antioxidant; coenzyme in oxygenation reactions (i.e., hydroxylation of collagen)	Scurvy

TABLE 32-3. Fat Soluble Vitamins

Name	Function	Deficiency
A (retinol; provitamin is β-carotene)	Needed to make rhodopsin	Night blindness; follicular hyperkeratosis; xerophthalmia
D (cholecalciferol)	Facilitates intestinal Ca^{2+} absorption; helps PTH mobilize Ca^{2+} from bone	Rickets in children; osteomalacia in adults
E (tocopherol)	Antioxidant	Hemolysis, neurologic damage
K (naphthoquinone group)	Promotes carboxylation of glutamate with prothrombin	Deficiencies of clotting factors 2,7,9,10; hemorrhage

[a]Oral intake: Recommended Daily Allowances from the National Research Council, 9th ed, Washington D.C. (revised 1980).
[b]Intravenous requirements: Guidelines of the American Medical Association/Nutritional Advisory Group, 1975.
[c]Estimated Safe Intake, NRC (1980).

ence. Subcutaneous fat present in skinfolds represents approximately 50% of total body fat. A commonly reported site of measurement is the tricep skinfold (TSF). Loss of these subcutaneous fat stores correlates with loss of total body fat.

Approximately 60% of total body protein is contained in skeletal muscle. This compartment is a representative fraction of total body protein reserves and can be estimated by anthropometric measurement. During malnutrition, skeletal muscle serves as a supply of amino acids for the synthesis of important proteins such as enzymes and γ-globulins and as an energy source. Depletion of muscle mass can be assessed by measurement of mid-arm muscle circumference (MAMC), mid-arm circumference (MAC), and mid-arm muscle area (MAMA):

$$\text{MAMC (cm)} = \text{MAC (cm)} - \frac{\text{TSF (mm)}}{10} * \pi$$

$$\text{MAMA (cm}^2) = \frac{(\text{MAMC})^2}{4}.$$

These derivations make several assumptions: (1) the adipose layer is evenly distributed about the arm; (2) the mid-arm muscle circumference approximates a circle; and (3) the bony contribution to arm composition is constant across populations. These assumptions have all been proven to be invalid to varying degrees. However, despite these limitations, anthropometry remains an important noninvasive test in nutritional assessment and is often used in combination with other nutritional tests or to serially evaluate nutritional status.

CIRCULATING SERUM PROTEINS

The circulating serum proteins are **synthesized and secreted by the liver.** Levels depend upon the presence of nutrient precursors and the adequacy of hepatic synthesis. A reduction in the supply of nutrient precursors results in a fairly rapid decrease in the synthetic rates of all the serum proteins. Circulating half-lives of these serum proteins are dependent on catabolic rate and distribution between the intravascular and extravascular spaces. While their serum level is influenced by changes in fluid balance, some of the serum proteins may also be affected by levels of vitamins and minerals: transferrin by iron and retinol binding protein by vitamin A. Clearly, serum protein levels are dependent on both **nutritional and non-nutritional factors.** In spite of these limitations, a number of serum proteins decline in response to starvation. The most commonly used serum proteins in nutritional assessment are albumin, transferrin, and prealbumin.

Albumin is the major serum protein synthesized by the liver. Approximately 40% of total body albumin can be found in the circulation. The primary functions of albumin are to maintain intravascular plasma oncotic pressure and to serve as a carrier for enzymes, drugs, hormones, and trace elements. The **20-day half-life** of albumin limits the use of serum levels in the detection of acute changes in nutrient intake, although serum levels will decline if nutrient deprivation is prolonged. The serum albumin level has been found to be the **best single predictor of adverse clinical outcome secondary to malnutrition.** However, there are limitations to its diagnostic accuracy: acutely malnourished patients may

have a normal serum albumin level owing to its long half-life; acute fluid overload may cause a dilutional decline in the serum concentration in well-nourished patients; and the malnourished patient who is dehydrated may have an artificially high level.

Transferrin is a serum globulin synthesized by the liver with a **half-life of eight days.** Transferrin transports iron in the plasma and aids in defense against bacteria by binding iron. The serum level of transferrin is markedly affected by nutritional status, however; significant changes in serum level may occur secondary to iron deficiency. The shorter half-life of transferrin should detect nutritional depletion and repletion at an earlier stage than albumin. However, studies have shown no advantage over albumin.

Prealbumin is a serum protein synthesized by the liver with a **half-life of two to three days.** Prealbumin functions in thyroxine transport and acts as a carrier for retinol-binding protein. Prealbumin is an early indicator of nutritional depletion and repletion, preceding the change in serum albumin. Measurable changes in prealbumin occur within seven days of a change in nutrient intake.

Other serum proteins proposed for use in nutritional assessment include retinol-binding protein, fibronectin, and somatostatin. A potential advantage of these proteins in nutritional assessment is their shorter serum half-life (e.g., 10 hours for retinol-binding protein). On the other hand, a previously healthy patient who sustains an acute decrease in nutrient intake of only a few days' duration may demonstrate a decline in these very short half-life proteins that does not indicate malnutrition.

MULTIPARAMETER INDICES

It is apparent that no single test is 100% sensitive and 100% specific in the diagnosis of clinically relevant malnutrition. The **Prognostic Nutritional Index** was developed to improve on our ability to predict postoperative complications linked to preoperative malnutrition. Four important parameters were identified and incorporated into the following predictive index:

$$\text{PNI (\% risk)} = 158 - 16.6(\text{ALB}) - 0.78(\text{TSF}) - 0.2(\text{TFN}) - 5.8(\text{DTH})$$

where PNI = prognostic nutritional index; ALB = serum albumin (g/dL); TSF = triceps skin fold measurement (mm); TFN = serum transferrin (mg/dL), DTH =

delayed-type hypersensitivity (area of induration; on a scale of 0 [anergic] to 4 [vigorous] reaction). The higher the PNI, the higher the predicted risk of postoperative complications.

BIOCHEMICAL PARAMETERS

Biochemical parameters that estimate skeletal muscle size include creatinine excretion, the creatinine-height index, and 3-methylhistidine. Creatinine is the breakdown product of creatine, a high-energy compound found in skeletal muscle. The quantity of creatinine in a 24-hour urine sample correlates well with body cell mass. For example, 1 g of urinary creatinine in a 24-hour urine represents approximately 18 kg of fat-free muscle. Renal excretion of creatinine may be compared to gender- and height-matched controls. This comparison forms the basis for the creatinine-height index. A creatinine-height index of 100% indicates a normal excretion of creatinine and a normal skeletal muscle mass; a creatinine-height index less than 80% of predicted defines skeletal muscle depletion.

3-Methylhistidine is an amino acid found primarily in skeletal muscle. Once catabolized, it is neither reused nor metabolized, and is excreted exclusively in the urine. These characteristics make 3-methylhistidine a potentially useful measure of the size of skeletal muscle stores, assuming a stable catabolic rate. The rate of excretion of 3-methylhistidine, like creatinine, is altered by dietary meat, exercise, sepsis, and other factors affecting catabolism.

IMMUNOLOGIC FUNCTION

While both cellular and humoral immune responses are affected by malnutrition, it appears that cell-mediated immunity is affected earlier and to a greater extent than humoral functions. However, alterations in immune function may occur secondary to concurrent disease and/or sepsis with no definite relationship to the degree of malnutrition as measured by other parameters.

SKELETAL MUSCLE FUNCTION AND NUTRITIONAL STATUS

All organ systems, including the skeletal muscle system, require a minimal nutrient supply to maintain normal physiologic function. Disease states that interfere with nutrient supply may manifest a measurable decline in skeletal muscle function before other organ system malfunction is evident or before malnutrition can be diagnosed by other tests. The technique involves nerve stimulation and quantitation of skeletal muscle function independent of voluntary effort. A decrease in the force of contraction and the maximal rate of muscle relaxation precedes measurable changes in body composition during periods of nutritional depletion.

Bibliography

Buzby GP, Mullen JL. Nutritional assessment. In: Caldwell M, Rombeau J, eds. *Clinical nutrition, vol I: enteral and tube feeding.* Philadelphia: WB Saunders, 1984.

Dempsey DT, Mullen JL. Prognostic value of nutritional indices. *JPEN* 1987;11:109s–114s.

Lukaski HC. Methods for the assessment of human body compositions traditional and new. *Am J Clin Nutr* 1987;46: 537–556.

Mullen JL, Buzby GP, Waldman TG, et al. Prediction of operative morbidity and mortality by preoperative nutritional assessment. *Surg Forum* 1979;30:80–82.

INDEX

Page numbers followed by t indicate tables. Page numbers followed by f indicate figures.